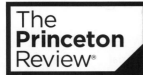

The Princeton Review

PCAT®
PREP

2nd Edition

The Staff of The Princeton Review

Penguin
Random
House

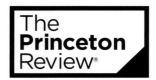

The Princeton Review
110 East 42nd St, 7th Floor
New York, NY 10017

Published in the United States by Penguin Random House, LLC, New York, and in Canada by Random House of Canada, division of Penguin Random House Ltd., Toronto.

Some material in this book was previously published in *AP Calculus AB Prep*, 2021 Edition, a trade paperback respectively published by Random House LLC.

ISBN: 978-0-525-57155-1
ISSN: 2767-8563

PCAT is produced by NCS Pearson, Inc.

The Princeton Review is not affiliated with Princeton University.

The material in this book is up-to-date at the time of publication. However, changes may have been instituted by the testing body in the test after this book was published.

If there are any important late-breaking developments, changes, or corrections to the materials in this book, we will post that information online in the Student Tools. Register your book and check your Student Tools to see if there are any updates posted there.

Editor: Orion McBean
Production Artist: Jennifer Chapman
Production Editors: Kathy Carter and Liz Dacey
Content Contributors: Patricia Eldredge, Jes Adams, and Eliz Markowitz

Printed in the United States of America.

10 9 8 7 6 5 4 3 2 1

2nd Edition

Editorial

Rob Franek, Editor-in-Chief
David Soto, Director of Content Development
Stephen Koch, Student Survey Manager
Deborah Weber, Director of Production
Gabriel Berlin, Production Design Manager
Selena Coppock, Director of Editorial
Aaron Riccio, Senior Editor
Meave Shelton, Senior Editor
Chris Chimera, Editor
Anna Goodlett, Editor
Orion McBean, Editor
Patricia Murphy, Editor

Penguin Random House Publishing Team

Tom Russell, VP, Publisher
Alison Stoltzfus, Senior Director
Brett Wright, Senior Editor
Emily Hoffman, Associate Managing Editor
Ellen Reed, Production Manager
Suzanne Lee, Designer
Eugenia Lo, Publishing Assistant

For customer service, please contact **editorialsupport@review.com**, and be sure to include:

- full title of the book
- ISBN
- page number

CONTRIBUTORS

The completion of this book would not have been possible without the help and dedication of several individuals. In particular, we would like to thank lead author Patricia Eldredge and co-authors Jes Adams, Dorothy Vandermolen, and Eliz Markowitz for their time and attention to revising this edition.

Special thanks to Christine Lindwall for her contributions to the online resources. Lastly, huge thanks to Jennifer Chapman, Kathy Carter, Liz Dacey, and Deborah Weber for their work on the production of this book.

CONTENTS

Get More (Free) Content
at PrincetonReview.com/prep

As easy as 1·2·3

1 Go to PrincetonReview.com/prep or scan the **QR code** and enter the following ISBN for your book: **9780525571551**

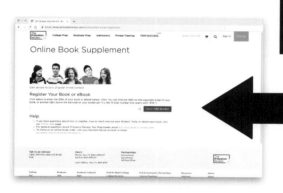

2 Answer a few simple questions to set up an exclusive Princeton Review account. *(If you already have one, you can just log in.)*

3 Enjoy access to your **FREE** content!

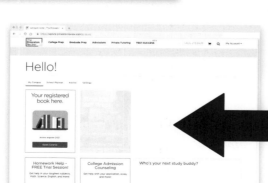

Once you've registered, you can...

- Access (2) online practice tests
- Download additional drill questions and a study plan
- Find useful information about taking the PCAT and applying to pharmacy school

- Check to see if there have been any corrections or updates to this edition
- Get our take on any recent or pending updates to the PCAT

Need to report a potential **content** issue?

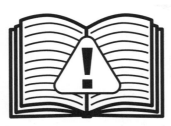

Contact **EditorialSupport@review.com** and include:

- full title of the book
- ISBN
- page number

Need to report a **technical** issue?

Contact **TPRStudentTech@review.com** and provide:

- your full name
- email address used to register the book
- full book title and ISBN
- Operating system (Mac/PC) and browser (Firefox, Safari, etc.)

Chapter 1

Test Basics

SO YOU WANT TO BE A PHARMACIST....

If you're like most pre-pharmacy students, you're interested in science and math and you really enjoy interacting with people. You look forward to having the opportunity to help people get the most out of their medicines. You're a good student and you'd much rather take biochemistry than another linguistics class. After years of preparation in high school and the beginning years of college, you're ready to apply to pharmacy school. There's just the small issue of...the PCAT.

A period of 3 hours and 40 minutes of essay writing, biology, chemistry, critical reading, math, and statistics can be quite a daunting task. And you know that getting a good score can make a good application for pharmacy school look great. Then there's the fact that the score you're given isn't just a scaled composite score, but also a percentile rank. That's right; they actually tell you exactly where you stand in comparison to other test-takers.

But as a first step in achieving your goal you've purchased this book, so you're off to a great start! We promise to demystify the PCAT for you, with clear descriptions of the different sections, how the test is scored, and what the test experience is like. We will help you understand general test-taking techniques as well as provide you with specific techniques for each section. We will review the science content you need to know as well as give you strategies for the Biology, Chemistry, Critical Reading, Quantitative Reasoning, and Writing sections. We'll show you the path to a good PCAT score and help you walk the path.

After all...you want to be a pharmacist. And we want you to succeed.

1.1 IMPORTANCE

The Pharmacy College Admissions Test (PCAT) is produced, administered, and scored by NCS Pearson, Inc. and was developed in cooperation with the American Association of Colleges of Pharmacy PCAT Advisory Committee to measure content knowledge and cognitive abilities considered essential for success in pharmacy programs. It is endorsed by the American Association of Colleges of Pharmacy (AACP), which is comprised of all accredited colleges and schools that have pharmacy degree programs. Current contact information for AACP is as follows:

American Association of Colleges of Pharmacy
www.aacp.org
email: mail@aacp.org

The exam is conducted at Pearson VUE Test Centers that are located throughout the United States and Canada. Registration for the PCAT is completed online at http://tpc-etesting.com/pcat/. While the PCAT is administered several times a year, registration is on a first-come, first-served basis. Within 24 hours of submitting your request, you will receive emailed instructions containing scheduling information. When visiting this site, notice that there are two registration deadlines: A "Registration and Schedule" deadline that affords you the greatest opportunity of obtaining your preferred testing date, time, and location, and a "Late Registration and Schedule" deadline that reduces the likelihood of obtaining your preferences and charges an additional fee. If after registering you choose to cancel your exam, first cancel your seat at Pearson VUE and then your registration at the testing site. The most up-to-date information on the locations of Pearson VUE centers, deadlines, and fees can be found on the PCAT website at https://www.pearsonassessments.com/graduate-admissions/pcat/about.html.

Nuts and Bolts of the PCAT

The following table highlights features of the PCAT exam.

Registration/Price	Online via http://tpc-etesting.com/pcat/. The price is $210. If you register late, you will incur extra fees and you may not be able to take the exam at the testing center of your choice.
Testing Centers	Pearson VUE centers
Security	Two forms of original, valid ID; one must be government issued and contain both your photograph and signature, and the other must contain your name. Names on the IDs must match exactly with the way your name appears on the registration.
Proctoring	Exam is proctored.
Frequency of Test	Select dates throughout the year
Format	Exclusively computer based; 192 multiple-choice questions, 1 writing prompt
Length of Test Day	3 hours and 40 minutes
Breaks	One 15-minute break
Essay Grading	Your essay is graded by two trained scorers, but the process may also include an electronic assessor.
Scoring	A composite score on a scale of 200–600 and a percentile rank against recent PCAT candidates

Allowed/Not Allowed	No timers/watches, earplugs or headphones, writing aids, calculators, phones, recording devices, cameras, food and beverages, reference materials, or other electronic devices. Erasable noteboard provided. Personal items may be stored in a secure area at the testing center.
Results: Timing and Delivery	Score report available online within 5 weeks of the end of the exam session. A printed unofficial preliminary score report is given at the testing center after completion of the exam.
Maximum Number of Retakes	Exam may be taken five times; if more are necessary, documentation verifying your applicant status at a school of pharmacy may be required.

1.2   TEST BREAKDOWN

The PCAT is 3 hours and 40 minutes long with one 15-minute break in the middle. The structure of the current test is shown below. Subtests are listed in order of appearance with the corresponding time allotted. The number of items in each subtest and the breakdown of content is also presented.

Test Breakdown:

Section	Subtest	Number of Items and Breakdown	Time Allotted (minutes)
Part 1	Writing	1 prompt	30
Part 2	Biological Processes	48	45
	General Biology	50%	
	Microbiology	20%	
	Anatomy and Physiology	30%	
Part 3	Chemical Processes	48	45
	General Chemistry	50%	
	Organic Chemistry	30%	
	Biochemistry	20%	
	Break		15
Part 4	Critical Reading	48	50
	Comprehension	30%	
	Analysis	40%	
	Evaluation	30%	
Part 5	Quantitative Reasoning	48	50
	Basic Math	25%	
	Algebra	25%	
	Probability and Statistics	18%	
	Precalculus	18%	
	Calculus	14%	
Total		192 multiple-choice +1 prompt	3 hrs 40 min +15 min break

Of the 48 questions in each section, only 40 count toward your PCAT score. Eight of the questions are experimental questions, which are being tested to see how they are handled by examiners. These experimental questions will not count toward your score.

Questions may be related to passages that are on a particular topic or may be discrete, free-standing questions. There are four questions per passage, and each passage is approximately 150–200 words long. If you are uncertain of your answer, you will be able to flag questions so that you can return to them later.

Scoring

Immediately following the completion of your test, you will receive a preliminary score report at the Pearson VUE Test Center. This report displays your multiple-choice scaled scores and preliminary percentile ranks. The Writing score is not included because it requires manual scoring.

The composite scaled score is an unweighted average of the four multiple-choice subsection scaled scores. Scales are comparable from year to year and range from 200–600. Typically, the median is about 400.

Percentile ranks are also reported. These are based on 2019 norms and range from 1–99. If you received a percentile score of 70, for example, you scored higher than 70% of those taking the test.

Writing scores are reported on a scale of 1.0–6.0. A mean Writing score is also reported, which shows the average of all candidate Writing scores during the 12-month period prior to the exam.

Be sure to check the admission standards for those programs in which you are interested so you are aware of their requirements. Pearson will send an Official Score Report to candidates and an Official Transcript to designated institutions. PCAT score data is sent to the Pharmacy College Application Service (PharmCAS) for distribution to subscribing institutions.

1.3 COMPUTER TEST-TAKING INFORMATION

The PCAT is a computer-based test (CBT). You need to be familiar only with basic keyboard and mouse commands to navigate through the exam, but be aware that you will not be able to strike-out or highlight. Instead, you will be given an erasable noteboard to use for scratch work. You will be able to answer questions for only one section at a time, and once you have completed that section, you will not be able to go back and change your answers. Your essay response will be typed into the space provided. Please keep in mind that you will not have access to the Internet or any outside references whatsoever, including online calculators.

Personal watches and clocks are not permitted while taking the test, but there will be a countdown timer in the corner of the screen.

1.4 DAY-OF STRATEGIES

On the day of the exam, plan to arrive at the testing center at least 30 minutes early. If you arrive more than 15 minutes late, you will not be allowed to take the exam, and you will lose your registration fee.

Pacing

Since the PCAT is a timed test, you must keep an eye on the timer and adjust your pacing as necessary. It would be terrible to run out of time at the end to discover that the last few questions could have been easily answered in just a few seconds each.

The multiple-choice sections are 45–50 minutes long, which gives you about 2 minutes per passage and 35 seconds per question.

Process of Elimination

1.4

Process of Elimination (POE) is probably the most useful technique you have to tackle PCAT questions. Since there is no guessing penalty, POE allows you to increase your probability of choosing the correct answer by eliminating those you are sure are wrong. If you are guessing between a couple of choices, consider the following:

1. Eliminate any choices that you are sure are incorrect or do not answer the issue addressed in the question.
2. Jot down some notes on your erasable noteboard to help clarify your thoughts.
3. Do not leave it blank! If you are not sure and you have already spent more than 60 seconds on that question, just pick one of the remaining choices.
4. Special Note: If all but one answer has been eliminated, the remaining choice must be the correct answer. Don't waste time pondering why it is correct; just click it and move on. The PCAT doesn't care if you truly understand why it's the right answer, only that you have the right answer selected. Moreover, if you know the correct answer, select it and move on. Don't try to understand why the other answers are wrong. Both of these strategies will save you valuable time.

Guessing

There is NO guessing penalty on the PCAT. NEVER leave a question blank! When you have two minutes remaining on your timer, go back to flagged questions and select the same letter for each of those questions. This letter is known as your Letter of the Day (LOTD).

Test Drive

Make sure you know where the test center is located and how to get there. It is a good idea to do a practice run so that you know where to park, what traffic will be like, and how long it will take to get to the test center.

Eat Healthy

Make sure that you are in top shape for the exam by eating healthy while studying and making sure to eat well on the day of the exam. Try to avoid excess caffeine and sugar in order to prevent jitteriness.

Break

Take advantage of the 15-minute break. Get up, stretch, and walk around. It will help you clear your head.

Sleep

Make sure to get plenty of sleep the night before the exam. Nothing makes a nearly four-hour exam tougher than a sleepy brain!

Chapter 2

Pharmacy Overview

2.1 PHARMACY SCHOOL PROGRAMS

As you'll soon learn, the road to the Doctor of Pharmacy (PharmD) can be quite complicated. The PCAT is just the beginning! The first thing you should do is acquaint yourself with the different pathways leading to the PharmD degree to decide which pathway is the best for you.

Pathway 1: 2–4 Years of Pre-pharmacy Study

Pre-pharmacy coursework can be completed at any accredited higher education institution. Generally, pharmacy programs do not require that students have a bachelor's degree as a prerequisite for entering a professional PharmD program. Some programs may offer early assurance pathways to pre-pharmacy students.

Pathway 2: 3–4 Years of a Pharmacy Curriculum

Most pharmacy programs in the United States require four years of study in a PharmD curriculum. Some institutions offer accelerated programs that allow you to complete the coursework in three years.

Pathway 3: Licensure Exam

To legally practice as a pharmacist in the United States, PharmD graduates must pass the North American Pharmacist Licensure Examination (NAPLEX). Additional licensure requirements may be imposed by a state board of pharmacy.

Other career development opportunities are available. These include residencies, fellowships, and other degrees.

Residency

This involves one to two years of postgraduate training that focuses on particular patient populations or diseases in a clinical setting.

Fellowships

Fellowships may include postgraduate training in academia, a research setting, or industry.

Other Degrees

After completing licensure requirements, pharmacists may choose to become board certified in specialty areas, such Critical Care, Infectious Diseases, Pharmacotherapy, and Cardiology, among others.

Pre-Pharmacy Coursework

All pre-pharmacy coursework must be completed before beginning the professional phase of the PharmD curriculum. The pre-pharmacy course requirements will vary by institution, but typically they include English Composition, Calculus, Statistics, Biology (with lab), Microbiology (with lab), General Chemistry (with lab), Organic Chemistry (with lab), Physics (with lab), Human Anatomy and Physiology, and Economics.

The Six-Seven Year Pharmacy School

This plan for graduation with a doctor of pharmacy degree includes two to three years of pre-pharmacy coursework followed by four years of professional studies, for a total of six to seven years. Students in this program attend directly from high school and may follow an expedited process into the professional phase of the program.

If not all PharmD seats are filled, six-year pharmacy schools usually accept transfer students beginning in the third year, which is the first professional year. Transfer students may be from other colleges within the same university or from other universities entirely. Most schools require that transfer students complete a list of prerequisite courses, which are equivalent to the courses required in the first two "pre-professional" years in the curriculum. Many schools require the PCAT, and some require an on-site interview.

Schools that use this format often have limited spots for transfer students, depending on the number of students already enrolled in their six-year program. In other words, if the class is already filled with students who began in the program straight out of high school, there may be no spaces available for transfer students.

The Two-Plus-Three Year Pharmacy School

Schools with this program structure include at least two years of pre-pharmacy coursework that is followed by three years of accelerated professional studies. The PharmD professional program is scheduled year-round, which shortens the PharmD degree timeframe.

The Two-Plus-Four-Year Pharmacy School

These schools follow much the same format as the six-year pharmacy schools, but in order for students to begin the first professional year (year 3), they must be accepted through a formal admissions process. Applications are generally accepted from both transfer students and students from within the university. Spots in the class are filled based on this admissions process. Students at these universities are not guaranteed admission into the professional years simply by maintaining a set GPA and completing required courses. Some of these schools require completion of a bachelor's degree in order to apply for admission into the professional program.

The Three-Plus-Four-Year Pharmacy School

This structure is similar to the Two-Plus-Four-Year program. These schools require at least three years of pre-pharmacy coursework, which is then followed by four years of professional study.

Early Assurance

Early assurance pathways are generally offered by invitation to select students during their first one to two years of college or university coursework. If early assurance students complete all of the program's pre-pharmacy and interview requirements, they may advance to the professional phase via an expedited process.

Whether you are a high school student, a transfer student, or someone who is looking at pharmacy as a second career, you should be aware of the type of program you are applying to and what its specific prerequisites are. These requirements are usually listed on the school's website, or they may be obtained by contacting the school's admissions department.

2.2 LIST OF PHARMACY SCHOOLS/ADMISSIONS INFORMATION

The number of pharmacy schools in the United States has increased dramatically from levels in the past. When considering which schools to apply to, you should consider many factors, including location, curriculum, faculty, and opportunities for specialized study, such as additional degree programs. In addition, consider the accreditation status of the school. The Accreditation Council for Pharmacy Education (ACPE) is the accrediting body for pharmacy schools. Newer schools may still be in the process of accreditation. Consult the ACPE website for further details on accreditation and to find out the accreditation status of schools you are interested in: www.acpe-accredit.org.

Pharmacy School Admissions

Admission requirements will differ depending on whether a student is applying for admission to the pre-professional or professional years. Admission to pre-professional years usually requires the following elements:

- Completed application
- Application fee
- High school transcript
- College transcripts, if any
- SAT/ACT scores
- Essay

Application for admission to the professional years requires careful attention. Most schools require the following elements:

- Completed application
- Application fee
- College transcript
- High school transcript
- PCAT scores
- Completion of prerequisite coursework, which mirrors the curriculum of that school's pre-professional years
- Onsite interview

Completion of prerequisite coursework can be challenging for students applying to multiple schools, as each school may have slightly different requirements. Early determination of the required courses can be helpful in deciding where to apply and what courses to take before applying.

Many pharmacy schools use the PharmCAS system to organize their admissions process. PharmCAS uses a standard application that can be submitted to multiple pharmacy schools. PharmCAS is run by the American Association of Colleges of Pharmacy (AACP) and is similar to the Common Application used by undergraduate schools. To find out which schools use PharmCAS, visit their website: www.pharmcas.org.

The PharmCAS system has a school directory that lists institutions alphabetically, their location, whether they are public or private, deadlines, and each program structure. Specific information can be obtained using the institution links. In addition, you can compare individual programs and apply filters that will help you in your search. The latest application information, which includes a school directory and application deadlines, can be found at https://www.pharmcas.org/sites/default/files/2020-07/2020-2021-pharmcas-application-instructions.pdf.

Pharmacy schools that use the PharmCAS system may have additional application requirements, so be sure to check each school's admissions packet.

2.3 POSTGRADUATE TRAINING AND CERTIFICATIONS

One of the advantages of obtaining a doctor of pharmacy degree is the career options that it provides. Fifty years ago, a pharmacist was thought of as simply the person behind the counter who was skilled at "counting by five" and who occasionally had tips on simple ailments such as bug bites or the common cold. Pharmacists today are viewed as more than the local "druggist" and have the skills not only to play an important role in public health, but also to serve in many capacities outside of the community pharmacy. Below is a list of just a few career opportunities for pharmacists:

- Community pharmacist
- Hospital pharmacist
- Academic pharmacist (faculty member)
- Consultant pharmacist
- Pharmacy manager
- Pharmaceutical industry pharmacist
- Medical writer
- Pharmaceutical sales representative
- Attorney (PharmD/JD)
- Physician (PharmD/MD)
- Research scientist (PharmD/PhD)
- Public health pharmacist
- Ambulatory care pharmacist
- Federal pharmacist (in agencies such as the FDA and NIH)

Many of these careers can be achieved simply with a doctor of pharmacy degree. However, there are many opportunities for further training after pharmacy school. This section will give details on the many postgraduate training opportunities available to pharmacists.

Residencies and Competency Areas

2.3

The majority of residencies are one-year positions that begin in July and end the following June. There are two "levels" of residency, post-graduate year one (PGY1) and post-graduate year two (PGY2). PGY1 residencies tend to focus on internal medicine with a goal of producing a well-rounded practitioner who is able to work in many different clinical areas. PGY2 residencies are usually specialized in a particular therapeutic area such as pediatrics, oncology, cardiology, or ambulatory care, just to name a few. Competency areas are summarized below.

PGY1

- Patient care
- Continuity of care during patient transitions
- Prepare, dispense, and manage medications to support safe and effective drug therapy
- Advancing practice and improving patient care
- Ability to evaluate and investigate practice, review data, and assimilate scientific evidence to improve patient care and/or the medical use system
- Leadership and management
- Management skills
- Teaching, education, and dissemination of knowledge
- Provide effective medication and practice related education
- Effectively employ effective preceptor's roles when engaged in teaching

PGY2

- Ambulatory care pharmacy
- Cardiology pharmacy
- Clinical pharmacogenomics
- Critical care pharmacy
- Emergency medicine pharmacy
- Geriatric pharmacy
- Health system pharmacy administration and leadership
- Infectious diseases pharmacy
- Informatics
- Internal medicine pharmacy
- Investigational drugs and research pharmacy
- Medication use safety and policy
- Neurology pharmacy
- Oncology pharmacy
- Pain management and palliative care pharmacy
- Pediatric pharmacy
- Pharmacotherapy
- Population health management and data analytics
- Psychiatric pharmacy
- Solid organ transplant pharmacy

Residencies are meant to prepare pharmacists with advanced training in pharmacotherapy. Graduates of residency programs usually take positions in hospitals or in academia, but the additional training can be helpful to prepare for almost any career in pharmacy.

The majority of residencies are offered by hospitals, though many community pharmacies now offer community practice residencies as well. For more information on residencies, and to access a directory of programs, see the American Society of Health-System Pharmacists (ASHP) website: www.ashp.org.

Fellowships

Similar to residencies, fellowships offer additional advanced training to pharmacists. Fellowships are usually longer than residencies, generally two to three years. Fellowships also tend to be more research-focused, and usually prepare graduates for a position in academia or in a pharmacy research career in the pharmaceutical industry. Some pharmacy schools offer fellowships in the pharmaceutical industry specifically, with part of the time being spent at the school, and part of the time at a pharmaceutical corporate site. For a directory of fellowship programs, visit the American College of Clinical Pharmacy (ACCP) website: www.accp.com.

Dual-Degree Programs

Dual degrees are gaining in popularity as students seek to specialize their degree in preparation for certain fields.

PharmD/PhD

Dual programs usually offer PhD's in pharmacology/toxicology, medicinal chemistry, or pharmaceutics. These programs allow students to complete both degrees usually within 9 or 10 years, rather than the 10 or 11 years it would normally take. Programs are designed for students who have a strong interest in research and plan for a career in academia or the pharmaceutical industry.

PharmD/MBA

Pharmacists who obtain MBA degrees are prepared to take on leadership roles in pharmacies, the pharmaceutical industry, or other industries that involve public health or project management. Schools that offer these degrees often offer summer or night classes to help fulfill the MBA requirements. Extra semesters of full-time or part-time classes may be required.

Other dual degrees that exist are the PharmD/MPH, PharmD/JD, and PharmD/MS.

Board of Pharmacy Specialties

The Board of Pharmacy Specialties (BPS) is an independent certification agency of the American Pharmacists Association (APhA). BPS oversees six specialty exams that pharmacists may apply to take if certain prerequisites are fulfilled. A passing score on one of these exams is known as "board certification." The current BPS exams include:

- Ambulatory care pharmacy
- Cardiology pharmacy
- Compounded sterile preparations pharmacy
- Critical care pharmacy
- Geriatric pharmacy
- Infectious diseases pharmacy
- Nuclear pharmacy
- Nutrition support pharmacy
- Oncology pharmacy
- Pediatric pharmacy
- Pharmacotherapy
- Psychiatric pharmacy
- Solid organ transplantation pharmacy

2.3

Unlike board certification exams, obtaining added qualifications involves submitting a portfolio of work completed, which is reviewed by a review board. Please see the BPS website for more information: www.bpsweb.org.

2.4   JOB OUTLOOK

Thanks to the aging population and the explosion of new drugs over the past few decades, the demand for pharmacists has grown tremendously. Pharmacists are needed not only in community pharmacies, but also in hospitals, where positions have increased due to the increased workload in hospital pharmacies. The ever-expanding career options for pharmacists, as detailed above, have also contributed to the increasing demand.

However, increasing numbers of pharmacy schools and pharmacy school graduates has affected the demand for pharmacists over the past few years, as reported in the 2019 National Pharmacist Workforce Survey. Changing demographics, the current health crises, the future economy as well as increasing specialization and recent healthcare legislation may impact this data.

Chapter 3

The Princeton Review Approach to Preparing for the PCAT

3.1   GOALS OF THIS BOOK

The Princeton Review is a leading test-preparation company with branches across the country and abroad. We've developed the techniques you'll find in our books, courses, and online resources by analyzing actual exams and testing their effectiveness with our students. What makes our techniques unique is our approach. We base our principles on the same ones used by the people who write the tests. We don't want you to waste your time with superfluous information; we'll give you just the information you'll need to get great score improvements. You'll learn to recognize and comprehend the relatively small amount of information that's actually tested. You'll also learn to avoid common traps, to think like the test-writers, to find answers to questions you're unsure of, and to budget your time effectively.

You need to do only two things: trust the techniques, and practice, practice, practice.

Myths

1. **If you've done well in your science and math courses, you don't need to study for the PCAT.**

    While good grades in science and math courses will certainly look good on your application to pharmacy school, you may not be as prepared for the PCAT as you think. First, it may have been a year or two since your last calculus class or general chemistry class. Second, learning good test-taking strategies (like those taught in this book) will help you handle difficult questions.

2. **The PCAT is a test of your science knowledge. Just focus your studying on the tough stuff like organic chemistry and you'll do fine.**

    While studying for organic chemistry will certainly be helpful on the PCAT, there's much more to the exam. The Biology and Chemistry sections take up only 90 minutes in the exam—that's 41%. Math, writing, and critical reading make up the rest. While organic chemistry might be the toughest part for you, don't forget to brush up on topics that are easier. If you're good at calculus, you want to make sure you get those questions right—it's easy points!

3. **There is a magic PCAT score that will guarantee your admission into pharmacy school.**

    The PCAT is only a part of your application packet to pharmacy school. While a good score can definitely help your application, there is no magic number that guarantees admission.

4. **Don't worry if you don't do as well as you'd like the first time. You can take the PCAT again.**

    You may take the PCAT five times. After the fifth time, you must submit a request in writing to retake the exam. Be sure to include your name and PCAT ID with your request.

5. **Don't worry if you get one bad score. Your transcript will list up to five test scores over a five-year period.**

    Your latest set of scores and test results from up to four other previous attempts over a five-year period will be sent to institutions if you apply to a PharmCAS school that requires the PCAT. Pharmacy schools have different requirements, so check with the institutions to find out their policies. Remember that if you choose the "No Score" option on the day of the exam, that score will not be reported to you or to any schools.

Tips

1. Start early. Studying for the PCAT the week before the exam won't get you far.
2. Make a schedule. Scheduling which topics you will review at different times will help you avoid cramming everything in the last few weeks before the exam.
3. Use this book. Read the chapters, and take the end-of-chapter drills. Focus your studying on areas of weakness.
4. Strive for a real understanding of chemistry and math equations rather than just memorization. This approach will help you keep your cool and answer questions in a reasonable amount of time.
5. Stay healthy. Weeks of all-nighters and junk food binges won't put your brain in the best state to take the PCAT. Eat healthy and get some sleep!
6. Study with a group. Some people find studying with a group to be helpful. Determine a schedule for meetings and stick to it. If you decide to create a study group, plan some time for individual study as well.

3.2   STUDYING TIMELINE/TOPIC OUTLINE

Below is a suggested studying timeline, but you need to figure out a schedule that works for you and fits your needs. For example, if you are finishing calculus right now and don't feel you need as much time in that area, alter your study schedule to reflect that.

Four Months Before the Test Date

Quantitative Skills
Week 1—Basic Math and Algebra
Week 2—Probability and Statistics
Week 3—Precalculus
Week 4—Calculus

Three Months Before the Test Date

Biology
Week 1—General Biology
Week 2—Microbiology
Week 3—Anatomy and Physiology
Week 4—Review areas of weakness in Biology

Two Months Before the Test Date

Critical Reading/Writing
Weeks 1 and 2—Critical Reading
Weeks 3 and 4—Writing

One Month Before the Test Date

Chemistry
Weeks 1 and 2—General Chemistry
Weeks 3 and 4—Organic Chemistry

The Test Date

Take the PCAT!

Chapter 4

Overall Strategies

4.1   CRACKING THE PCAT

This chapter contains some basic advice to get you into The Princeton Review mindset. You'll learn some core test-taking strategies to help you maximize your score. In addition, you'll see some of the different question formats you will probably encounter on test day. The PCAT is not an intelligence test; you can improve your score, in many cases substantially, by familiarizing yourself with the test and by practicing the techniques in this book. In many ways, taking a standardized test is a skill and, as with any skill, you can become more proficient at it by both practicing and following the advice of a good teacher. Think of your PCAT preparation as if you were practicing for a piano recital or a track meet; you wouldn't show up at the concert hall or track field without having put in hours of practice beforehand (at least we hope you wouldn't!). If you want to get a good score on the PCAT, you'll have to put in the necessary preparation time.

4.2   ANSWER THE EASY QUESTIONS FIRST

There will inevitably be questions you are great at and questions you don't like. The beauty of the PCAT is that you can answer questions in any order you like within a subtest. The question you can nail in 25 seconds is worth just as much as the question that will torture you for minutes on end. To maximize your score, leave the passages or free-standing questions you don't like for last. There is not enough time in any of the sections to work through every question, so if you are going to run out of time, make sure that the questions that get skipped are the ones it would have taken too long to answer anyway.

This method is called Answer the Easy Questions First. Doing so will result in two passes through each individual section. On the first pass, cherry pick. Answer the passage questions you like. Get all of those easy points in the bank before time starts running short. You know that the hard questions—or the ones that you don't like—are going to take more time. Also, although you should never rush, everyone starts to feel the pressure of the clock as time starts running low. This is often when mistakes happen. Leave those difficult, time-consuming questions for the end of the subtest. If you run out of time or make some mistakes at that point, it won't matter because these are low percentage questions for you anyway.

Move On

On your first pass through the questions, if you see a question you don't like, a question that looks hard, or a question that looks time consuming, skip it and leave it for the end. Sometimes, however, a question that looks easy turns out to be more troublesome than you thought. The question may be trickier than it first appeared. On the other hand, you may have simply misread the question, and it seems hard only because you're working with the wrong information. From start to finish, the PCAT takes about four hours to finish. Over four hours your brain is going to get tired. When that happens, misreading a question is virtually inevitable. Once you read a problem wrong, it is almost impossible to reread the problem and see it right. As long as you are still in the problem, you could read it 10 times in a row and you will read it the same wrong way each time.

Whether a question is harder than it first appeared, or made harder by the fact that you missed a key phrase or piece of information, the approach you've taken is not working. This is when you need to mark it, reset your brain, and come back to it. Do two or three other questions so you can refocus, and then return to the flagged problem.

When you skip the problem, your brain doesn't just forget the problem; it keeps on processing in the background. The distraction of the other questions helps your brain to consider the question from some other angles. When you return to the problem, you may find that the part that gave you so much trouble the first time is now magically clear. If the problem continues to give you trouble, skip it again.

Staying with a problem when you're stuck burns time but yields no points. You might spend two, three, five, or even six minutes on a problem but still be no closer to the answer. Spending five minutes to get one point will not get you enough points on a 30- or 45-minute section. In the five minutes you spend on a problem that you've misread, you could nail three or four easier questions. When you return to the question that gave you trouble, there is a good chance that you will spot your error, and the path to the correct answer will become clear. If it doesn't become clear, skip it again. Any time you encounter resistance on the test, do not keep pushing; bend like a reed and skip it. Skip early and often so that you always have questions to distract your brain when you get stuck.

Pacing

Speed kills on the PCAT. The clock has a way of infecting your brain. Just knowing that there is a ticking clock, however, provokes mistakes. The trick is to take each section as if there is no clock. As long as you are skipping the hard ones and coming back every time you run into trouble, you increase the likelihood of choosing the correct answer. Wrong answers drag your score down and often take up even more time than the right ones!

Remember that it is not the number of question that you answer that gives you your score; it is the number of questions you answer correctly. Accuracy is everything. Ignore the clock. Slow down and work for accuracy only. If you run into a brick wall, don't stay there; move onto an easier question and come back. The minute you try to go faster, however, your accuracy will go down and take your score along with it.

Accuracy is all that matters. Skip questions often.

There is only one exception to this, and that is the last two minutes of a section. A skipped question and a wrong answer count the same. In other words, there is no penalty for guessing on a question you don't know. When two minutes remain on your clock, stop what you're doing and answer any remaining unanswered questions using your Letter of the Day (LOTD). A few lucky guesses will pay off. If you don't get any of them right, no harm done.

To avoid careless mistakes and to make the best use of your time, we suggest the following:

1. **Be Aware of Your Personal Order of Difficulty (POOD).** Spend your time on the questions that are easiest for you. Work through them methodically and accurately and collect points.
2. **Use the Two-Pass System.** The Two-Pass system involves taking each section in two parts, or passes. During the first pass, focus on all the questions that you're comfortable with. On the second pass, return to the tougher questions and do the best you can on them in the remaining time.

4.3 POE—PROCESS OF ELIMINATION

After you've worked through the problems you know how to do, it's time for some Process of Elimination. With multiple-choice questions, there are many more wrong answers on the PCAT than there are right answers. Therefore, on some of the more difficult questions (those you do on your second pass), you'll actually be better served not by trying to find the *best* answer, but instead by finding the wrong answers and using POE, Process of Elimination.

It Doesn't Really Matter How You Get the Best Answer

Remember when you were in school, and even if you got a question wrong on a test, your teacher gave you partial credit? For example, maybe you used the right formula on a math question, but miscalculated and got the wrong result. Because you understood the concept, your teacher gave you some credit.

Well, those days are over. It doesn't matter how you get an answer or whether you understand why it's right. You simply have to click on the right answer choice. You might as well benefit from this by getting questions right without really knowing why they're right. POE is the way to go: learn it, live it, love it.

The Importance of Wrong Answers

By using POE on questions you find difficult, you will be able to improve your score on the PCAT by looking for wrong answers instead of right ones. Why? Because, once you've eliminated the wrong ones, picking the right one can be straightforward.

Wrong answers on standardized multiple-choice tests are known in the testing industry as "distractors," or "trap answers." They are called distractors because their purpose is to distract you away from correct choices. Trap answers are specifically designed to appeal to you. Oftentimes, they're the answers that seem to scream out "pick me!" as you work through a question. However, these attractive answers are often incorrect.

Remembering this simple fact can be an enormous help to you as you sit down to take the test. By learning to recognize distractors, you will greatly improve your score.

Improve Your Odds Indirectly

Every time you're able to eliminate an incorrect choice on a PCAT question, you improve your odds of finding the best answer; the more incorrect choices you eliminate, the better your odds.

For this reason, some of our test-taking strategies are aimed at helping you arrive at the correct answer indirectly. Doing this will make you much more successful at avoiding the traps laid in your path by the test-writers. This is because most of the traps are designed to catch unwary test-takers who try to approach the problems directly.

POE and Guessing

Guess, but guess intelligently.

If you guessed blindly on a four-choice PCAT problem, you would have a 1-in-4 chance of picking the correct answer. Eliminate one incorrect choice, and your chances improve to 1 in 3. Eliminate two, and you have a fifty-fifty chance of earning points by guessing. In other words, since you'll have to guess sometimes, why not improve your odds?

4.4 PRACTICE BY USING THAT NOTEBOARD!

In order for POE to work, it's crucial that you keep track of what choices you're eliminating. By crossing out a clearly incorrect choice, you permanently eliminate it from consideration. If you don't cross it out, you'll keep considering it. Crossing out incorrect choices can make it much easier to find the correct answer because there will be fewer places where it can hide.

Even though the PCAT answer choices have empty bubbles next to them, they are also labeled as A, B, C, and D. As you begin to work on multiple-choice questions and use POE, you will come to appreciate this labeling.

By crossing out a clearly incorrect choice, you permanently eliminate it from consideration.

A	A	A	A
B	B	B	B
C	C	C	C
D	D	D	D
A	A	A	A
B	B	B	B
C	C	C	C
D	D	D	D

Prepare your erasable noteboard like the one shown above. This method will give you distinct work areas per page. You should find this approach especially helpful on the Math section because it can keep your work on one question from running into your work on a previous question.

By having this erasable noteboard, you can physically cross off choices that you're eliminating. Use the pages every time you do a PCAT question, in this book or anywhere else. Get used to not writing near the question on paper since you won't be able to do so on test day.

Eliminating Choices on the PCAT

You will not have highlighting or strike-out capabilities on the computer-based test. Instead, you'll get a whiteboard or laminated sheets and a marker at the beginning of the test. Before you begin the test, ask for two markers in case one runs dry. You don't want to have to wait until a proctor notices your hand in the air and enters the testing room to give you a replacement. Valuable time will be lost.

Double-Check

By training yourself to avoid careless errors, you will raise your score.

Get into the habit of double-checking all of your answers before you click on your answer choice. Reread the directions and make sure you have done everything they asked you to—don't get the answer wrong just because you missed a word in the question.

The only way to reliably avoid careless errors is to adopt habits that make them less likely to occur. Always check to see that you've transcribed information correctly to your whiteboard. Always read the problem at least twice and note any important parts that you might forget later, such as *least, not, decreasing order,* and so on. Always check your calculations. And always read the question one last time before selecting your answer. This may seem like a lot to do since you generally have less than a minute per question, and that is why it's so important to practice, practice, and practice some more.

4.5   LET IT GO

Every time you begin a new section, focus on that section and put the last section you completed behind you. Don't think about that pesky chemistry question from an earlier section while a calculus question is on your screen. You can't go back, and besides, your impression of how you did on a section is probably much worse than reality.

The Week Before the Test

The week before the test is not the time for any major life changes. This is NOT the week to quit smoking, start smoking, quit drinking coffee, start drinking coffee, start a relationship, end a relationship, or quit a job. Business as usual, okay?

Now let's get cracking!

Chapter 5

Math Strategies

5.1 MAXIMIZE YOUR SCORE

As you're probably aware by now, doing well on the Math section will involve more than just knowing some math. It will also require the use of some good strategies. Let's go through some good strategies now; make sure you read this section carefully, because it will be important for you to keep these techniques in mind. The Quantitative Reasoning (Math) section is the last one of the test, and that means you will be tired and ready to just get through it, but that won't help your score.

The Two Roles of Techniques

The techniques are there to ensure that the questions that you should get right, you do get right. A couple of careless errors on easy questions will kill your score. The techniques are not just tools; they are proven standard approaches that save time and effort and guarantee points. Use these techniques on every question. Turn them into a habitual approach that you use every time.

5.2 READ CAREFULLY

For most people, a substantial number of their wrong answers in the Math sections are caused by nothing more than reading errors. As mentioned earlier, the PCAT is a nearly four-hour test, and at some point during these four hours your brain is going to get tired. When this happens you will read, see, or understand questions incorrectly. We've mentioned that once you see a problem wrong, it is nearly impossible to see it correctly. When this happens, even simple problems can become extremely frustrating. If you solve a problem and your answer is not one of the choices, this is what has happened. When you would swear that a problem can't be solved, this is what has happened. When you have absolutely no idea how to solve a problem, this is what has happened. If you find yourself with half a page full of calculations and are no closer to the answer, this is what has happened. You are in La La Land. Once you are in La La Land, you can continue to push on that problem all day and you won't get any closer.

There is a good chance that you are already familiar with this frustration. The first step is to learn to recognize it when it is happening. Here are some keys to recognizing when you are off track.

You know you are in La La Land when…

- You have spent more than three minutes on a single problem.
- Your hand is not moving.
- You don't know what to do next.
- Your answer is not one of the choices.
- You're spending lots of time working with some ugly numbers.

Once you recognize that you are in La La Land, get out. Continuing to push on a problem at this point is a waste of your time. You could easily spend three or four precious minutes on this problem and be no closer to the answer. Spend those three or four minutes on other questions. That time should be yielding you points, not frustration.

After you have completed two or three other questions, return to the one that was giving you trouble. Most likely, the reason it was giving you trouble is that you missed something or misread something the first time around. If the problem is still difficult, walk away again.

The minute you encounter any trouble with a question, walk away. There are plenty of other easier points for you to get with that time. Then return to the problem a few questions later. It's okay to take two or three runs at a tough problem. If you run out of time before returning to the question, so be it. Your time is better spent on easier problems anyway, since all problems count the same.

Forcing yourself to walk away can be difficult, especially when you have already invested time in a question. You will have to train yourself to recognize resistance when it occurs, to walk away, and then to remember to come back. Employ this technique anytime you are practicing for the PCAT. It will take some time to master. Be patient and give it a chance to work. With this technique, there are no questions that are out of your reach on the PCAT.

If you get really frustrated, take a few seconds to close your eyes and take a deep breath. You probably know how to do the math, but that won't help if you let the stress get to you. After a few seconds of de-stressing, read the question again carefully.

If you avoid reading mistakes, these questions may seem relatively easy, but that's exactly the point. You don't want to choose wrong answers when you know how to do the math. Careless mistakes can wreak havoc on your PCAT score.

There are several ways to decrease the number of reading mistakes you make in the Math section. Reread the question, particularly the stem, before selecting your answer. When you copy numbers and diagrams to your erasable noteboard, double-check your notes before working the problem. Finally, pay extra attention to key phrases such as "of the total" or "of the remaining" in word problems.

5.3 USING POE IN MATH

In the previous chapter, we explained Process of Elimination (POE). Use this method whenever you can on questions that are in standard multiple-choice format. Always read the answer choices before you start to solve a math problem because often they will help guide you—you might even be able to eliminate a couple of answer choices before you begin to calculate the answer.

Two effective POE tools are Ballparking and Trap Answers.

Ballparking

You Know More Than You Think

Say you were asked to find 30 percent of 50. Wait—don't do any math yet. Let's say that you glance at the answer choices and you see these:

> A. 5
> B. 15
> C. 30
> D. 80

Think about it. You know that 30 percent of 50 must be less than 50, right? So any answer choice that's greater than 50 can't be right. That means you should eliminate (D) before you even do any calculations! Thirty percent is less than half, so you can get rid of anything greater than 25, which means that (C) is gone too. What is 10% of 50? Eliminate (A). You're done. The only answer left is (B). This process is known as Ballparking. Remember that the answers are part of the question. There are a lot more wrong answers on the PCAT than there are right ones. If it were easy to find the right ones, you wouldn't need this book. It is almost always easier to identify and eliminate the wrong answers than it is to calculate the right one. Just make sure that you are using your whiteboard to eliminate answer choices instead of keeping track in your head.

Ballparking helps you eliminate answer choices and increases your odds of zeroing in on the correct answer. The key is to eliminate any answer choice that is "out of the ballpark."

Ballparking won't help you solve every question on the Quantitative section; you will need to do some calculations. However, the primary purpose of the PCAT is not to test your calculation abilities. In fact, you can often shortcut a problem to save some time or eliminate answers when you're unsure of how to solve a problem.

Even when you get stuck and can't completely solve a problem, you can often eliminate some answers. This won't necessarily lead you to the one and only right answer (although it might), but it will help you narrow down the possible answers before you guess. Approach the question on very simple terms and try to get a rough idea of what the answer is. Then eliminate answers that aren't very close.

The second aspect of Ballparking is saving time by approximating. Because time is precious, you don't want to waste it when you don't need to. On the PCAT, you can use approximations to make the calculations easier and faster. Whenever you see a calculation that looks difficult, try to round off the numbers to something you can handle easily. Then see which answers are "in the ballpark." If there's only one reasonably close answer, you don't need to calculate the precise answer. If there's more than one reasonably close answer, you'll want to go back and do the calculation to find the closest one. Wait a minute, isn't that a waste of time? Not really. The time you spend Ballparking is really short and it will save you from choosing the wrong answer by mistake. For example, you may misplace the decimal point, or accidentally multiply a fraction instead of dividing. However, you won't pick that trap answer if you already eliminated it through Ballparking. Simplifying the calculations will save you precious time.

Ballparking is particularly effective for questions with a drawn figure, including many geometry problems. Even if you don't know the formulas or how to set up the solution, you can make a rough estimate of the answer. Compare the thing the question wants (e.g., area or length of a line) to some known value in the diagram.

Try this method on the following example:

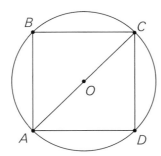

In the figure above, square *ABCD* has an area of 25. What is the area of the circle with center *O* ?

A. $\dfrac{5\sqrt{2}}{2}\pi$

B. $\dfrac{25}{4}\pi$

C. $\dfrac{25}{2}\pi$

D. 25π

Imagine that you have forgotten every geometry formula you've ever known. Just from "eyeballing" the diagram, you can see that the circle is bigger than the square, but less than twice as big. Since the square has an area of 25, the area of the circle is probably in the neighborhood of 35 or 40. The next step is to determine which answers are reasonably close to this estimate and which aren't, eliminating the latter.

Geometry answers often contain $\sqrt{2}$, $\sqrt{3}$, and π, so it's helpful to know some approximations for them: $\sqrt{2}$ is about 1.4, $\sqrt{3}$ is about 1.7, and π is about 3.

Using these approximations, you can find a value for each answer choice. Feel free to round off the numbers to make the calculation easier; after all, you're working with approximations anyway. Choice (A) is about 10 or 11, and (B) is about 18. These are both smaller than the square's area of 25, so you can eliminate them as possibilities for the circle's area. Choice (C) is about 36, which is in line with your estimate. Choice (D) is about 75, which is way too big. Given your rough estimate of 35 to 40, only (C) seems at all reasonable, and it is actually the correct answer.

Caution: On geometry problems, Ballparking depends on having an accurate diagram. If a diagram is labeled with something like, "Note: Figure not drawn to scale," you should not use a Ballparking approach.

Let's look at another problem:

A 100-foot rope is cut so that the shorter piece is $\frac{2}{3}$ the length of the longer piece. How many feet long is the shorter piece?

A. $66\frac{2}{3}$

B.   50

C.   40

D. $33\frac{1}{3}$

Here's How to Crack It

Now, before we dive into the calculations, let's use a little common sense. The rope is 100 feet long. If we cut the rope in half, each part would be 50 feet. However, we didn't cut the rope in half; we cut it so that there's a longer part and a shorter part. What has to be true of the shorter piece then? It has to be smaller than 50 feet. If it weren't, it wouldn't be shorter than the other piece. So looking at our answers, we can eliminate (A) and (B) without doing any real math. That's Ballparking. By the way, the answer is (C).

Trap Answers

Under such tight time constraints, it's easy to fall for "trap answers" in the answer choices to math problems. Remember that trap answers are answer choices that appear correct upon first glance, such as choice D in the previous example which is $\frac{1}{3}$ of 100. Often these answers will look so tempting that you'll choose them without actually bothering to complete the necessary calculations. For example, in the previous question on this page, one may simply cut the string into two pieces of $\frac{1}{3}$ the length and $\frac{2}{3}$ the length, leading to a trap answer of (D) $33\frac{1}{3}$ feet. Watch out for this! If a problem seems way too easy, be careful and double-check your work.

5.4 PLUGGING IN

Wouldn't it be wonderful if there were a way to get rid of those variables? Well, there is. It's a method called Plugging In. Whenever you see a problem with variables in the answer choices, you should consider this approach.

Why Plug In?

Plugging In is a powerful tool that can greatly enhance your math score, but you may be wondering why you should Plug In when algebra works just fine.

Some people are initially skeptical when they learn Plugging In. "That's not the real way to answer the question," they might say. Or, "Why should I learn another way to solve the problem, instead of using algebra?"

Well, there are several reasons that Plugging In is superior to algebra in most cases. First, you are much more likely to make a mistake when manipulating variables than when using "regular" numbers. Your brain simply processes "5 + 3" more easily than it does "$x + y$." In doing algebra, you have to concentrate on the variables, and that leaves you open to mistakes such as forgetting to convert units.

Here's why:

Plugging In converts algebra problems into arithmetic problems. No matter how good you are at algebra, you're better at arithmetic. Why? Because you use arithmetic every day, every time you go to a store, balance your budget, or tip a waiter. Chances are you rarely use algebra in your day-to-day activities.

Plugging In is more accurate than algebra. By plugging in real numbers, you make the problems concrete rather than abstract. Once you're working with real numbers, it's easier to notice when and where you've messed up a calculation. It's much harder to see where you went wrong (or to even know you've done something wrong) when you're staring at a bunch of x's and y's.

Finally, it's always a good idea to have plenty of tools at your disposal. If one way of attacking the problem doesn't work, you simply try another. Plugging In is a tool that works well in a variety of situations, making it a nice option when you're uncertain how to approach a particular question.

One of the best places to use Plugging In effectively is on algebra questions. Algebra questions are generally difficult for two reasons. First, they are often complicated, multistep problems. Second, the answer choices often involve "distractor" choices. These are answer choices that look right, but they are actually wrong. They're designed to tempt you or to influence how you think about a problem.

If you don't like algebra, you're in luck. You don't have to do it. Plugging In will take even the hardest, messiest problem and turn it into a simple arithmetic problem. It will never let you down.

Here Are the Steps

Step 1: **Recognize the Opportunity.** You can plug in on any problem that has variables in the answer choices. The minute you see variables in the answers, even before you have read the problem, you know you can plug in.

Step 2: **Engage the Hand.** You cannot solve Plugging In problems in your head. Even if it seems like an easy question of translating a word problem into an algebraic equation, remember that there are trap answer choices. When a question pops up, the minute you see variables, list your answer choices, A–D, on your whiteboard.

Step 3: **Plug In.** If the question asks for "*x* apples," come up with a number for *x*. The goal here is to make your life easier, so plug in something simple and happy, but avoid 1 or 0. If you plug in a number and the math starts getting creepy (anything involving fractions or negative numbers is creepy), don't be afraid to just change the number you plug in. Always label each variable on your whiteboard.

Step 4: **ID Target Number.** The target number is the value the problem asks you to solve for. Once you've arrived at a target number, write it down on your whiteboard and circle it.

Step 5: **Check All Answer Choices.** Anywhere you see a variable, plug in the number you have written down for that variable. Do any required math. The correct answer is the one that matches your target number. If more than one answer matches your target number, just plug in a different number for your variables and test the remaining answer choices.

Can I Just Plug In Anything?

Plug in numbers that will make the math EASY.

You can plug in any numbers you like, as long as they're consistent with any restrictions stated in the problem, but it's faster if you use easy numbers. What makes a number easy? That depends on the problem. In most cases, smaller numbers are easier to work with than larger numbers. Usually, it's best to start small, with 2, for example. As mentioned above, avoid choosing 0 and 1 since both of these numbers have special properties. Using either 0 or 1 will often make more than one answer choice appear correct. For example, if we plug in 0 for a variable, then the answers $2x$, $3x$, and $5x$ would all equal 0. If you avoid these bad number choices, you should also avoid these bad situations. Also, do not plug in any numbers that show up a lot in the question or answer choices. Let's look at an example so you can see how Plugging In works.

Try this one. Read through the whole question before you start to plug in numbers:

> The price of a certain stock increased 8 points, then decreased 13 points, and then increased 9 points. If the stock price before the changes was *x* points, which of the following was the stock price, in points, after the changes?
>
> A. $x - 5$
> B. $x - 4$
> C. $x + 4$
> D. $x + 5$

Here's How to Crack It

Let's use an easy number like 10 for the variable (write down "$x = 10$" on your whiteboard!). If the original price was 10, and then it increased 8 points, that's 18. Then it decreased 13 points, so now it's 5 (do everything out on the whiteboard—don't even add or subtract in your head). Then it increased 9 points, so now it's 14. So, it started at 10 and ended at 14. Circle 14 (our target answer) and plug in 10 for every x in the answer choices. Which one gives you 14?

(A) $10 - 5 = 5$—Nope.
(B) $10 - 4 = 6$—Nope.
(C) $10 + 4 = 14$—Bingo!
(D) $10 + 5 = 15$—Nope.

Pretty easy, huh?

> Don't skip steps! Use your whiteboard!
>
> 5.4

Good Numbers Make Life Easier

Small numbers aren't always the best choices for Plugging In, though. In a problem involving percentages, for example, 10 and 100 are good numbers to use. In a problem involving minutes or seconds, 30 or 120 are often good choices. (Avoid 60, however; it tends to cause problems.) You should look for clues in the problem itself to help you choose good numbers.

Let's work through the following problem, using the steps above:

> Always plug in when you see variables in the answer choices!

Mara has six more than twice as many apples as does Robert and half as many apples as does Sheila. If Robert has x apples, then, in terms of x, how many apples do Mara, Robert, and Sheila have?

A. $2x + 6$
B. $3x + 12$
C. $4x + 9$
D. $7x + 18$

> What's your target number?

Here's How to Crack It

Step 1:   **Identify the Opportunity.** What do you see? The variable, x, is in both the question and the answer choices. Good, so what do you do?

Step 2:   **Engage the Hand.** On the upper left-hand corner of your whiteboard, list answer choices (A) through (D).

Step 3:   **Plug In.** The problem tells us that Robert has x apples, so plug in a number for x. Make it something nice and happy. Try 4. On your whiteboard, write $x = 4$.

Step 4:   **ID Target Number.** The problem tells us that "Mara has six more than twice as many apples as does Robert." If Robert has 4 apples, then Mara must have 14. On your whiteboard, write $m = 14$. We are also told that Mara has "half as many apples as does Shelia." Ignoring the weird diction, that means that Shelia must have 28 apples. Write down $s = 28$. Now, what does the question ask you to find? It asks for the number of apples that Mara, Robert, and Shelia have. That's no problem; add the three up to come up with 46 apples. This is your target number. Write it down and circle it.

Step 5:   **Check All Answer Choices.** You are allowed to perform only one mathematical function in your head at a time. Anything more than that leads to trouble. For the first answer choice, therefore, you can do $2x$ in your head; that's 8, but write down $8 + 6$. You don't need to go any farther than that because this clearly will not add up to 46. Cross off (A). Choice (B) gives you $12 + 12$. This is also too small, so cross it off. Choice (C) gives you $16 + 9$. That gets you to 25, which is not your target number, so cross it off. Choice (D) is $28 + 18$. Do this on your whiteboard. Do NOT do it in your head. It equals 46, which is your target number.

(A) $2(4) + 6 = 14$ This is not 46, so eliminate it.

(B) $3(4) + 12 = 24$ Still not 46.

(C) $4(4) + 9 = 25$ This isn't 46 either.

(D) $7(4) + 18 = 46$ Bingo! This is your answer.

When a problem has variables in the answer choices, PLUG IN!

You can plug in any time the question has variables in the answer choices. You can usually plug in any number you wish, although you should always pick numbers that will be easy to work with. Some numbers can end up causing more trouble than they're worth.

When Plugging In, follow these rules:

1.   Don't plug in 0 or 1. These numbers, while easy to work with, have special properties.
2.   Don't plug in numbers that are already in the problem; this might confuse you as you work through it.
3.   Don't plug in the same number for multiple variables. For example, if a problem has x, y, and z in it, pick three different numbers to plug in for the three variables.

Finally, Plugging In can be a powerful tool, but you must remember to always check all four answer choices when you plug in. In certain cases, two answer choices can yield the same target number. This doesn't necessarily mean you did anything wrong; you just hit some bad luck. Plug in some new numbers, get a new target, and recheck the answers that worked the first time.

Hidden Variables

You've seen how Plugging In works when the answer choices contain variables, but sometimes the variable in the answers isn't quite so obvious. In fact, it may be invisible. If the answers contain fractions or percents, check the question. If it asks for a fraction or percent of some unknown amount, that unknown amount is the invisible variable. Plug in a number for that variable and use the steps you just learned.

Follow this example.

Marty spends $\frac{1}{3}$ of his weekly allowance on baseball cards. He spends $\frac{1}{4}$ of the rest on bubble gum. He spends $\frac{1}{6}$ of his allowance on soda pop. If Marty has no other expenses and saves the rest of his allowance in a piggy bank, what fraction of his allowance does he save in the piggy bank?

A. $\frac{1}{6}$

B. $\frac{1}{4}$

C. $\frac{1}{3}$

D. $\frac{5}{12}$

Here's How to Crack It

The question asks for a fraction of Marty's allowance, so Marty's allowance is the invisible variable in the answer choices. First, make up a number, say $60, for Marty's allowance. Second, work the problem using that number. Marty spends $\frac{1}{3} \times 60 = 20$ on baseball cards. That leaves 60 – 20 = 40 to spend. He spends $\frac{1}{4}$ *of the rest* or $\frac{1}{4} \times 40 = 10$ on bubble gum. That leaves 40 – 10 = 30 dollars. He spends $\frac{1}{6} \times 60 = 10$ on soda pop, leaving 30 – 10 = 20 dollars for his piggy bank. Third, you need to convert that number to match the answers. He saves 20 dollars out of the original 60 or $\frac{20}{60} = \frac{1}{3}$. The answer is (C).

Plugging In on Fraction and Percent Problems

When you come to questions that involve fractions or percents, you can simply plug in a number and work through the problem using that number. This approach works even when the problem doesn't have variables in it. Why? Because, as you know, fractions and percents express only a relationship between numbers—the actual numbers don't matter.

For example, look at the following problem:

Plugging in on fraction and percent problems is a great way to make your life easier.

---○---

A recent survey of registered voters in City x found that $\frac{1}{3}$ of the respondents support the mayor's property tax plan. Of those who did not support the mayor's plan, $\frac{1}{8}$ indicated they would not vote to reelect the mayor if the plan was implemented. Of all the respondents, what fraction indicated that it would not vote for the mayor if the plan is enacted?

What important information is missing from the problem?

A. $\frac{1}{16}$

B. $\frac{1}{12}$

C. $\frac{1}{6}$

D. $\frac{1}{3}$

Here's How to Crack It

Even though there are no variables in this problem, we can still plug in. On fraction and percent problems, there is often one key piece of information missing: the total. Plugging in for that missing value will make your life much easier. What crucial information is left out of this problem? The total number of respondents. So let's plug in a value for it. Let's say that there were 24 respondents to the survey. 24 is a good number to use because we'll have to work with $\frac{1}{3}$ and $\frac{1}{8}$, so we want a number that's divisible by both those fractions. Working through the problem with our number, we see that $\frac{1}{3}$ of the respondents support the plan. $\frac{1}{3}$ of 24 is 8, so that means 16 people do not support the plan. Next, the problem says that $\frac{1}{8}$ of those who do not support the plan will not vote for the mayor. $\frac{1}{8}$ of 16 is 2, so 2 people won't vote for the mayor. Now we just have to answer the question. Of all respondents, how many will not vote for the mayor? Well, there were 24 total respondents and we figured out that 2 aren't voting. So that's $\frac{2}{24}$ or $\frac{1}{12}$. Choice (B) is the one we want.

---○---

5.5 PLUGGING IN THE ANSWERS (PITA)

Some questions may not have variables in them but will try to tempt you into applying algebra to solve them. The technique for answering these questions is called Plugging In the Answers, or PITA for short. These are almost always difficult problems. Once you recognize the opportunity, however, they turn into simple arithmetic questions. In fact, the hardest part of these problems is often identifying them as opportunities for PITA. The beauty of these questions is that they take advantage of one of the inherent limitations of a multiple-choice test. The test-writers have actually given you the answers, and one of them must be correct. In fact, only one can work. The essence of this technique is to systematically Plug In the Answers into the question to see which answer choice works.

Here Are the Steps

Step 1:   **Recognize the Opportunity.** There are three ways to do this. The first triggers are the phrases "how much…," "how many…," or "what is the value of…." When you see one of these phrases in a question, you can plug in the answers. The second tip-off is specific numbers in the answer choices in ascending or descending order. The last tip-off is your own inclination. If you find yourself tempted to write your own algebraic formulas and to invent your own variables to solve the problem, it's a sure bet that you can just plug in the answers choices.

Step 2:   **Engage the Hand.** The minute you recognize the opportunity, list the numbers in the answer choices in a column in the upper left-hand corner of your whiteboard.

Step 3:   **Label the First Column.** What do these numbers represent? The question asks you to find a specific number. The answer choices are this number. At the top of the column, write down what these numbers represent.

Step 4:   **Start with (B) or (C).** If it's correct, you're finished. If it's incorrect, you can eliminate the choices above or below it, depending on the circumstances.

Step 5:   **Create Your Spreadsheet.** Suppose you start with (C). Use this number to work through the problem. It is always easier to understand the problem using a specific number. Work through the problem in bite-size pieces, and every time you have to do something with the number, make a new column. You can't have too many columns. Each column is a step in solving the problem.

Step 6:   **Rinse and Repeat.** On single-answer multiple-choice questions, only one answer choice can work. If (C) is correct, you are done. If it is not correct, you may be able to identify if it is too big or too small. If it is too big, you can eliminate it and every answer choice that is bigger. This very quickly improves your odds. It also gives you a little spreadsheet specifically designed to calculate the correct answer. When you need to check the remaining answer choices, let the spreadsheet do the thinking for you. All you need to do is to fill in the cells. As soon as you find an answer choice that works, you're done.

The following is an example of a PITA problem:

———————————◯———————————

An office supply store charged $13.10 for the purchase of 85 paper clips. If some of the clips were 16 cents each and the remainder were 14 cents each, how many of the paper clips were 14-cent clips?

A.   16
B.   25
C.   30
D.   35

Here's How to Crack It

Step 1:   **Recognize the Opportunity.** The question asks "how many of the paper clips...." That's your first sign. Additionally, you have specific numbers in the answer choices in ascending order.

Step 2:   **Engage the Hand.** The minute you recognize this as a PITA question, list your answer choices in a column on your whiteboard.

Step 3:   **Label the First Column.** What do those answer choices represent? They are the number of 14-cent clips, so label this column 14¢.

Step 4:   **For this problem, start with (C).** Assume that 30 of the clips were 14 cents each.

Step 5:   **Create Your Spreadsheet.** If 30 of the clips were 14 cents each, then the purchaser would have spent $4.20 on 14-cent clips. Label this column "amount spent." Now you know that there were 85 clips total, so if 30 of the clips were 14 cents each, there must have been 55 clips that were 16 cents each. Write down a 55 and label this column 16¢. The purchaser then spent $8.80 on 16-cent clips. Write this down and label this column "amount spent." You can now calculate the total spent. 4.20 + 8.80 = 13.00. Write this down and label this column "total."

Step 6:   **Rinse and Repeat.** You know that the purchaser spent $13.10 on paper clips. If (C) were correct, then the purchaser would have spent only $13.00 on paper clips. Since you know this is wrong, (C) cannot be correct. Cross it off. You also know that your total is too small. You need a greater portion of your clips to be the more expensive ones to get a higher total, so cross off (D). Now try (B). If 25 of the clips cost 14 cents each, the purchaser would have spent $3.50. There must have been 60 clips that cost 16 cents each (85 − 25 = 60). Then, the purchaser would have spent $9.60 on them. The total spent on clips, therefore, comes to $13.10, and you're done.

Make sure to keep your hand moving, to write down all steps. Here's what your whiteboard should look like after this problem:

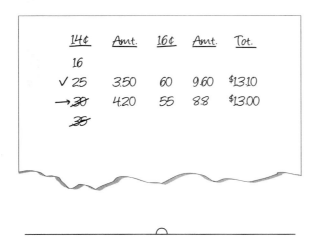

Are you tempted to do algebra? Are there numbers in the answer choices? Plug in the answers.

On PITA questions, you can stop once you've found the correct answer; you don't have to check all four answer choices. Just make sure you write EVERYTHING down when doing these questions (and, indeed, all math questions).

A Note on Plugging In and PITA

Plugging In and PITA are not the only ways to solve these problems, and it may feel weird using these methods instead of trying to do these problems "the real way." You may have even found that you knew how to work with the variables in Plugging In problems or how to write the appropriate equations for the PITA problems. If you can do either of those things, you're already on your way to a great Math score.

But think about it this way. We've already said that PCAT doesn't give any partial credit. So do you think doing it "the real way" gets you any extra points? It doesn't. On the PCAT, a right answer is a right answer, no matter how you get it. "The real way" is great, but unfortunately, it's often much more complex and offers many more opportunities to make careless errors.

The biggest problem with doing things the real way, though, is that it essentially requires that you invent a new approach for every problem. Instead, notice what we've given you here: two strategies that will work toward getting you the right answer on any number of questions. You may have heard the saying, "Give a man a fish and you've fed him for a day, but teach a man to fish and you've fed him for a lifetime." Now, don't worry. Our delusions of grandeur are not quite so extreme, but Plugging In and PITA are useful in a similar way. Rather than giving you a detailed description of how to create formulas and work through them for these problems, we're giving you a strategy that will help you to work through any number of similar problems.

5.6   HOW TO STUDY

Make sure you learn the content of each of the following chapters before you go on to the next one. Don't try to cram everything in all at once. It's much better to do a small amount of studying each day over a longer period; you will master both the math concepts and the techniques if you focus on the material a little bit at a time.

Practice, Practice, Practice

Practice may not make "perfect," but it will surely help. Use everyday math calculations as practice opportunities. Make sure your check has been added correctly at a restaurant, and figure out the exact percentage you want to leave for a tip. The more you practice simple adding, subtracting, multiplying, and dividing on a day-to-day basis, the more your arithmetic skills will improve for the PCAT.

After you work through this book, be sure to practice doing questions on our online tests and on real sample PCATs. There are sample exams at www.pcatweb.info and practice will rapidly sharpen your test-taking skills.

Finally, unless you trust our techniques, you may be reluctant to use them fully and automatically on the real PCAT. The best way to develop that trust is to practice before you get to the real test.

Chapter 6

General Biology

6.1   CELL BIOLOGY

Cell Membrane

The word **eukaryotic** refers to a cell that has a well-defined nucleus bound by a nuclear membrane, with a variety of organelles located outside the nuclear membrane. Some organelles have membranes around them while others do not. There are three types of eukaryotic cells: animal cells, plant cells, and fungal cells. **Prokaryotic** cells, on the other hand, are cells that lack membrane-bound organelles, including nuclei. Prokaryotes, which include bacteria, will be discussed in the next chapter.

There are several features of eukaryotic cells you should recognize. Let's start with these:

- a cell wall, which is *not* found in animal cells
- a cell membrane
- the **cytoplasm**, in which organelles are housed
- a **nucleus**, which is separated from the remainder of the cell by a **nuclear membrane**

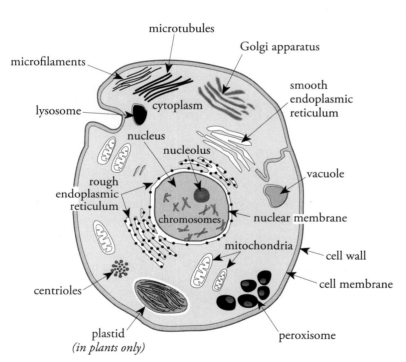

The **cell wall**, composed largely of carbohydrates, is found on the cells of many organisms, including plants, yeasts, and bacteria. Cell walls, however, are not found on animal cells.

Where present, the cell wall is the outermost structure of the cell. All cells, regardless of whether or not they have a cell wall, possess a cell membrane, composed primarily of protein and phospholipid.

Figure 1   Typical Eukaryotic Cell

Associated with the membrane are proteins. Proteins that are embedded in one of the two surfaces of the membrane are called **peripheral proteins**. Those that penetrate completely through the membrane are called **transmembrane proteins**.

The current understanding of membrane dynamics is termed the **fluid mosaic model**, because the membrane is seen as a mosaic of lipids and proteins which are free to move back and forth fluidly. According to this model, lipids and proteins are free to diffuse laterally, in two-dimensions, but are not free to flip-flop.

Phospholipid head groups and hydrophilic protein domains are restricted from entering the hydrophobic membrane interior just as hydrophilic molecules in the extracellular space are. Hence the membrane is said to have **polarity**. This just means that the inside face and the outside face remain different. A specific example of this is that all glycosylations are found on the extracellular face. So the "fluid" in "fluid mosaic" means that things are free to move back and forth, but in two dimensions only. One exception is that some proteins are anchored to the cytoskeleton and thus cannot move in any direction.

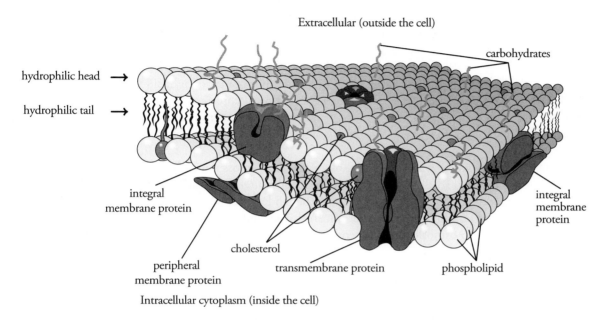

Figure 2 Lipid Bilayer

The **cell membrane** is permeable to some substances and impermeable to others. For that reason, it is termed **semipermeable**. Furthermore, the membrane's permeability is subject to modification; under some circumstances, it might be permeable to a given substance, and under others, it might be impermeable to that same substance. For that reason, it is termed **selectively permeable**. Since the cell membrane's permeability by and large determines which substances enter the cell and which do not, the membrane is said to regulate the cell's internal environment.

Simple Diffusion, Osmosis, and Tonicity

To understand these concepts, we are going to work through some hypothetical situations. First, put the cell membrane out of your mind for a bit and imagine a vessel filled with pure water. Imagine also that the vessel is divided into left and right halves by a membrane freely permeable to Solute X. Suppose now that Solute X is added to the vessel's left side but not to its right side.

Momentarily, the concentration of Solute X will be higher on the left than the right. Between the left and right sides of the vessel, Solute X will experience a concentration gradient (a difference in its concentration). The concentration gradient, however, will not endure. Rather, Solute X molecules will move naturally across the membrane from left to right until their concentration is uniform throughout the vessel. In other words, the solute will move "down" its concentration gradient (from an area of higher concentration to an area of lower concentration) until concentration is equalized.

The process just described is termed **simple diffusion**, which refers to this general phenomenon: in a given system of fluid, solute and solvent particles tend to disperse themselves so that solute concentration is uniform throughout the system. A variety of factors may prevent them from fully equalizing the concentration, but they have a natural tendency to do so. If circumstances allow solute particles to move freely throughout the system, they will move down their concentration gradient and thus distribute themselves in uniform concentration.

Imagine now another water-filled vessel with a membrane that separates its left and right sides. This time, suppose that (1) the vessel is expandable (like a balloon), (2) the membrane is freely permeable to water, and (3) the membrane is impermeable to Solute X.

Suppose now that Solute X is added to the vessel's left side (but not to its right side). The system will want to equilibrate concentration, but the membrane will not allow Solute X to cross. Yet, since the membrane is permeable to water, water will tend to move via simple diffusion from the vessel's right side to its left side in an effort to equalize the concentration of Solute X.

When simple diffusion causes water (and not solute) to move across a membrane, we use the word **osmosis.** Osmosis refers to simple diffusion in which water (not solute) moves across a membrane in an effort to equalize concentration. **Osmotic pressure** refers to the tendency of water to move across a membrane (via osmosis) in an effort to equilibrate concentration. In this second example, the addition of Solute X to the vessel's left side created an osmotic pressure tending to move water from right to left across the membrane.

When one solution (or one portion of a solution) has a higher concentration than another, the region of higher concentration is said to be hypertonic (or hyperosmotic) to the region of lower concentration. The region of lower concentration is said to be hypotonic (or hypoosmotic) to the one of higher concentration. Remember, this terminology is always used to describe a characteristic of one solution when it is being compared to another solution. Consider again the expandable (balloon-like) vessel described above. When Solute X was first added to its left side, the left side became hypertonic to the right (and the right became hypotonic to the left). By osmosis, water moved from the hypotonic region to the hypertonic region.

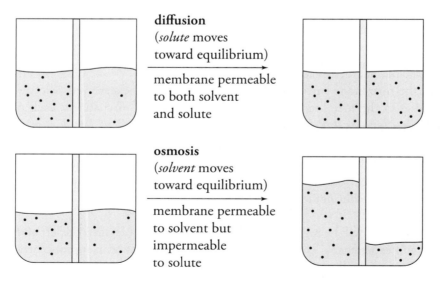

diffusion
(*solute* moves toward equilibrium)

membrane permeable to both solvent and solute

osmosis
(*solvent* moves toward equilibrium)

membrane permeable to solvent but impermeable to solute

In both diffusion and osmosis, the final result is that solute concentrations are the same on both sides of the membrane. The only difference is that in diffusion the membrane is permeable to solute and in osmosis it is not.

Figure 3   Diffusion and Osmosis

Now let's apply these examples to living cells. The cell membrane is freely permeable to many solutes, including most small, lipid-soluble substances (such as cholesterol), and small, uncharged molecules (such as oxygen and carbon dioxide). If any such solute should temporarily be in differing concentration inside and outside the cell (meaning that one side of the cell is hypertonic to the other), then, via simple diffusion, solute molecules will move across the cell membrane (inward or outward, as the situation may require) to "even out" the concentration. By simple diffusion, they will move across the membrane, down their concentration gradient, until concentrations are equal inside and outside the cell.

If a concentration gradient should develop across the cell membrane for a solute to which the membrane is not permeable, then water will tend to move from a hypotonic area to a hypertonic area, in an effort to equalize concentration. Water cannot pass through the plasma membrane via simple diffusion because it is too polar. However, it can freely pass through the plasma membrane with the help of transport channels that are always open and available; these are called **aquaporins.** These water pores are expressed on most eukaryotic cells.

So far, the examples we have talked about do not require the expenditure of energy. They are said to be passive, since molecules are passing down their gradients.

Facilitated Diffusion

Facilitated diffusion is the movement of a solute across a membrane, down a gradient, when the membrane itself (the pure lipid bilayer) is intrinsically impermeable to that solute. Specific integral membrane proteins allow material to cross the plasma membrane down a gradient in facilitated diffusion. For example, red blood cells (RBCs) require glucose, which they get from the bloodstream. However, glucose is a bulky hydrophilic molecule that cannot cross the RBC lipid bilayer. Instead, it must be shuttled across by a particular protein in the RBC plasma membrane. There are two well-characterized types of proteins that serve this sort of function: **channel proteins** and **carrier proteins**. Channels and carriers give the membrane its essential feature of **selective permeability**—permeability to *some* things despite impermeability to *most* things. The aquaporin channels we talked about earlier are also an example of facilitated diffusion.

Facilitated Diffusion: Channels

Channel proteins in the plasma membrane allow material that cannot pass through the membrane by simple diffusion to flow through the plasma membrane down a concentration gradient. Channels do this by forming a narrow opening in the membrane surrounded by the protein. Channels are very selective in what passes through the opening in the membrane. There are many kinds of ion channels, each of which allows the passage of only one type of ion through the channel down a gradient (see Figure 4). All cells have potassium ion channels, for example, that allow only potassium (and not sodium) to flow through the plasma membrane down a gradient. Some channels are open all the time; these are called unregulated channels or leak channels. Ion channels are said to be **gated** if the channel is open in response to specific environmental stimuli. A channel that opens in response to a change in the electrical potential across the membrane is called a **voltage-gated** ion channel. One that opens in response to binding of a specific molecule like a neurotransmitter is called a **ligand-gated** ion channel. The regulation of membrane potential by gated ion channels plays a key role in the nervous system.

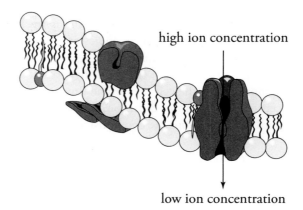

high ion concentration

low ion concentration

Figure 4   An Ion Channel

Facilitated Diffusion: Carriers

Carrier proteins also can transport molecules through membranes by facilitated diffusion, but they do so by a mechanism different from that of ion channels. Carrier proteins do not form a tunnel through membranes like ion channels do. Instead, carrier proteins bind the molecule to be transported at one side of the membrane and then undergo a conformational change to move the molecule to the other side of the membrane. Some carriers, called **uniports**, transport only one molecule across the membrane at a time. Other carriers termed **symports** carry two substances across a membrane in the same direction. **Antiports**, on the other hand, carry two substances in opposite directions.

Active Transport

Active transport is the movement of molecules through the plasma membrane against a gradient. Active transport requires energy input, since it is working against a gradient, and always involves a protein. Another way of saying that active transport requires energy input is to say that the transport process is coupled to a process that is thermodynamically favorable ($\Delta G < 0$). The gradient being pumped against is not necessarily just a concentration gradient. For charged molecules, like ions, it can also involve electric potentials that form a combined electrochemical gradient that must be pumped against. The form of energy input used to drive movement of molecules against an electrochemical gradient varies. In **primary active transport**, transport of a molecule is coupled to hydrolysis of adenosine triphosphate (ATP), the energy-carrying molecule found in cells. In **secondary active transport**, the transport process is not coupled *directly* to ATP hydrolysis. Instead, ATP is first used to create a gradient; then the potential energy in that gradient is used to drive the transport of some other molecule across the membrane. Since ATP is not used in the actual transport of the "other" molecule, the ATP use is described as *indirect*. For example, the transport of glucose into some cells is driven against the glucose concentration gradient by the cotransport of sodium ions down the sodium electrochemical gradient, previously established by an ATPase pump. A common mechanism driving secondary active transport of many different molecules involves coupling transport to the flow of sodium ions down a gradient.

The Na⁺/K⁺ ATPase and the Resting Membrane Potential

The **Na⁺/K⁺ ATPase** is a transmembrane protein in the plasma membrane of all cells in the body. It pumps 3 Na⁺ out of the cell, pumps 2 K⁺ into the cell, and hydrolyzes one ATP to drive the pumping of these ions against their gradients (Figure 5). The sodium that is pumped out of the cell stays outside, since the plasma membrane is impermeable to sodium ions. Some of the potassium ions that are pumped into the cell are able to leak back out through **potassium leak channels**. Potassium flows down its concentration gradient out of the cell through these leak channels. The movement of ions out of the cell helps the cell to maintain osmotic balance with its surroundings. As potassium leaves the cell through the leak channels, the movement of positive charge out of the cell creates an electric potential across the plasma membrane with a net negative charge on the interior of the cell. This potential created by the Na⁺/K⁺ ATPase is known as the **resting membrane potential**. The concentration gradient of high sodium outside of the cell established by the Na⁺/K⁺ ATPase is the driving force behind secondary active transport of many different molecules, including sugars and amino acids. To summarize, the activity of the Na⁺/K⁺ ATPase is important in three ways:

1. to maintain osmotic balance between the cellular interior and exterior
2. to establish the resting membrane potential
3. to provide the sodium concentration gradient used to drive secondary active transport

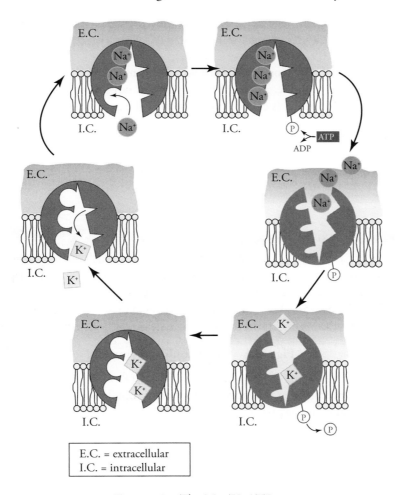

E.C. = extracellular
I.C. = intracellular

Figure 5   The Na⁺/K⁺ ATPase

Summary of Membrane Transport

Here is a summary of this section:

1. Passive diffusion is movement of lipid-soluble particles and some small uncharged molecules to which the cell membrane is freely permeable. Movement proceeds down a gradient (from areas of higher concentration to areas of lower concentration) and requires no expenditure of energy.
2. Facilitated diffusion is movement of lipid-insoluble substances and is mediated by channels or carrier proteins within the plasma membrane. Movement proceeds down a gradient and requires no expenditure of energy.
3. Active transport is movement against a gradient and, for that reason, requires the expenditure of energy. This energy can be provided directly by ATP hydrolysis (primary active transport) or indirectly (secondary active transport).

Endocytosis and Exocytosis

Another mechanism used to transport material across the plasma membrane is via membrane-bound vesicles that fuse with the membrane (see Figure 6). **Exocytosis** is a process to transport material outside of the cell; a vesicle in the cytoplasm fuses with the plasma membrane and the contents of the vesicle are expelled into the extracellular space. For example, the material released could be products secreted by the cell, such as hormones or digestive enzymes.

Endocytosis is the opposite of exocytosis: materials are taken into the cell by an invagination of a piece of the cell membrane to form a vesicle. Again, the cytoplasm is not allowed to mix with the extracellular environment. The new vesicle formed is called an **endosome**. There are three types of endocytosis:

1. phagocytosis
2. pinocytosis
3. receptor-mediated endocytosis

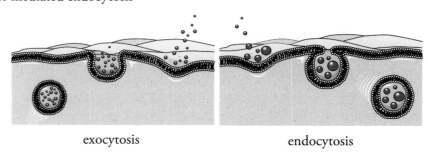

exocytosis   endocytosis

Figure 6   Endo- and Exocytosis

Phagocytosis means "cell eating." It refers to the nonspecific uptake of large particulate matter into a phagocytic vesicle, which later merges with a lysosome. Thus, the phagocytosed material will be broken down. The prime example of phagocytic human cells are macrophages ("big eaters") of the immune system, which engulf and destroy viruses and bacteria.

Pinocytosis (cell drinking) is the nonspecific uptake of small molecules and extracellular fluid via invagination. Primitive eukaryotic cells obtain nutrition in this manner, but virtually all eukaryotic cells participate in pinocytosis.

Receptor-mediated endocytosis is very specific. The site of endocytosis is marked by pits coated with the molecule clathrin (inside the cell) and with receptors that bind to a specific molecule (outside the cell).

Cellular Adhesions

While cells can be viewed as discrete living entities, those of the human body are organized into tissues. Cellular adhesions join cells together in various ways. In general, there are three types of cellular adhesions: tight junctions, gap junctions, and desmosomes.

Tight junctions link together portions of adjacent cell membranes to form a barrier. At a tight junction, there is no intercellular space. For example, tight junctions maintain the structural integrity of the small intestine's inner surface. There, they form the barrier that prevents the intestinal contents from leaking out between cells.

Gap junctions link together the cytoplasms of adjacent cells, and small particles, such as ions, can flow through them freely. They consist of protein channels that form a bridge between the two cells. Gap junctions are important in heart muscle contraction; they allow the heart's electrical signals to be passed quickly from cell to cell.

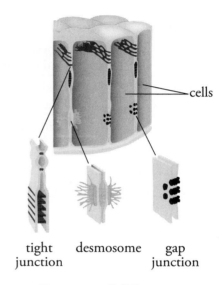

tight junction   desmosome   gap junction

Figure 7   Cell Junctions

Desmosomes are composed of plaque-like proteins embedded in the cell membrane to which the cytoskeleton is attached. Desmosomes are responsible for the structural integrity of most tissues in the human body.

Eukaryotic Cell Organelles

Here is a summary of some important eukaryotic organelles:

Organelle	Function	Number of Membranes
Nucleus	Contains and protects the DNA genome, transcription, partial assembly of ribosomes	2
Mitochondria	ATP production via the Krebs cycle, electron transport chain, and oxidative phosphorylation	2
Ribosomes	Synthesize proteins via translation	0
RER	Synthesis and modification of secretory and membrane-bound proteins	1
SER	Detoxification and glycogen breakdown in liver, steroid synthesis in gonads, calcium storage in skeletal muscle	1
Golgi apparatus	Modification and sorting of secretory and membrane-bound proteins	1
Lysosomes	Contain acid hydrolases that digest various substances	1
Peroxisomes	Metabolize lipids and toxins, producing H_2O_2	1

Table 1   Animal Cell Organelles

The **endomembrane system** of a cell consists of the:

1. outer membrane, located at the cell periphery
2. nuclear membrane, which encloses the nucleus
3. **endoplasmic reticulum,** found throughout the cytoplasm

We have already discussed the plasma membrane. Here we will discuss the other organelles. Let's start with the nucleus.

The **nucleus** of a eukaryotic cell houses the DNA (deoxyribonucleic acid) **genome.** The genome of each organism is divided across **chromosomes,** which are composed of DNA and structural proteins. Also located in the nucleus is a suborganelle called the **nucleolus.** This is the site of ribosomal ribonucleic acid (rRNA) synthesis and partial ribosome assembly. The nucleolus does not have an additional membrane around it; rather, it is a region of the nucleus. **Ribosomes** are made of both rRNA and proteins and are the site of translation. This is where an mRNA message is read to create a peptide chain. Ribosomes reside outside of the nucleus, in the cytoplasm of the cell. Some are free-floating and others are associated with the rough ER.

The network of channels that comprises the endoplasmic reticulum (ER) is of two types: **rough endoplasmic reticulum** (rough ER or RER) and **smooth endoplasmic reticulum** (smooth ER or SER). The rough ER is found in close association with ribosomes, which function in protein synthesis. The rough ER constitutes a principal site of cellular protein synthesis, specifically of proteins that are destined for the plasma membrane or the extracellular environment. The smooth ER is devoid of ribosomes; it does not participate in protein synthesis but is involved in lipid synthesis, drug detoxification, or calcium storage, depending on the tissue type.

The **Golgi apparatus** is a specialized derivative of the endoplasmic reticulum, consisting of a series of flattened sacs rather than channels. It is responsible for packaging and transporting proteins to the cell surface, where they are either expelled into the extracellular space or incorporated into the cell membrane. This transport is accomplished through **vesicles**, which pinch off from the Golgi and migrate to the cell surface. They then fuse with the cell membrane and release their contents through the process of exocytosis. The Golgi apparatus modifies some proteins before expelling them from the cell. The RER and the Golgi apparatus function together as the secretory protein pathway.

Lysosomes and **peroxisomes** contain many different types of enzymes and are important for degradation and detoxification. Peroxisomal enzymes degrade lipids and toxins, a metabolic process that produces hydrogen peroxide (H_2O_2). Peroxisomes contain catalase, an enzyme that breaks down hydrogen peroxide. Lysosomes contain hydrolytic enzymes that digest foreign particles and old organelles. In plant cells, lysosomes house certain toxins, including alkaloids (primary amines). **Vacuoles** constitute spaces or vacancies within the cytoplasm. Often they are fluid-filled. In protozoans, they function to expel wastes or excess fluid.

Mitochondria are double-membraned organelles that mediate the synthesis of ATP, the molecule associated with energy storage, and commonly termed the cell's "energy currency." The **inner mitochondrial membrane** is folded into convolutions called **cristae**. The interior of the inner mitochondrial membrane is termed the **matrix**. The Krebs cycle and oxidative phosphorylation occur within the mitochondria. These processes produce the bulk of the ATP generated in **aerobic** (oxygen-using) organisms. **Glycolysis** is a precursor step to these processes and produces a small amount of ATP. Glycolysis occurs in the cytosol of eukaryotic cells, which means that not all ATP is made in the mitochondria.

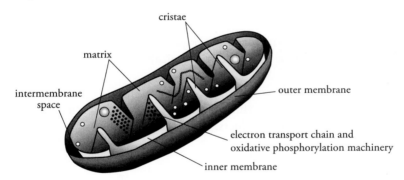

cristae

matrix

intermembrane space

outer membrane

electron transport chain and oxidative phosphorylation machinery

inner membrane

Figure 8 The Mitochondrion

Plastids, found almost solely in plant cells, contain **pigment** and function in **photosynthesis** as well as in other cellular processes. The most abundant of the plastids are **chloroplasts**, which contain the green pigment **chlorophyll**.

Cilia and Flagella

Cilia and **flagella** are associated with cellular locomotion, but depending on the cell site, they may serve other functions as well. In the human airway, cilia serve to propel foreign particles toward the throat, from which such particles can be expelled or swallowed. In protists, cilia and flagella serve as means of locomotion. The flagellum comprises the tail of a sperm cell and confers motility so that the sperm may reach and fertilize the ovum. In eukaryotic cells, both cilia and flagella are composed of a structured arrangement of **microtubules**.

6.2

Microtubules, Microfilaments, and Centrosomes

Microtubules are polymers made of the protein **tubulin.** In addition to being the structural basis of cilia and flagella, microtubules are also an important part of the cytoskeleton. Animal cells have an internal cytoskeleton composed of three types of proteins: microtubules, intermediate filaments, and **microfilaments.** All three are composed of noncovalently polymerized proteins; in other words, they are a massive example of quaternary protein structure. Microtubules are the thickest and microfilaments the thinnest. Microfilaments, which are composed of the protein actin, function in cellular movement.

Centrosomes are small organelles made of two **centrioles** and some surrounding proteins. They do not have a membrane. Centrosomes are located in the cytoplasm and anchor the microtubules. We will talk about centrosomes more when we get to mitosis.

6.2 METABOLISM AND ENERGY TRANSFORMATIONS

Enzyme Function

A cell's survival depends on the biochemical reactions it conducts. Most of these reactions would not proceed at a rate consistent with survival were it not for the availability of **catalysts.** In a biochemical context, **enzymes** catalyze reactions, so a cell's survival depends on its enzymes.

Whether a reaction is ultimately exothermic or endothermic, it requires energy at the outset. This energy is called the **activation energy.** Like all catalysts, enzymes reduce a reaction's activation energy. In so doing, they increase reaction rate. Like any catalyst, an enzyme itself undergoes no net change during the course of the reaction it catalyzes. An enzyme emerges from a chemical reaction unaltered in quantity and condition. Indeed, a single enzyme molecule will typically catalyze the same reaction over and over again.

Although an enzyme increases the rate at which a given reaction occurs, it does not affect the **equilibrium concentrations** of the reactants or products.

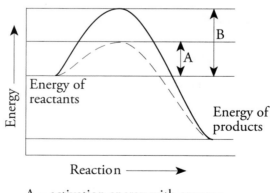

A = activation energy with enzyme
B = activation energy without enzyme
— — — catalyzed reaction
——— uncatalyzed reaction

Figure 9 Comparative Energies of Activation of a Reaction, Catalyzed and Uncatalyzed

Mechanism of Enzymatic Action

The first step in the functioning of an enzyme is the formation of a transient **enzyme-substrate complex**.

Each enzyme associates with its substrate at an **active site**, meaning a site on the enzyme's surface that is physically structured to accommodate the substrate molecule. For example, if a reaction involves two substrate molecules, the enzyme's active site can draw them close together and allow them to interact. Substrates are able to react when they are incorporated into an enzyme-substrate complex. Therefore, while an enzyme-substrate complex is formed from enzyme and substrates, its dissociation liberates enzyme and product(s):

Substrate A + Substrate B + Enzyme → Enzyme-Substrate Complex → Enzyme + Product(s)

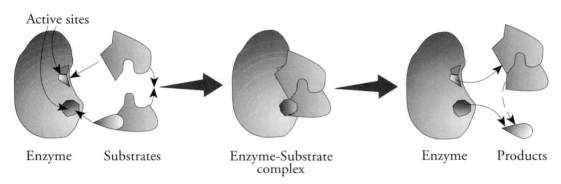

Active sites

Enzyme   Substrates   Enzyme-Substrate   Enzyme   Products
complex

Figure 10   Enzymatic Activity

Enzyme specificity refers to the fact that an enzyme is usually specific to one reaction. An enzyme functions because of the relationship of its physical conformation to the substrate(s) on which it acts. Generally, the active site is structurally unreceptive to any molecules except those substrates to which the enzyme is specific; therefore, only reactions involving those substrates will be catalyzed. An early theory proposed to explain this specificity was called the **lock-and-key** hypothesis, which states that the enzyme's shape accommodated precisely the shape of the substrate. This hypothesis has been elaborated upon in the **induced fit** hypothesis, which states that the enzyme's shape compels the substrate to take on the shape of the reaction's transition state. This hypothesis is now the prevailing model for enzyme activity.

Limitations of Enzymatic Activity

Most enzymes are proteins. Any condition that affects the stability of a protein molecule, therefore, potentially affects an enzyme's stability and its ability to function. Such conditions include pH and temperature. A given enzyme will function only within particular ranges of pH and temperature.

In fact, an enzyme will function only within a very small pH range. For most enzymes, this pH is between 6.5 and 8.0 (which is the normal physiological pH range), but there are enzymes whose optimum pH falls outside this range. For example, pepsin, the proteolytic enzyme that operates in the stomach, works best in the pH range of the stomach, which is approximately 1.5 to 2.5. Similarly, most enzymes work best at physiological temperatures (around 37°C). Below this temperature, enzymatic activity slows, but the structure of the enzyme remains intact. Above this temperature, the enzyme's three-dimensional structure begins to break down. Since the enzyme's shape is critical to its proper function, enzymatic activity falls off dramatically at temperatures exceeding 37°C by a significant amount. This breakdown in

6.2

the enzyme's shape is called **denaturation**, and it occurs under conditions that disrupt hydrogen bonds, which function in maintaining the protein molecule's secondary and tertiary structures. Denaturation also explains the drop-off in enzymatic activity that occurs at pH values outside an enzyme's optimum range. If favorable pH and temperature conditions are restored, the enzyme will usually renature, or return to its functional conformation.

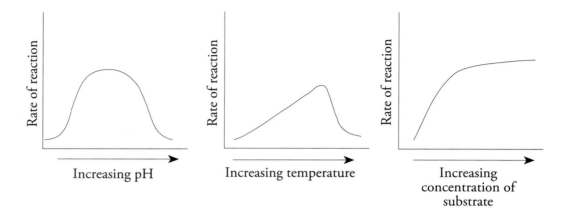

Figure 11   Factors That Affect Enzyme Function

The rate of a catalyzed reaction depends on both the concentration of substrate and the concentration of enzymes. When substrate is first added to a reaction system, only a few molecules will be required to catalyze the reaction. In other words, only a few enzyme molecules are involved in enzyme-substrate complexes (ES); most remain as free enzyme molecules (E). As the concentration of substrate is increased, the proportion of ES will increase while the proportion of free E decreases. With continued addition of substrate, eventually all of the enzymes in the system will be involved in ES complexes; the addition of more substrate will not increase the overall rate of the reaction, since there is no more available enzyme to accommodate the additional substrate. At this point, the only way to increase the overall rate of reaction (assuming that external conditions, e.g., temperature, remain constant) is to add more enzyme to the system.

For their activity, certain enzymes require the availability of **cofactors** or **coenzymes**. Cofactors are inorganic substances, such as Fe^{2+} or Cu^{2+} ions. Coenzymes are organic substances, such as vitamins.

Enzyme Inhibition

Enzymes exert control over the cell's activities by determining which reactions occur and which do not. This means that the activity of enzymes themselves must be closely controlled. There are several ways to do this, but one common example is a process called **feedback inhibition.** This is when an enzyme's activity may be inhibited by accumulation of the product. Some reaction products are toxic in high concentrations; feedback inhibition prevents the cell from producing an excessive quantity of product. Also, accumulating too much product can be a waste of energy.

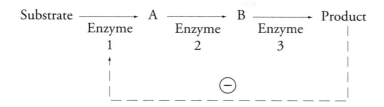

Figure 12 Feedback Inhibition of Enzyme Action

Competitive inhibition occurs when two molecules, one of which is the substrate and one of which is called the **inhibitor**, compete for an enzyme's active site. If bound to the enzyme, the substrate will participate in the reaction, but the inhibitor will not. Assuming that substrate concentration does not change, then for the time during which the inhibitor is bound to the enzyme, the enzyme is essentially nonfunctional. By effectively diluting the concentration of enzyme in a reaction system, it suppresses the rate of reaction.

Energy Production in the Cell: ATP

Most cellular processes rely on energy that is stored in the cell until it is needed and available for conversion to a usable form. **Adenosine triphosphate (ATP)** is the form in which most cells store their energy just before use. ATP is dubbed the cell's "energy currency." In a molecule of ATP, adenine (a nitrogenous base) is linked to ribose (a sugar), which is also linked to a chain of three phosphate (PO_4) groups. The bonds that link the two phosphate groups farthest from the adenosine moiety are **high-energy bonds.** Their disruption releases more energy than does disruption of other bonds in the molecule. (Remember that no bond releases energy when broken. The energy from disruption actually comes from the subsequent formation of bonds that are more stable.)

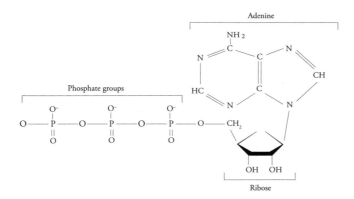

Figure 13 Adenosine Triphosphate (ATP)

Although removal of both the second and third phosphate groups yield about the same amount of free energy under standard conditions, it is the third phosphate group that is removed most often in physiological systems. The liberated energy is then used to drive otherwise unfavorable processes.

The energy required to synthesize ATP is derived from glucose molecules stored in the cell. Glucose is a six-carbon monosaccharide. The chemical bonds within the molecule are broken by a series of reactions. The energy released by the formation of more stable bonds is an energy source for ATP production.

ATP is produced anaerobically via the process of glycolysis. Depending on the cell type and its oxygen supply, glycolysis might be followed, in turn, by

a. **fermentation**, another anaerobic process, which facilitates the continuity of glycolysis, or

b. certain aerobic processes that produce additional ATP.

Glycolysis

Glycolysis is a series of enzymatic reactions that breaks down a glucose molecule to yield two molecules of pyruvate (a three-carbon molecule). This process requires an initial input of two ATP molecules, but it leads to the production of four ATP molecules, for a net gain of two ATP molecules. Glycolysis also generates two molecules of NADH, which constitute the reduced form of two NAD^+ molecules. In this reduced form, NADH stores energy that will ultimately generate additional ATP if oxygen is present.

In net chemical terms, glycolysis (which involves a number of steps and substeps) may be represented like this:

$$1 \text{ Glucose} + 2\text{ADP} + 2P_i + 2\text{NAD}^+ \rightarrow 2 \text{ pyruvate} + 2\text{ATP} + 2\text{NADH} + 2H_2O + 2H^+$$

Note that:

- Glycolysis occurs in the cell's cytoplasm, where the substrates and enzymes necessary for its several steps are available.
- Glycolysis is an **anaerobic** process that occurs in both aerobic and anaerobic cells.
- For each molecule of glucose that undergoes glycolysis, the cell enjoys a net gain of 2ATP molecules (from two ADP molecules and two phosphate ions) and 2NADH molecules (from 2NAD$^+$ molecules, 2 hydrogen ions, and 4 electrons). Here is a summary:

  (a) $2\text{ADP} + 2P_i \rightarrow 2\text{ATP}$

  (b) $2\text{NAD}^+ + 2H^+ + 4e^- \rightarrow 2\text{NADH}$

Glycolysis represents a primitive process that arose very early in the evolution of life. All cells harbor the enzymes necessary to conduct this anaerobic process, and some prokaryotes depend on it as their sole means of producing ATP. Such cells are known as obligate or tolerant anaerobes because they either require low oxygen conditions to survive, or can put up with oxygen being present but don't use it in ATP production. Eukaryotes, including animal cells, depend predominantly on aerobic respiration (to be discussed shortly) but will resort to glycolysis as a kind of "emergency process" when oxygen is in short supply.

Fermentation

If oxygen is unavailable, or for a cell that cannot conduct aerobic respiration, the pyruvate produced through glycolysis undergoes fermentation. **Fermentation** is an anaerobic process in which some organic molecule accepts (is reduced by) the hydrogen atoms produced during glycolysis. In most animal cells, the hydrogen acceptor is pyruvate itself, the very molecule produced by glycolysis. Pyruvate is converted to lactate, and NAD^+ is regenerated from NADH.

$$\text{pyruvate} + \text{NADH} + H^+ \rightarrow \text{lactate} + NAD^+$$

In humans undergoing vigorous exercise, the cardiovascular system may be unable to supply actively metabolizing muscle with enough oxygen to sustain aerobic cellular respiration. This results in an oxygen debt, and the affected muscle cells conduct glycolysis, anaerobically, in order to sustain some degree of ATP production. Glycolysis is followed by fermentation, which produces lactate. Lactate, and the decreased pH it produces, causes the pain associated with muscle fatigue.

For each pyruvate produced via glycolysis, fermentation yields one molecule of lactate and regenerates one molecule of NAD^+ from NADH. For each molecule of glucose undergoing glycolysis, therefore, fermentation produces two molecules of lactate and regenerates two molecules of NAD^+.

Fermentation does not produce ATP. Yet under anaerobic conditions, fermentation is essential to the continuity of glycolysis; without it, glycolysis would grind to a halt. That is because NAD^+, which is essential to glycolysis, is a relatively limited chemical resource within the cell. Fermentation serves to regenerate NAD^+—to prevent its depletion—so that glycolysis may continue.

Glycolysis

$$\text{1 glucose} + \text{2ADP} + 2P_i + \textbf{2NAD}^+ \rightarrow \text{2 pyruvate} + \text{2ATP} + \text{2NADH} + 2H_2O + 2H^+$$

Fermentation

$$\text{2 pyruvate} + \text{2NADH} + 2H^+ \rightarrow \text{2 lactate} + \textbf{2NAD}^+$$

In yeasts, the hydrogen acceptor that mediates fermentation is not pyruvate, but rather acetaldehyde, which is produced when pyruvate loses a terminal CO_2 group. The acetaldehyde molecule accepts the hydrogen produced via glycolysis, producing NAD^+ and ethyl alcohol. For that reason, fermentation in yeasts is among the processes long exploited by humankind to produce alcoholic beverages.

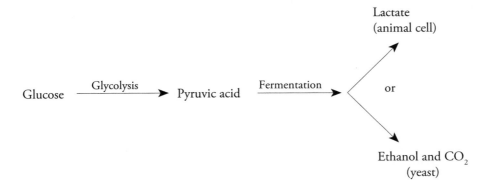

Figure 14 Anaerobic Pathways

Aerobic Processes

When adequate oxygen is available, aerobic organisms do not conduct fermentation. Rather, following glycolysis, they direct pyruvate toward aerobic respiratory processes, in which they use molecular oxygen as a final oxidizing agent—a final electron acceptor. In terms of harvesting energy from glucose (measured in terms of ATP production), aerobic respiration is far more efficient than glycolysis followed by fermentation. Glycolysis and fermentation, as already noted, yield a net production of 2ATP molecules per molecule of glucose. In aerobic respiration, on the other hand, a molecule of glucose produces between 30 and 32 molecules of ATP.

Aerobic or cell respiration involves several phases. After glycolysis, each pyruvic acid molecule is transported into the matrix and converted to acetyl-CoA. Next come the Krebs cycle, the electron transport chain (ETC), and finally oxidative phosphorylation (OP). The Krebs cycle and ECT/OP require oxygen and are therefore aerobic. The mitochondria is where aerobic respiration and all aerobic reactions occur.

PDC and Krebs Cycle

Pyruvate produced during glycolysis is channeled to the Krebs cycle via the multienzyme complex pyruvate dehydrogenase (PDC), located in the mitochondrial matrix. In a reaction known as oxidative decarboxylation, pyruvate dehydrogenase catalyzes the release of carbon dioxide from pyruvate, and the resulting molecule is oxidized (two electrons are transferred to NAD^+ to produce NADH). The acetyl group that is produced is then combined with coenzyme A to yield acetyl-CoA.

$$pyruvate + CoA + NAD^+ \rightarrow acetyl\text{-}CoA + CO_2 + NADH$$

The **Krebs cycle** (also called the **citric acid cycle** or the **tricarboxylic acid cycle**) represents eight reactions designed to harness energy released from the stepwise oxidation of pyruvate (deprotonated pyruvic acid). You should know the fundamental principles of the Krebs cycle and be able to identify some critical steps.

In the first step of the Krebs cycle, acetyl-CoA, a two-carbon molecule, reacts with the four-carbon oxaloacetate molecule to produce a six-carbon citrate molecule deprotonated (citric acid).

$$acetyl\text{-}CoA + oxaloacetate \rightarrow citrate$$

Citrate then undergoes a series of oxidation-reduction reactions that lead to removal of two carbon groups as CO_2. The energy released during these redox reactions is used to reduce four **electron carrier molecules**. Specifically, three molecules of NAD^+ and one FAD molecule are reduced, as shown in the following reactions:

$$NAD^+ + 2e^- + 2H^+ \rightarrow NADH + H^+$$

$$FAD^+ + 2e^- + 2H^+ \rightarrow FADH_2$$

These reduced electron carriers store energy and are oxidized in a later stage of aerobic respiration, thereby releasing their energy into a process that generates ATP. For now, think of NADH and $FADH_2$ as high energy electron carriers that are temporarily storing some of the energy that started in glucose.

The Krebs cycle regenerates the four-carbon oxaloacetate, which can then recombine with another molecule of acetyl-CoA to initiate another turn of the cycle.

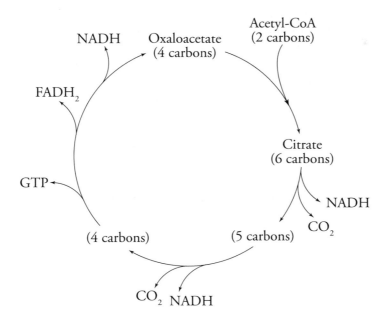

Figure 15 The Krebs Cycle

In addition to the reduced electron carriers, one molecule of GTP (guanosine triphosphate) is produced from GDP (guanosine diphosphate) and inorganic phosphate during each turn of the Krebs cycle. The phosphate bonds in GTP are essentially equivalent in energy to those in ATP. Indeed, GTP can transfer its third phosphate group to ADP to produce ATP. Some cells and certain cell processes can use GTP directly as an energy currency; they do not have to convert it to ATP first.

Overall, each turn of the Krebs cycle oxidizes citric acid in a stepwise fashion and stores the liberated energy in NADH, $FADH_2$, or GTP. The products of each cycle are:

- three molecules of NADH
- one molecule of $FADH_2$
- one molecule of GTP
- two molecules of CO_2
- one molecule of oxaloacetate (regenerated for the next turn of the cycle)

Glycolysis generates two molecules of pyruvate per glucose, and the PDC converts each into a molecule of acetyl-CoA. This means that each glucose molecule requires two turns of the Krebs cycle. In other words, per glucose, the Krebs cycle produces:

- six molecules of NADH
- two molecule of $FADH_2$
- two molecule of GTP
- four molecules of CO_2
- two molecules of oxaloacetate

Here is a summary of how the six carbons in a molecule of glucose have transitioned through cell respiration:

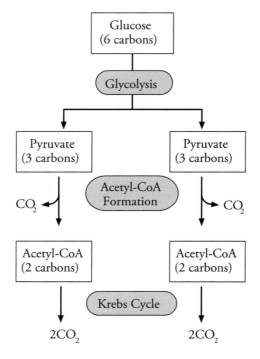

Figure 16 Carbon Atoms in Cell Respiration

Electron Transport Chain and Oxidative Phosphorylation

To understand the electron transport chain (ETC) and oxidative phosphorylation (OP), you must recall the structure of a mitochondrion. Each mitochondrion contains two membranes, an outer membrane and an inner membrane, each composed of a lipid bilayer. The outer membrane is smooth and contains large pores formed by porin proteins. The inner membrane is impermeable, even to very small items like H^+, and is densely folded into structures termed cristae. Cristae extend into the matrix, which is the innermost space of the mitochondrion. The space between the two membranes, the intermembrane space, is continuous with the cytoplasm due to large pores in the outer membrane. Enzymes of the Krebs cycle and the pyruvate dehydrogenase complex are located in the matrix, and those of the electron transport chain and oxidative phosphorylation are bound to the inner mitochondrial membrane.

There are two goals of ETC/OP:

1. reoxidize all the electron carriers reduced in glycolysis, PDC, and the Krebs cycle
2. store energy in ATP

NADH created in the cytoplasm via glycolysis are transported into the mitochondria before they can be passed along the electron transport chain. All the other molecules of NADH and $FADH_2$ were produced inside the mitochondrial matrix, so they are in the right place to donate electrons to the electron transport chain.

The electron transport chain is a group of five electron carriers. Each member of the chain reduces the next member down the line. Three members are large protein complexes found embedded in the inner mitochondrial membrane. The others are smaller electron carriers. The chain is organized so that the first large carrier receives electrons from NADH as it is oxidized to NAD^+. $FADH_2$ is oxidized at the second member of the ETC. The electrons released by these oxidation reactions are transferred through the chain, and each of the three large membrane-bound proteins pumps protons across the inner mitochondrial membrane (out of the matrix and into the intermembrane space) every time electrons flow past. This creates a large proton gradient that is harnessed by an enzyme called **ATP synthase.** This large protein complex contains a proton channel that spans the inner membrane. As protons pass through ATP synthase, ATP is synthesized from ADP + P_i. Thus, ATP production is dependent on a proton gradient. Once the electrons reach the end of the electron transport chain, they combine with protons and oxygen (the ultimate electron acceptor) to form water.

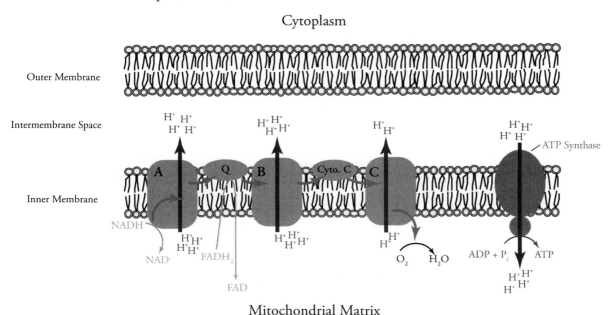

Figure 17   The Electron Transport Chain

In summary:

*   Oxidative phosphorylation is the oxidation of the high-energy electron carriers NADH and $FADH_2$ coupled to the phosphorylation of ADP to produce ATP.
*   Energy released through oxidation of NADH and $FADH_2$ by the electron transport chain is used to pump protons out of the mitochondrial matrix.
*   This proton gradient is the source of energy used to drive the phosphorylation of ADP to ATP.

Here is a summary of energy flow through cell respiration:

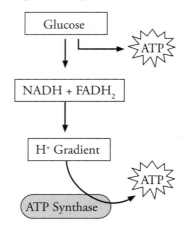

Figure 18 Energy Flow in Cell Respiration

How does all this work out to a total ATP yield per glucose? Let's start with a summary of what we've made:

Process	Location	Net Output	
		Carbon Products (per glucose)	Other Products (per glucose)
Glycolysis	Cytoplasm	2 pyruvate	2NADH 2ATP
PDC	Mitochondrial matrix	2 acetyl-CoA 2CO_2	2NADH
Krebs Cycle	Mitochondrial matrix	4CO_2	6NADH 2FADH$_2$ 2ATP

You can convert this into ATP by doing some calculations. NADH and $FADH_2$ are not equivalent to each other in terms of ATP yield, and it costs something to bring cytoplasmic NADH into the mitochondria. Overall:

- each cytoplasmic NADH = 1.5ATP
- each mitochondrial NADH = 2.5ATP
- each mitochondrial $FADH_2$ = 1.5ATP

The conversions look like this:

Process	Output (per glucose)	Conversion	ATP (per glucose)
Glycolysis	2NADH	× 1.5	3
	2ATP	× 1	2
PDC	2NADH	× 2.5	5
Krebs Cycle	6NADH	× 2.5	15
	2FADH$_2$	× 1.5	3
	2ATP	× 1	2
Total			30

Overall, this means that each glucose yields 30 molecules of ATP in a eukaryotic cell.

Other Metabolic Pathways of the Cell

There are several other metabolic pathways that play important roles in maintaining sugar and energy levels.

Glycogenolysis vs. Gluconeogenesis

Glycogenolysis is the term for glycogen breakdown. Glycogen, a polymer of glucose found in muscle and liver cells, is the main form of carbohydrate storage in animals. **Glycogenesis** (the synthesis of glycogen) and glycogenolysis are opposing processes, controlled by hormones that regulate blood sugar levels and energy. Glycogenolysis occurs in response to glucagon, when blood sugar levels are low. It results in glucose being released into the blood.

Gluconeogenesis occurs when dietary sources of glucose are unavailable, and when the liver has depleted stores of glucose. This process, which occurs primarily in the liver (with a small amount occurring in the kidneys), involves converting non-carbohydrate precursor molecules (such as lactate, pyruvate, Krebs cycle intermediates, and the carbon skeletons of most amino acids) into oxaloacetate and then glucose.

β-Oxidation

Fatty acids are made in the cytoplasm of **hepatocytes** (liver cells) via fatty acid biosynthetic pathways. They are stored in **adipocytes** (fat cells) as **triglycerides** (triacylglycerol or TAG). Fatty acids can be broken down in the hepatocyte mitochondria via **fatty acid β-oxidation** in response to metabolic need. This process involves removing two carbons at a time from the fatty acid and converting these carbons to acetyl-CoA. β-oxidation generates one NADH and one FADH$_2$ for each 2-carbon group removed. The acetyl-CoA can then enter the Krebs cycle. The glycerol backbone of the TAG can be converted into glucose and can enter cellular respiration at glycolysis.

Amino Acid Catabolism

Proteins in cells are constantly being made, kept for a certain period of time (minutes to weeks), and then degraded back into amino acids. In addition, humans absorb amino acids from dietary proteins. These free amino acids can be catabolized via several pathways. The amino group is removed and converted into urea for excretion. The remaining carbon skeleton (also called an α-keto acid) can be either broken down into water and CO_2 or converted to glucose or acetyl-CoA.

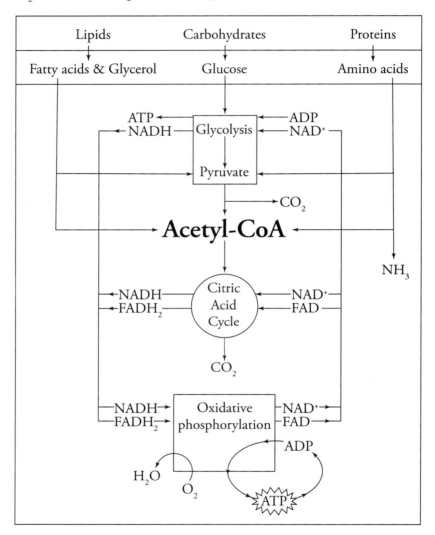

Figure 19   Metabolic Pathways

6.3 MOLECULAR BIOLOGY

Genome

Within the nucleus of a eukaryotic cell are the chromosomes, which are composed of **deoxyribonucleic acid (DNA)**. A full complement of the organism's chromosomes is present in all of its **somatic** cells; a somatic cell is any cell of the body except sperm and egg cells. Human chromosomes and those of other higher order eukaryotes generally exist in pairs. Because of this, the organism is termed **diploid,** or $2n$. Most of the pairs are homologous, which means that they are the same size and length as each other and contain the same genes in the same locations. However, the alleles of these genes can be different so their sequences can be different.

Every human somatic cell has 46 chromosomes ($2n = 46$), or 23 pairs of chromosomes. One such pair constitutes the **sex chromosomes** and can be a **hemizygous** pair; this means that the two chromosomes are different from each other. Hemizygous sex chromosomes are found in males only; they are XY. These two chromosomes are different sizes and contain different genes. This means that males have only one copy of the genes on each of these chromosomes, which is pretty unique in a diploid organism. Females have homologous sex chromosomes; they are XX. The remaining 22 pairs (sometimes called **autosomes**) are also homologous. Overall then, we say:

Within the human somatic cell nucleus are 46 chromosomes organized into 22 pairs of homologous chromosomes (or autosomes) and either one pair of hemizygous sex chromosomes (XY) or one pair of homologous sex chromosomes (XX).

The phenomenon of paired chromosomes follows from the fact that eukaryotic organisms generally arise by sexual reproduction (each individual having two parents). For example, chromosome 1 in humans is the largest chromosome, and since humans are diploid, each somatic cell has two copies of chromosome 1: one copy came from an individual's mother and the other came from an individual's father. The same is true for the other chromosomes. Of the 46 human chromosomes, therefore, 23 derive from the father and 23 derive from the mother.

It is important to remember that prokaryotic cells (bacteria) have a genome also, but bacterial genomes have a different structure. In prokaryotic cells, the genome is also composed of double stranded (ds) DNA, but there is only one highly coiled, circular chromosome, which is not enclosed in a membrane or nucleus.

Chromosome Structure

DNA molecules are very long. They fit within the eukaryotic cell nucleus only because they are wrapped and coiled. More specifically, they wrap themselves in a complicated arrangement around packaging proteins called **histones**. Near the time of cell division, chromosomes wrap around their histones in a highly condensed form that makes the histones visible as discrete units that resemble beads on a string. The visible units of histone are called **nucleosomes**.

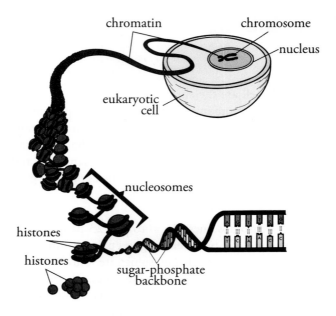

Figure 20 DNA Packaging

DNA Structure and the Double Helix

Picture an ordinary ladder; horizontal rungs run between two long, parallel upright sides. Now, imagine that someone twists the ladder so that the two upright sides become spirally shaped, each one winding around the other. You have just conceived a rudimentary picture of the DNA molecule; it looks like a twisted ladder. It has two spirally shaped strands, with rungs running between them. Recall now that another word for a spirally shaped object is **helix**. For example, the groove that runs up the shaft of a corkscrew is a helix. That means that each of the DNA molecule's two strands constitutes a helix. Since the molecule embodies two such helices, each one wound around the other, we say:

The DNA molecule is a double-stranded molecule in which the two strands form a double helix.

In your mind, unwind the double helix and picture it again as a ladder. Each of the two strands comprises a series of **2′ deoxy-D-ribose** molecules (often called deoxyribose) bound to one another by **phosphodiester bonds**. In other words, the backbone strands of DNA are made of alternating units of deoxyribose and phosphate, so that in a schematic diagram, they look like this:

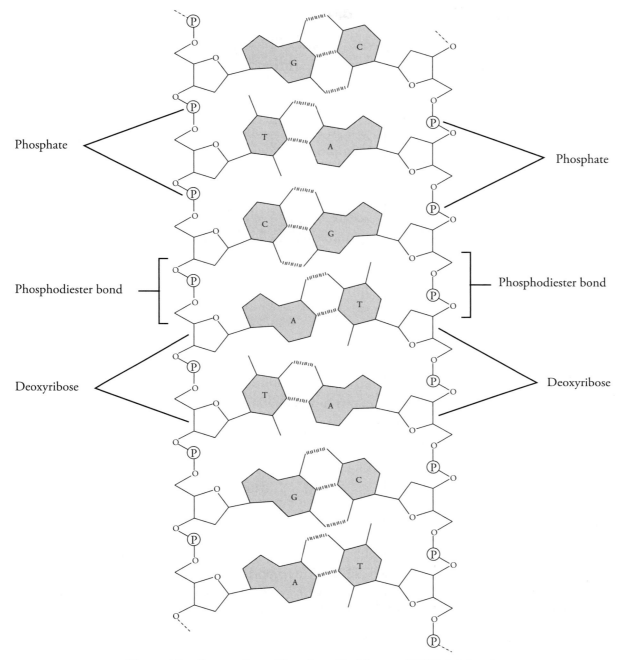

Figure 21　Deoxyribose-Phosphate Backbone of DNA Molecule

Deoxyribose is a sugar or carbohydrate, so this part of DNA is sometimes called its **sugar-phosphate backbone.** The orientation of deoxyribose is the way in which we name the direction of a DNA strand. The end of each backbone is called either 5′ or 3′, depending on the orientation of this sugar group. In double-stranded DNA, one strand runs in the 5′ to 3′ direction, and the other complementary strand runs in the 3′ to 5′ direction. This means that the two DNA strands are antiparallel.

Running between opposing units on each strand (analogous to the ladder's rungs) are pairs of nitrogenous heterocyclic bases, one base attached to each strand. A **nucleotide** is made of one phosphate group, a deoxyribose sugar, and a nitrogenous base.

6.3

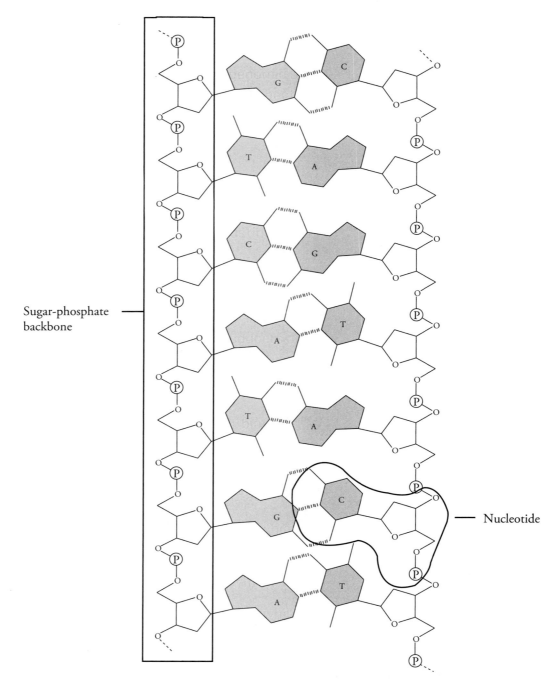

Sugar-phosphate backbone

Nucleotide

Figure 22 Nucleotides in DNA

The DNA molecule features four different nitrogenous bases. Two are **purines** and two are **pyrimidines**. In alphabetical order, the four nucleotides found in DNA are

1. adenine (A)   — a purine
2. cytosine (C)   — a pyrimidine
3. guanine (G)   — a purine
4. thymine (T)   — a pyrimidine

A useful way to remember the purines and pyrimidines is the following:

- **Pure** silver (silver is Ag on the periodic table): the **pur**ines are **A**denine and **G**uanine
- You **CUT** a "pye": the pyrimidines are **C**ytosine, **U**racil (in RNA), and **T**hymine

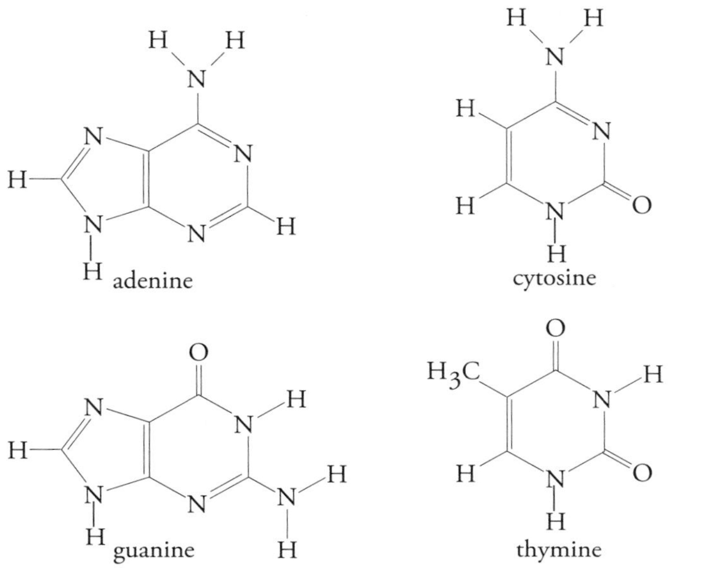

Figure 23   DNA Bases: Adenine, Cytosine, Guanine, Thymine

Base-Pairing Between Purines and Pyrimidines

On each strand of the DNA molecule, a nitrogenous base (either purine or a pyrimidine) is bound to each deoxyribose-phosphate unit. Across the rungs of the ladder, nucleotides pair according to this simple rule: each purine pairs with (or is complementary to) a pyrimidine:

- the purine **adenine (A)** pairs with the pyrimidine **thymine (T)**
- the purine **guanine (G)** pairs with the pyrimidine **cytosine (C)**

These are the rules of base-pairing (or nucleotide pairing), and you can remember them by listing the four nucleotides in alphabetical order and by remembering that the one at the top of the list pairs with the one at the bottom, while the two in the middle of the list pair with each other. The rules of base-pairing arise partly from **steric hindrance**, or size restrictions regarding the structure of the different bases and the spaces available to them. Since the purines are composed of two rings and the pyrimidines have just one ring (see Figure 23), complementary bases across the rungs of the ladder must always have one of each for the backbone to be parallel. If a purine is paired with a purine, the backbone of DNA would have to kink outward to accommodate four rings; if a pyrimidine is paired with a pyrimidine, the DNA backbone would have to kink inward.

A small sequence of a DNA molecule (untwisted) might, therefore look like this:

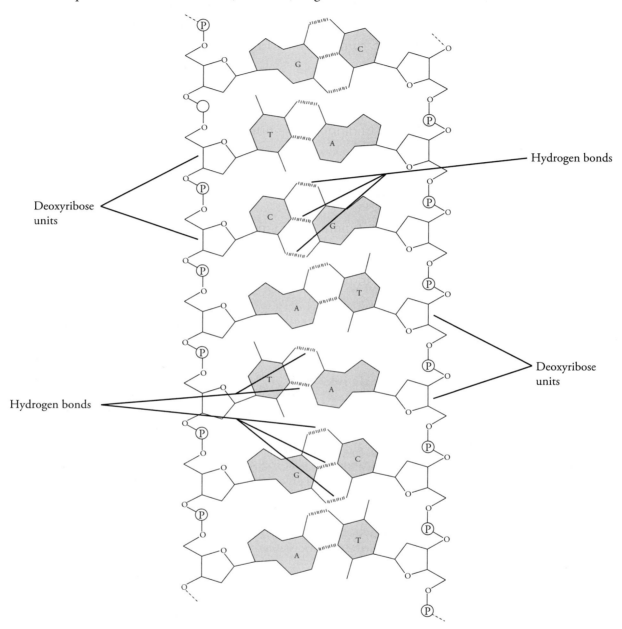

Figure 24   Base-Pairing of a Double-Stranded DNA Molecule

Each base pair is joined by hydrogen bonds (represented in Figure 24 by the hatched lines between nucleotide pairs). When adenine and thymine pair, two hydrogen bonds form to join them. When guanine and cytosine pair, three hydrogen bonds form to join them. Hydrogen bonds do not offer the strength of true covalent bonds, but by their large number, they impart considerable support to the DNA molecule (just as they produce a high degree of surface tension for aggregation of water molecules).

The backbone of every strand of a DNA molecule is the same: it is made of deoxyribose units joined by phosphodiester bonds. DNA molecules can differ from each other in the ordering of the nitrogenous bases bound to the strands (and, consequently, the ordering of nucleotide pairs). For example, if a DNA molecule had the nucleotide sequence:

$$(5') - T \quad A \quad G \quad T \quad G - (3')$$

according to the base-pairing rules discussed above, the other deoxyribose-phosphate strand of that same DNA molecule would carry a complementary nucleotide sequence:

$$(3') - A \quad T \quad C \quad A \quad C - (5')$$

This is the conventional way to write out double-stranded DNA sequences: the top strand is written 5′ to 3′ (left to right) and the bottom strand is written in an antiparallel way with 3′ on the left and 5′ on the right. If a single-stranded sequence is being shown, it is written with the 5′ on the left and 3′ on the right.

DNA Replication

Cells must duplicate their genome (or chromosomes) prior to mitosis. Replication of a chromosome requires the replication of DNA. **DNA replication** (also called DNA synthesis) occurs in the S phase of the cell cycle and begins at an **Origin of Replication** (or Ori), a specific sequence of nucleotides that are the signal to start DNA synthesis. First, the DNA strands must be unwound; this is facilitated by **helicase** enzymes. The hydrogen bonds that join base pairs rupture, and the molecule's two strands are separated. The two deoxyribose-phosphate strands do not fully separate before daughter strands begin to form. Rather, they partially diverge at what is called a **replication bubble**, which has two **replication forks** (Figure 25).

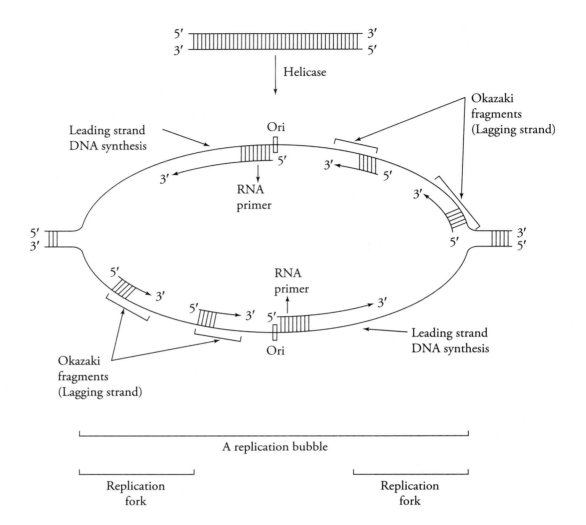

Figure 25 DNA Replication

Each strand, sometimes called a parent strand, then serves as a **template** for the production of a new daughter strand complementary to it. Synthesis of the new strand is accomplished by a family of enzymes called **DNA polymerases**, which read the template strand and synthesize a new complementary daughter strand. In order to begin synthesis, DNA polymerases require a primer. This is accomplished by an enzyme named **primase**, which lays down short RNA primers so DNA polymerases can begin.

DNA polymerases are one-way enzymes; they read the DNA template in the 3′ to 5′ direction and synthesize DNA in the 5′ to 3′ direction (that is to say, DNA polymerases make the 5′ end of the new DNA strand first, and add new nucleotides onto the 3′ end of a strand). Nucleotides (composed of phosphate-deoxyribose-nitrogenous base) are aligned along the template according to the base-pairing rules discussed earlier. Then, deoxyribose units are joined by phosphodiester bonds, paired nucleotides are joined by hydrogen bonds, and for each template there results a new double-stranded molecule. Because each of the newly formed molecules contains half of the original DNA molecule, replication is said to be **semi-conservative.**

The Polarity Problem and Its Solution

There are three directional concepts to keep in mind:

(1) Recall that the DNA molecule's two deoxyribose-phosphate strands lie in antiparallel orientation. As depicted in Figure 25, the top strand runs in the 5′ to 3′ direction from left to right, and the bottom strand runs in the 5′ to 3′ direction from right to left (this is the convention when drawing double stranded DNA).

(2) The replication forks at either end of the replication bubble open in opposite directions; the fork on the left will continue opening to the left and the fork on the right will continue opening to the right.

(3) DNA polymerases synthesize DNA in one direction only: 5′ to 3′. A newly growing nucleotide chain does NOT take on new nucleotide units at its 5′ end; DNA polymerases will add nucleotide units only to the 3′ end of the growing chain. On the top strand in Figure 25, DNA polymerases will read from right to left because they must read the template from 3′ to 5′. On the bottom strand of Figure 25, DNA polymerases will read from left to right.

These three directional concepts lead to the difference between leading strand synthesis and lagging strand synthesis. Return to Figure 25: For DNA synthesis from the top strand template and to the left of the Ori, there are no issues; the replication fork is opening to the left and DNA synthesis is happening in this direction also. For DNA synthesis from the bottom strand template and to the right of the Ori, the same is true; the replication fork is opening to the right and DNA synthesis via DNA polymerases is happening in the same direction. We call these two the **leading strands**. For leading strand synthesis, the 3′ of the new strand (the end of that is being added onto by DNA polymerases) is leading into the replication fork.

This is not the case for the other two strands (top template to the right of the Ori, and bottom template to the left of the Ori). For these two strands, the cell faces a polarity problem: The replication fork is opening one direction and DNA can be synthesized only in the opposite direction. These strands are presenting the 5′ end of the new daughter strand to the replication fork but DNA polymerases cannot add nucleotides to this end. For example, the replication fork on the right of Figure 25 is opening to the right. However, synthesis from the top strand template must occur from right to left.

The only way around this is to synthesize the new DNA in fragments. Primase lays down a short primer and DNA polymerases create a new fragment of DNA by reading away from the replication fork (still synthesizing in the 5′ to 3′ direction). As the fork opens, another primer is laid down and another fragment is synthesized. These fragments, called **Okazaki fragments**, constitute the **lagging strand**; this mechanism of synthesis solves the polarity problem. Fragments are then joined by **DNA ligase** to generate a continuous DNA strand.

In summary, DNA replication occurs in the following steps:

1. The Ori is recognized on the DNA strand.
2. DNA strands are separated via helicase.
3. A replication bubble is formed, with two replication forks.
4. RNA primers are laid down by primase.
5. DNA polymerases read the template strand (in the 3′ to 5′ direction) and synthesize a new complementary strand (in the 5′ to 3′ direction). This can occur in a continuous way (as in the leading strand) or discontinuously (as in the lagging strand).
6. The leading strand and Okazaki fragments of the lagging strand are joined by DNA ligase.
7. RNA primers are removed and replaced with DNA (this is done by DNA polymerases).

RNA Versus DNA

Chromosomes serve their critical function within the cell (and the organism) by mediating the synthesis of **ribonucleic acid (RNA)**. Both DNA and RNA are nucleic acids, polymers composed of nucleotide monomers. However, there are some differences between them:

Characteristic	DNA	RNA
Sugar in the backbone	Deoxyribose (no OH on the 2′ carbon of ribose)	Ribose (has an OH on the 2′ carbon of ribose)
Pyrimidines	Cytosine and thymine	Cytosine and uracil
Strandedness	Usually double-stranded (except in some viruses)	Usually single-stranded
Stability	More stable	Less stable
Lifespan in the cell	Permanent	Transient

Table 2

RNA, therefore, is a nucleic acid composed of a sugar-phosphate backbone in which the sugar component is ribose. Bound to each ribose unit of the backbone is one of the four nitrogenous bases:

1. adenine (A)   —a purine
2. cytosine (C)   —a pyrimidine
3. guanine (G)   —a purine
4. uracil (U)   —a pyrimidine

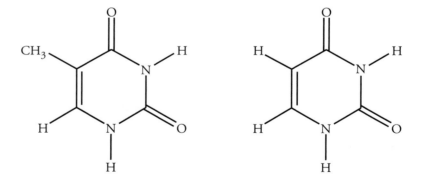

Figure 26 Thymine (left) is in DNA, While Uracil (right) is in RNA

There are three common forms of RNA, each differing from the other in their function(s). Beyond the three well-recognized types, there are additional forms of RNA that serve enzymatic roles. The three predominant types of RNA are:

1. ribosomal RNA (rRNA)
2. transfer RNA (tRNA)
3. messenger RNA (mRNA)

Transcription: From DNA to RNA

In the synthesis of any of the three types of RNA, DNA serves as a template, and the process is termed **transcription**. Transcription is similar (but not identical) to DNA replication. Both DNA replication and transcription begin with separating the DNA molecule's two strands. In DNA replication, *both* strands serve as templates for the synthesis of a new DNA strand. In transcription, *one* of the strands serves as a template for the synthesis of an RNA molecule. The same base-pairing rules apply to DNA replication and transcription, except in DNA replication thymine is used, and in transcription, uracil is used. For example, if some portion of a DNA template carries the nucleotide sequence:

$$(5') - \quad T \quad G \quad A \quad C \quad A \quad - (3')$$

then the complementary sequence of the newly formed RNA molecule would be:

$$(3') - \quad A \quad C \quad U \quad G \quad U \quad - (5')$$

or, expressed in conventional 5′ to 3′ direction:

$$(5') - \quad U \quad G \quad U \quad C \quad A \quad - (3')$$

Because RNA is a single-stranded molecule, it results from the reading of only one DNA strand; between the two strands of DNA, only one serves as a template for RNA synthesis. The other one is complementary to the template, just like the RNA will be complementary to the template. Because of this, the DNA strands are given names: The one that serves as a template and is actually read and transcribed is called the template, the **non-coding strand** or the **anti-sense strand**. The other strand that does *not* serve as template is called the **coding strand** or **sense strand**. This is because RNA and the coding strand are both complementary to the template, and thus have the same sequence or code as each other (except for the T/U switch of course).

Recall that DNA polymerases generated the new daughter strands in DNA replication. In transcription, formation of an RNA polymer is catalyzed by enzymes called **RNA polymerases**. These two enzymes are similar in their mechanism of action; both DNA polymerases and RNA polymerases add nucleotides to the 3′ end of the growing chain. Therefore, the template DNA is read in the 3′ to 5′ direction and the new nucleic acid molecule is synthesized in the 5′ to 3′ direction.

Transcription occurs in three steps:

1. initiation
2. elongation
3. termination

During **initiation,** RNA polymerase binds the DNA template at a region called the **promoter.** The promoter is a particular sequence of DNA; it determines which DNA strand is the template, where transcription starts, and the direction of transcription. One common example of a promoter is called a **TATA box**. Next, RNA polymerase unwinds the template strand (there is no need for helicase here) and starts reading it in the 3′ to 5′ direction. Once it reaches a region called the **start site,** RNA polymerase starts creating an RNA transcript by reading the template DNA.

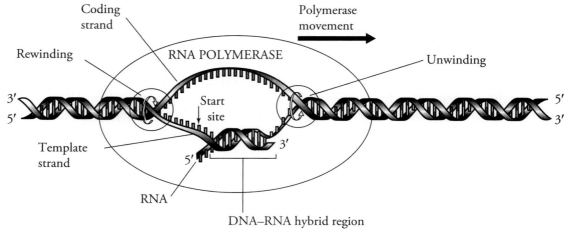

Figure 27   Transcription

It is customary to say that transcription starts at a point and proceeds **downstream,** which means toward the 3′ end of the coding strand and transcript. **Upstream** means toward the 5′ end of the coding strand, beyond the 5′ end of the transcript. Upstream nucleotide sequences are referred to with negative numbers, and downstream sequences are referred to with positive numbers. The first nucleotide that is actually transcribed is given the number +1.

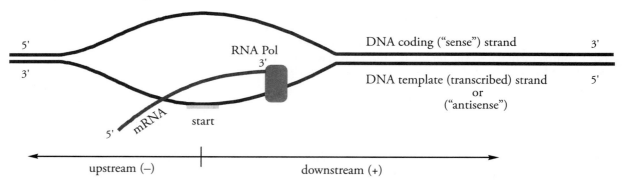

Figure 28   Reference Points in Transcription

During **elongation,** RNA polymerase builds RNA by adding nucleotides onto the 3′ end of the new molecule, as in DNA replication. RNA polymerase catalyzes the creation of a phosphodiester bond between the 5′ end of the one nucleotide and the 3′ end of the next, releasing pyrophosphate (PP$_i$). RNA polymerase moves along the template, adding additional nucleotides to the growing chain of RNA. This continues until the enzyme reaches a sequence called the **terminator,** or **termination signal.** Here, RNA polymerase and the newly synthesized RNA transcript dissociate and transcription is complete. This is the last step of transcription, **termination.**

Eukaryotic transcript occurs in the nucleus because this is where the DNA is located. After an RNA transcript has been synthesized, it undergoes post-transcriptional modification. First it is spliced to remove unnecessary sequences. The spliceosome removes introns and connects exons. In other words, introns go in the trash and exons are kept and expressed. A 5′ cap and a 3′ poly-A tail are added to the RNA transcript for stability. Finally, the RNA molecule is exported out of the nucleus and into the cytoplasm where it can be bound and read by ribosomes in the process of translation.

Because bacterial cells do not have a nucleus, they can perform transcription and translation at the same time. As soon as the 5′ end of an RNA transcript has been created, it can be bound by a ribosome and read to create a peptide chain. In other words, in a bacterial cell it is possible to both synthesize and read one molecule of RNA at the same time!

Translation: From mRNA to Protein

Generally speaking, translation is a process in which mRNA issues orders that are read by the ribosome and carried out by molecules of tRNA coupled to amino acids. Translation is generally a process in which:

1. The ribosome recognizes some portion of the mRNA molecule and binds it.
2. The ribosome reads the mRNA molecule, three nucleotides at a time (these three nucleotides are called a **codon**).
3. When read by the ribosome, each codon on the mRNA orders that some particular amino acid be brought to the ribosome.
4. Molecules of tRNA within the cytosol bring amino acids to the ribosome, as instructed by mRNA.
5. Amino acids brought to the ribosome, one by one, in a sequence ordered by the mRNA molecule, are connected via peptide bonds to form a polypeptide.

Ribosome, tRNA, and Amino Acid Activation

Because translation involves ribosomes and tRNA, we first look at the nature of these complexes, and then at the thermodynamics tied to the bonding of tRNA with amino acid, a process called amino acid activation.

A prokaryotic ribosome embodies two subunits, a large one and a small one, sometimes called the **50S** and **30S** subunits, respectively. The total ribosome is **70S**. In eukaryotes, the small subunit is **40S**, the large subunit is **60S**, and the total ribosome is **80S**. The "S" represents the unit "Svedberg" and denotes sedimentation rate; a higher value indicates a higher sedimentation rate and larger mass. Each subunit is a complex of rRNA and proteins. The ribosome also features three tRNA binding sites called the **A site** (or aminoacyl-tRNA site), the **P site** (or peptidyl-tRNA site), and the **E site** (or exit-tRNA site). In both prokaryotes and eukaryotes, many ribosomes synthesizing the same protein simultaneously associate with one another to form a **polyribosome**.

Transfer RNA, or tRNA, is a single-stranded molecule of RNA. Because there are regions where the tRNA molecule is complementary to itself, tRNAs fold into a cloverleaf structure that is composed of stems (areas of internal complementarity) and loops. tRNAs have two functional sites, the **anticodon** and the **amino acid acceptor site**.

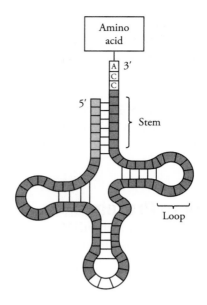

Figure 29 Transfer RNA (tRNA)

The tRNA anticodon is a sequence of three nucleotides. Since the anticodon is three nucleotides in length and since there are four nucleotide options for each site (A, C, G, or U), there are 64 different anticodons (this comes from 4 × 4 × 4). Like any set of nucleotides, those of the tRNA anticodon have complements according to the base-pairing rules described in earlier sections. The anticodon on tRNA is complementary to the codon on the mRNA transcript.

The tRNA molecule's amino acid acceptor site is a site at which the molecule binds (accepts) an amino acid. A given tRNA molecule with its particular anticodon has a binding site for one particular amino acid. However, since there are 64 anticodons and only 20 amino acids, there might be more than one tRNA molecule specific to a given amino acid. For example, the anticodon (3') - C G G - (5') is specific to alanine; it binds alanine and only alanine. On the other hand, the anticodons (3') - C G A - (5'), (3') - C G U - (5'), and (3') - C G C - (5') are also specific to alanine. They, too, bind alanine and only alanine.

The amino acid acceptor site of any tRNA molecule is the same as that of any other, which raises this question: On what basis does tRNA recognize the amino acid to which it is specific? For each amino acid, there exists (at least) one enzyme called an **aminoacyl-tRNA synthetase**. The synthetase enzyme recognizes both the tRNA carrier and the amino acid to which it is specific. Recognition between tRNA and amino acid, therefore, is mediated not by tRNA, but by the relevant aminoacyl-tRNA synthetase.

The binding of an amino acid to its tRNA to produce the corresponding aminoacyl-tRNA is called **amino acid activation**. The word "activation" comes from the thermodynamics of this process. The reaction in which an amino acid is bound to its tRNA is endergonic (meaning ΔG is positive). It involves the cleavage of two high-energy phosphate bonds (ATP → AMP + 2P$_i$), and the reaction looks like this:

$$\text{Amino Acid + ATP + tRNA} \rightarrow \text{Aminoacyl-tRNA + AMP + PP}_i$$

Subsequent cleavage of the pyrophosphate (PP_i) by pyrophosphatase drives the equilibrium forcefully to the right. The ester linkage between the amino acid and the tRNA is a relatively high-energy bond, and for that reason, the amino acid is said to be activated; the energy stored within this bond is later used to drive peptide bond formation.

The principal functions of tRNA are to bind amino acids, bring them to the ribosome, line them up according to an order dictated by the mRNA codons, and facilitate the formation of peptide bonds to form proteins. Transfer RNA, therefore, mediates the process of translation.

Steps of Translation

Like transcription, translation proceeds in three steps:

1. initiation
2. elongation
3. termination

During **initiation,** the small ribosomal subunit (30S in prokaryotes and 40S in eukaryotes) binds near the 5′ end of an mRNA. It scans the transcript sequence until it finds the AUG start codon. Next, a tRNA molecule (with the anticodon UAC and bound to the amino acid methionine) interacts with the AUG codon on the mRNA. These three molecules together (small ribosomal subunit, tRNA-Met, and a molecule of mRNA) are called the initiation complex. Finally, the large ribosomal subunit (50S in prokaryotes and 60S in eukaryotes) is recruited. The first amino acid added will be the N-terminus of the peptide chain.

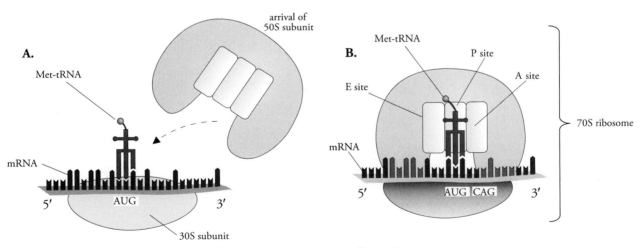

Figure 30 Initiation of Translation

During elongation, the ribosome reads the mRNA codons, tRNA molecules bearing appropriate anticodons bring amino acids to the ribosome, and peptide bonds form between the adjacent amino acids to form a polypeptide. The amino acid sequence of the polypeptide is dictated by the mRNA codons.

In more detailed terms, elongation involves this series of events:

1. An mRNA codon is exposed at the A site of the ribosome.
2. An aminoacyl-tRNA, whose anticodon is complementary to the codon, arrives at the A site and forms hydrogen bonds with the codon. This step requires the hydrolysis of one phosphate from GTP.
3. A peptide bond is formed between the two amino acids. The bond between the amino acid and the tRNA in the P site is broken.
4. The ribosome moves, or translocates, a distance of three nucleotides along the mRNA molecule in the 5′ to 3′ direction. Translocation moves the growing polypeptide anchored to a tRNA molecule to the P site of the ribosome, moves the old tRNA to the E site, and exposes the next mRNA codon at the A site. This step requires the hydrolysis of one GTP.

These steps repeat and the polypeptide chain grows, one amino acid at a time. The E site always contains a tRNA that has lost its amino acid to the growing peptide chain. This tRNA exits the ribosome and is recycled to the cytoplasm where it can be joined with another amino acid. The P site always contains a tRNA hydrogen bonded to the mRNA transcript, and this anchors the peptide chain to the ribosome. The A site is always where the next aminoacyl-tRNA arrives.

Overall, it costs four high-energy phosphate bonds to add an amino acid. Two high energy bonds are required by aminoacyl-tRNA synthetase to join the tRNA with its amino acid, one phosphate bond is required to bring the aminoacyl-tRNA into the A site of the ribosome, and a final phosphate bond is required to translocate the ribosome so the next codon can be read. This means that for a cell to translate a short 250 amino acid peptide chain, it would require 1,000 molecules of ATP! Making proteins is highly expensive for the cell.

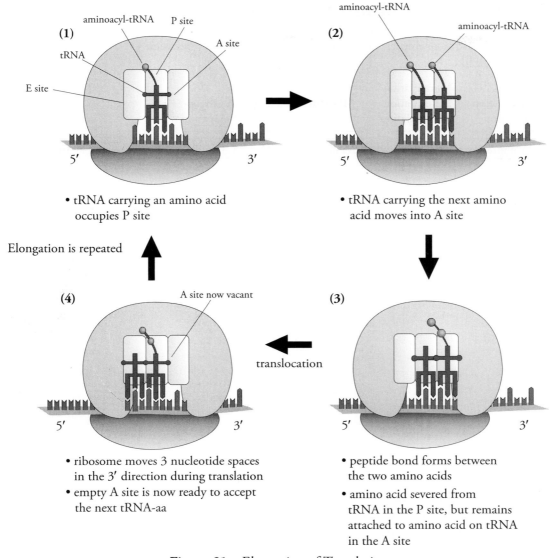

Figure 31   Elongation of Translation

The last amino acid added will be the C-terminus of the peptide chain. **Termination** occurs when a stop codon appears in the ribosomal A site. There are three stop codons (UAG, UGA, UAA), which can be remembered using the three phrases "You (U) Are Gone, U Go Away, U Are Away." Stop codons do not code for tRNA molecules. Rather, their arrival at the A site causes **release factors** (proteins) to stop the elongation process and to release the newly formed polypeptide from the ribosome. The ribosome dissociates into large and small subunits ready to begin the process of translation anew.

Not all of the mRNA transcript codes for a protein. The region of the transcript before the start codon is called the **5′ untranslated region** (or 5′ UTR). There is also some extra sequence on the other end of the RNA called the **3′ untranslated region** (or 3′ UTR). The 5′ UTR contains upstream regulatory sequences that help with initiation; the 3′ UTR contains downstream regulatory sequences that help with termination.

DNA Replication vs. Transcription vs. Translation

Now that we have covered all of molecular biology, let's review. Recall that transcription involved a small portion of DNA from promoter to terminator. The relationship between DNA, RNA, and a peptide chain might look like this:

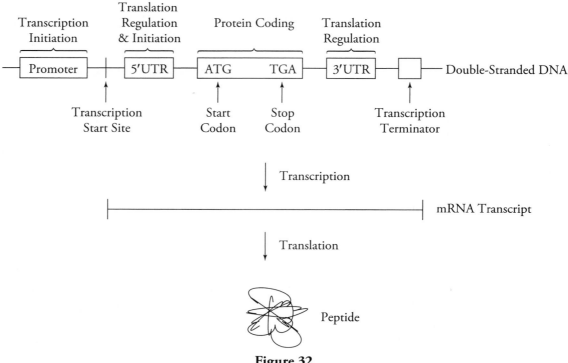

Figure 32

Notice that transcription is initiated at the promoter, starts at the start site (downstream from the promoter), and ends at the terminator. The protein coding region is within the mRNA transcript, but is not the entire mRNA transcript; mRNA also contains regulatory regions at the 5′ and 3′ ends (the 5′UTR and 3′UTR). Translation is initiated at the 5′UTR, starts at the start codon (ATG on the DNA coding strand or AUG on the mRNA transcript), and ends at one of the stop codons (UAG, UGA, UAA).

It is important to remember the similarities and differences between DNA replication, transcription, and translation. In summary:

	DNA Replication	Transcription	Translation
Signal to get ready	Ori	Promoter	5′ UTR
Signal to start	Ori	Start site	AUG start codon
Key enzyme	DNA polymerase	RNA polymerase	Ribosome (made of rRNA and peptides)
Other enzymes	Helicase Primase Ligase	Spliceosome (eukaryotes only)	Aminoacyl tRNA synthetases
Template molecule	DNA	DNA	mRNA
Read direction	3′ to 5′ on the DNA template	3′ to 5′ on the DNA template	5′ to 3′ on the RNA template
Molecule synthesized	DNA	RNA	Peptides
Build direction	5′ to 3′	5′ to 3′	N-terminus to C-terminus
Prokaryotic location	Cytoplasm	Cytoplasm	Cytoplasm
Eukaryotic location	Nucleus	Nucleus	Cytoplasm
Signal to stop	When the replication bubbles or newly synthesized strands meet and are ligated together	Terminator	Stop codon (UAG, UGA, UAA)

Table 3

6.4 MITOSIS AND MEIOSIS

Cell Cycle

Cells reproduce through the process of mitosis. The period of the cell's life cycle between mitotic divisions is called interphase. Interphase has three subphases: (1) **G_1 phase**, also called **gap phase 1**; (2) **S phase**, also called the **synthesis phase**; and (3) **G_2 phase**, also called **gap phase 2**.

- During G_1, the cell grows, runs metabolic pathways such as cell respiration, and builds proteins and organelles.
- During the S phase the cell reproduces its genome in preparation for division. This is done via DNA replication, which we reviewed earlier.
- During G_2, the cell continues to grow and synthesize proteins and organelles. It also prepares for mitosis.
- Mitosis (or the M phase) involves nuclear division.
- Cytoplasmic division is also called **cytokinesis.**

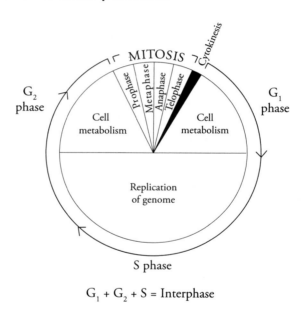

$$G_1 + G_2 + S = \text{Interphase}$$

Figure 33   The Cell Cycle

Replication of the Genome

During the S phase of interphase, all 23 pairs of the cell's chromosomes replicate. When replication is complete, each chromosome has a duplicate. Each pair of duplicates is joined at a **centromere**. These duplicates are called sister chromatids and because they are the product of DNA replication, sister chromatids are identical to each other.

Before a chromosome duplicates itself, it is, of course, one chromosome. Even after it duplicates itself (and the DNA quantity is doubled), the duplicated unit is still considered one chromosome. Here is another way to think about this: before DNA replication, each of your 46 chromosomes is present in a single copy.

This means there is one chromatid per chromosome. Each chromosome has a centromere that divides it into two arms, and each chromosome is made of one long piece of double-stranded DNA. After DNA replication, each chromosome is made of two identical chromatids, connected together at the centromere. Now there are two identical pieces of DNA and four arms coming out of the centromere, so each chromosome looks like the letter X (once it is condensed).

This section is pretty confusing for most people, so let's look at this another way:

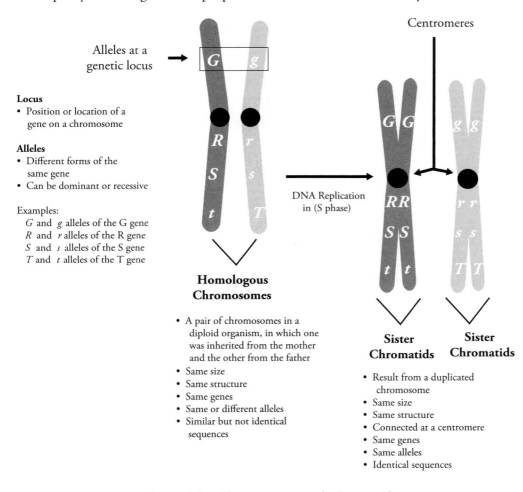

Figure 34   Chromosomes and Chromatids

Before DNA replication, a human cell has 23 pairs of chromosomes. Even after replication, for as long as duplicated pairs are joined at their centromeres, the cell still has only 23 pairs of chromosomes, each chromosome comprising a pair of sister chromatids. Each pair of sister chromatids (joined at a centromere) represents what *will* become two separate chromosomes. It is very important that you're clear on all this terminology before getting into mitosis, so you may want to go back and read that section again.

Mitosis

Interphase is followed by mitosis, a process that is customarily divided into four phases—**prophase**, **metaphase**, **anaphase**, and **telophase**—and results in division of the nucleus. Mitosis is followed by the division of the cytoplasm, called cytokinesis.

During prophase, chromosomes condense to the point that they are visible under the light microscope as an X-shaped structure. The nucleolus slowly disappears. Centrosomes move to opposite poles of the cell. Star-shaped fibers, called **aster fibers**, form around the centrosomes. Microtubules give rise to a mitotic spindle, which spans the cell from pole to pole. The nuclear membrane begins to dissolve.

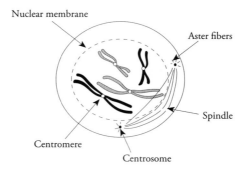

Figure 35   The Cell at Prophase of Mitosis

During metaphase, **kinetochore fibers** associated with the centromeres interact with the mitotic spindle, allowing movement of chromosomes. Chromosomes align on the **metaphase plate** so that centromeres lie in a plane along an axis at the cell's midpoint. Kinetochore fibers help to align and maintain the chromosomes on the metaphase plate.

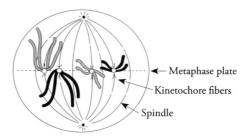

Figure 36   The Cell at Metaphase of Mitosis

During anaphase, sister chromatids separate as a result of the splitting of the centromere and move toward opposite poles of the cell along the path marked by the spindle apparatus. With the separation of sister chromatids, each chromatid is called a **daughter chromosome.** The following diagram is worth considering for a moment before you move on. In the prophase and metaphase diagrams, we were looking at a cell with four X-shaped chromosomes. Look at Figure 37. Now the cell has eight linear chromosomes. When sister chromatids separate from each other, each becomes a chromosome; the number of chromosomes doubles. This means that during anaphase, the cell goes from being $2n$ with duplicated chromosomes, to being $4n$ (tetraploid) with single copy chromosomes. For example, human cells at this point contain 96 chromosomes.

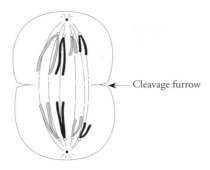

Figure 37   The Cell at Anaphase of Mitosis

At telophase, daughter chromosomes are positioned at opposite poles of the cell, and kinetochore fibers disappear. A nuclear membrane forms around each set of daughter chromosomes. The chromosomes decondense and are no longer visible by light microscopy. Nucleoli then reappear; mitosis and nuclear division are complete.

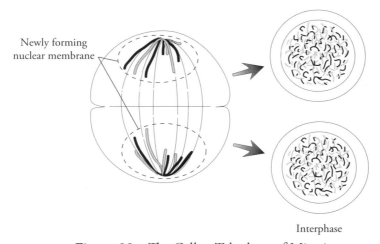

Figure 38   The Cell at Telophase of Mitosis

Cytokinesis can begin during the last part of anaphase or the early part of telophase. A **cleavage furrow** forms along the equator of the cell. This furrow deepens until it ultimately divides the cell, forming two daughter cells. Each daughter cell possesses a diploid number of chromosomes. The daughter cells then enter the interphase period of the cell cycle.

Meiosis

Reduction division refers to the generation of haploid daughter cells by a diploid parent cell. Reduction division is accomplished by meiosis and is the basis of **gametogenesis** (discussed shortly). Like mitosis, meiosis involves nuclear division and cytokinesis. Nuclear division in meiosis includes the same four stages as mitosis: prophase, metaphase, anaphase, and telophase. Meiosis, however, involves two divisions (or two cycles) instead of one. The first meiotic division/cycle consists of prophase I, metaphase I, anaphase I, and telophase I; the second meiotic division/cycle consists of prophase II, metaphase II, anaphase II, and telophase II.

The First Meiotic Division

The first phase of the first meiotic division is termed prophase I. Prophase I follows interphase, during which the cell duplicates its chromosomes. As in mitosis, chromosomes condense during prophase I, the nucleolus begins to disassemble and disappear, and centrioles move to opposite poles of the cell. Aster fibers form around the centrioles. The mitotic spindle forms and spans the cell from pole to pole. The nuclear membrane begins to break down.

Prophase I differs from mitotic prophase in that homologous pairs of duplicated chromosomes align in proximity to one another, forming **tetrads**. The association of homologous pairs of duplicated chromosomes to form the tetrad is termed **synapsis**.

The proximity between homologous chromosomes during synapsis allows chromatids from one homologue to swap segments with the other homologue. This is a process called crossing over, and this form of genetic recombination is specific to meiosis.

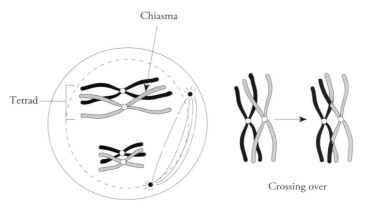

Figure 39   Synapsis and Crossing Over During Meiosis I

Meiotic metaphase I differs from mitotic metaphase in that pairs of homologous chromosomes (instead of single chromosomes) align on the spindle apparatus. That is, tetrads (composed of four chromatids) align along the spindles. By comparison, in mitotic metaphase a double-stranded chromosome composed of two sister chromatids aligns on the metaphase plate.

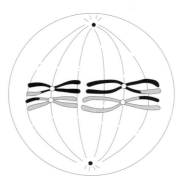

Figure 40   Alignment of Chromosome Pairs on Metaphase Plate During Metaphase I of Meiosis

In meiotic anaphase I, homologous chromosome pairs move to opposite poles of the cell. Centromeres, however, do not split. The two chromatids belonging to a chromosome remain attached. Each pole of the cell, therefore, contains one chromosome from each pair of homologous chromosomes.

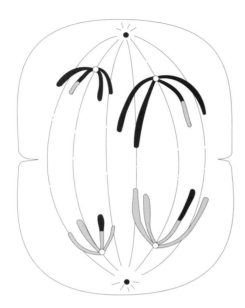

Figure 41　The Cell at Anaphase of Meiosis I

At meiotic telophase I, the chromosomes form two clusters at either end of the cell. The cell cytoplasm divides, leaving two daughter cells, each with genetic material from only one member of each pair of homologous chromosomes. This is a crucial point and one a lot of people forget: by the end of meiosis I, the cell is haploid! It still has duplicated chromosomes (with two sister chromatids each), but each cell has only one of each chromosome. For example, human cells at this point contain 23 chromosomes.

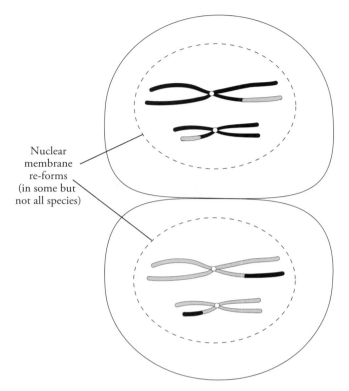

Figure 42   Telophase I

The Second Meiotic Division

Each daughter cell that arises from the first meiotic division has half of the full complement of chromosomes, but it has two copies of that half. The two copies of each chromosome are joined by a centromere. During the second meiotic division, each daughter cell undergoes prophase II, metaphase II, anaphase II, and telophase II in much the same manner as a cell that undergoes mitosis. At anaphase II, centromeres divide, and the two chromatids are pulled to opposite poles of the cell. Cytokinesis follows, and two daughter cells result, each of which has one of the four chromatids from each original tetrad. Because the process just described occurs in each of the two daughter cells produced in the first meiotic division, a total of four daughter cells is produced. Each of the four daughter cells produced by meiosis is haploid.

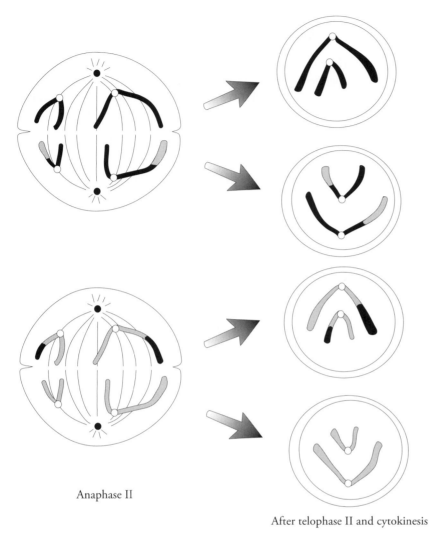

Anaphase II

After telophase II and cytokinesis

Figure 43   Anaphase II through Telophase II and Cytokinesis

Mitosis and Meiosis: Fundamental Differences

Mitosis generates two diploid daughters and meiosis generates four haploid daughters. The difference in ploidy and number of daughter cells arises from an initial difference in the alignment of chromosomes on the spindle apparatus and in the subsequent separation of chromosomes to form new daughter nuclei. In mitosis, chromosomes align without pairing with their homologues. Centromeres then divide, and each daughter is provided with one copy of all chromosomes.

In the first meiotic division, chromosomes align on the spindle apparatus in association with their homologues. Centromeres do not then divide. Rather, homologous chromosomes separate, and each daughter cell is provided with two copies of one half of the original genome. That is, each receives two copies of only one member of each homologous pair. Each daughter then undergoes the second meiotic division, in which centromeres divide. Each daughter produces two new daughters (for a total of four daughters). Each daughter cell has one copy of one member of each homologous pair.

Gametogenesis

Gametogenesis refers to the generation of **gametes** through meiosis. More specifically, **spermatogenesis** is formation of **sperm cells**, which is the male gamete, and **oogenesis** denotes the formation of an **ovum**, which is the female gamete. Spermatogenesis occurs in the **seminiferous tubules** of the **testes** (male gonads), and oogenesis in the **ovaries** (female gonads). Ova and sperm are haploid cells, and their fusion at fertilization forms the diploid **zygote**. The zygote gives rise to a new diploid organism.

Spermatogenesis

Within the seminiferous tubules of the testes reside relatively undifferentiated diploid cells called **spermatogonia**.

Some spermatogonia multiply, enlarge, and undergo genomic replication to produce a large number of primary spermatocytes, each of which then undergoes a first meiotic cycle to yield two secondary spermatocytes. Each secondary spermatocyte then undergoes a second meiotic cycle to produce two haploid spermatids. Each primary spermatocyte, therefore, produces four haploid spermatids.

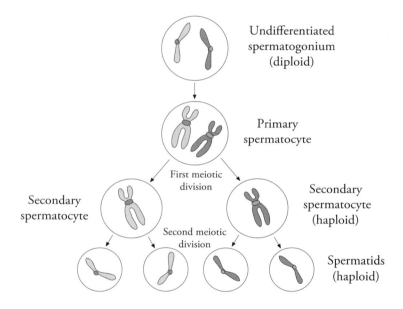

Figure 44   Spermatogenesis

Oogenesis

Oogenesis produces a single mature haploid ovum. The process begins in the ovary, where a diploid **oogonium** begins meiosis to produce a **primary oocyte**. The primary oocyte undergoes the first meiotic division. Unlike the first meiotic division that accompanies spermatogenesis, this division divides cytoplasm unequally between the progeny, producing one larger and one smaller daughter cell. The larger one is called a **secondary oocyte**, and the smaller a **polar body**. The polar body is simply a way to get rid of half the genetic material; the polar body will disintegrate and die. If fertilization occurs, the secondary oocyte undergoes a second meiotic division. This produces two daughter cells, which are also haploid. Again the cytoplasm is allocated unequally, producing one small haploid polar body and one haploid

ootid. The ootid then matures to become a large haploid ovum. The point of this is the conservation of cytoplasm; almost all the cytoplasm from the original oogonium ends up in the secondary oocyte and then the ootid. The net products of oogenesis, then, are two small haploid polar bodies, which degenerate, and one large haploid ovum.

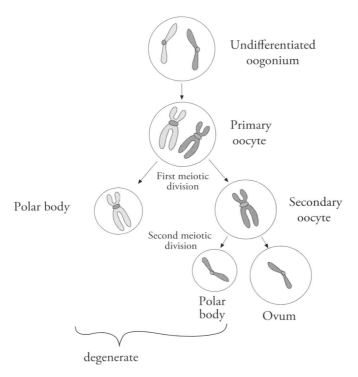

Figure 45 Oogenesis

6.5   GENETICS

Common Genetics Definitions

What Is a Gene?

A gene is a sequence of DNA on a chromosome, which codes for a gene product. There are three common gene products:

1. rRNA, made via transcription
2. tRNA, made via transcription
3. polypeptide, made via transcription and translation. The polypeptide for which a gene codes might represent a discrete functional protein or one subunit of a protein, which is functional when all of its subunits are fully assembled. As a general rule, one gene codes for one polypeptide, but there may be different forms of the polypeptide in eukaryotes due to alternative splicing.

Most DNA in a chromosome does not constitute genes; much of the DNA housed within a chromosome serves to regulate the function of other DNA sequences that code directly for polypeptides. In eukaryotes, there are also non-protein-coding DNA sequences called introns. Moreover, some chromosomal DNA sequences serve no (presently) known function at all; according to current understanding, only about one percent of the DNA found on a given human chromosome directly codes for polypeptide formation. In other words, all genes contain chromosomal DNA sequences, but not all chromosomal DNA sequences constitute genes. For the rest of this chapter, keep these three important points in mind:

1. Genes are composed of DNA on chromosomes and usually code for one of three final gene products: rRNA, tRNA, or a polypeptide.
2. Proteins formed via transcription and translation are encoded by DNA on the chromosomes.
3. An organism's genetic traits are traceable, largely due to the proteins formed by its cells via the processes of transcription and translation.

What Is a Locus?

The area on a chromosome on which a gene is physically located is called a **genetic locus**; the locus of a gene is its address on the chromosome and in the genome.

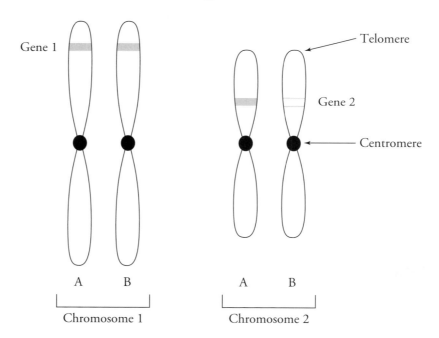

Figure 46 Two Genes, Located at Two Different Loci on Two Different Chromosomes

Recall that in diploid organisms, chromosomes ordinarily exist in homologous pairs, with each parent contributing one chromosome to each pair. As we've mentioned before, homologous chromosomes are the same size and contain the same genes at the same location. However, they may not code for the same versions of each gene. At any given genetic locus, the two chromosomes of a given homologous pair might be:

- identical in DNA sequence and code for the same form of the gene (shown on Chromosome 1 in Figure 46)
- different in DNA sequence and code for different versions of the same gene (shown on Chromosome 2 in Figure 46)

What Is an Allele?

Different forms or versions of a gene are called **alleles**. Alleles have different DNA sequences and a given gene can have numerous alleles. (For example, more than 400 alleles of the *GLA* gene have been published! Many of these cause a rare genetic disorder called Fabry disease.) However, since humans are diploid, their genome can at most contain two alleles of a given single-copy gene. Some humans contain only one allele of some genes, if both their homologous chromosomes contain the same allele.

Figure 46 shows two chromosomes, 1 and 2. For each chromosome, two copies are shown (A and B), as would be present in a diploid organism. The individual that has these chromosomes in their genome would have received or inherited one Chromosome 1 and one Chromosome 2 from their mother and one Chromosome 1 and one Chromosome 2 from their father. The two homologous pairs of Chromosome 1 are the same size and code for the same genes in the same location. The same is true of Chromosome 2.

For Gene 1 on Chromosome 1, the same form of the gene is shown (grey). The DNA sequences of these two copies of Gene 1 are identical and the gene codes for the same gene product. The individual would be called **homozygous** at this locus. In contrast, this individual contains two different alleles of Gene 2 on Chromosome 2 (one grey and one white). These two forms of Gene 2 code for different versions of the gene product and have different DNA sequences. Since this individual has two different alleles at this locus, they would be called **heterozygous** for Gene 2. The full complement of alleles possessed by an organism represents its **genotype**.

Genotype and Phenotype

The ultimate significance of a genotype lies in the **traits** it produces, meaning the features, attributes, or characteristics that it imparts to an organism. Height, color-blindness, and lactose intolerance all constitute "traits." When we discuss an organism's traits, we refer to its **phenotype**. For example, we might say that one individual's phenotype is blue eye color and that another's phenotype is green eye color; eye color is a trait and blue and green are phenotypes that would be associated with different alleles in the genotype. An organism's phenotype is governed by its genotype—by its overall inventory of alleles. More specifically, phenotype comes about according to the way in which combined alleles interact to produce traits.

Consider hypothetical Trait X and two parents—a father who is positive for Trait X and a mother who is negative for Trait X. Depending on the nature of the two inherited alleles and the way in which they interact, the offspring might manifest:

a. Trait X fully
b. Trait X not at all
c. Trait X in some intermediate, attenuated, or hybrid form

The dynamics through which an individual's genotype creates its phenotype are intimately tied to the phenomena of homozygous and heterozygous genotypic states.

Homozygous and Heterozygous Genotypes

With respect to a given genetic locus, an individual's two alleles might be identical, meaning that the two alleles inherited from its two parental gametes were identical. Such an individual is homozygous with reference to that genetic locus. The essence of the word *homozygous* refers to an organism whose two alleles for a given locus, or gene, are identical.

On the other hand, if, for some genetic locus, an organism carries two different alleles on corresponding sites of homologous chromosomes, it is said to be heterozygous. The phenomena of homozygous and heterozygous genotypes give phenotypic effect to dominant and recessive alleles.

Dominant and Recessive Alleles

Consider a hypothetical trait T. Assume that trait T appears when the organism manufactures protein T and does not appear when the organism fails to manufacture protein T. Finally, suppose that the production or failure to produce protein T is governed by a particular allele that exists in two forms:

1. allele *T* codes for protein T
2. allele *t* does not code for protein T

Imagine that a particular individual is homozygous for the allele that produces protein T. We designate her genotype as *TT,* meaning that at the relevant homologous pair, both chromosomes code for the production of protein T. The cells of this individual will manufacture protein T and she will, therefore, manifest trait T; her genotype is *TT,* and her phenotype for trait T is positive.

Imagine another individual who is homozygous for the allele that does not code for protein T. We designate his genotype as *tt,* meaning that at the relevant homologous pair, both chromosomes fail to code for protein T. This individual will fail to produce protein T and fail to manifest trait T. His genotype is *tt* and his phenotype for trait T is negative.

Now, imagine an individual who is heterozygous for the allele under discussion. We designate the genotype as *Tt,* meaning that at the relevant chromosomal pair, one chromosome carries the allele that codes for protein T and the other carries the allele that does not code for protein T. Since one of the two alleles codes for protein T, this individual will produce protein T and will consequently manifest trait T. His genotype is *Tt* and his phenotype for trait T is positive.

In the example of trait T, if the individual carries one allele that codes for Protein T (*T*) and one that does not (*t*), that individual will manifest trait T. This means the *T* allele is **dominant** over the *t* allele. In the heterozygous individual (*Tt*), the *T* allele (positive for the trait) expresses itself over the phenotype of the *t* allele (negative for the trait). The *t* allele expresses itself only when present on both alleles, or when the individual is homozygous for that allele (*tt*).

When two alleles interact in the way just described, we say that they exhibit **classical dominance.** This is based on Mendel's Law of Dominance (that one trait can mask the effects of another trait), and so can also be called Mendelian inheritance. The essential features and phenomena associated with classical dominance are:

1. Dominant alleles are denoted by a capital letter and recessive traits are denoted by a lowercase letter.
2. When an individual is either homozygous for the dominant allele (such as *TT*) or heterozygous (such as *Tt*), that individual expresses the dominant phenotype (such as T positive).
3. When an individual is homozygous for the recessive allele (such as *tt*), that individual expresses the recessive trait (such as T negative).

Mendelian Genetics

Gregor Mendel described the statistical behavior of inheritance of traits in pea plants long before the nature of DNA and chromosomes was known. Unlike Mendel, however, we are now familiar with the molecular basis of genetics in meiosis and genes, and the laws of genetics that Mendel formulated can now be presented with insight based on this knowledge. Although Mendelian genetics generally involves only the simplest patterns of inheritance, it forms the foundation for understanding more complicated situations.

Mendel observed that traits were governed by pairs of hereditary material (alleles). The first of Mendel's laws, the **Law of Segregation**, states that the two alleles of an individual are separated and passed on to the next generation singly. Mendel's second law, the **Law of Independent Assortment**, states that the alleles of one gene will separate into gametes independently of alleles for another gene. We will illustrate these principles using the garden pea plant, but the principles apply equally well to humans and many other organisms.

A trait that can be studied in the pea plant is the color of the pea. We can call *G* the allele for green color, while *g* is the allele for yellow pea color. Mating between plants, a **cross**, is used as a tool in genetics to discern genotypes by looking at the phenotypes of progeny from a cross. A **pure-breeding strain** of yellow or green peas consistently yields progeny of the same color when mated within the strain. For example, if mating yellow plants with yellow plants always produces yellow progeny, yellow is a pure-breeding strain. Let's assume that G is the dominant allele of the color gene, and g is the recessive allele. If a green plant is encountered, to deduce the genotype of the plant, one can do a **testcross**. The progeny of a testcross are called the **F_1 generation**. The results of a testcross depend on statistics and follow Mendel's laws.

The principle of segregation can be illustrated with the color gene described above for the pea. If a pea is heterozygous Gg, its gametes will contain either the G allele or the g allele, but never both. The probability that a gamete in the heterozygote will contain one allele or the other is 50%, completely random. To illustrate the Law of Independent Assortment, we need to introduce a second gene, one that controls the shape of the pea. W is the dominant allele, resulting in wrinkled peas, while w is the recessive allele, resulting in smooth peas in homozygous ww plants. According to the Law of Independent Assortment, the genes for the color of peas and the shape of peas are passed from one generation to another independently. The nature of the shape gene in a given gamete does not depend on and is not influenced by the color gene, if independent assortment is true.

Here is a summary of Mendel's principles of genetics:

Law of Dominance	One trait can mask the effects of another trait	
Law of Segregation	Alleles of a gene are distributed randomly but equally in gametes	
Law of Independent Assortment	Traits can segregate and recombine independently of other traits	

Table 4

The Punnett Square

It is possible to predict the results of a cross between two individuals using Mendel's Laws of Segregation and Law of Independent Assortment. Determining the result can be complex, however, so a visual tool called the **Punnett square** is sometimes used to make the process simpler. Let's look at a simple square first:

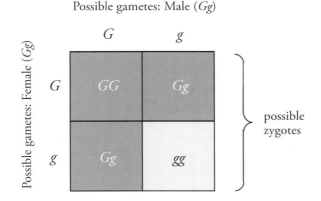

Figure 47   A Punnett Square Involving One Gene

Here, a Punnett square depicts a cross between two pea plants that are heterozygous for the color gene, with *G* the dominant green allele and *g* the recessive yellow allele. To draw a Punnett square, the following steps are involved:

Step 1:   Determine the gametes that are possible from each parent in the cross.

Step 2:   Draw a square with the possible gametes from each parent on two sides.

Step 3:   Fill in the square with the zygote genotypes that would result from each possible combination of gamete.

Step 4:   Determine the phenotype of each genotype.

Step 5:   Find the probability of each genotype and each phenotype.

If you have to work a probability question more complicated than this on the PCAT (for example one that involves two different genes), you are better off using some basic rules of probability and doing a small amount of math. Let's look at how to do this quickly and accurately.

Common Monohybrid and Dihybrid Crosses

Although Punnett squares are useful to understand the biology behind genetic crosses, they are time-consuming and error prone, especially on a standardized test like the PCAT. Another way to answer genetic cross questions is to know some common crosses and two probability rules. Let's look at the monohybrid crosses first; these are crosses that involve only one gene:

Parental Cross	Genotypic Ratio of Offspring	Phenotypic Ratio of Offspring
AA × *aa*	100% *Aa*	100% dominant A phenotype
AA × *Aa*	50% *AA* 50% *Aa*	100% dominant A phenotype
Aa × *aa*	50% *Aa* 50% *aa*	50% dominant A phenotype 50% recessive a phenotype
Aa × *Aa*	25% *AA* 50% *Aa* 25% *aa* This is also called a 1:2:1 ratio	75% dominant A phenotype 25% recessive a phenotype

Table 5

It is also useful to know some probability rules for two common dihybrid genetic crosses (those that involve two genes). They are:

Parental Cross	Genotypic Ratio of Offspring	Phenotypic Ratio of Offspring
AaBb × *aabb**	25% *AaBb* 25% *Aabb* 25% *aaBb* 25% *aabb*	25% A and B phenotypes 25% A and b phenotypes 25% a and B phenotypes 25% a and b phenotypes
AaBb × *AaBb*	n/a**	A 9:3:3:1 ratio of: 9 offspring have A and B phenotypes 3 offspring have A and b phenotypes 3 offspring have a and B phenotypes 1 offspring has a and b phenotypes

Table 6

*This cross can also be called a **testcross**, because one of the individuals is homozygous recessive.

**It is quite complicated to predict genotypic ratios in a heterozygous dihybrid cross. Instead, you would break the cross down into two separate genes, calculate the probabilities associated with each, and then multiply these two numbers, since you want to include the results from gene 1 *and* gene 2 in your final answer. Let's look at how to do this.

The Rule of Multiplication and the Rule of Addition

The **Rule of Multiplication** states that the probability of both of two independent events happening can be found by multiplying the odds of either event alone. For example, if the probability of being struck by lightning is 1 in a million (10^{-6}) and the probability of winning the lottery is 10^{-7}, then the probability of both happening is the product: $10^{-6} \times 10^{-7} = 10^{-13}$.

The **Rule of Addition** can be used to calculate the chances of either of two events happening. The chance of either A or B happening is equal to the probability of A added to the probability of B, minus the probability of A and B occurring together. For example, the chance of either getting hit by lightning *or* winning the lottery is $10^{-6} + 10^{-7} = 1.1 \times 10^{-6}$. (*Note*: The product of 10^{-6} and 10^{-7} is so small that it can be neglected from the equation.)

These rules can be a shortcut to using a Punnett square in many genetics problems.

6.5

Non-Mendelian Genetics

Linkage

The traits that Mendel studied and based the Law of Independent Assortment on were located on separate chromosomes. Genes that are located on the *same* chromosome may not display independent assortment, however. The failure of genes to display independent assortment is called **linkage**.

If genes are located very close to each other on the same chromosome, they will probably *not* be inherited independently of each other. Let's illustrate this with a pea gene for height and two alleles of the height gene, tall (*T*) and short (*t*), with the *T* allele dominant and the *t* allele recessive. If the height gene and the color gene are very near each other on the same chromosome, then the alleles of these genes on a specific chromosome will probably assort together into gametes during meiosis (Figure 48). This can limit the possible combinations of alleles in gametes or change their relative probabilities.

1. *TtGg* individual with independent assortment between the two genes

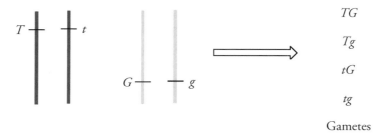

2. *TtGg* individual with complete linkage of the two genes

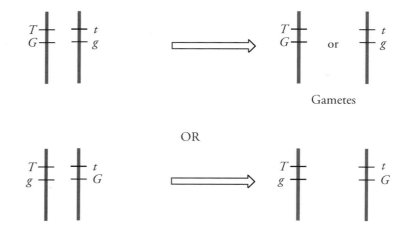

Figure 48   Linkage of Alleles during Meiosis

In the first example, although the genes are on the same chromosome, they are far apart. Recombination can occur between them and each of the resultant gametes will be present 25% of the time. This example is following Mendel's rules.

In the second example, the two genes are right beside each other with no space in between; they are 0 map units apart. They are completely linked and will be inherited as a unit. To know how linked alleles will assort during meiosis, it is necessary to know which alleles are on a chromosome together. As seen in Figure 48, there are two possible ways the height and color genes could be linked. The dominant alleles of two different genes can be linked together on the same chromosome (*TG*), the recessive alleles of two different genes can be linked (*tg*) on the other chromosomes. The other option is that one dominant and one recessive allele can be linked (*Tg* and *tG*). In either case, the genes are inherited as a unit, in the same allele combinations as in the parental cell.

There is also an intermediate option, in which genes are on the same chromosome as each other and more than 0 but less than 50 map units apart. In this case, some recombination can occur between the genes, but not as much as if the genes were far apart and unlinked. In this instance, parental combinations of alleles occur at a higher frequency and the products of recombination occur at a lower frequency.

Incomplete Dominance

Alternative alleles do not always (or even usually) interact to exhibit classic dominance. For some traits, alleles interact to produce an intermediate phenotype or a blended phenotype. In this case, we say that the trait exhibits **incomplete dominance**. For example, suppose flower color in plants exhibits incomplete dominance, plants with an *RR* genotype have red flowers, and plants with a *WW* genotype have white flowers. In this case, plants with an *RW* genotype would have pink flowers. For alleles that display incomplete dominance, different capital letters are used for alleles of a gene (e.g., *R* and *W* instead of *R* and *r*).

6.5

Codominance

In other cases, two different alleles for the same locus might express themselves not as an intermediate phenotype, but as two distinct phenotypes both present in a single individual. Alleles for the human blood groups (which determine your blood type) exhibit this form of interaction, known as **codominance.**

Human blood is commonly typed as A, B, or O, and either positive or negative. Blood type is determined by the expression of antigens on the surface of red blood cells (also called **erythrocytes).** An antigen is a molecule that is recognized by an antibody.

The blood group (A, B, AB, or O) is governed by three alleles designated I^A, I^B, and i at one locus:

- The I^A allele codes for an enzyme that adds the sugar galactosamine to the lipids on the surface of red blood cells. People with this allele express antigen A on their erythrocytes.
- The I^B allele codes for an enzyme that adds the sugar galactose to the lipids on the surface of red blood cells. People with this allele express antigen B on their erythrocytes.
- The i allele does not add any sugar to the surface of red blood cells.

An individual of genotype:

1. $I^A I^A$ or $I^A i$ shows the addition of galactosamine to the surface lipids of the red blood cells (or expresses antigen A); this person has blood type A.
2. $I^B I^B$ or $I^B i$ shows the addition of galactose to the surface lipids of the red blood cells (or expresses antigen B); this person has blood type B.
3. $I^A I^B$ shows the addition of *both* galactose and galactosamine to the surface lipids of the red blood cells (or expresses both antigens A and B); this person has blood type AB.
4. *ii* shows the addition of no sugar to the surface lipids of the red blood cells (expresses neither antigen A nor antigen B); this person has type O blood.

Note that the alleles I^A and I^B exhibit codominance. The individual who carries both alleles exhibits the trait tied to each. Neither allele is recessive in relation to the other. At the same time, however, the i allele, which does not code for the addition of any sugar on the red blood cell surface, *is* recessive in relation to both the I^A and I^B alleles. Only the genotype *ii* produces the blood type O phenotype.

Positive or negative blood type is determined by a separate gene called the Rh factor or antigen D, which exhibits classical dominance. Individuals who express antigen D have positive blood (genotype *DD* or *Dd*). If they do not express antigen D, they have negative blood (genotype *dd*).

Genetic Alteration and Diversity

Genes generally undergo alteration via two mechanisms: recombination and mutation.

Recombination

Genetic recombination generally refers to a process in which genetic information on one chromosome is moved to either a:

a. chromosome that belongs to some other cell
b. different chromosome within the same cell (often but not always a homologous chromosome)

The human immunodeficiency virus (HIV), for example, transfers a segment of its genome to a human chromosome, and the human cell thereby undergoes (severely pathologic) genetic recombination. Crossing over between homologous chromosomes in prophase I of meiosis is another example of recombination.

Mutation

Mutation refers to the process of changing a DNA sequence on a chromosome. This introduces genetic variation that can have a deleterious effect, improve an organism's adaptability, or have no effect at all.

Mutations in cells destined to produce gametes (the germ cells) potentially affect the genome of off-spring. Mutation of germ cells, therefore, is critical to the genetic variability that underlies evolution and natural selection. Mutation of a somatic (non-gametic) cell is less significant to the evolutionary process but may have serious consequences for the affected individual. Mutation of a single somatic cell, for example, may be the first event in the genesis of cancer.

Causes of mutation include mistakes in replication of the genome during cell division, chance chemical malformations (such as spontaneous deamination, which means loss of a nitrogen group), and environmental agents such as chemicals and ultraviolet light. For example, compounds that look like purines and pyrimidines (with large flat aromatic ring structures) cause mutations by inserting themselves between base pairs or by intercalating, thereby causing errors in DNA replication. Any compound that can cause mutations is called a **mutagen.**

Point mutations are single base pair substitutions (A in place of G, for example). There are three subclassifications of point mutations:

1. **Missense mutations** cause one amino acid to be replaced with a different amino acid.
2. **Nonsense mutations** cause a stop codon to replace a regular codon.
3. **Silent mutations** change a codon into a new codon for the same amino acid so there is no change in protein amino acid sequence.

If a missense mutation leads to little change in the structure and function of the gene product (protein), it is referred to as a **conservative mutation.**

There are five kinds of **gene rearrangement mutations:**

1. Insertion
2. Deletion
3. Inversion
4. Amplification or duplication
5. Translocation

Insertion refers to the addition of one or more extra nucleotides into a DNA sequence. Deletion is the removal of one or more nucleotides from a DNA sequence. Both of these mutations can cause a shift in the reading frame. For example, AAACCCACC can be read as AAA, CCC, ACC. It would code for the tripeptide Lys-Pro-Thr. Inserting an extra G into the first codon could produce this: AGAACCCACC. This would be read AGA, ACC, CAC, C. It now codes for Arg-Thr-His (plus there's an extra C nucleotide). Not only has the first codon changed, but the whole piece of DNA will be read differently from that point on. Mutations causing a change in the reading frame are called **frameshift mutations.** Generally speaking, frameshift mutations are serious, especially if they occur early on in the gene. Frameshift mutations often lead to a premature stop codon, where early termination of translation yields an incomplete polypeptide.

In addition to insertions and deletions (sometimes called **indels**), there are three other types of gene rearrangement mutations:

Mutation	Definition	Example
Inversion	Chromosome section is flipped	
Amplification or Duplication	Chromosome section is duplicated	
Translocation	Chromosome segment is swapped with another (nonhomologous) chromosome	

Table 7

Sex Determination and Inheritance Patterns

Sex Determination

We've already introduced the concept of autosomes and sex chromosomes.

Now consider the meiotic processes of spermatogenesis and oogenesis. At anaphase of the first meiotic division, all chromosomal pairs separate, including the sex chromosomes. In the case of oogenesis, both the secondary oocyte and the first polar body take an X chromosome (since the parent diploid cell has no Y chromosome to donate). Consequently, all mature ova carry an X chromosome; none carry a Y chromosome. In the case of spermatogenesis, one secondary spermatocyte takes the X chromosome and the other takes the Y chromosome. Consequently, half of the mature spermatozoa carry an X chromosome and half carry a Y chromosome.

Sex is determined when a spermatozoon fertilizes the ovum. If the ovum is fertilized by an X-bearing spermatozoon, the zygote is XX (female). If the ovum is fertilized by a Y-bearing spermatozoon, the zygote is XY (male). Since 50 percent of spermatozoon carry a Y chromosome and 50 percent carry an X chromosome, there is a 50 percent chance of a zygote being male and a 50 percent chance of the zygote being female.

Inheritance Patterns

In the human population, most traits are carried by autosomes (the 22 pairs of chromosomes that are not X or Y). In addition, some traits are carried by the mitochondrial genome, some are carried by the X chromosomes, and some are carried by the Y chromosome.

Autosomal traits can be recessive (the affected individual needs two copies of the affected allele to show the trait) or dominant (one copy of the affected allele is enough to show the trait). Autosomal traits affect males and females with equal frequency.

Mitochondrial traits are passed onto offspring from the mother and only the mother. This is because spermatozoon pass only 23 nuclear chromosomes to the zygote. The ovum also donates 23 nuclear chromosomes and all the other cellular components, including organelles. Since there is a very small and separate genome in the matrix of the mitochondria, all individuals inherit their mitochondrial genome (and any associated traits) from their mother. These traits are not recessive or dominant, since there is only one copy of the mitochondrial genome; they are either present or absent.

Y-linked traits are very rare. They never affect females (since females have no Y chromosome) and are passed from father to son. Similar to mitochondrial traits, there is no issue of dominance with these traits. Males have only one copy of the Y chromosome, so the trait is either present or absent.

There are also some traits that are carried on the X chromosome. These traits, which are termed **sex-linked** (or sometimes **X-linked**), can be dominant or recessive. Two very common recessive X-linked traits are red/green color blindness and hemophilia. Let's look at an example.

The dominant *CB* allele is associated with the normal phenotype (no red/green color blindness) and the recessive *cb* allele is associated with color blindness. This means that:

1. Any male who carries the color-blind allele ($X^{cb}Y$) will be color-blind. Even though the gene is recessive, the male has no second X chromosome to dominate it. The recessive gene is free to express itself and will do so.
2. A female who carries the color-blind gene on both X chromosomes ($X^{cb}X^{cb}$) will be color-blind. The gene is recessive, but if it is carried on two X chromosomes, the genotype has no allele that will dominate it. The recessive gene will express itself.
3. A female who carries the color-blind gene on one of her X chromosomes but not on the other ($X^{CB}X^{cb}$) will not be color-blind. The color-blind allele is recessive; the X chromosome that carries the dominant allele (*CB*) will prevent the recessive allele (*cb*) from expressing itself. Females with this genotype are called **carriers** of the trait because they carry the X^{cb} allele and can pass it onto any offspring they may have.
4. Males with an $X^{CB}Y$ and females with an $X^{CB}X^{CB}$ genotype will have normal vision and will not pass the X^{cb} color-blindness allele to any offspring they may have.

Because a sex-linked trait is carried on the X chromosome, and because a male receives a Y chromosome from his father (not an X chromosome), it follows that a sex-linked trait cannot pass from a male to a male. Rather, a male who carries a sex-linked recessive gene has always inherited it from his mother.

Because a male passes his X chromosome to his daughters, it follows that any male who carries a sex-linked recessive gene will pass it to all of his daughters. The daughter will not be positive for the trait, however, unless she has also inherited the affected and recessive allele from her mother and is homozygous for the gene.

Because a female passes one of her two X chromosomes to each of her offspring, it follows that any female who carries a sex-linked recessive allele will pass it to 50 percent of her offspring, regardless of their sex. All of her sons who inherit the affected allele will be positive for the phenotype. Her daughters who inherit the affected allele will not be positive for the trait, unless they also inherit the allele from their father and are homozygous.

There are six common modes of inheritance. They are summarized here:

Inheritance Pattern	Identification	Unaffected Genotypes	Affected Genotypes
Autosomal recessive	• can skip generations • # of affected males ~# of affected females • unaffected parents can have affected offspring	*AA* *Aa*	*aa*
Autosomal dominant	• does not skip generations • # of affected males ~# of affected females • affected parents pass the trait to either all or half of their offspring	*aa*	*AA* *Aa*
Y- Linked	• affects males only; females never have the trait • affected male has all affected sons • unaffected male cannot have an affected son	XY^a	XY^A

Table 8

6.5

Inheritance Pattern	Identification	Unaffected Genotypes	Affected Genotypes
Mitochondrial	• material inheritance • all humans receive their mitochondrial genome from their mother; sperm contribute only nuclear chromosomes • affected female has all affected children • affected male cannot pass the trait onto his children • unaffected female cannot have affected children	a	A
X-linked recessive	• can skip generations • tends to affect males more than females • unaffected female can have affected sons • affected female has all affected sons, but can have both affected and unaffected daughters	$X^A X^A$ $X^A X^a$ $X^A Y$	$X^a X^a$ $X^a Y$
X-linked dominant	• hardest to identify • does not skip generations • usually affects males more than females • affected male has all affected daughters • affected female can have unaffected sons, and give the trait equally to sons and daughters	$X^a X^a$ $X^a Y$	$X^A X^A$ $X^A X^a$ $X^A Y$

Table 8 (continued)

Pedigrees

It is possible you may see a small and straightforward pedigree on the PCAT, so we will review some basics here. Typically pedigrees on the PCAT have three generations and fewer than 12 individuals.

Often it is not possible to perform controlled genetic crosses to ascertain the nature of inheritance of a trait, particularly when people are involved. In these cases, families can be studied to determine the pattern of inheritance. Researchers organize the information learned from families into **pedigrees**, which are charts depicting inheritance of a trait (Figure 49). By studying the pedigree of families, researchers can determine the pattern of inheritance of a gene, whether it is linked to other genes, and whether individuals are likely to pass on a trait to their offspring. Pedigrees follow certain conventions in how they are drawn:

1. Males are represented by squares and females by circles.
2. A cross (mating) between a male and female is represented by a horizontal line connecting them.
3. Offspring from a cross are connected to their parents by a vertical line, and to each other by a horizontal line with vertical branches for each sibling.
4. Offspring of unknown gender (unborn children) are represented by a diamond shape.
5. Individuals affected by a trait being studied are shaded in; unaffected or normal individuals are not shaded in.

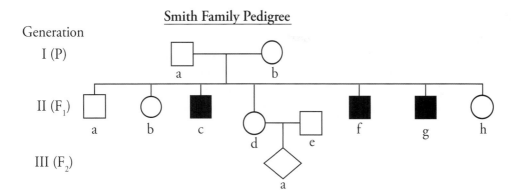

Figure 49 A Pedigree

Many pedigrees make a common assumption: individuals mating into the family (i.e., individuals for which you have no information on their parents or grandparents) are assumed to be homozygous normal unless their phenotype tells you differently. The basis of this assumption is that the traits being studied are usually relatively rare in the human population, and therefore it is likely that a non-family member is homozygous for the **wild type allele**; this allele encodes the phenotype most common in a particular natural population. In many instances, the terms wild type allele and normal allele are used interchangeably.

A pedigree can be analyzed as follows:

1. Figure out the mode of inheritance for the trait:
    A. Check for mitochondrial inheritance. Affected females will have all affected children but affected males cannot pass the trait on.
    B. Check for Y-linked inheritance. Diseases linked to the Y chromosome affect only males and will show father-to-son transmission.
    C. Is the allele that causes the trait dominant or is it recessive? Recessive traits commonly skip generations, but dominant traits do not.
    D. Is the gene involved carried on the X chromosome? If so, there tends to be an unequal distribution of affected males vs. affected females.
2. Assign alleles and write down on your noteboard which letters stand for which alleles. For example, D = normal, d = affected.
3. You may want to also write down genotypes. For example, DD and Dd = normal, dd = affected.
4. Start with the individual you're being asked about and work backward up the pedigree. Figure out genotypes as you go.
5. Calculate probabilities of inheritance where necessary.
6. It is highly unlikely you will have to look at two different traits on one pedigree, but if you do, repeat the steps above for the other trait.

The following are example pedigrees for six modes of inheritance (X-linked recessive, X-linked dominant, autosomal recessive, autosomal dominant, mitochondrial, and Y-linked). For each pedigree, determine which mode of inheritance is displayed.

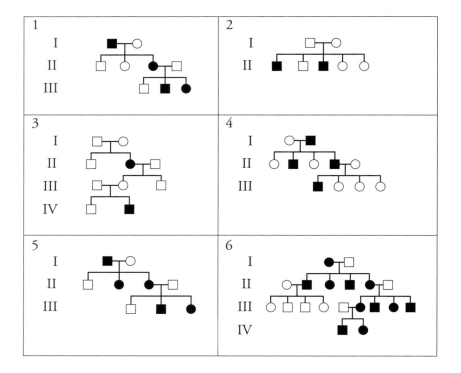

Answers
1. autosomal dominant
2. X-linked recessive
3. autosomal recessive
4. Y-linked
5. X-linked dominant
6. mitochondrial inheritance

Explanations

The easiest inheritance patterns to spot are mitochondrial (passed from mothers to all offspring) and Y-linked (passed from fathers to sons, and females are never affected). Let's start by finding these two. Since Pedigree 6 shows a trait with maternal inheritance, this must be mitochondrial inheritance. The affected father in generation II does not pass the trait to any of his children, but the affected mothers in generations I, II, and III pass the trait onto all their offspring. Pedigree 4 shows a trait with Y-linked inheritance. The trait is passed from father to all sons and does not affect females.

Next, both Pedigree 2 and Pedigree 3 show traits that skip generations. That is, there are individuals on the pedigree that are affected by the trait but who have unaffected parents. Therefore, these two pedigrees must be for recessive traits. One is autosomal and the other is X-linked.

Since the trait on Pedigree 2 affects males more than females, it is likely X-linked, and since the trait on Pedigree 3 affects males and females equally, it is probably autosomal. Let's verify this by looking more closely at Pedigree 3. If this trait is X-linked recessive, then the affected female in generation II must have the genotype $X^a X^a$, and would have had to receive the allele for the trait from both her parents. However, for an X-linked recessive, the unaffected male in generation I would have the genotype $X^A Y$, and would only have X^A to donate to his daughter. Therefore this pedigree cannot represent an X-linked recessive trait;

it must represent an autosomal recessive trait. The male in generation I must have the genotype *Aa*, the female in generation I must have the genotype *Aa*, and the affected female in generation II must have the genotype *aa*. The remaining pedigree, Pedigree 2, must be X-linked recessive.

Finally, Pedigrees 1 and 5 show traits that do not skip generations. That is, affected individuals have affected parents. These are pedigrees for dominant traits; one is X-linked and one is autosomal. The only difference between these two pedigrees is the middle daughter in the second generation; in Pedigree 1 she is unaffected and in Pedigree 5 she is affected. Let's focus on her father (the male in generation I) since this is where she gets the allele for the trait. If the trait is X-linked dominant, the male in generation I would be $X^A Y$; thus all females in generation II would inherit X^A from their father, and all of them would be affected. Since the middle daughter in Pedigree 1 is not affected, Pedigree 1 must show autosomal dominance and the pedigree for the X-linked dominant trait must be Pedigree 5.

6.6 EVOLUTION

Population Genetics

Mendelian genetics describes the inheritance of traits in the progeny of specific individuals. For the purposes of topics such as natural selection and evolution, however, the more relevant issue is not the inheritance of traits from individuals but in a whole population from one generation to another. **Population genetics** describes the inheritance of traits in populations over time. The word population has a specific meaning in this setting: a **population** consists of members of a species that mate and reproduce with each other. To a population geneticist, each individual is merely a temporary carrier of the alleles in a population.

In population genetics, the units of genetic inheritance are alleles of genes, just as in Mendelian genetics. However, in population genetics, alleles are examined across the entire population rather than in individuals. The sum total of all genetic information in a population is called the **gene pool**. The frequency of an allele in a population is a key variable used to describe the gene pool.

Hardy-Weinberg in Population Genetics

Population genetics does not simply describe the gene pool of a population but attempts to predict the gene pool of a population in the future. The **Hardy-Weinberg Law** states that frequencies of alleles in the gene pool of a population will not change over time, provided that these five assumptions are true:

1. There is no mutation.
2. There is no migration.
3. There is no natural selection.
4. There is random mating.
5. The population is sufficiently large to prevent random drift in allele frequencies.

At the molecular level, this means that segregation of alleles, independent assortment, and recombination during meiosis can alter the combinations of alleles in gametes. However, these processes will not change the frequency of an allele in the population as a whole.

The Hardy-Weinberg Law has also been translated into mathematical terms. Assuming that there are two alleles of a gene in a population, the letter p is used to represent the frequency of the dominant allele, and the letter q is used to represent the frequency of the recessive allele. Since there are only two alleles, the following fundamental equation must be true:

$$p + q = 1$$

Based on these allele frequencies, it is possible to calculate the proportion of each genotype in a population (or genotype frequencies). Remember that the frequency of a dominant allele, G, equals p and the frequency of a recessive allele, g, equals q. This means that:

1. p^2 = the frequency of the GG genotype
2. $2pq$ = the frequency of the Gg genotype
3. q^2 = the frequency of the gg genotype

If G and g are the only two alleles for this gene, these are the only three genotypes possible. This means that:

$$p^2 + 2pq + q^2 = 1$$

Let's look at an example. If the frequency of the G allele is 0.25 in a population of 1,000 mice, determine the number of individuals who are Gg heterozygotes if there is random mating but no migration, mutation, random drift, or natural selection.

If the frequency of the G allele (p) is 0.25, then the frequency of the g allele (q) must be 0.75, since $p + q = 1$. The frequency of the heterozygotes in the population will be $2pq = 2(0.25)(0.75) = 0.375$. Therefore, the number of individuals in this population who are heterozygotes will be $0.375 \times 1,000 = 375$.

After one generation, a population will reach **Hardy-Weinberg equilibrium**, in which allele frequencies no longer change. Since allele frequencies do not change, and genotype frequencies can be calculated from allele frequencies, it follows that genotype frequencies also do not change over time.

Hardy-Weinberg in the Real World

Hardy-Weinberg requires a number of assumptions in order to be true; it describes a highly idealized set of conditions required to prevent alleles from being added or removed from a population. In reality, it is not possible for a population to meet all of the conditions required by Hardy-Weinberg.

1. Mutation: Mutation is inevitable in a population. Even if there are no chemical mutagens or radiation, inherent errors by DNA polymerase would over time cause mutations and introduce new alleles in a population.
2. Migration: If migration occurs, animals leaving or entering the population will carry alleles with them and disturb the Hardy-Weinberg equilibrium.
3. Natural Selection: For there to be no natural selection, there would have to be unlimited resources, no predation, no disease, and so on. This is not a set of conditions encountered in the real world.
4. Non-random mating: If individuals pick their mates preferentially based on one or more traits, alleles that cause those traits will be passed on preferentially from one generation to another.
5. Random drift: If a population becomes very small, it cannot contain as great a variety of alleles. In a very small population, random events can alter allele frequencies significantly and have a large influence on future generations.

Origin of Life

Based on radioisotope dating, the Earth is thought to be 4.5 billion years old. All life evolved from pro-karyotes. The oldest fossils are 3.5 billion-year-old outlines of primitive prokaryotic cell walls found in stromatolites (layered mats formed by colonies of prokaryotes). Even older life forms certainly existed but lacked cell walls and thus left no fossil record (at least none have yet been discovered). Hence life on Earth is older than 3.5 billion years, nearly as old as the planet itself.

The atmosphere of the young Earth was different from today's atmosphere. The predominant gases then were probably H_2O, CO, CO_2, and N_2. The most important thing to note here is the absence of O_2. It is thought that the early atmosphere was a **reducing environment**, where electron donors were prevalent. Oxygen is an electron acceptor, and thus tends to break organic bonds. In this early world, simple organic molecules, or monomers ("single units") could form spontaneously. The energy for this synthesis was provided by lightning, radioactive decay, volcanic activity, or the Sun's radiation, which was more intense than it is today due to the thinner atmosphere. Laboratory recreations of the early environment result in the spontaneous formation of amino acids, carbohydrates, lipids, and ribonucleotides, as well as other organic compounds.

Spontaneous polymerization of these monomers can also be observed in the lab (including spontaneous polymerization of ribonucleotides). No enzymes were present when this was occurring for the first time in nature, but it is thought that metal ions on the surface of rocks and especially clay acted as catalysts. This is known as **abiotic synthesis**. Polypeptides made in this way are called **proteinoids**.

Proteinoids in water spontaneously form droplets called **microspheres**. When lipids are added to the solution, **liposomes** form, with lipids forming a layer on the surface of proteins. A more complex particle known as a **coacervate** includes polypeptides, nucleic acids, and polysaccharides. Coacervates made with pre-existing enzymes are capable of catalyzing reactions. Microspheres, liposomes, and coacervates are collectively referred to as **protobionts**.

Protobionts resemble cells in that they contain a protected inner environment and perform chemical reactions. They can also reproduce to a certain extent: when they grow too large, they split in half. What is lacking, however, is an organized mechanism of heredity. This was first provided by RNA. As noted above, RNA chains form spontaneously in the appropriate solution. Even more interesting is the observation that single-stranded (ss) RNA chains can be self-replicating. A daughter chain lines up on the parent by base pairing and then spontaneously polymerizes with a surprisingly low error rate. A nonspecific catalyst such as a metal ion can further increase the efficiency of RNA self-replication. Furthermore, it is now known that RNA has catalytic activity in modern cells. For example, in primitive eukaryotes, introns are spliced out of the mRNA by **ribozymes**, which are RNA enzymes.

Somehow a mechanism evolved for polypeptides to be copied from early RNA genes. You already know about the inherent tendency for phospholipids to form lipid bilayers. Given all this information, it's not too hard to imagine true cells evolving from a primordial soup at the dawn of time. The last step in the evolution of the earliest cells would have been the switch from RNA to DNA as the genetic material. DNA is more stable due to its 2′-deoxy structure and also due to the fact that it spontaneously forms a compact double-stranded helix.

6.6

Evolution by Natural Selection

At one time, life on Earth was generally viewed as static and unchanging, but we now know that this is not the case. Over the geologic span of Earth's history, many species have arisen, changed over millions of years, given rise to new species, and died out. These changes in life on Earth are called **evolution**. Although he did not arrive at his theory alone, Charles Darwin played an important role in shaping modern thought by proposing natural selection as the mechanism that drives evolution. **Natural selection** is an interaction between organisms and their environment that causes differential reproduction of different phenotypes and thereby alters the gene pool of a population. In essence, the Theory of Evolution by natural selection is this:

1. In a population, there are heritable differences between individuals.
2. Heritable traits (alleles of genes) produce traits (phenotypes) that affect the ability of an organism to survive and have offspring.
3. Some individuals have phenotypes that allow them to survive longer, be healthier, and have more offspring than others.
4. Individuals with phenotypes that allow them to have more offspring will pass on their alleles more frequently than those with phenotypes that have fewer offspring.
5. Over time, those alleles that lead to more offspring are passed on more frequently and become more abundant, while other alleles become less abundant in the gene pool.
6. Changes in allele frequency are the basis of evolution in species and populations.

To put it simply, evolution occurs when natural selection acts on genetic variation to drive changes in the genetic composition of a population. A key term in evolution is **fitness** (sometimes called Darwinian fitness). In evolutionary terms, fitness is not how well an animal is physically adapted to a niche in the environment, or how well it can feed itself, but how successful it is in passing on its alleles to future generations. The way to have greater fitness is by having more offspring that pass on their alleles to future generations of the population. Some species achieve greater fitness through sheer numbers of progeny produced, who are then left to fend for themselves. Other species have fewer progeny but protect and nurture the young to maturity.

Sources of Genetic Diversity

Natural selection acts on the genetic diversity in a population to alter allele frequencies, causing evolution. Genetic diversity in a population is a requirement for natural selection to occur. Natural selection does not introduce genetic diversity, however; it can act only on existing diversity to alter allele frequencies.

There are two sources of genetic variation in a population: new alleles and new combinations of existing alleles. New alleles are the result of mutations in the genome. New combinations of alleles are generated during sexual reproduction as a result of independent assortment, recombination, and segregation during meiosis. By increasing and maintaining genetic variation in a population, sexual reproduction allows for greater capacity for adaptation of a population to changing environmental conditions.

Modes of Natural Selection

Natural selection can occur in many different ways and have different effects in a population. The following are a few examples:

1. Directional Selection: Some traits follow a bell-shaped curve of expression, with most individuals clustered around the average and some members of a population trailing off in either direction away from the average. If natural selection removes those at one extreme, the population average over time will move in the other direction. Example: Giraffes get taller as all short giraffes die for lack of food.

2. Divergent Selection: Rather than removing the extreme members in the distribution of a trait in a population, natural selection removes the members near the average, leaving those at either end. Over time divergent selection will split the population in two and perhaps lead to a new species. Example: Small deer are selected because they can hide, and large deer are selected because they can fight, but mid-sized deer are too big to hide and too small to fight.

3. Stabilizing Selection: Both extremes of a trait are selected against, driving the population closer to the average. Example: Birds that are too large or too small are eliminated from a population because they cannot mate.

4. Artificial Selection: Humans intervene in the mating of many animals and plants, using artificial selection to achieve desired traits through controlled mating. Example: The pets and crop plants we have are the result of many generations of artificial selection.

5. Sexual Selection: Animals often do not choose mates randomly but have evolved elaborate rituals and physical displays that play a key role in attracting and choosing a mate. Example: Some birds have bright plumage to attract a mate, even at the cost of increased predation.

6.6

Species Concept and Speciation

A species is a group of organisms capable of reproducing with each other sexually. Two individuals are not members of the same biological species if they cannot mate and produce fit offspring. The creation of new species is known as **speciation**. An important premise in modern evolutionary biology is that all species come from pre-existing species. **Cladogenesis** is branching speciation (*clado* is from the Greek for branch), in which one species diversifies and becomes two or more new species. For example, if individuals of a species become geographically isolated, there can be no gene flow between them. Over time each population will accumulate mutations and new combinations of alleles. The two populations will end up genetically different from each other, which can lead to reproductive isolation. Eventually, the two populations will not be able to breed with each other and will have therefore become different species.

Speciation has left traces which taxonomists use to classify organisms. **Homologous structures** are physical features shared by two different species as a result of a common ancestor. For example, bird wings have five bony supports that resemble distorted human fingers, and dog paws also resemble distorted human hands. The explanation is that dogs, birds, and people all have a common ancestor that had five-toed feet. **Analogous structures** serve the same function in two different species, but not due to common ancestry. The flagellum of the human sperm and bacterial flagella are examples; they have entirely different structures in different organisms yet play the same role in motility.

Convergent evolution occurs when two different species come to possess many analogous structures due to similar selective pressures. For example, bats and birds appear very similar even though bats are mammals. The opposite of convergent evolution is divergent evolution, in which divergent selection causes cladogenesis. Parallel evolution describes the situation in which two species go through similar evolutionary changes due to similar selective pressures. For example, in an ice age, all organisms would be selected for their ability to tolerate cold.

Diversity of Life and Taxonomy

Taxonomy is the science of biological classification, originated by Carolus Linnaeus in the 18th century. He devised the binomial classification system we use today, in which each organism is given two names: genus and species. The binomial name of an organism is written in italics (or is underlined) with the genus capitalized and the species not, as in *Homo sapiens* (man the wise). Taxonomy is an important part of biology because it is used to determine the evolutionary relationship of organisms to one another. There are eight principal taxonomic categories: domain, kingdom, phylum, class, order, family, genus, and species. For example, humans are:

- Domain: Eukarya
- Kingdom: Animalia
- Phylum: Chordata
- Class: Mammalia
- Order: Primates
- Family: Hominidae
- Genus: Homo
- Species: sapiens

The largest taxonomic division is the **domain**. There are three recognized domains: Bacteria, Archaea, and Eukarya. Domains Bacteria and Archaea include prokaryotic organisms, and Domain Eukarya includes eukaryotic organisms. Each domain can be further subdivided into **kingdoms**. Currently there are three well-recognized eukaryotic kingdoms (Animalia, Plantae, and Fungi), and great debate over the number of kingdoms that should be present in the other prokaryotic domains and in the single-celled eukaryotes (protists).

Table 9 is a chart summarizing domains and kingdoms. Bacteria, fungi, and protists will be discussed in greater detail in the next chapter because they have important roles in human health and disease. You do not need to be familiar with plant biology (beyond what is in the table) for the PCAT.

Domain	Bacteria	Archaea	Eukarya			
Kingdom	**Formerly Monera**		**Protista**	**Fungi**	**Plantae**	**Animalia**
Cell Wall	Peptidoglycan	Chain mail proteins	Optional and varied	Chitin	Cellulose	None
Membrane-Bound Organelles	None	None	Typical eukaryotic organelles such as nucleus, RER, SER, Golgi, peroxisomes, lysosomes, chloroplasts, vacuoles, mitochondria, etc.			
Chromosomes	1 circular ds DNA	1 circular ds DNA	Several linear ds DNA chromosomes			
Life cycle and Reproduction	Asexual repro. (binary fission)	Asexual repro. (binary fission)	Varied (sexual and asexual)	Varied (sexual and asexual)	Mostly sexual repro.	Mostly sexual repro.
Cellularity	Unicellular	Unicellular	Mostly unicellular	Mostly multicellular	Multicellular	Multicellular
Ploidy	Haploid	Haploid	Haploid or diploid	Mostly haploid	Alternate between haploid and diploid	Diploid
Cellular motility	Flagella	Flagella	Amoeboid or flagellar	Non-motile	Some flagellated sperm	Amoeboid or flagellar
Cilia	None	None	Characteristic 9 + 2 arrangement of microtubules			
Flagella	Bacterial flagellin proteins	Archaeal flagellin proteins				
Nutrition	Varied, absorptive	Varied, absorptive	Varied	Chemotroph Heterotroph Absorptive	Autotroph via photosynth.	Chemotroph Heterotroph Ingestive
Glycolysis/ATP	All living organisms perform glycolysis and use ATP. All kingdoms contain at least some members which perform oxidative phosphorylation.					
Examples	Bacteria *E. coli* Blue-green algae	Extremophiles	Amoeba Euglena Paramecium *Plasmodium* Seaweed	Yeasts Molds Mushrooms	Trees Flowers Mosses Ferns	Sponges Worms Mollusks Insects Chordates

Table 9 Taxonomic Characteristics

6.6

CHAPTER 6 KEY TERMS

2′ deoxy-D-ribose
30S
3′ untranslated region
40S
50S
5′ untranslated region
60S
70S
80S
abiotic synthesis
activation energy
active site
active transport
adenine (A)
adenosine triphosphate (ATP)
adipocytes
aerobic
alleles
amino acid acceptor site
amino acid activation
aminoacyl-tRNA synthetase
anaerobic
analogous structures
anaphase
anticodon
antiports
anti-sense strand
aquaporins
A site
aster fibers
ATP synthase
autosomal traits
autosomes
carrier proteins
catalysts
cell membrane
cellular adhesions
cell wall
centrioles
centromere
centrosomes
channel proteins
chlorophyll
chloroplasts
chromosomes
cilia
citric acid cycle
cladogenesis
classical dominance
clathrin

cleavage furrow
coacervate
coding strand
codominance
codon
coenzymes
cofactors
competitive inhibition
conservative mutation
convergent evolution
cristae
cross
cytokinesis
cytoplasm
cytosine (C)
daughter chromosome
denaturation
deoxyribonucleic acid (DNA)
desmosomes
diploid
divergent evolution
DNA ligase
DNA polymerases
DNA replication
domain
dominant
downstream
electron carrier molecules
elongation
endocytosis
endomembrane system
endoplasmic reticulum
endosome
enzymes
enzyme specificity
enzyme-substrate complex
equilibrium concentrations
erythrocytes
E site
eukaryotic
evolution
exocytosis
F_1 generation
fatty acid β-oxidation
feedback inhibition
fermentation
fitness
flagella
fluid mosaic model
frameshift mutations

gametes

gametogenesis

gap junctions

gap phase 1 (G$_1$ phase)

gap phase 2 (G$_2$ phase)

gated

gene pool

gene rearrangement mutations

genetic locus

genetic recombination

genome

genotype

gluconeogenesis

glycogenesis

glycogenolysis

glycolysis

Golgi apparatus

guanine (G)

Hardy-Weinberg equilibrium

Hardy-Weinberg Law

helicase

helix

hemizygous

hepatocytes

heterozygous

high-energy bonds

histones

homologous structures

homozygous

incomplete dominance

indels

induced fit

inhibitor

initiation

inner mitochondrial membrane

kinetochore fibers

kingdoms

Krebs cycle

lagging strand

Law of Independent Assortment

Law of Segregation

leading strands

ligand-gated

linkage

liposomes

lock-and-key

Lysosomes

matrix

metaphase

metaphase plate

microfilaments

microspheres

microtubules

missense mutations

mitochondria

mutagen

mutation

Na$^+$/K$^+$ ATPase

natural selection

non-coding strand

nonsense mutations

nuclear membrane

nucleolus

nucleosomes

nucleotide

nucleus

Okazaki fragments

oogenesis

oogonium

ootid

origin of replication

osmosis

osmotic pressure

ovaries

ovum

parallel evolution

pedigrees

peripheral proteins

peroxisomes

phagocytosis

phenotype

phosphodiester bonds

photosynthesis

pigment

pinocytosis

plastids

point mutations

polar body

polarity

polyribosome

population

population genetics

potassium leak channels

primary active transport

primary oocyte

primase

prokaryotic

promoter

prophase

proteinoids

protobionts

P site

Punnett square

pure-breeding strain

purines

pyrimidines

pyrimidines
receptor-mediated endocytosis
receptors
reducing environment
reduction division
release factors
replication bubble
replication forks
resting membrane potential
ribonucleic acid (RNA)
ribosomes
ribozymes
RNA polymerases
rough endoplasmic reticulum
Rule of Addition
Rule of Multiplication
secondary active transport
secondary oocyte
selectively permeable
selective permeability
semi-conservative
seminiferous tubules
semipermeable
sense strand
sex chromosomes
sex-linked
silent mutations
simple diffusion
smooth endoplasmic reticulum
somatic
speciation
spermatogenesis
spermatogonia

sperm cells
start site
steric hindrance
sugar-phosphate backbone
symports
synapsis
synthesis phase (S phase)
TATA box
taxonomy
telophase
template
termination
termination signal
terminator
testcross
testes
tetrads
thymine (T)
tight junctions
traits
transcription
transmembrane proteins
tricarboxylic acid cycle
triglycerides
tubulin
uniports
upstream
vacuoles
vesicles
voltage-gated
wild type allele
X-linked
zygote

GENERAL BIOLOGY DRILL

1. Which of the following is a correct matching of eukaryotic organelle to function?

   A. Rough ER—surrounded by a double membrane
   B. Nucleus—present in eukaryotes but absent in prokaryotes
   C. Mitochondria—inner membrane has a large surface area due to cristae
   D. Lysosome—digest foreign particles and old organelles

2. The process of movement of ions through a carrier protein is described in the following steps:

   I. An ion present in a cell binds to a carrier protein.
   II. A phosphate group from ATP transfers energy to the carrier protein.
   III. The carrier protein undergoes conformational change and releases the ion outside the cell membrane against the concentration gradient.

   What is this process called?

   A. Diffusion
   B. Active transport
   C. Osmosis
   D. Facilitated diffusion

3. Which of the following processes describes the role of mitochondria in energy transformation?

   A. ATP is released during the conversion of glucose to pyruvate.
   B. ADP and P_i form 4 ATP molecules in a ten-step process.
   C. ATP is released by the breakdown of a three-carbon compound to CO_2.
   D. Coenzyme NADH, formed during glycolysis, is converted to NAD^+.

4. Which step connects glycolysis to the citric acid cycle?

   A. Isocitrate undergoes decarboxylation, resulting in a five-carbon compound α-ketoglutarate.
   B. Pyruvate loses a carbon atom, resulting in a two-carbon compound acetyl-CoA.
   C. Fructose 1, 6-bisphosphate splits into phosphate and glyceraldehyde 3-phosphate.
   D. Malate undergoes oxidation in the presence of malate dehydrogenase and forms oxaloacetate.

5. When *Pseudomonas aeruginosa* enters body tissues, it produces the virulence factor exotoxin A, which inhibits the elongation factor eEF2. Which of the following processes is blocked by exotoxin A?

   A. Pyruvate dehydrogenase complex
   B. Membrane transport
   C. Meiosis
   D. Protein synthesis

6. The central dogma of molecular biology states that:

   A. RNA is a template for DNA synthesis via transcription, then RNA is a template for protein synthesis via translation.
   B. RNA is a template for protein synthesis via both transcription and translation.
   C. DNA is a template for RNA synthesis via transcription, then RNA is a template for protein synthesis via translation.
   D. DNA is a template for RNA synthesis via translation, then RNA is a template for protein synthesis via transcription.

7. What is the role of microtubules during a cell cycle?

   A. They are involved in DNA replication during the S phase.
   B. They pull apart the sister chromatids during anaphase.
   C. They stop a cell from dividing before cytokinesis.
   D. They form enzymes during the G_1 phase.

8. There are several stages of the cell cycle in a typical eukaryotic cell. At which stage are enzymes required for DNA replication synthesized?

    A. G_1 phase
    B. S phase
    C. M phase
    D. G_2 phase

9. Which of the following is a true statement regarding meiosis?

    A. Daughter cells formed are always diploid.
    B. The number of chromosomes in daughter cells is the same as that in parent cells.
    C. Pairing of homologous chromosomes takes place.
    D. Daughter cells are used in growth and replacement of damaged cells.

10. Sickle cell anemia is a disorder that occurs because of a recessive autosomal gene. If one parent has sickle cell anemia and the other is a carrier of the disorder, which of the following summarizes the chance of the disorder occurring in their offspring?

    A. 50% normal and 50% carriers
    B. 50% carrier and 50% having sickle cell anemia
    C. 25% normal, 25% having sickle cell anemia, and 50% carriers
    D. 25% carriers, 25% having sickle cell anemia, and 50% normal

11. Which of the following summarizes a Mendelian genetic pattern?

    A. Two golden Labrador retrievers breed to produce puppies with either black, brown, or golden fur.
    B. Two parents with Rh-positive type blood have a child with Rh-negative blood.
    C. The *JRV32* and *NCA80* genes are close together and on the same chromosome, so they are inherited as a pair instead of independently.
    D. Individuals with an $I^A I^B$ genotype have blood type AB.

12. Natural selection:

    A. acts on genetic diversity in a population.
    B. has no effect on allele frequency.
    C. introduces genetic diversity.
    D. is caused by evolution.

13. Which of the following describes evolutionary fitness?

    A. How well an organism is physically adapted to a niche in the environment
    B. How well an organism can feed itself
    C. How successful an organism is in passing on its alleles to future generations
    D. How successful an organism is during times of drought or famine

Want More Practice?
Register your book online for more drill questions!

Answers and Explanations

1. **D** The rough ER is surrounded by a single membrane, not a double membrane (eliminate choice A). While choices (B) and (C) are true statements, they don't describe organelle *function*. Lysosomes digest foreign particles and old organelles (choice D is correct).

2. **B** Diffusion does not require ATP (eliminate choice A). The example in the question stem uses ATP to transport ions against a concentration gradient, so active transport (choice B) is correct. Osmosis is the movement of water (or solvent) across a semipermeable membrane from an area of higher concentration to an area of lower concentration (eliminate choice C). Facilitated diffusion does not require ATP for the transport of molecules (eliminate answer choice D).

3. **C** Conversion of glucose into pyruvate happens in glycolysis and this occurs in the cytoplasm (eliminate choice A). Choice (B) is also describing glycolysis, in which ADP and P_i form 4 ATP molecules in 10 steps (eliminate choice B). In the mitochondria, ATP is released by the breakdown of a three-carbon compound (pyruvate) to CO_2 (via the pyruvate dehydrogenase complex and Krebs cycle). Energy in pyruvate is transferred to GTP and the electron carriers NADH and $FADH_2$; the electron transport chain harnesses energy from NADH and $FADH_2$ to create a proton gradient, which powers ATP synthase as it builds ATP from ADP and P_i (choice C is correct). Fermentation recycles the coenzyme NADH that is formed during glycolysis back to NAD^+ (eliminate choice D).

4. **B** There are many distracting answer choices here; focus on what you know and don't be intimidated by all the biochemistry in this question. Each molecule of pyruvate, produced in glycolysis, loses a carbon atom resulting in a two-carbon compound (acetyl-CoA). This two-carbon compound is used in the beginning of the Krebs cycle (choice B is correct). Choices (A) and (D) describe steps in the citric acid cycle and neither connects glycolysis to the citric acid cycle (eliminate choices A and D). Choice (C) is one of the steps in glycolysis and does not connect glycolysis to the citric acid cycle (eliminate choice C).

5. **D** Elongation is a step in translation, while a cell is making proteins (choice D is correct). The pyruvate dehydrogenase complex (or PDC), membrane transport, and meiosis do not include a step or process called elongation (eliminate choices A, B, and C).

6. **C** The process of reading DNA and creating RNA is termed transcription (eliminate choices A and D). RNA serves as a messenger from the nucleus to the cytoplasm. In the cytoplasm, RNA is read and used to create a protein in a process called translation (eliminate choice B). The overall process is DNA → RNA → protein and this unidirectional flow represents the central dogma (fundamental law) of molecular biology (choice C is correct).

7. **B** DNA replication during S phase requires many different enzymes, but not microtubules (eliminate choice A). During anaphase, microtubules (made of the protein tubulin) pull apart sister chromatids and move them to opposite poles of the cell (answer choice B is correct). Cytokinesis begins with the formation of a cleavage furrow, which is accomplished by a ring of microfilaments encircling the cell and contracting. This process is not inhibited by microtubules (eliminate choice C). Microtubules do not function as enzymes during the G_1 phase (eliminate choice D).

8. **A** The G$_1$ phase of a cell cycle takes place before the S phase, and DNA replication takes place during the S phase. Enzymes used during DNA replication must be synthesized during the G$_1$ phase (choice A is correct).

9. **C** The meiotic mother cell is diploid, whereas daughter cells are always haploid (eliminate choice A). This means that during meiosis, the number of chromosomes in daughter cells is half that of the parent cell (eliminate choice B). Pairing of homologous chromosomes takes place during prophase I of meiosis (choice C is correct). Meiosis results in the formation of gametes. Cells produced by mitosis (not meiosis) are used in the growth and replacement of damaged cells (eliminate choice D).

10. **B** Start by assigning alleles: *S* = wild type or normal, and *s* = sickle cell anemia. This means the parental cross is *ss* × *Ss*. All offspring will insert the recessive *s* allele from the first parent. The other parent will pass on the dominant normal allele 50% of the time (leading to *Ss* offspring, who are called carriers) and the recessive disease-causing allele the other 50% of the time (leading to *ss* offspring with sickle cell anemia). Therefore, offspring of this cross will be 50% carrier and 50% having the disorder (choice B is correct).

11. **B** Mendelian inheritance patterns apply to traits with two phenotypes that are caused by one gene with two alleles, one dominant and the other recessive. There are three phenotypes in choice A (eliminate this option). Positive and negative blood type is determined by a gene called the Rh factor or antigen D, which exhibits classical dominance. If individuals express antigen D, they have positive blood (genotype *DD* or *Dd*). If they do not express antigen D, they have negative blood (genotype *dd*). If two parents are both heterozygotes (*Dd*), they will both have Rh-positive type blood but could have a child with Rh-negative blood (choice B is correct). Choice C describes two genes that are linked and would therefore display non-Mendelian inheritance (eliminate choice C). Individuals with AB blood express both I^A and I^B; this is an example of codominance, which is not Mendelian inheritance (eliminate choice D).

12. **A** Natural selection acts on the genetic diversity in a population (choice A is correct) to alter allele frequencies (eliminate choice B), causing evolution (eliminate choice D). Genetic diversity in a population is a requirement for natural selection to occur. Natural selection does not introduce genetic diversity however (eliminate choice C); it can act only on existing diversity to alter allele frequencies.

13. **C** In evolutionary terms, fitness is not how well an animal is physically adapted to a niche in the environment (eliminate choice A), or how well it can feed itself (eliminate choices B and D), but how successful it is in passing on its alleles to future generations (choice C is correct).

Quick Review

Cell Biology

- All cellular membranes are made of lipid bilayers with distinct hydrophobic and hydrophilic regions.

- Membranes act as selective barriers that regulate which molecules can cross into or out of the cell.

- Molecules naturally want to move from regions of higher concentration to regions of lower concentration (with respect to that particular molecule).

- Diffusion is the movement of particles down their concentration gradient.

- Osmosis is the movement of water down its concentration gradient.

- Hydrophobic molecules (e.g., O_2, CO_2, steroids) cross the cell membrane by simple diffusion.

- Hydrophilic, polar molecules (e.g., ions, glucose, water) must cross the membrane with the help of a membrane protein (channel or carrier); this is called facilitated diffusion.

- Active transport uses energy to move molecules against their concentration gradients (from low concentration areas to higher concentration areas).

- Primary active transport uses ATP directly, while secondary active transport relies on gradients previously established by a primary active transporter.

- The Na^+/K^+ ATPase is a primary active transporter that moves three Na^+ ions out of the cell for every two K^+ ions it moves into the cell. This helps establish the resting membrane potential of the cell, helps maintain osmotic balance in the cell, and sets up an Na^+ gradient that can be used for secondary active transport.

- Exocytosis transports material out of the cell via a vesicle fusing with the plasma membrane; endocytosis transports material into the cell via a similar mechanism.

- Tight junctions help form a seal between cells so that the flow of molecules across the entire cell layer is regulated.

- Desmosomes form general adhesions between cells.

- Gap junctions form connections between cells that allow the flow of cytoplasm from cell to cell.

- For PCAT, you should know the structures and functions of the following eukaryotic organelles:

Organelle	Function	Number of Membranes
Nucleus	Contains and protects the DNA genome, transcription, partial assembly of ribosomes	2
Mitochondria	ATP production via the Krebs cycle, electron transport chain, and oxidative phosphorylation	2
Ribosomes	Synthesize proteins via translation	0
RER	Synthesis and modification of secretory and membrane-bound proteins	1
SER	Detoxification and glycogen breakdown in liver, steroid synthesis in gonads, and calcium storage in skeletal muscle	1
Golgi apparatus	Modification and sorting of secretory and membrane-bound proteins	1
Lysosomes	Contain acid hydrolases that digest various substances	1
Peroxisomes	Metabolize lipids and toxins, producing H_2O_2	1

- Cilia and flagella are made of microtubules in a 9 + 2 arrangement. Both are associated with cellular locomotion.

- Microtubules are polymers of the protein tubulin.

- Centrosomes (made of two centrioles and proteins) anchor microtubules.

- Cytoskeleton is made of microtubules, intermediate filaments, and microfilaments.

Metabolism and Energy Transformations

- Enzymes are biological catalysts, which increase the rate of a reaction by lowering activation energy (E_a).

- Enzymes are controlled in many ways; common examples are negative feedback and competitive inhibitors.

- Adenosine triphosphate (ATP) contains two high-energy bonds and is how cells store and use energy.

- Cellular respiration is oxidation of carbohydrates, reduction of electron carriers, and generation of ATP.

- Glycolysis occurs in the cytoplasm and generates two pyruvate molecules, two ATP, and two NADH per glucose.

- Under anaerobic conditions, cells perform fermentation to regenerate NAD^+; this allows glycolysis to continue in the absence of oxygen and the electron transport chain.

- The pyruvate dehydrogenase complex (PDC) functions in the mitochondrial matrix, converts pyruvate into acetyl-CoA, and generates an NADH (or two per glucose).

- Krebs cycle in the mitochondrial matrix generates six NADH, two $FADH_2$, and two GTP per glucose.

- The electron transport chain in the inner mitochondrial membrane starts with oxidation of electron carriers, NADH and $FADH_2$, and ends with reduction of oxygen. It generates a proton gradient across the inner mitochondrial membrane.

- ATP synthase in the inner mitochondrial membrane uses the proton gradient to generate ATP (2.5ATP per NADH from the mitochondrial matrix, 1.5ATP per NADH from the cytoplasm, and 1.5ATP per $FADH_2$).

- There are several other metabolic pathways in the cell and many of them converge on the Krebs cycle: glycogenolysis, glycogenesis, gluconeogenesis, β-oxidation of fatty acids, and amino acid catabolism.

Molecular Biology

- DNA is the fundamental unit of inheritance in cells.

- DNA and RNA are polymers, made of nucleotide monomers.

- A nucleotide contains phosphate group(s), a sugar (deoxyribose in DNA and ribose in RNA), and a nitrogenous base.

- Nitrogenous bases are categorized as purines (adenine or guanine) or pyrimidines (thymine, cytosine, or uracil).

- Adenine always pairs with thymine via two hydrogen bonds; cytosine always pairs with guanine via three hydrogen bonds.

- Uracil replaces thymine in RNA, and the ribose in RNA has an OH group on carbon 2.

- Eukaryotic DNA is packaged around histone proteins.

- DNA replication:
  - occurs in the S-phase of the cell cycle
  - is semiconservative in nature
  - occurs in a replication bubble, which has two replication forks
  - starts at an origin of replication (ORI)

- Several enzymes are involved in DNA replication:

  - Helicases unwind parental DNA at the origin of replication.
  - Primases synthesize a short RNA primer.
  - DNA polymerase synthesizes new DNA, proofreads, and replaces the RNA primer.
  - DNA ligase attaches segments of DNA (e.g., Okazaki fragments in the lagging strand).

- Template strand is read 3' to 5' and the new strand is synthesized 5' to 3'.

- Each replication bubble has two leading strands and two lagging strands with Okazaki fragments.

- Central dogma of molecular biology says that DNA is read to make RNA via transcription, and RNA is read to make a peptide chain via translation.

- Transcription is the first part of protein synthesis; it is the creation of an RNA transcript by an RNA polymerase that reads the DNA template.

- Like in DNA replication, the template strand is read 3' to 5' and the new strand is synthesized 5' to 3' in transcription.

- In eukaryotes, the RNA transcript is modified before translation:

  1. Introns are removed during splicing.
  2. A 5' cap and a 3' poly-A tail are added for stability.
  3. RNA transcript is transported from the nucleus to the cytoplasm.

- Both transcription and translation occur in three steps each: initiation, elongation, termination.

- Translation is the second part of protein synthesis; it is the creation of a polypeptide chain by ribosomes that read an mRNA transcript.

- Ribosomes are 30S + 50S = 70S in prokaryotes, and 40S + 60S = 80S in eukaryotes.

- tRNA molecules are bound to amino acids and carry them to the ribosome.

	DNA Replication	Transcription	Translation
Signal to get ready	Ori	Promoter	5'UTR
Signal to start	Ori	Start site	AUG start codon
Key enzyme	DNA polymerase	RNA polymerase	Ribosome (made of rRNA and peptides)
Other enzymes	Helicase Primase Ligase	Spliceosome (eukaryotes only)	Aminoacyl tRNA synthetases
Template molecule	DNA	DNA	mRNA
Read direction	3' to 5' on the DNA template	3' to 5' on the DNA template	5' to 3' on the RNA template
Molecule synthesized	DNA	RNA	Peptides
Build direction	5' to 3'	5' to 3'	N-terminus to C-terminus
Prokaryotic location	Cytoplasm	Cytoplasm	Cytoplasm
Eukaryotic location	Nucleus	Nucleus	Cytoplasm
Signal to stop	When the replication bubbles or newly synthesized strands meet and are ligated together	Terminator	Stop codon (UAG, UGA, UAA)

Mitosis and Meiosis

- Cell cycle has four phases:

G_1	Cell growth and metabolism
S phase	DNA replication of the genome
G_2	Cell growth and metabolism, preparation for mitosis
M phase	Mitosis via prophase, metaphase, anaphase, telophase Nuclear division and then cytoplasmic division via cytokinesis

- Mitosis results in two daughter cells that are identical to each other and identical to the original parent cell.

    o Prophase: chromosomes condense, nuclear membrane and nucleolus disappear, centrosomes migrate to opposite ends of the cell, mitotic spindle starts to form (aster fibers).
    o Metaphase: chromosomes line up on metaphase plate.
    o Anaphase: chromosomes separate, and sister chromatids (each is now a chromosome) are pulled to opposite ends of the cell.
    o Telophase: opposite of prophase.

- From a single diploid precursor cell, meiosis generates four haploid cells (gametes) with a random mix of alleles; this is due to crossing over (recombination) in prophase I and separation of homologous chromosomes in anaphase I.

  - Crossing over happens in prophase I.
  - Homologous chromosomes pair up on either side of the metaphase plate in metaphase I.
  - Homologous chromosomes move to opposite ends of the cell in anaphase I.
  - Meiosis II is similar to mitosis.

	Mitosis	Meiosis
Purpose	Cell replication	Reproduction
Products	Somatic cells	Gametes (eggs and sperm)
# cell divisions	1	2
G_1	$2n, 1x$	$2n, 1x$
S	$2n, 1x \rightarrow 2n, 2x$	$2n, 1x \rightarrow 2n, 2x$
G_2	$2n, 2x$	$2n, 2x$
Anaphase I	$2n, 2x \rightarrow 4n, 1x$ Sister chromatids are pulled apart Number of chromosomes doubles	$2n, 2x \rightarrow 2n, 2x$ Homologous chromosomes are moved to opposite sides of cell
Telophase I (after cytokinesis)	$2n, 1x$	$1n, 2x$
Anaphase II	n/a	$1n, 2x \rightarrow 2n, 1x$ Sister chromatids are pulled apart Number of chromosomes doubles
Telophase II (after cytokinesis)	n/a	$1n, 1x$
# daughter cells	2	4
DNA in parents vs. daughter	Same	Daughter cells have half the DNA
Daughter ploidy	Diploid	Haploid

Legend:

$1n$ = haploid (e.g., 23 chromosomes in a human cell)

$2n$ = diploid (e.g., 46 chromosomes in a human cell)

$4n$ = tetraploid (e.g., 92 chromosomes in a human cell)

$1x$ = single copy chromosomes with one sister chromatid/chromosome (e.g., before DNA replication)

$2x$ = double copy (replicated) chromosomes with two sister chromatids/chromosome (e.g., after DNA replication)

- Gametogenesis is the generation of gametes via meiosis.

- Spermatogenesis is the formation of four sperm cells from a spermatogonia.

- Oogenesis is the formation of one ovum and two polar bodies from an oogonia.

Genetics

- A gene is a segment of DNA that codes for a gene product (e.g., protein, rRNA, tRNA).

- Different forms of genes are called alleles.

- Each person has one or two alleles for each gene, but a population can have hundreds of different alleles of a gene.

- Organisms express phenotypes (physical characteristics) according to their genotypes (combinations of alleles).

- Genetic generations are P, F_1, F_2, etc.

- Mendel's principals of genetics include the Law of Dominance, Law of Segregation, and Law of Independent Assortment.

- Classical (Mendelian) inheritance occurs when a phenotype or trait is determined by one gene with two alleles; one allele is dominant (expressed) and the other is recessive (silent).

- Common monohybrid crosses:

Cross	Phenotype Ratio	Genotype Ratio
$AA \times aa$	100% Aa	100% A
$Aa \times AA$	50% AA 50% Aa	100% A
$Aa \times aa$	50% Aa 50% aa	50% A 50% a
$Aa \times Aa$	25% AA (1) 50% Aa (2) 25% aa (1)	75% A (3) 25% a (1)

- Common dihybrid crosses:

  - $AaBb \times aabb$ (a testcross) gives a genotypic and phenotype ratio of 1 $AaBb$: 1 $Aabb$: 1 $aaBb$: 1 $aabb$.
  - $AaBb \times AaBb$ gives a phenotypic ratio of 9 A–B– : 3 A–bb : 3 aaB– : 1 $aabb$.

- Rules of probability can be used to determine genotypes and phenotypes of offspring from given crosses, or the probability of having offspring with certain traits:

  ○ Rule of multiplication: probability of A **and** B occurring is P(A) × P(B).
  ○ Rule of addition: probability of A **or** B occurring is P(A) + P(B) − P(A and B together).

- There are several exceptions to classical dominance, including linkage, incomplete dominance, and codominance.

- Linkage occurs when two genes are close together (< 50 map units apart) on the same chromosome; it leads to alleles being inherited together (less recombination) instead of independently.

- Incomplete dominance occurs when two different alleles for a single trait result in a blended phenotype.

- Codominance occurs when two different alleles for a single trait are expressed simultaneously, but independently (no blending).

- Genetic diversity comes from recombination and mutation.

- Point mutations are classified according to their effect on the DNA (transition/transversion) or their effect on the amino acid sequence (missense, nonsense, or silent).

- There are five kinds of gene rearrangement mutations: insertion, deletion, inversion, amplification or duplication, and translocation.

- Indels can cause frameshift mutations; because they change the reading frame of a gene, these affect every amino acid from the point of the mutation on and are generally serious.

- Pedigrees can be used to analyze the patterns of inheritance of different traits. There are six primary modes of inheritance: autosomal recessive, autosomal dominant, mitochondrial, Y-linked, X-linked recessive, and X-linked dominant.

Evolution

- Hardy-Weinberg Law can be used to study population genetics.

  - It assumes classical dominance with only two alleles and unchanging allele frequencies.
  - It is based on five assumptions: no mutation, no natural selection, no migration, large populations, and totally random mating.

- Earth is more than 4 billion years old and the early atmosphere was a reducing environment.

- Life on Earth started more than 3 billion years ago and the origin of life likely followed this pattern: amino acids → proteinoid → microsphere → liposome → coacervate → protobiont → cell.

- Natural selection drives evolution by allowing individuals with random, beneficial mutations to survive and pass those beneficial mutations on to their offspring.

- Natural selection can occur in many different ways, such as directional selection, divergent selection, stabilizing selection, artificial selection, and sexual selection.

- The creation of new species is known as speciation.

- Homologous structures are the result of divergent evolution to form new species.

- Analogous structures are the result of convergent evolution, in which different species must meet similar environmental challenges.

- Taxonomy, the science of biological classification, determines the evolutionary relationship of organisms to one another.

- There are eight principal taxonomic categories: domain, kingdom, phylum, class, order, family, genus, and species.

Chapter 7

Microbiology and Immunology

7.1 MICROBIOLOGY IN CONTEXT

Introduction to Pharmaceuticals and Disease

Pharmacists dispense prescription drugs, which are also called medications, medicines, or pharmaceuticals. There are many different classifications of medications and innumerable reasons for requiring them. Pharmaceuticals can be classified by their chemical properties, route of administration, mechanism of action, the biological system they affect, or their therapeutic effect.

One classification system has to do with the source of the therapeutic:

- **Small-molecule drugs** are derived from chemical synthesis.
- **Biopharmaceuticals** (also called biologics) are made in or extracted from a biological source.

Let's look at a few examples. Acetaminophen ($C_8H_9NO_2$) is a medication used to treat pain and fever. Ibuprofen ($C_{13}H_{18}O_2$) is a nonsteroidal anti-inflammatory drug (NSAID) that is used to treat pain, fever, and inflammation. Both of these drugs are small-molecule drugs and taken orally.

Biopharmaceuticals include recombinant proteins, vaccines, gene therapy, monoclonal antibodies, and cell therapy. For example, people with Fabry disease have a mutation that causes low levels of the enzyme α-galactosidase A in their lysosomes. This disorder can be treated by administering a biologic version of the missing enzyme. This enzyme can be synthesized by cells or tissues grown in a lab and then extracted for use. Another example is insulin, a protein hormone used to treat diabetes. There are many ways to make medicinal insulin, such as using genetically altered *E. coli* to synthesize it in a lab.

Drugs are typically used to treat or manage the symptoms of a disease. A **disease** is an abnormal condition that negatively affects the structure or function of an organism. Diseases are associated with signs and symptoms and may be caused by either an external factor, such as a **pathogen**, or by an internal dysfunction. In this chapter we will explore microbiology and the world of pathogens. Your physiological systems and some examples of how they can malfunction will be reviewed in the next chapter.

Public health is a large field of science that aims to improve the health of populations. **Epidemiology** is more focused; it is the study and analysis of the distribution, patterns, and determinants of health and disease in certain populations. Public health and epidemiology shape policy and healthcare.

Infectious Diseases

Infectious diseases are caused by **pathogenic microorganisms** (or microbes), such as bacteria, viruses, parasites, or fungi. These diseases can spread to individuals from the environment or from one person to another. **Transmission,** or spread of the disease, can happen via direct or indirect contact:

- Direct contact results when a disease is spread by physical contact.
- Indirect contact results when a disease is spread by droplets, an intermediate living organism, food, water, or soil.

Sterilization and disinfection are used to limit the spread of infectious disease by nonliving objects. **Sterilization** kills all microbes present, while **disinfection** kills many but not all microbes present. Both of these processes use chemicals, heat, or radiation.

Once a disease has been transmitted, there are additional ways to limit its spread and treat the individuals affected. **Immunization,** a crucial aspect of protecting global populations against infectious disease, will be discussed later in this chapter. **Antimicrobial agents** are natural or synthetic substances that kill or inhibit the growth of microorganisms. Many target one species of pathogen, but **broad-spectrum antimicrobials** target many species of similar microbes. There are four major classes of antimicrobial agents, and we will see some examples of each throughout this chapter:

- **Antibacterial drugs** or **antibiotics** are used to treat bacterial infections. They kill or inhibit the growth of a bacterium.
- **Antifungal drugs** are used to treat fungal infections. They kill or inhibit the growth of a fungus.
- **Antiviral drugs** are used to treat viral infections.
- **Antiparasitic drugs** are used to treat parasitic infections. They destroy the parasite, inhibit its growth, or expel it from the host.

The suffix *-icide* is used if an antimicrobial agent kills the pathogen (e.g., bactericide, fungicide, virucide, parasiticide). The suffix *-static* is used if the antimicrobial agent inhibits the growth of the pathogen (e.g., bacteriostatic, virustatic, fungistatic, parasitistatic).

Antimicrobial resistance occurs when microbes evolve over time to develop resistance to a drug used to target them. It is important to note that microbes, not humans, become antimicrobial resistant. Resistance makes infections harder to treat because the patient being treated with a drug will no longer respond to that medicine. Resistance is thus a major public health concern. Global increases in antimicrobial resistance are due to overuse and misuse of antimicrobial drugs.

7.2 BACTERIA

Prokaryotes vs Eukaryotes

All living organisms (which does not include viruses) can be classified as either **prokaryotes** or **eukaryotes**. The classification of organisms into these groups is based on examination of their internal cellular structure. Representatives from both groups are able to carry out the basic biochemical processes of photosynthesis, the Krebs cycle, and oxidative phosphorylation to produce ATP. The primary feature of prokaryotes that distinguishes them from eukaryotes is that prokaryotes do not contain **membrane-bound organelles** (nucleus, mitochondria, lysosomes, etc.). *Prokaryote* means "before the nucleus," and the lack of a nucleus indicates that prokaryotes are evolutionarily the oldest kingdom. Unlike viruses, however, prokaryotes possess all of the machinery required for life. They are true cells and living organisms. Prokaryotes include **bacteria** and **archaea** (extremophiles).

Bacterial Structure

In this section we will review bacterial cell structure. Unlike a eukaryotic cell, there are no membrane-bound organelles in prokaryotic cells. Ribosomes are not membrane-bound organelles and are found in bacteria. The prokaryotic genome is a single double-stranded circular DNA chromosome. It is not located in a nucleus and is not associated with histone proteins, as the eukaryotic genome is. In bacteria, transcription and translation occur in the same place, at the same time. Ribosomes begin to translate mRNA before it is completely transcribed.

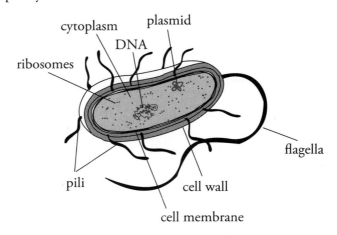

Figure 1   A Prokaryote

Remember that the bacterial ribosome is structurally different from the eukaryotic ribosome, though both function the same way. These differences allow us to prescribe various antibiotics that interfere with bacterial translation without disrupting our own. For example streptomycin and tetracycline are antibiotics that bind only to bacterial ribosomes.

One last genetic element that can be found in prokaryotic cells is the **plasmid**. This is a circular piece of double-stranded DNA that is much smaller than the genome. Plasmids are referred to as extrachromosomal genetic elements. They often encode gene products that may confer an advantage upon a bacterium carrying the plasmid. For example, plasmids frequently carry antibiotic-resistance genes; these are genes that encode proteins which can break down antibiotics. When these antibiotic-resistant bacteria infect humans, they are harder to kill than non-resistant bacteria. This means they cause infections that are harder to treat.

Cell Membrane and Cell Wall

The bacterial cytoplasm is bounded by a lipid bilayer that is similar to our own plasma membrane. Outside the lipid bilayer is a rigid cell wall. It provides support for the cell, preventing lysis due to osmotic pressure. The bacterial cell wall is composed of **peptidoglycan**, a complex polymer unique to prokaryotes. The bacterial cell wall is the target of many antibiotics, such as penicillin. The enzyme **lysozyme,** which is found in tears and saliva and made by lytic viruses, destroys peptidoglycan in the bacterial cell wall, resulting in an osmotically fragile structure called a **protoplast**.

Capsule

Another attribute which only some bacteria have is the **capsule** or **glycocalyx**. This is a sticky layer of polysaccharide "goo" surrounding the bacterial cell and often surrounding an entire colony of bacteria. It makes bacteria more difficult for immune system cells to eradicate. It also enables bacteria to adhere to smooth surfaces such as rocks in a stream or the lining of the human respiratory tract.

Flagella

Another item only some bacteria have are long, whip-like filaments known as **flagella**, which are involved in bacterial motility. A bacterium that possesses one or more flagella is said to be **motile**, because flagella are the only means of bacterial locomotion.

The structure of a flagellum is fairly complicated and includes a **filament** or rod, the **hook**, and the **basal structure** (Figure 2). The basal structure anchors the flagellum to the inner and outer membranes (for a Gram-negative bacterium; more to come on this later) and rotates the rod in either a clockwise or counter-clockwise manner. Rotation of the rod requires a large amount of energy or ATP. It is important to remember that the prokaryotic flagellum structure is different from that of the eukaryotic flagellum (which contains a "9 + 2" arrangement of microtubules).

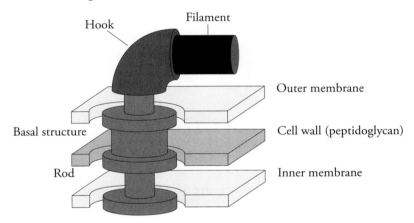

Figure 2   The Prokaryotic Flagellum

Bacterial Classification

Bacterial Shape

How we target bacteria when treating diseases caused by pathogenic bacteria depends on their characteristics and classification. Bacteria are often classified according to their shape. The three shapes and their proper names are organized in the following table:

Shape	Proper name (plural)	Proper name (singular)
round	cocci	coccus
rod-shaped	bacilli	bacillus
spiral-shaped	spirochetes or spirilla	spirochete, spirillum

Table 1   Bacterial Classification by Shape

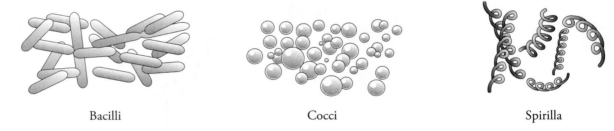

Bacilli   Cocci   Spirilla

Figure 3

Gram Staining of the Cell Wall

This method of classification is derived from the extent to which bacteria turn color in a procedure termed **Gram staining**. The two groupings are **Gram-positive** bacteria, which stain strongly (a dark purple color), and **Gram-negative** bacteria, which stain weakly (a light pink color).

Gram-positive bacteria have a thick peptidoglycan layer outside of the cell membrane and no other layer beyond this. Gram-negative bacteria have a thinner layer of peptidoglycan in the cell wall but have an additional outer layer containing lipopolysaccharide. The intermediate space in Gram-negative bacteria between the cell membrane and the outer layer is termed the **periplasmic space**, in which are sometimes found enzymes that degrade antibiotics (see Figure 4). The increased protection of Gram-negative bacteria from the environment is reflected in their weak staining, as well as in their increased resistance to antibiotics.

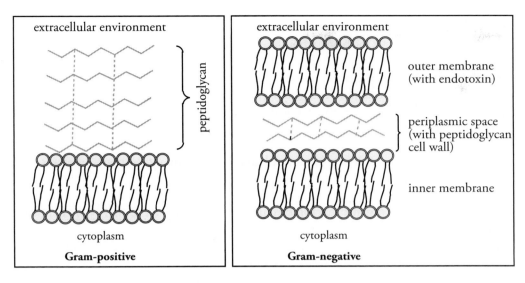

Figure 4   Gram-Positive Versus Gram-Negative Bacteria

Now that we have reviewed Gram staining, it is a good time to compare endotoxins and exotoxins. **Endotoxins** are normal components of the outer membrane of Gram-negative bacteria that aren't inherently poisonous. However, they cause our immune system to have such an extreme reaction that we may die as a result. Endotoxins cause the most trouble when many bacteria die and their disintegrated outer membranes are released into the circulation. When this occurs, cells of the immune system release so many chemicals that the patient goes into what is called septic shock. In such a condition, much of the aqueous portion of the blood is leaked into the tissues, causing a drop in blood pressure and other problems that may be fatal. Endotoxins can have various chemical structures including lipopolysaccharide, which contains sugars bound to lipids.

Exotoxins are very toxic substances secreted by both Gram-negative and Gram-positive bacteria into the surrounding environment. Exotoxins help the bacterium compete with other bacterial species, such as normal inhabitants of the mammalian gut. Some diseases that are caused by exotoxins are botulism, diptheria, tetanus, and toxic shock syndrome.

Temperature

Another characteristic of bacteria used to categorize them is their ability to tolerate environmental variables, such as temperature. Though bacteria as a group can grow at a wide range of temperatures, each species has an optimal growth temperature. If the temperature is too high or too low, bacteria fail to grow and may be killed, hence the use of boiling to kill bacteria and refrigeration to slow bacterial growth and prevent food spoilage. Most bacteria favor mild temperatures similar to the ones that humans and other organisms favor (30°C); they are called **mesophiles** (moderate temperature lovers). **Thermophiles** (heat lovers) can survive at temperatures up to 100°C in boiling hot springs or near geothermal vents in the ocean floor. Bacteria that thrive at very low temperatures (near 0°C) are termed **psychrophiles** (cold lovers).

Nutrition

Bacteria can be classified according to their carbon source and their energy source:

- **Autotrophs** use CO_2 as their carbon source.
- **Heterotrophs** rely on organic nutrients (such as glucose) created by other organisms.
- **Chemotrophs** get their energy from chemicals.
- **Phototrophs** get their energy from light.

Each bacterium is either a chemotroph or a phototroph and is either an autotroph or a heterotroph. Thus, there are four types of bacteria:

1. **Chemoautotrophs** build organic macromolecules from CO_2 using the energy of chemicals. They obtain energy by oxidizing inorganic molecules like H_2S.
2. **Chemoheterotrophs** require organic molecules such as glucose made by other organisms as their carbon source and for energy. We are chemoheterotrophs.
3. **Photoautotrophs** use only CO_2 as a carbon source and obtain their energy from the Sun. Plants are photoautotrophs.
4. **Photoheterotrophs** are odd in that they get their energy from the Sun, like plants, but require an organic molecule made by another organism as their carbon source.

Oxygen Use and Tolerance

Remember that oxygen metabolism is aerobic metabolism. Bacteria which require oxygen are called **obligate aerobes**. Bacteria which do not require oxygen are called **anaerobes**. There are three subcategories: **facultative anaerobes** use oxygen when it's around, but don't need it. **Tolerant anaerobes** can grow in the presence or absence of oxygen but do not use it in their metabolism. **Obligate anaerobes** are poisoned by oxygen. This is because they lack certain enzymes necessary for the detoxification of free radicals that form spontaneously whenever oxygen is around. Obligate anaerobes commonly infect wounds.

Bacterial Life Cycle

Bacteria reproduce asexually. In asexual reproduction, there is no meiosis, no meiotic generation of haploid gametes, and no fusion of gametes to form a new individual organism. Instead, each bacterium grows in size until it has synthesized enough cellular components for two cells rather than one, replicates its genome, and then divides in two. This process in bacteria is also known as **binary fission** (fission means "to split").

Genetic Exchange Between Bacteria

Bacteria reproduce asexually, but genetic exchange is evolutionarily favorable because it fosters genetic diversity. Bacteria have three mechanisms of acquiring new genetic material: transduction, transformation, and conjugation. Note that none of these has anything to do with reproduction! **Transduction** will be reviewed in the virus section of this chapter because it is the transfer of genomic DNA from one bacterium to another by a lysogenic phage. **Transformation** occurs when a bacterial cell obtains DNA from the environment. This DNA can be a plasmid or a segment of a chromosome. **Conjugation** is most important for you to understand, so we will review it in more detail.

Conjugation

In conjugation, bacteria make physical contact and form a bridge between the cells. One cell copies its DNA, and this copy is transferred to the other cell. The key to bacterial conjugation is an extrachromosomal element known as the **F (fertility) factor.** The F factor contains several genes, many of which are involved in conjugation itself. Bacteria that have the F factor in a plasmid are male, or F^+, and will transfer the F factor to female cells. Bacteria that do not contain the F factor are female, F^-, and will receive the F factor from male cells to become male.

Conjugation starts when the male cell produces a sex pilus and contacts a female cell. This forms a conjugation bridge. DNA transfer between the two bacteria cells is unidirectional; it occurs in one direction only, from male to female cell (see Figure 5).

The F factor can sometimes become integrated into the bacterial chromosomes through recombination. A cell with the F factor integrated into its genome is called an **Hfr (high frequency of recombination) cell**. When an Hfr cell performs conjugation, it copies its chromosomal DNA and passes some to all of it over to a female cell. The amount of DNA that is transferred depends on how long the two cells stay connected. In order for the recipient cell to keep the new genetic information, it must recombine the DNA into the genome or retain it in a plasmid. It is worth noting that both male and Hfr cells can only mate with female bacterial cells.

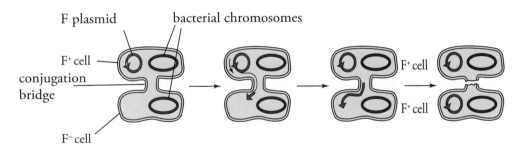

Figure 5   Conjugation and transfer of an F plasmid from an F^+ donor to an F^- recipient

Antibiotics

Antibacterial drugs target something in the bacterial cell that is different from the host cell. Because bacteria are prokaryotic and we are eukaryotic, there are many options; antibiotics can target cell wall synthesis, protein synthesis, or metabolic pathways not present in eukaryotes. For example, penicillin kills bacteria by inhibiting peptidoglycan synthesis. This blocks remodeling of the bacterial cell wall and causes cell lysis and death.

Microbial Ecology

The Earth is inhabited by millions of different species, populations, and communities. We reviewed the definition of a species in the previous chapter. A **population** is a group of individuals of a single species that live in the same general area and are thus subject to the same environmental factors and resources. Many different populations existing together make up a **community.** Within each community, different organisms have different roles:

- **Producers** (or autotrophs) are photosynthetic organisms that can produce their own food and provide a source of food for other organisms.
- **Consumers** (or heterotrophs) are organisms that rely on the food made by the producers. They eat either producers or other consumers.

Nutrient Cycles

Because raw materials on Earth are limited resources, it makes sense to recycle them. Inorganic molecules are taken up by various organisms and converted into biologically useful forms; after these organic versions of the molecules cycle through the community, they are returned to their inorganic forms by decomposers. For the PCAT, you should be familiar with how bacteria contribute to the carbon cycle and the nitrogen cycle.

Carbon Cycle

The **carbon cycle** is a repeating cycle of processes that shuttle carbon atoms around the Earth, through living and nonliving things. Carbon atoms cycle between:

- Biomass: carbon is present in organic molecules of all living things and in dead organic matter that is undergoing decomposition.
- Atmosphere: carbon is present as carbon dioxide (CO_2) and methane (CH_4) gas.
- Ocean: carbon is found dissolved in ocean water as bicarbonate (HCO_3^-).
- Inside the Earth: carbon is present deep in the Earth as sediment of marine organisms from millions of years ago. This contributes to fossil fuels.

Bacteria move carbon atoms through the carbon cycle by performing photosynthesis, cell respiration, fermentation, and decomposition.

Photosynthesis

Organisms that perform **photosynthesis** are called autotrophs; some examples are plants, cyanobacteria, and some protists. These organisms use chlorophyll to absorb solar energy and also use water and CO_2. The goal is to produce sugar, which is used as an energy source for the cell or organism. Oxygen is released as a by-product.

Nitrogen Cycle

The **nitrogen cycle** is a repeating cycle of processes that shuttle nitrogen atoms around the Earth, through living and nonliving things. Nitrogen is present in the atmosphere as N_2, but most organisms on Earth can't use nitrogen in this form. This is one of the reasons bacteria are important in microbial ecology. **Nitrogen fixation** is a process by which bacteria convert N_2 into ammonia (NH_3), and then ammonium (NH_4^+) or nitrate (NO_3^-), which can be used by plants. Nitrogen enters animals when they eat plants. Nitrogen returns to the soil through waste products (such as urine) or when organisms die, and their decaying matter is broken down by decomposers. Nitrogen can also be recycled back into the atmosphere by denitrifying bacteria that convert nitrate back into N_2.

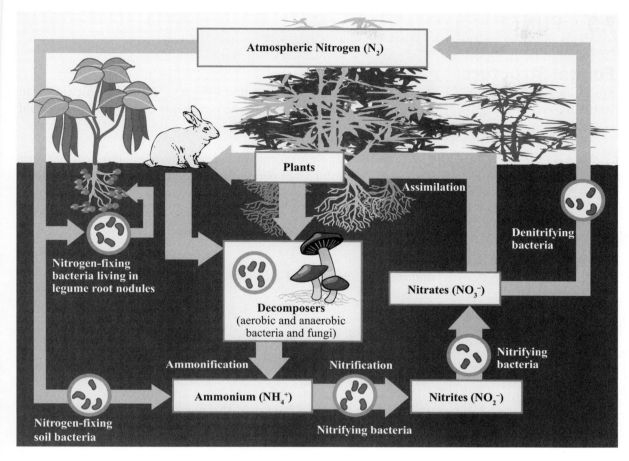

Figure 6 Nitrogen Cycle

Symbiotic Relations

Living organisms interact with each other in their community. **Symbiosis** is a close biological relationship between two species, in which at least one species benefits from the interaction. There are three types:

- In **commensalism,** is when one member of the pair is helped by the association and the other member is unaffected. For example, many species of bacteria and fungi live on your skin as part of its natural flora. The bacterium *Staphylococcus epidermidis* does not affect you but uses the dead cells of your skin as nutrients.
- In a **mutualistic** relationship, both partners benefit from the association. For example, bacteria in your digestive tract out-compete harmful bacteria and in return, they get a steady supply of food.
- **Parasitic** relationships are those in which one partner benefits and the other is harmed. For example, an intestinal tapeworm harms its human host. The tapeworm receives nutrients at the expense of the host, who develops nutritional deficiencies.

7.3 FUNGI

Fungal Structure

Most fungi are nonmotile, multicellular eukaryotes; one exception is yeast, which is unicellular. In addition to all the typical eukaryotic organelles we discussed in the last chapter, fungi also have a rigid cell wall made of **chitin.**

Fungi are heterotrophs; they must consume other organisms for energy. Most fungi are either **saprophytes,** meaning they feed off dead plants and animals, or parasites that feed off living organisms, doing harm to the host.

Fungal Reproduction

Fungi are haploid and can reproduce both sexually and asexually. Asexual reproduction of fungi can occur one of four ways:

- In **budding,** a new smaller organism or single cell grows outward from an existing one. It detaches and grows into a new fungus.
- In **fragmentation,** the fungus breaks into small pieces and each one develops into a new fungus.
- **Asexual spores** are formed via mitosis, germinate, and grow into a new fungus.
- During **fission,** a parent cells grows and then splits in two. This process is similar to the way in which bacterial cells divide.

Fungi can also reproduce sexually. First, haploid gametes are made via mitosis. Fusion of haploid fungal gametes produces a diploid zygote, as in humans. In fungi, however, the diploid zygote quickly enters meiosis to produce haploid cells once again. These haploid cells repeatedly divide by mitosis to produce a new haploid adult.

Antifungal Drugs

Because both humans and fungi are eukaryotic, antifungal drugs can be hard to design; human cells and pathogenic fungi use many of the same cell components and processes. Some antifungal drugs target the fungal cell wall. Others target fungal-specific components of the plasma membrane or cell cycle machinery.

For example, fluconazole ($C_{13}H_{12}F_2N_6O$) is an antifungal medication used to treat a number of fungal infections. It inhibits an enzyme that converts lanosterol to ergosterol, an essential component of the fungal plasma membrane. Fluconazole is primarily fungistatic but has been shown to be fungicidal against certain organisms.

7.4   VIRUSES

Viruses infect all life forms on Earth, including plants, animals, protists, and bacteria. Viruses are **obligate intracellular parasites**. This means that they are only able (*obligated*) to reproduce within (*intra*) cells. While within cells, viruses have some of the attributes of living organisms, such as the ability to reproduce; but outside cells, viruses are without activity. Viruses on their own are unable to perform any of the chemical reactions characteristic of life, such as synthesis of ATP and macromolecules. Therefore, viruses are not cells or even living organisms. To reproduce, they commandeer the cellular machinery of the host they infect and use it to manufacture copies of themselves. In the final analysis, a virus is nothing more than a package of nucleic acid that says, "Pick me up and reproduce me."

Viral Structure and Function

The structure of viruses reflects their reproductive cycle. In general, all viruses have a nucleic acid genome packaged in a protein shell. The exterior protein packaging helps convey the genome from one cell to infect other cells. Once in a cell, the viral genome directs production of new copies of the genome and of the protein packaging needed to produce more virus. However, the nature of the genome, the protein packaging, and the viral reproductive cycle vary tremendously between different viruses.

A viral genome may consist of either DNA *or* RNA that is either single- *or* double-stranded and is either linear *or* circular. Viruses use virtually every conceivable form of nucleic acid as their genome. However, a given type of virus can have only one type of nucleic acid as its genome, and a mature virus does not contain nucleic acid other than its genome.

Surrounding the viral nucleic acid genome is a protein coat called the **capsid**. The capsid provides the external morphology of the virus, protects the viral genome, allows the virus to attach to the host, and gets the viral genome into the host cell.

The T4 bacteriophage virus is commonly used in research; its host is the bacterium *E. coli*. This virus has a relatively complicated structure and a DNA genome.

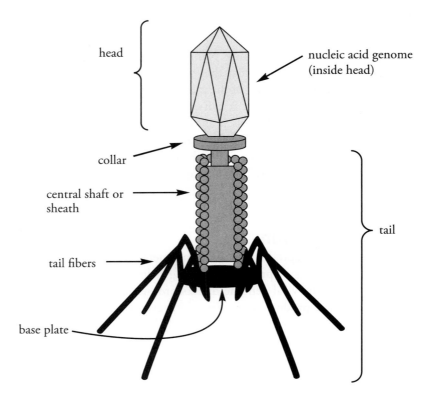

Figure 7   Bacteriophage T4

Many animal viruses also possess an **envelope** that surrounds the capsid. This is a membrane on the exterior of the virus derived from the membrane of the host cell. It contains phospholipids, proteins, and carbohydrates from the host membrane, in addition to proteins encoded by the viral genome. Enveloped viruses acquire this covering by budding through the host cell membrane. To infect a new host, some enveloped viruses fuse their envelope with the host's plasma membrane, which leaves the de-enveloped capsid inside the host cell.

The surface of a virus determines what host cells it can infect. Viral infection is not a random process, but highly specific. A virus binds to a specific receptor on the cell surface as the first step in infection. After binding, the virus will be internalized, either by fusion with the plasma membrane or by receptor-mediated endocytosis. Only cells with a receptor that matches the virus will become infected, explaining why only specific species or specific cell types are susceptible to infection. The viral surface is also important for recognition by our immune system.

Viral Reproduction

Most viruses reproduce via either the lytic cycle or the lysogenic cycle. Either way, the first step is binding to the exterior of a host cell. This is called **attachment** or **adsorption.** Next, the viral genome is injected into the host cell in a process termed **penetration** or **eclipse.** From here, a virus enters either the lytic cycle or the lysogenic cycle.

Lytic Cycle

As soon as the viral genome has entered the host cell, host polymerases and/or ribosomes begin to rapidly transcribe and translate it. The virus uses host cell machinery and resources to create many copies of viral proteins and viral genomes. Often, the virus uses a specific enzyme to degrade the host cell genome, thus creating a large pool of nucleotides that can be used to build viral genomes. The viral capsid assembles around the viral genome, and viruses finally burst out of the host cell. Here is a common example, showing a phage attacking a bacterial host:

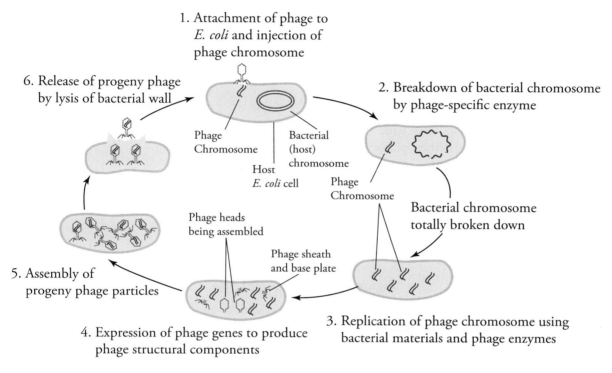

Figure 8 The Lytic Cycle

Lysogenic Cycle

The lytic cycle is an efficient way for a virus to rapidly increase its numbers. It presents a problem though: all host cells are destroyed. This is an evolutionary disadvantage. Some viruses are cleverer: they enter the **lysogenic cycle**. Upon infection, the viral genome is incorporated into the host genome. The virus is now referred to as a **prophage** if the host is a prokaryote or a **provirus** if the host is a eukaryote. Once hidden in the host genome, the prophage/provirus is silent; its genes are not expressed, and viral progeny are not produced. The cleverness of the lysogenic cycle lies in the fact that every time the host cell reproduces itself, the prophage is reproduced too. Eventually, the prophage becomes activated. It now removes itself from the host genome (in a process called **excision**) and enters the lytic cycle.

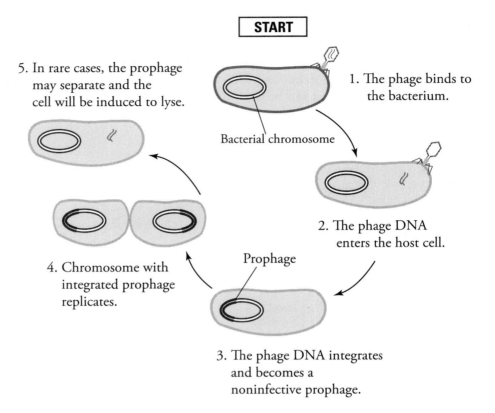

START

5. In rare cases, the prophage may separate and the cell will be induced to lyse.

1. The phage binds to the bacterium.

Bacterial chromosome

2. The phage DNA enters the host cell.

4. Chromosome with integrated prophage replicates.

Prophage

3. The phage DNA integrates and becomes a noninfective prophage.

Figure 9   The Lysogenic Cycle

One potential consequence of the lysogenic cycle is that when the viral genome activates, excising itself from the host genome, it may accidentally take part of the host genome along with it. In subsequent infections, the virus will integrate the "stolen" host DNA along with its own genome into the new host's genome. This process is called transduction and is one way for genetic exchange to happen between host cells (such as bacteria), using the virus as a shuttle for DNA.

Antiviral Drugs

Most antiviral agents aim to block the virus from getting into the host cell, inhibit viral synthesis once in the host, block viral assembly, or inhibit viral release from the host cell. Like the other antimicrobial agents, antiviral drugs aim to target the virus but not harm the host. Designing safe and effective antiviral agents is challenging because viruses use a host cell to replicate.

In addition, viruses evolve quickly and this can make them resistant to currently available treatments. They replicate quickly so they evolve on a shorter timescale than their hosts. In addition, viruses with an RNA genome have a high mutation rate, which leads to increased variation.

Oseltamivir ($C_{16}H_{28}N_2O_4$) is an example of an antiviral medication used to treat and prevent influenza A and influenza B. Oseltamivir competitively inhibits neuraminidase, an enzyme found on the surface of the influenza virus. Neuraminidase helps virus particles exit the host cell, so oseltamivir prevents new viruses from being released.

7.5   PARASITES

As we saw earlier in this chapter, a parasite is an organism that lives on or in a host organism. There are three main classes of parasites that can cause disease in humans: protozoa, helminths, and ectoparasites.

Protozoa

Protozoa are microscopic, one-celled organisms. They are sometimes called animal-like **protists** because they are heterotrophs and most are capable of moving. Protozoa can live in human intestines, blood, or other tissues; they can also multiply in humans, which means that a serious infection can start with just one parasitic cell. Protozoa that infect humans are classified according to their method of motility. Some examples are **flagellates** that move using flagella, **ciliates** that move via cilia, **amoebas** that move via pseudopodia, and *Plasmodium* whose adult stage is not motile.

Helminths

Helminths are large, multicellular parasitic worms. Like protozoa, helminths can live in human intestines, blood, or other tissues. Some examples are **roundworms** (or **nematodes**) and **flatworms** (also called **platyhelminths**), such as **trematodes (flukes)** and **cestodes (tapeworms)**.

Ectoparasites

An **ectoparasite** is a parasite that lives on the outside of its host. They can attach or burrow into the skin and remain there for weeks to months. Some examples are ticks, fleas, lice, and mites. While these organisms can cause diseases on their own, they are also important as **vectors,** or transmitters, of different pathogens. For example, Lyme disease is a common vector-borne illness and is caused by the bacterium *Borrelia burgdorferi,* which is transmitted by the deer tick.

Parasitic Infections

Parasitic infections cause a tremendous burden of disease, especially in the tropics and subtropics. They are typically spread through contaminated water, food, waste, soil, or blood. For example, transmission of *Entamoeba histolytica,* which causes amebic dysentery, typically occurs through a fecal-oral route, such as ingesting contaminated food or water.

Protozoa that live in human blood or tissue are often transmitted to other humans by an insect vector. For example, the malaria-causing parasite *Plasmodium,* is transmitted through *Anopheles* mosquitoes. If a female mosquito feeds on a human with malaria, the *Plasmodium* parasite can be transmitted to the next person bitten by that mosquito.

Antiparasitic Drugs

Because pathogenic parasites are very diverse, there are many different types of antiparasitic drugs. Each has a unique mechanism of action that targets a particular parasite or class of parasites. Like all the other antimicrobial treatments, antiparasitic drugs target an aspect of the pathogen that is distinct from the host cells.

For example, giardiasis is a parasitic disease caused by *Giardia duodenalis,* a flagellated protozoa. Giardia is one of the most common parasitic human diseases globally. Metronidazole ($C_6H_9N_3O_3$) is an antibiotic and antiprotozoal medication used to treat giardiasis. Metronidazole is reduced in anaerobic bacteria and protozoans, where it then forms radicals that inhibit nucleic acid synthesis of the pathogen.

7.6 IMMUNOLOGY

The Immune System

The interior of the body provides a warm, protective, nourishing environment where microorganisms can flourish. We could not survive without a versatile and efficient immune system to destroy invaders without destroying the body itself. There are three types of immunity, which we will review in this chapter: innate, humoral, and cell-mediated. All three branches aim to attack and eliminate pathogens. The humoral and cell-mediated branches together make up our **adaptive** or **acquired immune system**.

In addition, we will be discussing many different types of immune cells in this chapter. These **leukocytes** or **white blood cells (WBCs)** are all derived from hematopoietic stem cells (HSCs), which reside in your bone marrow. Here is a summary of important immune cells:

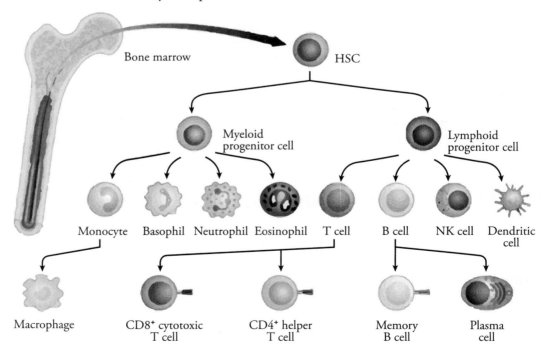

Figure 10   Types of Leukocytes

All WBCs are large, complex cells with all the normal eukaryotic cell structures (nucleus, mitochondria, etc.). Some white blood cells (such as macrophages and neutrophils) move by amoeboid motility (crawling). This is important because they are able to squeeze out of capillary intercellular junctions (spaces between capillary endothelial cells) and can therefore roam free in the tissues, hunting for foreign particles and pathogens. Some WBCs exhibit **chemotaxis,** which means movement directed by chemical stimuli. The chemical stimuli can be toxins or waste products released by pathogens, or can be chemical signals released from other white blood cells.

Basophils, neutrophils, and eosinophils are types of **granulocytes.** These white blood cells are important in the innate immune system and are characterized by the presence of specific granules in their cytoplasm. These cells are attracted to injury sites via chemotaxis, and phagocytize antigens to neutralize them. **Phagocytosis** is a type of endocytosis, in which a cell uses its plasma membrane to engulf a large particle. Once inside the cell, the engulfed material is neutralized, killed, or degraded.

Innate Immunity

Innate immunity refers to the general, nonspecific protection the body provides against various invaders. The principal components of innate immunity include the following:

1. The skin is an excellent barrier against the entry of microorganisms. It prevents many types of pathogens from infecting us and is the most important part of our innate immune system; skin is our barrier to the outside world.
2. Tears, saliva, and blood contain lysozyme, an enzyme that kills some bacteria by destroying their cell walls.
3. The extreme acidity of the stomach destroys many pathogens which are ingested with food or swallowed after being passed out of the respiratory tract.
4. **Macrophages** and **neutrophils** indiscriminately phagocytize microorganisms.
5. **Basophils** and **eosinophils** fight parasites and help mediate the allergic response.
6. **Natural killer (NK) cells** provide a fast response to virus-infected cells and tumor formation. They quickly recognize and kill stressed cells (usually within 3 days), acting as a first line of defense while the adaptive immune system is preparing for attack.
7. **Inflammation,** which occurs when cells or tissues have been injured, is triggered by **histamine** release. This results in dilation and increased permeability of blood vessels, which causes increased blood flow to the site of damage.
8. The **complement system** is a group of about 20 blood proteins that can nonspecifically bind to the surface of foreign cells, leading to their destruction.

The innate immune system is preprogrammed to react to common broad categories of pathogens. It is not specific and has no immunological memory.

Humoral Immunity, Antibodies, and B Cells

Humoral immunity refers to specific protection by proteins in the plasma called **antibodies (Ab)** or **immunoglobulins (Ig).** Antibodies specifically recognize and bind to microorganisms (or other foreign particles), leading to their destruction and removal from the body. Each antibody molecule is composed of two copies of two different polypeptides, the **light chains** and the **heavy chains**, joined by disulfide bonds (Figure 11). In addition, each antibody molecule has two regions, the **constant region** and the **variable (antigen binding) region**. There are several different classes of immunoglobulins: IgG, IgA, IgM, IgD, and IgE. The classes of immunoglobulins have slightly different functions, with most of the antibodies circulating in plasma in the IgG class. The variable regions are responsible for the specificity of antibodies in recognizing foreign particles.

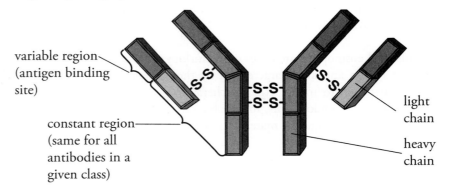

Figure 11   Antibody Structure

Each antibody forms a unique variable region that has a different binding specificity. The molecule that an antibody binds to is known as an **antigen (Ag)**. Examples of antigens are viral capsid proteins, bacterial surface proteins, and toxins in the bloodstream (such as tetanus toxin). The specificity of antigen binding is determined by the fit of antigen in a small three-dimensional cleft formed by the variable region of the antibody molecule (Figure 11). Antigens are often large molecules which have many different recognition sites for different antibodies. The small site that an antibody recognizes within a larger molecule is called an **epitope**. Very small molecules often do not elicit the production of antibodies on their own but will when bound to an antigenic large molecule like a protein. The protein in this case is called a **carrier**, and the small molecule that becomes antigenic is known as a **hapten**.

When an antibody binds to an antigen, the following can contribute to removal of the antigen from the body:

1. Binding of an antibody may directly inactivate the antigen. For example, binding of an antibody to a viral coat protein may prevent the virus from binding to cells.
2. Binding of an antibody can induce phagocytosis of a particle by macrophages and neutrophils.
3. The presence of antibodies on the surface of a cell can activate the complement system to form holes in the cell membrane and lyse the cell.

Antibodies are produced by a type of lymphocyte called **B cells**. Antibodies produced by an individual B cell can recognize only one specific antigen, but B cells in general produce antibodies that recognize an immense array of antigens. How do B cells produce such a broad array of antibodies? Does the genome encode a gene for every possible antibody molecule, a million genes for a million different potential antibodies? No. Immature B cells are derived from precursor stem cells in the bone marrow. The genes that encode antibody proteins are assembled by recombination from many small segments during B cell development. Thus, there are many different B cell clones, each with a different variable region. The immature B cells express antibody molecules on their surface. When antigen binds to the antibody on the surface of a specific immature B cell, that cell is stimulated to proliferate and differentiate into two kinds of cells: plasma cells and memory cells. **Plasma cells** actively produce and secrete antibody protein into the plasma. **Memory cells** are produced from the same clone and have the same variable regions, but do not secrete antibody; they are like pre-activated, dormant B cells. The memory cells remain dormant, sometimes for years, waiting for the same antigen to reappear. If it does, the memory cells then become activated, and start producing antibody very quickly, so quickly that no symptoms of illness appear. This method of selecting B cells with specific antigen binding is called **clonal selection**.

The first time a person encounters an antigen during an infection, it can take a week or more for B cells to proliferate and secrete significant levels of antibody. This process, known as the **primary immune response**, is too slow to prevent symptoms of the infection from occurring. It usually takes 7–14 days. The immune response to the same antigen the second time a person is exposed, the **secondary immune response**, is much swifter and stronger, so much so that symptoms never develop, and the person is said to "be immune." This immunity can last for years and is due to the presence of the memory cells produced during the first infection. Memory cells are formed in both the B cell lineage and the T cell lineage. **Vaccination** is used to improve the response to infection by exposing the immune system to an antigen associated with a virus or bacterium, thus building up the secondary immune response if the live pathogen is encountered in the future.

Cell-Mediated Immunity and the T Cell

There are two main types of **T cells**: **T helpers** (CD4$^+$ cells) and **T killers** (cytotoxic T cells, CD8$^+$ cells). The role of the T helper is to activate B cells, T killer cells, and other cells of the immune system. Hence, the T helper is the central controller of the whole immune response. It communicates with other cells by releasing special hormones called **lymphokines** and **interleukins**. The T helper cell is the host of HIV, the virus that causes AIDS.

The role of the T killer cell is to destroy abnormal host cells, namely:

1. Virus-infected host cells
2. Cancer cells
3. Foreign cells such as the cells of a skin graft given by an incompatible donor

The "T" in T cell stands for **thymus,** because they develop in this gland during childhood. Trillions of different T cells are produced in the bone marrow during childhood. Each of these is specific for a particular antigen, just as with B cells. The protein on the T cell surface that can bind antigen is the **T cell receptor (TCR)**.

The production of these trillions of different T cells with different T cell receptors is random. As a result, many of them will be specific for normal molecules found in the human body, or self antigens. It is very important to get rid of all T cells specific for self antigens, because such T cells can cause an **autoimmune reaction**, in which the immune system attacks the host. The role of the thymus in T cell development is to destroy all self-specific T cells. The result is that billions of T cells survive, but billions of others do not. The ones that survive go on to proliferate if stimulated by antigen in the proper context, each producing a group of identical T cells, all specific for a particular antigen. Such a group is known as a **T cell clone.** Clonal selection in response to antigen recognition is similar in B and T cells.

The function of T cells is exceedingly complex. As a brief introduction, the way a T cell recognizes a bad cell is by "examining" (binding to) proteins on its surface. One important group of cell-surface proteins is known as the **major histocompatibility complex (MHC)**. Our cells are programmed to have MHC proteins on their surfaces so that the immune system can keep an eye on what is going on inside every cell.

There are two kinds of MHCs, known as MHC class I and MHC class II, or simply **MHC I** and **MHC II**. MHC I proteins are found on the surface of every nucleated cell in the body. Their role is to randomly pick up peptides from the inside of the cell and display them on the cell surface. This allows T cells to monitor cellular contents. For example, if a cell is infected with a virus, one of its class I MHC complexes will display a piece of a virus-specific protein. When a T killer cell detects (binds to) the viral protein displayed on the cell's MHC I, it becomes activated and will proliferate.

The role of MHC II is more complex. Only certain special cells have MHC II. These cells are known as **antigen-presenting cells** (**APCs**). The antigen-presenting cells include macrophages and B cells. Their role is to phagocytize particles or cells, chop them up, and display fragments using the MHC II display system, which T helpers then recognize (bind to). After a T helper is activated by antigen displayed in MHC II, it will activate B cells and stimulate proliferation of T killer cells that are specific for that antigen. The activated B cells mature into plasma cells and secrete antibodies specific for the antigen. The complexity of this process helps explain why the primary immune response takes a week or more.

Dendritic cells are also antigen-presenting cells; they process antigen material and present it on their surface to T cells. Therefore, they act as messengers between the innate and the adaptive immune systems. Dendritic cells are present in tissues that are in contact with the external environment, such as the skin, the respiratory tract, and the digestive tract. Once activated, they migrate to lymph nodes and interact with T cells and B cells to initiate the adaptive immune response. There are at least a few different types of dendritic cells; some are lymphocytes and others are more similar to monocytes.

Other Tissues Involved in the Immune Response
There are several additional tissues and organs that contribute to our immunity:

- **Bone marrow** is where all blood cells are synthesized from a common progenitor. The cell that gives rise to all other blood cells is the bone marrow stem cell (also called the hematopoietic stem cell).
- The **spleen** filters blood and is a site of immune cell interactions, just like **lymph nodes.** The spleen also destroys aged red blood cells (RBCs).
- The thymus is the site of T cell maturation. The thymus shrinks in size in adults since maturation of the immune system and creation of T cells happen mostly in children.
- **Tonsils** are masses of lymphatic tissue in the back of the throat that help "catch" pathogens entering the body through respiration or ingestion. Tonsils are not required for survival and are sometimes removed if they become infected, especially in children.
- The **appendix,** which is found near the beginning of the large intestine, is very similar to the tonsils, both in structure and function. Like tonsils, the appendix is not required for survival and is often removed if it becomes infected.

CHAPTER 7 KEY TERMS

acquired immune system
adaptive immune system
adsorption
amoebas
anaerobes
antibacterial drugs
antibiotics
antibodies (Ab)
antifungal drugs
antigen (Ag)
antigen-presenting cells (APCs)
antimicrobial agents
antimicrobial resistance
antiparasitic drugs
antiviral drugs
appendix
archaea
asexual spores
attachment
autoimmune reaction
autotrophs
bacteria
basal structure
basophils
B cells
binary fission
biopharmaceuticals
bone marrow
broad-spectrum antimicrobials
budding
capsid
capsule
carbon cycle
carrier
cestodes (tapeworms)
chemoautotrophs
chemoheterotrophs
chemotaxis
chemotrophs
chitin
ciliates
clonal selection
commensalism
community
complement system
conjugation
constant region
consumers (or heterotrophs)
dendritic cells

disease
disinfection
eclipse
ectoparasite
endotoxins
envelope
eosinophils
epidemiology
epitope
eukaryotes
excision
exotoxins
facultative anaerobes
F (fertility) factor
filament
fission
flagella
flagellates
flatworms
fragmentation
glycocalyx
gram-negative
gram-positive
gram staining
granulocytes
hapten
heavy chains
helminths
heterotrophs
Hfr (high frequency of recombination) cell
histamine
hook
humoral immunity
immunization
immunoglobulins (Ig)
inflammation
innate immunity
interleukins
leukocytes
light chains
lymph nodes
lymphokines
lysogenic cycle
lysozyme
macrophages
major histocompatibility complex (MHC)
membrane-bound organelles
memory cells
mesophiles

MHC I
MHC II
motile
mutualistic
natural killer (NK) cells
nematodes
neutrophils
nitrogen cycle
nitrogen fixation
obligate aerobes
obligate anaerobes
obligate intracellular parasite
parasitic
pathogen
pathogenic microorganisms
penetration
peptidoglycan
periplasmic space
phagocytosis
photoautotrophs
photoheterotrophs
photosynthesis
phototrophs
plasma cells
plasmid
plasmodium
platyhelminths
population
primary immune response
producers (or autotrophs)
prokaryotes

prophage
protists
protoplast
protozoa
provirus
psychrophiles
public health
roundworms
saprophytes
secondary immune response
small-molecule drugs
spleen
sterilization
symbiosis
T cell clone
T cell receptor (TCR)
T cells
T helpers (CD4$^+$) cell
thermophiles
thymus
T killers (CD8$^+$) cell
tolerant anaerobes
tonsils
transduction
transformation
transmission
trematodes (flukes)
vaccination
variable (antigen binding) region
vectors
white blood cells (WBCs)

MICROBIOLOGY AND IMMUNOLOGY DRILL

1. APX452 is a new chemical agent currently in development. This compound is thought to destroy viruses but has minimal to no effect on bacteria or fungi. This agent is most likely a:

    A. biocide.
    B. detergent.
    C. virucide.
    D. virustatic.

2. Which of the following statements is true for Gram positive bacteria?

    A. They have a thick cell wall made up of peptidoglycan.
    B. They have a periplasmic space between the outer and inner membranes.
    C. They have lipopolysaccharides bound to the cell wall.
    D. They have an additional outer membrane.

3. *Escherichia coli* are rod-shaped prokaryotes. These cells are:

    A. bacilli and contain mitochondria for cell respiration.
    B. cocci and perform photosynthesis.
    C. bacilli and contain 70S ribosomes for protein synthesis.
    D. cocci and have many flagella made of a 9 + 2 arrangement of microtubules.

4. Livestock stir up various insects while grazing. Cattle egrets, who follow the livestock, feed upon these insects. Which form of interdependence exists between the livestock and the egrets?

    A. Mutualism
    B. Opportunism
    C. Parasitism
    D. Commensalism

5. During peptidoglycan biosynthesis, penicillin inhibits transpeptidase action. This causes:

    A. bursting of the cell due to loss of osmotic pressure.
    B. enhanced DNA replication.
    C. genomic integration of a viral genome.
    D. limited binary fission rates.

6. Fungi are eukaryotic heterotrophs and most are either saprophytes or parasitic. Which of the following is an incorrect matching of one of these terms to its definition?

    A. Eukaryote—cells with membrane-bound organelles
    B. Heterotrophs—must consume other organisms for energy
    C. Saprophytes—feed off dead plants and animals
    D. Parasites—feed off living organisms, doing no harm to the host

7. Which of the following is a correct pairing of parasite to example?

    A. Ectoparasites—lice and ticks
    B. Helminths—amoeba and cestodes
    C. Protozoa—flatworms and roundworms
    D. Protozoa—trematodes and *Plasmodium*

8. Which of these is least likely to happen when a virus replicates in a host cell and viral antigens are expressed on the host's cell surface?

    A. B cell number increases to form more plasma cells.
    B. Killer T cells bind viral antigens expressed on MHC I.
    C. Helper T cells allow cross talk between NK cells and B cells.
    D. T lymphocytes recognize these antigens as foreign.

9. Which statement could correctly describe the role of a vaccine in preventing a disease?

    A. A vaccine stops B cell response, thus preventing disease.
    B. A vaccine releases antibodies into the blood and this binds pathogenic antigens.
    C. A vaccine carries surface antigens from pathogens, thus activating the immune response.
    D. A vaccine contains B and T lymphocytes that neutralize pathogenic antigens.

10. *Staphylococcus aureus* produces coagulase that results in the clotting of fibrin. As a consequence, fibrin is deposited on the surface of bacterial cells. What immunological effect is likely to be caused by this action?

    A. Pathogenicity of *S. aureus* will decrease.
    B. *S. aureus* will no longer be identified as an antigen.
    C. *S. aureus* will bind with a larger number of antibodies.
    D. There will be no change in the immune response.

Want More Practice?
Register your book online for more drill questions!

Answers and Explanations

1. **C** A biocide is a substance that kills living organisms (eliminate choice A). Detergents are water-soluble cleansing agents but this is not relevant to the question stem (eliminate choice B). A virucide is an antimicrobial agent that destroys viruses (choice C is correct). Virustatic agents inhibit proliferation of viruses but do not necessarily destroy them (eliminate choice D).

2. **A** Gram positive bacteria have a thick layer of peptidoglycan that makes up their cell wall (choice A is correct). Gram negative bacteria have an additional outer membrane (eliminate choice D), which contains lipopolysaccharides (eliminate choice C) and is separated from the inner membrane by the periplasmic space (eliminate choice B).

3. **C** Rod-shaped bacteria are called bacilli (eliminate choices B and D). Bacteria (or prokaryotes) do not contain any membrane-bound organelles, including mitochondria (eliminate choice A). Bacteria contain 70S ribosomes with 30S and 50S subunits. Ribosomes perform translation, the second part of protein synthesis (choice C is correct).

4. **D** Commensalism occurs when only one symbiont is benefitted and the other symbiont is not affected in any way. The correct answer is choice (D). Mutualism occurs when all symbionts are benefitted from each other, so eliminate choice A. Opportunism is not a type of interdependence, so eliminate choice (B). Parasitism occurs when one symbiont is benefitted and the other symbiont is harmed, eliminating choice (C).

5. **A** The bacterial cell wall is composed of peptidoglycan, a complex polymer unique to prokaryotes. It provides support for the cell, preventing lysis due to osmotic pressure. If penicillin inhibits peptidoglycan biosynthesis, the cell will burst (choice A is correct). DNA replication, infection by a virus, and bacterial cell division via binary fission are not relevant to the bacterial cell wall (eliminate choices B, C, and D).

6. **D** Eukaryotic cells contain membrane-bound organelles such as a nucleus and mitochondria (choice A is true, so eliminate it). Fungi are heterotrophs; they must consume other organisms for energy (choice B is true, so eliminate it). Most fungi are either saprophytes, meaning they feed off dead plants and animals (eliminate choice C), or parasites that feed off living organisms, doing harm to the host (choice D is incorrect and thus the right answer).

7. **A** There are three main classes of parasites that can cause disease in humans: protozoa, helminths, and ectoparasites. Some examples of protozoans are flagellates that move using flagella, ciliates that move via cilia, amoebas that move via pseudopodia (eliminate choice B), and *Plasmodium* whose adult stage is not motile. Some examples of helminths are roundworms (or nematodes) and flatworms (also called platyhelminths), such as trematodes (flukes) and cestodes (tapeworms). This means you should eliminate choices (C) and (D). Some examples of ectoparasites are ticks, fleas, lice, and mites (choice A is correct).

8. **C** During viral infection, B cells are activated and differentiate into plasma and memory cells (choice A occurs and is not the answer). Killer T cells bind viral antigens expressed on MHC I (eliminate choice B) and recognize these antigens as foreign (eliminate choice D). Helper T cells allow cross talk between cell-mediated and humoral immune systems. They have a minimal role in activating NK cells (choice C is least likely and is the correct answer).

9. **C** A vaccine triggers an immune response; it does not stop the B cell response (eliminate choice A). Vaccines do not releases antibodies into the blood (eliminate choice B) or contain B and T lymphocytes (eliminate choice D). Vaccination works by exposing the immune system to an antigen associated with a virus or bacterium. This improves the response to infection by activating the fast secondary immune response if the live pathogen is encountered in the future. The antigen in a vaccine could be a surface protein from a pathogen, since the immune system would recognize that molecule as foreign and mount an immune response (choice C is correct).

10. **B** Clotting and deposition of fibrin on the surface of bacterial cells will hide antigens present on the cell surface of *S. aureus*. This will increase pathogenicity of *S. aureus* since the bacterial cells will be hidden from the immune system (choice A is wrong). This extracellular coating will prevent *S. aureus* from being identified as a foreign antigen (choice B is correct, eliminate choice D). Antibodies will be less likely to bind the bacterial cells (eliminate choice C).

Quick Review

Infectious Diseases and Prevention

- Public health aims to improve the health of populations.

- Epidemiology is the study and analysis of the distribution, patterns, and determinants of health and disease in certain populations.

- A disease is an abnormal condition that negatively affects the structure or function of an organism.

- Infectious diseases are caused by pathogenic microorganisms (or microbes), such as bacteria, fungi, viruses, or parasites.

- Sterilization and disinfection are used to limit the spread of infectious disease by nonliving objects.

Bacteria

- Prokaryotes have no membrane-bound organelles (e.g., nucleus, mitochondria, etc.); all their cellular processes occur in the cytosol.

- Bacteria have cell walls made out of peptidoglycan.

- Some bacteria have flagella, which are used for motility and are distinct from eukaryotic flagella in structure.

- Bacteria can be classified by:

  - Shape: round = coccus; rod = bacillus; spiral = spirillum.
  - Gram staining: Gram positive = thick cell wall, stain dark purple; Gram negative = thinner cell wall, outer membrane, stain light pink.
  - Temperature: mesophiles = room temperatures or body temperatures; thermophiles = high temperatures such as $100^\circ C$; psychrophiles = low temperatures such as $0^\circ C$.
  - Carbon source: autotrophs = CO_2; heterotrophs = organic nutrients.
  - Energy source: chemotrophs = chemicals; phototrophs = light.
  - Oxygen use: obligate aerobes = need O_2; facultative anaerobes = can use O_2; tolerant anaerobes = put up with O_2; obligate anaerobes = poisoned by O_2.

- Bacteria reproduce via asexual binary fission; this increases the population size exponentially but does not increase genetic diversity of the population.

- Bacteria have three methods to increase genetic diversity:

  ○ Transformation is uptake of environmental DNA.
  ○ Transduction is sharing genomic DNA via a lysogenic phage.
  ○ Conjugation occurs between bacteria; plasmid or genomic DNA is exchanged via a conjugation bridge.

Microbial Ecology

- A population is a group of individuals of a single species that live in the same general area and are thus subject to the same environmental factors and resources.

- Many different populations existing together make up a community.

- Producers (or autotrophs) are photosynthetic organisms that can produce their own food and provide a source of food for other organisms.

- Consumers (or heterotrophs) are organisms that rely on the food made by the producers. They eat either producers or other consumers.

- Carbon and nitrogen atoms are cycled through the community via living and non-living things.

- Carbon atoms cycle between biomass, the atmosphere, oceans, and inside the Earth.

- Bacteria move carbon atoms through the carbon cycle by performing photosynthesis, cell respiration, fermentation, and decomposition.

- Photosynthesis is the process by which autotrophs such as plants, cyanobacteria, and some protists use energy from the Sun to produce food.

- Summary equation for photosynthesis is $6\ CO_2 + 6\ H_2O + energy \rightarrow C_6H_{12}O_6 + 6\ O_2$.

- Nitrogen fixation is a process by which bacteria convert N_2 into ammonia (NH_3), and then ammonium (NH_4^+) or nitrate (NO_3^-), which can be used by plants.

- Three types of symbiosis: commensalism = ☺ + ☺; mutualism = ☺ + ☺; parasitism = ☺ + ☹.

Fungi

- Fungi are eukaryotic, heterotrophs, and have a cell wall made of chitin.

- Asexual reproduction options are budding, fragmentation, asexual spores, or fission.

- Fungi can sexually reproduce via spores.

Viruses

- All viruses are made up of nucleic acids (either RNA or DNA) surrounded by a protein coat (capsid).

- Viruses are obligate intracellular parasites that must rely on host cells to reproduce.

- Animal viruses may also have an envelope (lipid bilayer) surrounding the capsid. The envelope is derived from the host cell and is acquired by budding through the host cell membrane.

- Viral infection is specific; molecules on the viral surface determine which type of host cell it will infect.

- Viruses replicate via two major reproductive cycles:

  - Both start with attachment and penetration.
  - Lytic cycle: more virus is made very quickly via taking over host cell machinery, making viral components, assembly, bursting out of host cell (lysis; kills host cell).
  - Lysogenic cycle: virus becomes dormant by integrating into the host cell genome to be replicated with host genome, can excise from the genome and enter the lytic cycle.

Parasites

- Three classes of parasites can cause disease in humans: protozoa, helminths, and ectoparasites.

- Protozoa: microscopic, one-celled organisms; animal-like protists.
  - Examples: flagellates, ciliates, amoebas, and *Plasmodium* (cause malaria).

- Helminths: large, multicellular parasitic worms.
  - Examples: roundworms (nematodes), flatworms (platyhelminths) such as trematodes (flukes), and cestodes (tapeworms).

- Ectoparasites: live on the outside of their hosts, cause disease and/or act as vectors.
  - Examples: ticks, fleas, lice, and mites.

- Parasitic infections typically spread through contaminated water, food, waste, soil, or blood.

Medical Microbiology

- Immunization or vaccination exposes the immune system to an antigen associated with a virus or bacterium and facilitates a fast and effective secondary immune response.

- Antimicrobial agents kill or inhibit the growth of microorganisms.

- Antibacterial drugs or antibiotics kill or inhibit the growth of a bacterium.

- Antifungal drugs kill or inhibit the growth of a fungus.

- Antiviral drugs are used to treat viral infections.

- Antiparasitic drugs destroy a parasite, inhibit its growth, or expel it from the host.

- Antimicrobial resistance occurs when a microbe evolves over time to develop resistance to a drug used to target it. This makes infections harder to treat.

Immune System

- Immunity is driven by white blood cells or leukocytes, including:

Cell	Class	Role
Macrophage	Monocyte	• phagocytose debris, dead cells, microorganisms, pathogens • amoeboid motility • exhibit chemotaxis
Neutrophil	Granulocyte	• phagocytose bacteria • amoeboid motility • exhibit chemotaxis
Basophil	Granulocyte	• store and release histamine • destroy parasites such as bacteria, fungi, viruses • function in allergic response and inflammation
Eosinophil	Granulocyte	• destroy parasites such as bacteria, fungi, viruses • function in allergic response and inflammation
CD8$^+$ cytotoxic T cell	Lymphocyte	• kill cells marked for destruction, e.g., virus-infected cell or tumor cell, tissue graft
CD4$^+$ helper T cell	Lymphocyte	• activate other immune cells • control and coordinate the immune response, e.g., cross talk between humoral and cell-mediated immune responses
Memory cell [B and T]	Lymphocyte	• can survive for decades • repeatedly generate an accelerated and robust immune response when an antigen is seen a second time • responsible for the fast secondary immune response and long-term immunity • created in response to vaccination
Plasma cell	Lymphocyte	• mature B cell • produce antibodies
NK cell	Lymphocyte	• kill cells marked for destruction, e.g., virus-infected cell or tumor cell, tissue graft
Dendritic cell	Monocyte or lymphocyte	• antigen-presenting cells • activate other immune cells • cross talk between innate and adaptive immune responses

- Macrophages and neutrophils are phagocytes.

- Basophils, neutrophils, and eosinophils are granulocytes.

- B cells, T cells, and NK cells are lymphocytes.

- Innate immunity is nonspecific and includes the skin, lysozyme, stomach acid, phagocytes, basophils, eosinophils, NK cells, inflammation, and the complement system.

- Adaptive or acquired immunity is divided into humoral and cell-mediated branches.

- Humoral immunity is driven by B cells and their production of antibodies.

- Immature B cells differentiate into plasma cells and memory cells.

- Antibodies (immunoglobulins) are highly specific for particular antigens (foreign molecules).

- Cell-mediated immunity is handled by T cells.

- Killer (cytotoxic) T cells (CD8$^+$) destroy "self" cells that are displaying abnormal antigen on MHC I.

- Helper T cells (CD4$^+$) are activated by antigen displayed on MHC II and secrete chemicals to help activate and stimulate the proliferation of killer T cells and B cells.

- Primary immune response is slow (7–14 days); secondary immune response is due to the presence of memory cells and is fast (1–2 days).

Chapter 8

Human Anatomy and Physiology

8.1 CARDIOVASCULAR AND CIRCULATORY SYSTEMS

Overview of the Circulatory System

The cells of a multicellular organism have the same basic requirements as unicellular organisms. Living so close to billions of other cells has many advantages, but there are drawbacks too. Each cell must compete with its neighbors for nutrients and oxygen and must also cope with the waste products that are inevitable in so dense a civilization. Other requirements of multicellular living are efficient communication and **homeostasis**. The circulatory system addresses these problems by accomplishing the following goals:

1. Distributing nutrients from the digestive tract, liver, and adipose (fat) tissue
2. Transporting oxygen from the lungs to the entire body and carbon dioxide from the tissues to the lungs
3. Transporting metabolic waste products from tissues to the excretory system (i.e., the kidneys)
4. Transporting hormones from endocrine glands to targets and providing feedback
5. Maintaining homeostasis of body temperature
6. Maintaining **hemostasis** (blood clotting). This does not address a need of a multicellular organism *per se*, but rather is necessitated by the presence of the circulatory system itself.

The flow of blood through a tissue is known as **perfusion**. Inadequate blood flow, known as **ischemia**, results in tissue damage due to shortages of O_2 and nutrients, and buildup of metabolic wastes. When adequate circulation is present but the supply of oxygen is reduced, a tissue is said to suffer from **hypoxia**.

Components of the Circulatory System

Functions of the circulatory system involve transport of blood throughout the body and exchange of material between the blood and tissues. The **heart** is a muscular pump that forces blood through a branching series of vessels to the lungs and the rest of the body. Vessels that carry blood away from the heart at high pressure are **arteries**, and vessels that carry blood back toward the heart at low pressure are **veins**. As arteries pass farther from the heart, the pressure of blood decreases, and they branch into increasingly smaller arteries called **arterioles**. The arterioles then pass into the **capillaries**, very small vessels, often just wide enough for a single blood cell to pass. Arterioles have smooth muscle in their walls that can act as a control valve to restrict or increase the flow of blood into the capillaries of tissues. The capillaries have thin walls made of a single layer of cells. They are designed to allow the exchange of material between the blood and tissues. After passing through capillaries, blood collects in small veins called **venules**, and then into the veins leading back to the heart. From the heart, the blood can be pumped out once again through the arteries to the capillaries in the tissues.

To achieve both efficient oxygenation of blood in the lungs and transport of oxygenated blood to the tissues, the human heart has evolved to have two sides separated by a thick wall; this allows the heart to pump blood in two separate circuits. The right side of the heart pumps blood to the lungs, and the left side of the heart pumps blood to the rest of the body. The flow of blood from the heart to the lungs and back to the heart is the **pulmonary circulation**, and blood flow from the heart to the rest of the body and back again is the **systemic circulation**. Figure 1 summarizes pulmonary circulation; you can see flow of deoxygenated blood from the right ventricle to the pulmonary circulation via right and left pulmonary arteries. You can also track the return of oxygenated blood from the pulmonary circulation to the left atrium via right and left pulmonary veins.

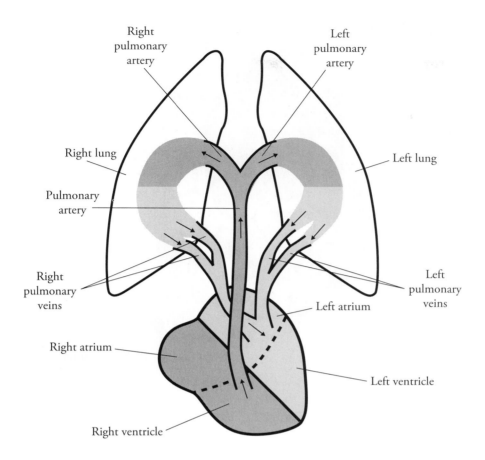

Right pulmonary artery

Left pulmonary artery

Right lung

Left lung

Pulmonary artery

Right pulmonary veins

Left pulmonary veins

Left atrium

Right atrium

Left ventricle

Right ventricle

Figure 1   Pulmonary Circulation

By having two separate circulations, most blood passes through only one set of capillaries before returning to the heart. There are exceptions to this, however: **portal systems**. In the hepatic portal system, blood passes first through capillaries in the intestine, and then collects in veins to travel to the liver, where the vessels branch and the blood passes again through capillaries. Another example is the hypothalamic-hypophysial portal system, in which blood passes through capillaries in the hypothalamus to the portal veins, then to capillaries in the pituitary. Portal systems evolved as direct transport systems, to transport nutrients directly from the intestine to the liver or hormones from the hypothalamus to the pituitary, without passing through the whole body.

The Heart

The heart has two kinds of chambers involved in pumping blood, the **atria** and the **ventricles** (Figure 2). The atria are reservoirs or "waiting rooms" where blood can collect from the veins before getting pumped into the ventricles. The muscular ventricles pump blood out of the heart at high pressures into the arteries. The systemic circulation and the pulmonary circulation are separated within the heart, so the right and left sides of the heart each have one atrium and one ventricle. The right atrium receives deoxygenated blood from the systemic circulation (via the large veins, the **inferior vena cava,** and **superior vena cava**) and pumps it into the right ventricle. From the right ventricle, blood passes through the pulmonary artery to the lungs. Oxygenated blood from the lungs returns through the pulmonary veins to the left atrium and is pumped into the left ventricle before being pumped out of the heart in a single large artery, the **aorta**, to the systemic circulation.

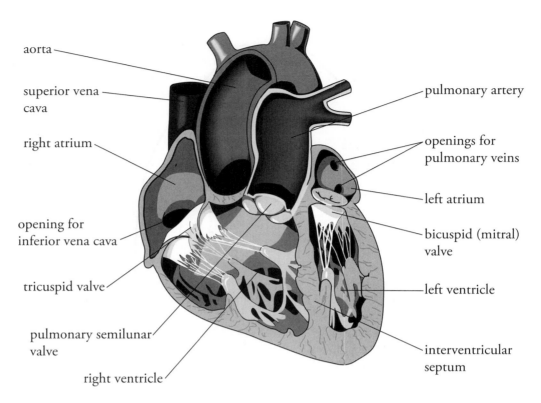

Figure 2   The Heart

The heart is a large muscular organ which requires a blood supply of its own. The very first branches from the aorta are **coronary arteries** which branch to supply blood to the wall of the heart. They are called "coronary" because they encircle the heart forming a crown shape. Deoxygenated blood from the heart collects in **coronary veins**, which drain into the right atrium.

Valves

Valves are necessary to ensure one-way flow through the circulatory system. Valves in the heart are especially important, since the pressure differentials there are so extreme; ventricular pressure is very high and atrial pressure is lower. Hence, an **atrioventricular (AV) valve** between each ventricle and its atrium is necessary to prevent backflow.

The AV valve between the left atrium and the left ventricle is the **bicuspid** (or **mitral**) **valve**. The AV valve between the right atrium and the right ventricle is the **tricuspid valve**.

Another set of valves is needed between the large arteries and the ventricles; these are the **pulmonary** and **aortic semilunar valves**. Together these two valves are known simply as the semilunar valves.

There are also valves throughout the venous system. These valves are necessary because in passing through capillaries, blood loses its pressure. Hence there is not much of a driving force pushing it toward the heart. Contraction of skeletal muscle becomes important, because normal body movements push and squeeze the veins, pressurizing venous blood and pushing it along. Venous valves prevent backflow; as long as the valves hold up, the blood moves toward the heart.

Cardiac Cycle

The heart contracts, then relaxes, in a cycle which ends only in death. The left and right sides of the heart proceed through the same cycle at the same time. The cardiac cycle is divided into two periods, **diastole** and **systole** (pronounced dy-AS-toe-lee and SIS-toe-lee). During diastole, the ventricles are relaxed, and blood is able to flow into them from the atria. In fact, the atria contract during diastole, to propel blood into the ventricles more rapidly. At the end of diastole, the ventricles contract, initiating systole. The ensuing buildup of pressure causes the AV valves to slam shut. Over the next few milliseconds, the pressure in the ventricles increases rapidly, until the semilunar valves fly open and blood rushes into the aorta and pulmonary artery. Systole is the period of time during which the ventricles are contracting, beginning at the "lub" sound and ending at the "dup." At the end of systole, the ventricles are nearly empty and stop contracting. As a result, the pressure inside falls rapidly, and blood begins to flow backward, from the pulmonary artery into the right ventricle, and from the aorta into the left ventricle. But very little back-flow actually occurs, because the semilunar valves slam shut when the pressure in the ventricles becomes lower than the pressure in the great arteries. At this point, the heart has completed a full cardiac cycle and is back in diastole.

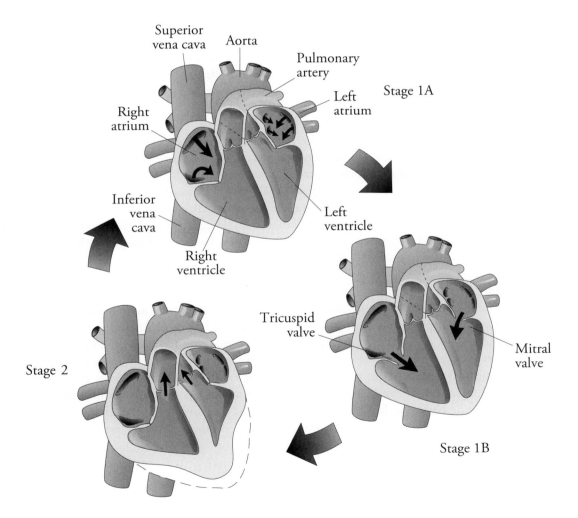

Figure 3   Blood Flow During Stages of Heart Contraction

Heart Sounds, Heart Rate, and Cardiac Output

The "lub-dup" of the heartbeat is produced by valves slamming shut. The "lub" results from the closure of the AV valves at the beginning of systole, and the "dup" is the sound of the semilunar valves closing at the end of systole.

The **heart rate** (HR) or **pulse** is the number of times the "lub-dup" cardiac cycle is repeated per minute. The normal pulse rate is about one beat per second, ranging from 45 to 80 beats per minute (b.p.m.) The amount of blood pumped with each systole is known as the **stroke volume (SV)**. The total amount of blood pumped per minute is termed the **cardiac output (CO)**, defined by the equation

$$\text{cardiac output (L/min)} = \text{stroke volume (L/beat)} \times \text{heart rate (beats/min)}$$
$$\text{CO} = \text{SV} \times \text{HR}$$

Rhythmic Excitation of the Heart

Interestingly, the heart is *not* stimulated to contract by neuronal or hormonal influences, although these can change the rate and strength of contraction (the **contractility** of the heart). Instead, initiation of each action potential that starts each cardiac cycle occurs automatically from within the heart itself, in a special region of the right atrium called the **sinoatrial (SA) node**. Under normal circumstances, the cells of the SA node act as the **pacemaker of the heart**. SA node cells transmit their action potential to cardiac muscle cells (or **myocytes**) of the atrium, and to the rest of the conduction cells in the heart. We will discuss each of these routes.

The signal from the SA node causes both atria to contract simultaneously and fill the ventricles with blood. An action potential (and thus contraction) spreads throughout the cardiac muscle because cardiac muscle is a **functional syncytium.** A syncytium is a tissue in which the cytoplasm of different cells can communicate via gap junctions. In cardiac muscle, gap junctions are found in intercalated disks, the connections between cardiac muscle cells. Depolarization of a cardiac muscle cell can be communicated directly through the cytoplasm to neighboring cardiac muscle cells through these gap junctions. As a result, once an action potential starts, it spreads in a wave of depolarization throughout the cardiac muscle tissue in the atria or the ventricles. The atria and the ventricles are separate syncytia.

The action potential also spreads down the special conduction pathway, which transmits action potentials very rapidly without contracting. The pathway connects the SA node to the **atrioventricular (AV) node**. Since this pathway connects two nodes, it is referred to as the **internodal tract**. Note that while the impulse travels to the AV node almost instantaneously, it spreads through the atria more slowly, because contracting heart muscle cells pass the impulse more slowly than specialized conduction fibers. At the AV node, the impulse is delayed slightly; it then passes from the node to the ventricles via the conduction pathway again. This part of the conduction pathway is known as the **AV bundle (bundle of His)**. The AV bundle divides into the **right** and **left bundle branches**, and then into the **Purkinje fibers**, which allow the impulse to spread rapidly and evenly over both ventricles. As the ventricles contract, blood is pushed up and out of the heart.

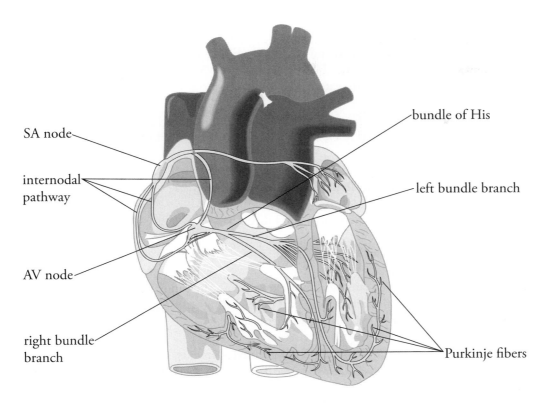

SA node

internodal pathway

AV node

right bundle branch

bundle of His

left bundle branch

Purkinje fibers

Figure 4   Cardiac Conduction System

Regulation of the Heart by the Autonomic Nervous System

The autonomic nervous system regulates the rate of contraction. The intrinsic firing rate of the SA node is about 120 beats per minute, but the normal heart rate is only about 60–80 beats/minute because the parasympathetic nervous system continually inhibits depolarization of the SA node.

The sympathetic system can also influence the heart. It kicks in when increased cardiac output is needed during a "fight or flight" response. First, sympathetic postganglionic neurons directly innervate the heart, releasing norepinephrine. Second, epinephrine secreted by the adrenal medulla binds to receptors on cardiac muscle cells. The effect of sympathetic activation is stimulatory: heart rate increases, and so does the force of contraction.

Blood

Blood has a liquid portion called **plasma**, and a portion which is composed of cells. The cellular elements of blood are known as **formed elements**. Plasma accounts for 55 percent of the blood volume and consists of the following items dissolved in water:

- Electrolytes, such as Na^+, K^+, Cl^-, Ca^{2+}, and Mg^{2+} ions
- Buffers, such as bicarbonate (HCO_3^-), to maintain a constant pH of 7.4
- Sugars, mainly glucose
- Blood proteins, most of which are made by the liver
- Lipoproteins, which transport lipids in the bloodstream
- CO_2 and O_2
- Metabolic waste products, such as urea and bilirubin

Some examples of blood proteins include:

- **albumin**: essential for maintaining osmotic pressure in the capillaries
- immunoglobulins (or antibodies): a key part of the immune system
- **fibrinogen**: essential for blood clotting (or hemostasis)

Centrifuging whole blood separates plasma from formed elements, as shown below. The volume of blood occupied by erythrocytes (also known as red blood cells or RBCs) is known as the **hematocrit** (Figure 5). White blood cells (**leukocytes**) and platelets account for a small volume (about 1 percent). Remember from the previous chapter that all formed elements of the blood develop from cells in the bone marrow, known as bone marrow stem cells or hematopoietic stem cells.

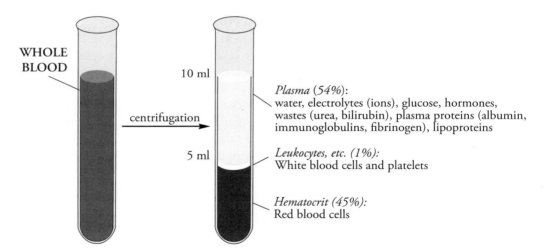

Figure 5 Hematocrit and Components of Blood

If whole blood is allowed to clot, one is left with a solid clot plus a clear fluid known as **serum**. Hence, serum is similar to plasma except that it lacks all the proteins involved in clotting.

Erythrocytes

The hormone **erythropoietin** (made in the kidney) stimulates RBC production in the bone marrow. Aged RBCs are eaten by phagocytes in the spleen and liver.

The erythrocyte is a cell, but it has no nucleus or other organelles such as mitochondria. However, it does require the energy of ATP for processes such as ion pumping and basic maintenance of cell structure during its 120-day lifetime in the bloodstream. Lacking mitochondria, the RBC relies on glycolysis for ATP synthesis. The purpose of the RBC is to transport O_2 to the tissues from the lungs and CO_2 from the tissues to the lungs. Hence it requires a large surface area for gas exchange. A high surface-to-volume ratio is achieved by the RBC's flat, biconcave shape (like a deflated basketball or a throat lozenge). The RBC is able to carry oxygen because it contains millions of molecules of hemoglobin, which we will talk about shortly.

Blood Typing

Blood typing is the classification of a person's blood based on the presence or absence of certain surface antigens on their red blood cells. The two most important blood group antigens are the **ABO blood group** and the **Rh blood group**.

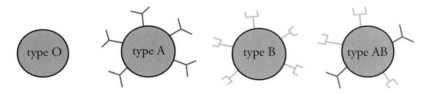

Figure 6   RBC Surface Antigens

Antibodies against A and B antigens are produced early in infancy and can cause clumping and destruction of red blood cells bearing an unfamiliar antigen; this is called a **transfusion reaction**. For example, a person with blood type AB has both A and B antigens on their RBCs and recognizes both as "self." Neither will be seen as foreign, so people with blood type AB can receive blood from all other blood types; they are universal recipients.

People with type A blood recognize only the A antigen as "self"; the B antigen is flagged as foreign. Therefore, people with type A blood can receive type A blood and type O blood, but they cannot receive type B blood or type AB blood because it would cause a transfusion reaction.

People with type O blood can receive only type O blood. They do not express A or B antigens, so their immune system doesn't recognize these antigens as "self" and instead flags them as foreign. Type A blood, type B blood, and type AB blood will all cause transfusion reactions in a type O person. However, type O blood can be given to any other blood type. Type O RBCs express no antigens, so there is nothing to be seen as foreign to a donor. For this reason, type O blood is the universal donor.

Here's a summary table:

Blood Type	Genotype	Can Receive from	Can Donate to
A	$I^A I^A$ or $I^A i$	A or O	A or AB
B	$I^B I^B$ or $I^B i$	B or O	B or AB
O	ii	O only	O, A, B, or AB (universal donor)
AB	$I^A I^B$	O, A, B, or AB (universal recipient)	AB only

Table 1　Human Blood Type

Antibodies to the Rh antigen do not develop unless a person with Rh– blood is exposed to Rh+ blood, an event called "sensitization." Subsequent exposure to Rh+ blood can then result in a transfusion reaction. This is particularly dangerous in the case of an Rh– mother carrying an Rh+ baby. Typically, if it is the first baby, there are no complications (unless the mother had been previously sensitized); the mother's blood and the baby's blood do not mix during pregnancy. However, on delivery, some Rh+ cells from the child can mix with the mother's Rh– blood and lead to her sensitization. Future Rh+ babies are then at risk, since the anti-Rh antibodies can cross the placental barrier to clump and/or destroy the Rh+ baby's red blood cells. This condition, known as **hemolytic disease of the newborn** or **erythroblastosis fetalis,** can be fatal. Injection of the mother at the time of birth with anti-Rh antibodies can clump and lead to the destruction of any stray Rh+ cells from the baby; this can prevent sensitization of the mother and protect future unborn Rh+ children.

Leukocytes

White blood cells fight infection and dispose of debris. We discussed these cells in the previous chapter but will review them again here.

Cell	Class	Role
Macrophage	Monocyte	• phagocytose debris, dead cells, microorganisms, pathogens • amoeboid motility • exhibit chemotaxis
Neutrophil	Granulocyte	• phagocytose bacteria • amoeboid motility • exhibit chemotaxis
Basophil	Granulocyte	• store and release histamine • destroy parasites such as bacteria, fungi, viruses • function in allergic response and inflammation
Eosinophil	Granulocyte	• destroy parasites such as bacteria, fungi, viruses • function in allergic response and inflammation
CD8$^+$ cytotoxic T cell	Lymphocyte	• kill cells marked for destruction, e.g., virus-infected cell or tumor cell, tissue graft
CD4$^+$ helper T cell	Lymphocyte	• activate other immune cells • control and coordinate the immune response, e.g., cross talk between humoral and cell-mediated immune responses
Memory T cell	Lymphocyte	• can survive for decades • repeatedly generate an accelerated and robust immune response when an antigen is seen a second time • responsible for the fast secondary immune response and long-term immunity • created in response to vaccination
Plasma cell	Lymphocyte	• mature B cell • produce antibodies
Memory B cell	Lymphocyte	• can survive for decades • repeatedly generate an accelerated and robust antibody-mediated immune response when an antigen is seen a second time • responsible for the fast secondary immune response and long-term immunity • created in response to vaccination
NK cell	Lymphocyte	• kill cells marked for destruction, e.g., virus-infected cell or tumor cell, tissue graft
Dendritic cell	Monocyte or lymphocyte	• antigen-presenting cells • activate other immune cells • cross talk between innate and adaptive immune responses

Table 2   Roles of Leukocytes

Platelets and Hemostasis

Like red blood cells, platelets have no nuclei and a limited lifespan. They are derived from the fragmentation of large bone marrow cells called **megakaryocytes**, which are derived from the same stem cells that give rise to red blood cells and white blood cells. The function of platelets is to aggregate at the site of damage to a blood vessel wall, forming a **platelet plug**. This immediately helps stop bleeding. Hemostasis is a term for the body's mechanism of preventing bleeding.

The other component of the hemostatic response is **fibrin**. This is a threadlike protein which forms a mesh that holds the platelet plug together. When the fibrin mesh dries, it becomes a scab, which seals and protects the wound. When bleeding occurs, the plasma protein fibrinogen is converted into fibrin by a protein called **thrombin**. A blood clot, or **thrombus**, is a scab circulating in the bloodstream. Calcium as well as many accessory proteins are necessary for the activation of thrombin and fibrinogen. Several of the proteins depend on vitamin K for their function. Defects in these proteins result in **hemophilia** ("loving to bleed"), an X-linked recessive group of diseases involving excessive bleeding.

Transport of Gases

Oxygen

Oxygen is too hydrophobic to dissolve in the plasma in significant quantities. Hence, RBCs are used to bind and carry O_2. RBCs are able to carry oxygen because they contain millions of molecules of **hemoglobin** (Hb). This is a complex protein composed of four polypeptide subunits. Each subunit contains one molecule of **heme**, which is a large multi-ring structure that has a single iron atom bound at its center. The role of heme with its iron atom is to bind O_2. Since each hemoglobin has four subunits and each subunit has one heme, each molecule of hemoglobin can carry four molecules of oxygen. Hemoglobin has some important properties that make it an excellent oxygen carrier.

The four subunits of hemoglobin do not bind oxygen independently of each other. When one of the subunits binds oxygen, its conformation changes and this change in three-dimensional structure is communicated to the other subunits through contacts between the polypeptides. As a result, the other subunits alter their conformation and increase their affinity for oxygen as well. Thus, hemoglobin is said to bind oxygen **cooperatively**.

Carbon Dioxide

Carbon dioxide is transported in the blood in three ways:

1. 73% of CO_2 transport is accomplished by the conversion of CO_2 to **carbonic acid**, which can dissociate into **bicarbonate** and a proton according to this reaction:
    $$CO_2 + H_2O \rightleftharpoons H_2CO_3 \rightleftharpoons HCO_3^- + H^+$$
    These compounds are extremely water-soluble and are thus easily carried in the blood. The conversion of CO_2 into carbonic acid is catalyzed by an RBC enzyme called **carbonic anhydrase**. This reaction is also important as the principal plasma pH buffer.
2. Some CO_2 (~ 20%) is transported by simply being stuck onto hemoglobin. It does not bind to the oxygen-binding sites, but rather to other sites on the protein.
3. CO_2 is somewhat more water-soluble than O_2, so about 7% can be dissolved in the blood and carried from the tissues to the lungs. Virtually no oxygen can be dissolved in the blood.

8.2 LYMPHATIC SYSTEM

The lymphatic system is a one-way flow system. It begins with tiny lymphatic capillaries in all the tissues of the body that merge to form larger lymphatic vessels. These merge to form large lymphatic ducts. Lymphatic vessels have valves, and the larger lymphatic ducts have smooth muscles in their walls. As a result, the lymphatic system acts like a suction pump to retrieve water, proteins, and white blood cells from the tissues. The fluid in lymphatic vessels is called **lymph**. The lymph is filtered by numerous **lymph nodes**. The large lymphatic ducts merge to form the **thoracic duct**, which is the largest lymphatic vessel, located in the chest. The thoracic duct empties into a large vein near the neck.

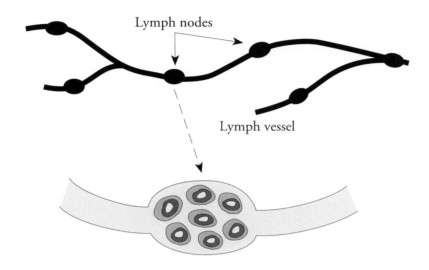

Figure 7

Lymph Nodes

Numerous lymph nodes are found along each lymph vessel. They are an important part of the immune system because they contain millions of white blood cells that can initiate an immune response against anything foreign that may have been picked up in the lymph. Infection in one part of the body causes swelling of regional lymph nodes as lymphocytes in the nodes multiply to combat the infection.

Other Lymphatic Organs

The spleen and thymus are also components of the lymphatic system. The spleen, located under the stomach, functions much like a large lymph node, except that the spleen acts as a lymphatic filter for blood while lymph nodes filter the lymph fluid. In addition, the spleen destroys old erythrocytes.

Found in the middle of the upper chest, the thymus is a small lymphoid organ that is especially active between birth and puberty. T lymphocytes mature in the thymus, which degenerates during adolescence and adulthood, becoming largely nonfunctional.

8.3   ENDOCRINE SYSTEM

Endocrine vs. Exocrine Glands

The endocrine system controls body homeostasis over hours and days by promoting communication among various tissues and organs through the secretion of hormones. Hormones are secreted by endocrine organs, more commonly called **endocrine glands**. Hormones usually act at considerable distances from the sites of their release. They are released from an endocrine gland into the bloodstream, by which they are carried to their target cells. In contrast, **exocrine organs** secrete their products into the external environment (including the lumen of the gut) via ducts. These secretions can be mucus-based or serous (watery secretions that usually contain enzymes). Some example of exocrine organs are the salivary glands, mammary glands, pancreatic acinar cells, or sweat glands.

Most endocrine hormones act slowly and for a long period of time (i.e., minutes to years) to maintain homeostasis. Their secretion is modulated by changes in bodily needs and conditions. Because they are secreted directly into the bloodstream, endocrine hormones come into contact with nearly every cell of the body. Despite that fact, a given hormone may not have any effect on a given cell type. Most hormones affect a cell only if the cell has a receptor that binds them, either on the surface of the cell or inside the cell. A hormone's target cells, then, are those cells that have receptors for it. A given cell type might be the target of one hormone, many hormones, or no hormones, depending on the number and kind of receptors it expresses.

Types of Hormones

Hormones can be generally grouped into one of three classes: peptide hormones, steroid hormones, or amino acid derivatives. These chemical classes of hormones are made differently, travel in the blood differently, function at the target cell differently, and affect the target cell differently. Below is a summary table of the key features of peptide and steroid hormones. Most amino acid derivatives act like peptide hormones (for example, epinephrine), but some can act like steroid hormones (for example, thyroid hormone).

	Peptide Hormone	**Steroid Hormone**
Chemical Class	Hydrophilic	Hydrophobic
Synthesis	Made in RER, Golgi apparatus	Made from cholesterol in SER
Storage	Stored in vesicles	Secreted right away; no storage
Blood travel	Dissolve in the plasma (because they are hydrophilic)	Travel in the blood bound to proteins (because they are hydrophobic)
Receptor binding	Bind to receptors on surface of the target cell; because they are hydrophilic, they cannot diffuse across the plasma membrane	Diffuse across the plasma membrane and bind to receptors in the cytoplasm of the target cell
Effect on target	Induce second messenger cascades that result in modifying the existing enzymes and proteins	Go to nucleus and alter transcription; change amount and types of proteins in the target cell
Length of effect	Rapid but short-lived	Slow but long-lasting

Table 3   Key Features of Peptides vs. Steroid Hormones

Organization and Regulation of the Endocrine System

The endocrine system has many different roles. Hormones are essential for gamete synthesis, ovulation, pregnancy, growth, sexual development, and overall level of metabolic activity. Despite this diversity of function, endocrine activity is harmoniously orchestrated. Regulation of the endocrine system is generally automatic and relies on feedback regulation.

An example of feedback regulation is the interaction between the hormone **calcitonin** and serum $[Ca^{2+}]$. The function of calcitonin is to prevent serum $[Ca^{2+}]$ from peaking above normal levels, and the amount of calcitonin secreted is directly proportional to increases in serum $[Ca^{2+}]$ above normal. When serum $[Ca^{2+}]$ becomes elevated, calcitonin is secreted. Then when serum $[Ca^{2+}]$ levels fall, calcitonin secretion stops. The falling serum $[Ca^{2+}]$ level (*that which is regulated*) feeds back to the cells which secrete calcitonin (*regulators*). The serum $[Ca^{2+}]$ level is a physiological endpoint which must be maintained at constant levels. This demonstrates the role of the endocrine system in maintaining homeostasis, or physiological consistency.

An advantage of the endocrine system and its feedback regulation is that very complex arrays of variables can be controlled automatically. It's as if the variables controlled themselves. However, some integration (a central control mechanism) is necessary. Superimposed upon the hormonal regulation of physiological endpoints is another layer of regulation: hormones that regulate hormones. Such meta-regulators are known as **tropic hormones**.

For example, **adrenocorticotropic hormone (ACTH)** is secreted by the anterior pituitary. The role of ACTH is to stimulate increased activity of the portion of the adrenal gland called the **adrenal cortex**, which is responsible for secreting cortisol (among other steroid hormones). ACTH is a tropic hormone because it does not directly affect physiological endpoints, but merely regulates another regulator (cortisol). Cortisol regulates physiological endpoints, including cellular responses to stress and serum [glucose]. Feedback regulation applies to tropic hormones as well as to direct regulators of physiological endpoints; the level of ACTH is influenced by the level of cortisol. When cortisol is needed, ACTH is secreted, and when the serum [cortisol] increases sufficiently, ACTH secretion slows.

You may have noticed that in both of our examples, the effect of feedback was inhibitory: the result of hormone secretion inhibits further secretion. Inhibitory feedback is called **negative feedback** or **feedback inhibition**. Most feedback in the endocrine system (and if you remember, most biochemical feedback) is negative. There are few exceptions (examples of **positive feedback**), which will be reviewed later in this chapter.

There is a final layer of control. Many functions of the endocrine system depend on instructions from the brain. The portion of the brain which controls much of the endocrine system is the **hypothalamus**, located at the center of the brain. The hypothalamus controls the endocrine system by releasing tropic hormones that regulate other tropic hormones, called **releasing and inhibiting factors** or **releasing and inhibiting hormones**.

For example (Figure 8), the hypothalamus secretes corticotropin releasing hormone (CRH, also known as CRF, where "F" stands for factor). The role of CRH is to cause increased secretion of ACTH. Just as ACTH secretion is regulated by feedback inhibition from cortisol, CRH secretion, too, is inhibited by cortisol. You begin to see that regulatory pathways in the endocrine system can get pretty complex.

8.3

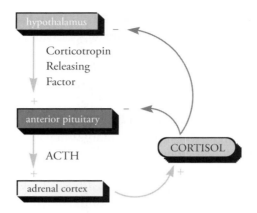

Figure 8   Feedback Regulation of Cortisol Secretion

Understanding that the hypothalamus controls the anterior pituitary and that the anterior pituitary controls most of the endocrine system is important. Damage to the connection between the hypothalamus and the pituitary is fatal, unless daily hormone replacement therapy is given. This endocrine control center is given a special name: **hypothalamic-pituitary control axis** (Figure 9). The hypothalamus exerts its control of the pituitary by secreting its hormones into the bloodstream, just like any other endocrine gland; what's unique is that a special miniature circulatory system is provided for efficient transport of hypothalamic releasing and inhibiting factors to the anterior pituitary. This blood supply is known as the **hypothalamic-pituitary portal system**.

One more bit of background information is necessary before we can delve into specific hormones. The pituitary gland has two halves: front (anterior) and back (posterior); see Figure 9. The **anterior pituitary** is also called the **adenohypophysis** and the **posterior pituitary** is also known as the **neurohypophysis**. It is important to understand the difference. The anterior pituitary is a normal endocrine gland, and it is controlled by hypothalamic releasing and inhibiting factors (essentially tropic hormones). The posterior pituitary is composed of axons which descend from the hypothalamus. These hypothalamic neurons that send axons down to the posterior pituitary are an example of **neuroendocrine cells**, neurons which secrete hormones into the bloodstream.

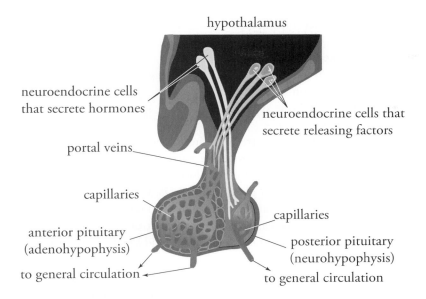

Figure 9   The Hypothalamic-Pituitary Control Axis

Principal Endocrine Organs

There are eight major endocrine glands in humans: pancreas, adrenal glands, thyroid gland, parathyroid glands, hypothalamus, pituitary, ovaries, and testes. This is not an exhaustive list; there are other organs (such as the thymus, heart, and kidney) that can also be classified as endocrine glands, but these will not be focused on here. In this section, we will focus on the six major endocrine glands, discussing the hormones they release and how this affects human physiology and homeostasis. The sexual hormones of the ovaries and testes and control of reproduction will be covered later in this chapter.

Pancreas

The **pancreas** is both an endocrine gland and an exocrine gland. It is an exocrine organ because it secretes digestive enzymes and bicarbonate into the lumen of the duodenum. Exocrine secretions of the pancreas come from acinar cells and empty via ducts into the gastrointestinal tract. The pancreas is an endocrine organ because it secretes hormones, three of which are **insulin, glucagon,** and **somatostatin**. All three are secreted by pancreatic islet cells located in the **islets of Langerhans**. Insulin (secreted by the β cells) and glucagon (secreted by the α cells) regulate glucose transport, storage, and metabolism. Somatostatin (secreted by the δ cells) inhibits many digestive processes.

Glucose in our body comes from two major sources. First, polysaccharides that we eat are chemically broken down and then absorbed by the gastrointestinal tract. Second, glucose can be produced by the liver and released into the blood. In the absence of insulin, all body cells—except those of the brain and liver—are relatively impermeable to glucose. Glucose in the blood tends to remain in the blood when insulin secretion is low. When insulin secretion is high, however, circulating glucose is taken up by cells throughout the body, lowering blood glucose levels. The cells that receive the glucose either store it or metabolize it to produce ATP. It is important to note that the brain takes up glucose from the blood whether or not insulin is secreted. When the liver takes up glucose, it converts large quantities of it to **glycogen**, a long carbohydrate polymer that serves as a storage form of glucose. This biochemical process is called **glycogenesis**.

Overall, insulin has four main functions in the human body. These are:

1. increasing cellular uptake of glucose
2. promoting formation of glycogen from glucose in the liver
3. reducing glucose concentration in the blood
4. increasing protein and triglyceride synthesis

In many respects, glucagon has effects that are opposite to the those of insulin; glucagon promotes the breakdown of glycogen in the liver through a process termed **glycogenolysis**. The breakdown of glycogen produces glucose, which is, in turn, released into the blood. Glucagon also promotes the manufacture of glucose in the liver through a process called **gluconeogenesis**. Gluconeogenesis involves the synthesis of glucose—not from glycogen, but from lactate, amino acids, and triglycerides. This newly formed glucose is also released into the blood. The most easily detectable effect of glucagon, therefore, is an increase of the blood's glucose levels. Glucagon also increases **lipolysis** (lipid breakdown). It is important to note that glucagon does not decrease cellular uptake of glucose.

In the service of homeostasis, a high blood glucose level normally stimulates the secretion of insulin. The insulin causes the body cells to take up glucose, thus lowering the blood glucose level. A low blood glucose level tends to decrease insulin secretion and raise glucagon secretion. The increased glucagon secretion causes the release of glucose from the liver and raises the blood glucose level.

Hyperglycemia refers to excessively high levels of glucose in the blood and is typically due to diminished insulin secretion or activity. **Hypoglycemia** refers to excessively low levels of glucose in the blood and may result from elevated levels of insulin or insufficient glucagon levels in the body.

Adrenal Glands

An **adrenal gland** sits on each kidney; humans have a left and a right adrenal gland. Each gland has two distinct regions that are developmentally and functionally distinct. The two regions are related more in name than in function, and are termed the adrenal cortex and the **adrenal medulla**.

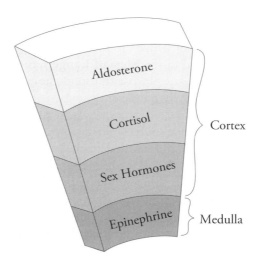

Figure 10   The Adrenal Gland and the Hormones It Releases

Adrenal Cortex

The adrenal cortex is the outer portion of the adrenal gland. It produces a class of endocrine hormones called corticosteroids, which are subdivided into three groups: the **mineralocorticoids**, the **glucocorticoids**, and the **sex hormones**.

Mineralocorticoids affect levels of the minerals sodium and potassium in the body. The main mineralocorticoid secreted by the adrenal cortex is the steroid hormone **aldosterone**, which acts primarily at the distal convoluted tubule of the kidney. Aldosterone increases the interstitial concentration of solutes, and so promotes the movement of water from tubule to interstitium. The ultimate effects of aldosterone are to increase:

1. urinary excretion of potassium
2. interstitial sodium concentration
3. water conservation (as an effect secondary to the increase of interstitial sodium concentration)

As a result, it is not surprising that aldosterone secretion is stimulated by high levels of extracellular potassium, low levels of extracellular sodium, and low fluid levels (blood volume).

The glucocorticoids affect plasma glucose concentrations. They have a wide range of effects on many organ systems. One such effect is similar to that of glucagon: they increase blood glucose levels, especially in response to environmental stressors. The glucocorticoids also strengthen cardiac muscle contractions, increase water retention, and have anti-inflammatory and anti-allergic activities. The main glucocorticoid secreted by the adrenal cortex is the steroid hormone **cortisol**. Cortisol is released as part of the long-term stress response and affects most tissues in the body. It increases plasma glucose levels (mainly via increasing gluconeogenesis), and inhibits immune activity. Cortisol release is controlled by the hypothalamus and the anterior pituitary, and cortisol causes negative feedback to both these areas of the brain.

Finally, the adrenal cortex secretes low levels of the sex steroids, mostly the androgens (the sex hormones that are dominant in men). The adrenal cortex is the main source of androgens in women (since women have no testes) and plays a role in sex drive.

Adrenal Medulla

The adrenal medulla secretes **catecholamines**, mostly **epinephrine** (also known as **adrenaline**). Epinephrine is an amino acid derivative that acts like a peptide hormone. Receptors for norepinephrine and epinephrine are widely distributed throughout the body. It is normally released in very small quantities and is largely reserved for stressful situations in which the body prepares for the so-called "fight or flight" response. In general, epinephrine increases heart rate, raises blood pressure, and increases alertness.

Thyroid

The **thyroid** is a flat gland located in the neck, in front of the larynx. It synthesizes and secretes two hormones: calcitonin and the thyroid hormones.

Thyroid hormones include **thyroxine** (also known as thyroid hormone, T4) or its analog, **triiodothyronine** (thyroid hormone, T3). Most cells of the body have receptors for thyroxine and triiodothyronine. Both of these hormones are synthesized in the follicles of the thyroid gland from the amino acid tyrosine.

8.3

Although thyroid hormones are amino acid derivatives, they are hydrophobic, travel in the plasma bound to plasma proteins, and affect target cells by binding receptors in the nucleus. Overall, thyroid hormones act like steroid hormones.

Thyroxine contains four atoms of iodine, while triiodothyronine contains three atoms of iodine. Thyroid hormones produce a generalized increase in metabolism throughout the body; they stimulate increased oxygen demand and heat production as well as growth and development. The release of thyroid hormones is controlled by the hypothalamus and anterior pituitary.

Hypothyroidism refers to an inadequate production of thyroid hormone. A patient with hypothyroidism tends to be overweight and slowed down in physical (and sometimes mental) activities. Although rare in areas where modern medicine is available, **cretinism** arises from a deficiency of thyroid hormone in the first six months of life.

Thyroid hormones require iodine. Insufficient dietary iodine intake produces a decrease in thyroid hormone production. A feedback mechanism stimulates the thyroid to increase its function, and as a result, the thyroid undergoes excessive growth (hypertrophy), producing the condition known as **goiter**. Goiter manifests as a large prominence in the anterior aspect of the neck. The prominence is the overgrown thyroid itself.

The peptide hormone calcitonin is produced in the **parafollicular cells** of the thyroid. Calcitonin reduces blood calcium concentration and inhibits the normal process of bone resorption. It has the opposite effect as parathyroid hormone.

Parathyroid Glands

The parathyroids are a set of four small glands located on the posterior aspect of the thyroid gland. The peptide hormone **parathyroid hormone** (**PTH**, also known as **parathormone**) exerts effects opposite to those of calcitonin. It is secreted in response to low blood levels of calcium, and through actions on various organs, it increases levels of blood calcium. It acts to:

1. increase bone resorption and consequent calcium release
2. increase intestinal calcium uptake
3. promote calcium re-uptake at the kidney

Hypothalamus

The hypothalamus is a portion of the diencephalon of the forebrain. It releases several hormones that control secretions from the pituitary gland. The hypothalamus provides neural input and central control of the endocrine glands outside of the brain. The hypothalamus serves as a high-level coordinating and regulating center for both the endocrine system and the autonomic nervous system. It integrates a variety of information from the **cerebral cortex** and **limbic systems**, and regulates output from the pituitary glands.

Pituitary Gland

The pituitary gland is a small structure on the underside of the brain; like the hypothalamus, it is part of the diencephalon of the forebrain. The pituitary gland has two halves. The front half is called the anterior pituitary and the back half is called the posterior pituitary.

Anterior Pituitary

The anterior pituitary secretes six peptide hormones you should be familiar with. Four of them play a key role in controlling other endocrine secretions; these tropic hormones act as chemical switches, stimulating or inhibiting other endocrine glands:

1. **Thyroid-stimulating hormone (TSH)**: Stimulates the thyroid gland to secrete thyroid hormone.
2. Adrenocorticotropic hormone (ACTH): Stimulates the adrenal cortex to secrete cortisol.
3. **Luteinizing hormone (LH)**: Stimulates the gonads (ovaries or testes) to promote sex hormone secretion and gamete production.
4. **Follicle stimulating hormone (FSH)**: Stimulates the gonads (ovaries or testes) to promote sex hormone secretion and gamete production.

In addition to hormones that regulate the release of other hormones at a distant gland, the anterior pituitary secretes two other hormones that interact directly with certain target organs:

5. **Growth hormone (GH)**: Influences the development of skeletal muscle, bone, and organs in infants and children. Without growth hormone, children fail to develop normally. GH is also known as **somatotropin (STH).**
6. **Prolactin**: Directly targets the female breasts, where it stimulates breast development and milk production.

Posterior Pituitary

The posterior pituitary secretes two peptide hormones. These hormones are not synthesized in the posterior pituitary; they are made in neural soma in the hypothalamus and transported via vesicles down axons to the posterior pituitary. They are stored in the posterior pituitary, from which they are released directly into the bloodstream as needed. The two hormones secreted by the posterior pituitary are:

1. **Antidiuretic hormone (ADH)**: Causes the kidney to retain water during times of thirst. It is also known as **vasopressin.**
2. **Oxytocin**: Released at childbirth (parturition), causing the uterus to contract and push the fetus through the birth canal. It also causes milk letdown for nursing.

Gland	Hormone (class)	Target/effect
Hypothalamus	releasing and inhibiting factors (peptides)	anterior pituitary/modify activity
Anterior pituitary	growth hormone (GH) (peptide)	↑ bone & muscle growth, ↑ cell turnover rate
	prolactin (peptide)	mammary gland/milk production
tropic	thyroid stimulating hormone (TSH) (peptide)	thyroid/↑ synthesis & release of TH
	adrenocorticotropic hormone (ACTH) (peptide)	↑ growth & secretory activity of adrenal cortex
gonadotropic	luteinizing hormone (LH) (peptide)	ovary/ovulation, testes/testosterone synth.
	follicle stimulating hormone (FSH) (peptide)	ovary/follicle development, testes/spermatogenesis
Posterior pituitary	antidiuretic hormone (ADH, vasopressin) (peptide)	kidney/water retention
	oxytocin (peptide)	breast/milk letdown, uterus/contraction
Thyroid	thyroid hormone (TH, thyroxine) (modified amino acid)	child: necessary for physical & mental development; adult: ↑ metabolic rate and temp.
thyroid C cells	calcitonin (peptide)	bone, kidney; lowers serum $[Ca^{2+}]$
Parathyroids	parathyroid hormone (PTH) (peptide)	bone, kidney, small intestine/raises serum $[Ca^{2+}]$
Thymus	thymosin (children only) (peptide)	T cell development during childhood
Adrenal medulla	epinephrine (modified amino acid)	sympathetic stress response (rapid)
Adrenal cortex	cortisol ("glucocorticoid") (steroid)	long-term stress response; ↑ blood [glucose]; ↑ protein catabolism; ↓ inflammation and immunity
	aldosterone ("mineralocorticoid") (steroid)	kidney/↑ Na^+ reabsorption to ↑ blood pressure
	sex steroids	not normally important, but an adrenal tumor can overproduce these, causing masculinization or feminization
Endocrine pancreas (islets of Langerhans)	insulin (β cells secrete) (peptide)—absent or ineffective in diabetes mellitus	↓ blood [glucose]/↑ glycogen and fat storage
	glucagon (α cells secrete) (peptide)	↑ blood [glucose]/↓ glycogen and fat storage
	somatostatin (SS—δ cells secrete) (peptide)	inhibits many digestive processes
Testes	testosterone (steroid)	male characteristics, spermatogenesis
Ovaries/placenta	estrogen (steroid)	female characteristics, endometrial growth
	progesterone (steroid)	endometrial secretion, pregnancy
Heart	atrial natriuretic factor (ANF) (peptide)	kidney/↑ urination to ↓ blood pressure
Kidney	erythropoietin (peptide)	bone marrow/↑ RBC synthesis

Table 4   Summary of the Hormones of the Endocrine System

8.4 INTEGUMENTARY SYSTEM

Structure and Layers of the Skin

The skin is the largest organ in the body, by size and by weight (Figure 11). Its role is to protect us from pathogens, to prevent excessive evaporation of water, and to regulate body temperature. The outermost layer of the skin is called the **epidermis**; it lies upon the deeper **dermis**, which rests on **subcutaneous tissue** or **hypodermis**. The hypodermis is a protective, insulating layer of fat (adipose tissue).

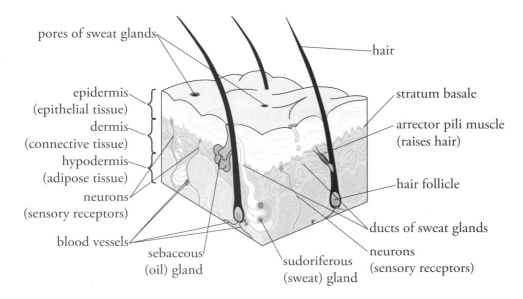

Figure 11   Skin Layers

The epidermis is composed of stratified (many layers of) squamous epithelial cells. These cells are constantly sloughed off and then replenished by mitosis of cells at the deepest part of the epidermis, the **stratum basale**. A cell in this layer divides, and one of the resulting daughter cells moves outward. Soon this cell will die and be pushed farther and farther outward by continued mitosis below, until it flakes away from the surface of the body. The significance of many layers of epithelial cells is that they provide a strong protective structure.

Another important facet of the stratified squamous cells of the epidermis is that they are **keratinized**. This means that as they die, they become filled with a thick coating of the tough, hydrophobic protein **keratin**. Keratin helps make the skin waterproof.

Epidermal epithelial cells also contain **melanin**. This is a brown pigment, produced by **melanocytes,** specialized cells in the epidermis. Melanin helps absorb the ultraviolet light of the Sun to prevent damage to underlying tissue.

8.4

Beneath the epidermis lies the **dermis**. The dermis consists of various cell types embedded in a connective tissue matrix. It contains blood vessels that nourish both the dermis and the epidermis (the epidermis has no blood vessels of its own). The dermis also contains **sensory receptors**, which convey information about touch, pressure, pain, and temperature to the central nervous system. Also found in the dermis are **sudoriferous (sweat) glands**, **sebaceous (oil) glands**, and **hair follicles**. Hairs consist of dead epithelial cells bound tightly together. Some specialized regions of skin contain **ceruminous (wax) glands** (e.g., external ear canal).

The sudoriferous gland is composed of a tube-like structure that originates in the dermis and leads through the epidermis to a pore on the surface of the skin. The purpose of sweat is to allow loss of excess heat by evaporation. Sweat contains water, electrolytes, and urea. Sweat glands are responsive to aldosterone. People living in hot climates must sweat a lot. In order to conserve sodium, they have a high level of aldosterone, and thus their sweat does not waste salt.

Temperature Regulation by the Skin

Humans are **homeotherms**, meaning our body temperature is relatively constant. Heat is generated by metabolic processes and muscle contraction. We have four strategies to cope with cold weather:

1. Contraction of skeletal muscles produces heat, whether it is involuntary (shivering) or voluntary (jumping up and down).
2. Our skin insulates us so that we conserve heat generated by metabolism. Subcutaneous (beneath the skin) tissue contains a layer of insulating fat, which helps.
3. Heat loss by conduction is minimized by constriction of blood vessels in the dermis; this is called **cutaneous vasoconstriction** and occurs in response to cold weather or upon activation of the sympathetic nervous system. This is why the skin becomes cold and pale when one is frightened.
4. We use items like clothing and blankets to help us conserve heat.

A mechanism for dissipation of excess heat is also necessary. This is accomplished by two mechanisms in the skin:

1. Sweating allows heat loss by evaporation.
2. Dilation of blood vessels in the dermis (**cutaneous vasodilation**) results in heat loss by conduction.

8.5 NERVOUS SYSTEM AND SENSES

The Neuron

Nerves, ganglia, and the brain are composed of clusters of nerve cells, or **neurons.**

Neuron Structure and Function

The neuron is the fundamental cellular unit of the nervous system. In addition to the organelles normally found in eukaryotic cells, the neuron contains a number of unique organelles specialized for the transmission of electrical impulses. Cytoplasmic extensions of the cell, called **dendrites**, act like antennae, or sensors: they receive stimuli. A single, elongated cytoplasmic extension, known as the **axon** (or nerve fiber), is specialized to transmit signals. The distal end of the axon bears small extensions called **synaptic terminals**, which contain **synaptic vesicles**. The synaptic vesicles store **neurotransmitters**, the molecules that transmit chemical signals from one neuron to the next. In some situations, a neurotransmitter will exert an excitatory effect on a neuron, while in others, it will have an inhibitory effect.

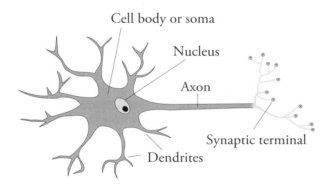

Figure 12   Specialized Features of the Neuron

Neuronal Resting Potential

Like all human cells, neurons express and constantly operate an energy-dependent sodium-potassium pump (Na^+/K^+ ATPase) that moves two potassium ions into the cell and three sodium ions out of the cell, across the plasma membrane. Across the neuronal membrane, then, there exists an imbalance of ion concentrations and an imbalance of charge. As in other cells:

1. Na^+ concentration is higher outside the cell than inside.
2. K^+ concentration is higher inside the cell than outside.
3. The cell's interior cell is electrically negative relative to its exterior.

In an ordinary motor neuron, the imbalance of charge (or the charge gradient) gives the neuronal interior a charge of approximately –70 millivolts (mV) relative to the exterior. For that reason, we say that such a neuron's **resting membrane potential** (**RMP**) is approximately –70 millivolts.

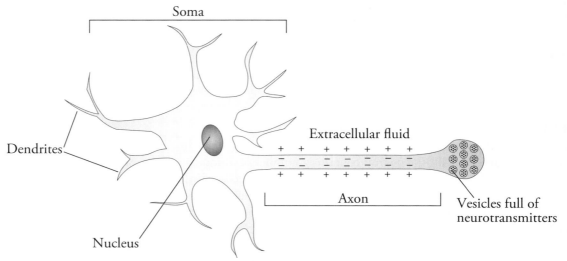

Figure 13   The Interior of a Resting Neuron Is Negative Relative to Its Exterior

Action Potential

Initiation

When a neuron is in its resting, unexcited state, its membrane is largely impermeable to sodium and somewhat permeable to potassium due to the presence of **potassium leak channels.** If some electrical, chemical, or mechanical event causes the dendritic membrane to increase its sodium permeability, sodium ions flow down their gradient and into the cell.

Since sodium ions are positively charged, their inward movement tends also to eliminate the membrane's charge gradient, and the cell's interior thus begins to lose its relative negativity. As the electrical potential within the cell rises from its resting potential of –70 mV toward zero, it crosses a critical **threshold** (–50 mV). When the internal charge reaches the threshold potential, **voltage-gated sodium channels** open.

Voltage-Gated Sodium Channels and Depolarization

Voltage-gated sodium channels are membrane channels, composed of a protein complex. They open and close in response to changes in membrane potential. Voltage-gated sodium channels have three conformations:

1. Closed: In this conformation, the channel does not allow sodium into the cell.
2. Open: In this conformation, the channel is activated and open wide, which allows sodium into the cell. The channel opens when the plasma membrane reaches the threshold potential of –50 mV.
3. Inactivated: When the cell has **depolarized** to +35 mV, the voltage-gated sodium channels inactivate. In this conformation, they do not allow sodium into the cell but they are also unable to open. The channel must be reset to the closed conformation before they can open again, which occurs during the absolute refractory period.

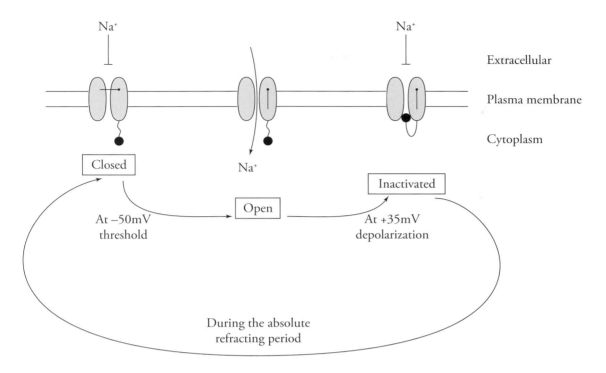

Figure 14   The Voltage-Gated Sodium Channel

When voltage-gated sodium channels are wide open, sodium ions pour into the cell, rapidly raising the potential of the interior above zero to approximately +35 mV. This reversal of membrane potential from –70 mV to +35 mV (due to the influx of sodium ions through the voltage-gated sodium channels) constitutes the first part of an **action potential.**

The depolarization just described occurs at one small portion of the dendritic membrane. Yet the whole of the neuronal membrane, from dendrite through distal axon, houses voltage-gated sodium channels. When depolarization occurs at some small area of the dendrite, electrical positivity at that small area causes nearby sodium channels to open as well. Sodium rushes into an adjacent portion of the cell, and that portion of the cell depolarizes as well. The positive charge in that portion causes sodium channels in the next nearby region to open wide, and so that region, too, undergoes depolarization. The whole process propagates itself rapidly down the neuron from dendrite to axon, and in this way, the whole neuron fires an action potential.

It is frequently said that neurons discharge according to an "all-or-nothing" rule, meaning that neurons do not have the capacity to fire with variable intensity. A neuron has no option to fire strongly or weakly. In other words, it cannot depolarize more or less. Neurons either fire an action potential (from –70 mV to +35 mV) or they do not. Whether or not a neuron generates an action potential depends on whether the initial increase in sodium permeability at the dendrite (however it is caused) produces sufficient change in the membrane potential to reach the threshold. If it does not, then the voltage-gated sodium channels remain closed and no dramatic depolarization occurs. If membrane potential does rise to threshold level (–50 mV), sodium channels open and dramatic depolarization occurs at a small site and rapidly propagates itself along the whole neuron.

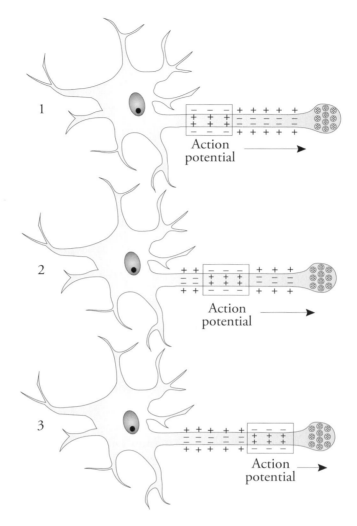

Figure 15   Propagation of a Nerve Impulse Along the Axon

Voltage-Gated Potassium Channels and Repolarization

At the peak of an action potential (when the cell potential is +35mV), voltage-gated sodium channels become inactivated. At just about the same time, **voltage-gated potassium channels** have finished opening up; they actually start doing this around –50mV but take a while to complete the process. With the potassium channels open, potassium ions rush out of the cell along their concentration gradient (created initially by the sodium-potassium ATPase pump).

By moving outward across the neuronal cell membrane, positively charged potassium ions reduce electrical potential within the cell. The cell's interior once again becomes negative and is then said to be **repolarized.** During this time, the voltage-gated sodium channels are resetting from the inactivated state back to closed. When the potential of the cell reaches –70mV once again, the voltage-gated potassium channels close. However, there is a delay between when these channels should close and when they actually close; voltage-gated potassium channels are effectively slow to open and slow to close. Because the voltage-gated potassium channels stay open a little too long, too many potassium ions flow out of the cell and the potential drops to approximately –90mV. During this time, the cell is said to be **hyperpolarized.**

After the voltage-gated potassium channels close, the sodium-potassium ATPase and the potassium leak channels steadily bring the membrane back to the resting potential of –70mV.

The phrase "action potential" is therefore used to describe a combination of two sequential events:

1. depolarization (–70mV to +35mV) due to sodium inflow
2. repolarization (+35mV to –70mV) due to potassium outflow

Refractory Periods

From +35 mV to –70 mV, the neuron cannot fire an additional action potential. This is called the **absolute refractory period** and arises because sodium channels are inactivated and cannot reopen until they have reset (or undergo a conformational switch from inactive form to the closed conformation).

Just after the cell passes the –70mV threshold and is hyperpolarized due to the delay of the voltage-gated potassium channels, the cell is susceptible to another action potential but requires a stimulus stronger than the one normally needed by a resting cell. This phenomenon, called the **relative refractory period,** arises because the potential of the cell is below that of a resting cell.

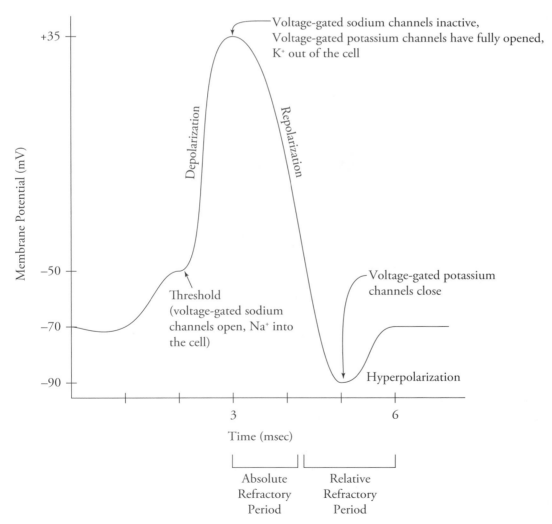

Figure 16   Principal Stages and Ion Flows Associated with an Action Potential

Saltatory Conduction: Myelin Sheath

Certain neurons can conduct an impulse faster and more efficiently due to **myelination** of their axons. **Schwann cells** encase long, discrete sections of the axons of neurons in the **peripheral nervous system (PNS)** by wrapping layers of their plasma membranes around the axon, creating **myelin sheaths**. A similar function is served by **oligodendrocytes** in the **central nervous system (CNS).** Small areas of the axon remain unmyelinated at regular intervals along the axon's length. These unsheathed areas are called the **nodes of Ranvier.** The highly insulating properties of the myelin serve to block transmission of the depolarizing nerve impulse where myelin sheaths cover the axon, leaving the exposed nodes of Ranvier as the only sites available for electrical propagation along the axon. It is not necessary, then, for depolarization to occur along the entire membrane, a process that would consume a relatively long period of time. Myelin insulation significantly accelerates transmission of an impulse as depolarization jumps from one node of Ranvier to the next (**saltatory conduction**), effectively skipping across the long, insulated portions of the axon.

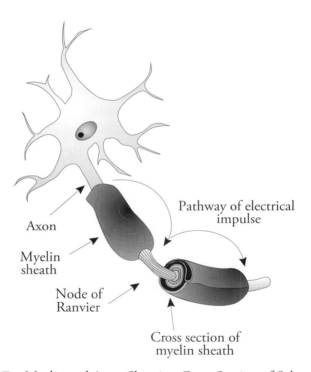

Figure 17   Myelinated Axon Showing Cross Section of Schwann Cell Layers

Schwann cells and oligodendrocytes are types of glial cells: specialized, non-neuronal cells that provide structural and metabolic support to neurons. Glia maintain a resting membrane potential but do not generate action potentials. There are several types:

Cell Type	Location	Primary Functions
Schwann cells	PNS	Form myelin, increase action potential conduction speed along axons
Satellite cells	PNS	Cover the surface of neuron cell bodies in ganglia of the PNS
Oligodendrocytes	CNS	Form myelin, increase action potential conduction speed along axons
Microglia	CNS	Remove dead cells and debris
Ependymal cells	CNS	Produce and circulate cerebrospinal fluid
Astrocytes	CNS	Maintain the blood-brain barrier, guide neuronal development, regulate synaptic communication via regulation of neurotransmitter levels

Table 5   Types of Glial Cells and Their Functions

8.5

Impulse Transmission at the Synapse

When the action potential impulse arrives at the end of the axon, it triggers **voltage-gated calcium channels** to open; Ca^{2+} flows into the cell, binds with regulatory proteins and causes exocytosis of neurotransmitter-containing synaptic vesicles. The vesicles fuse with the plasma membrane and neurotransmitter molecules are released from the cell.

The neuron that releases neurotransmitters is called the **presynaptic neuron**. Neurotransmitters are released from synaptic vesicles into the **synaptic cleft**—the space between the presynaptic membrane and the postsynaptic membrane. At the **synapse**, the distance between the two cells is minute enough to permit rapid diffusion of a neurotransmitter from the first neuron to either a second neuron or a tissue such as a muscle, gland, or organ. Synaptic transmission is the way in which a neuron can communicate with another cell.

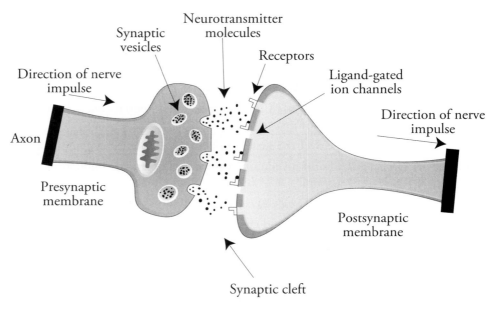

Figure 18

After neurotransmitters diffuse across the synaptic cleft, they bind to receptors on the postsynaptic membrane. These receptors are specific to the neurotransmitter. Each postsynaptic neuron can receive signals from many presynaptic neurons, each releasing a different neurotransmitter. For this reason, postsynaptic neurons express receptors for many types of neurotransmitters.

Most postsynaptic receptors are **ligand-gated ion channels**, with specific neurotransmitters serving as ligands. Binding of the neurotransmitter to its receptor induces a conformational change in the receptors that opens ion channels within the membrane. The resulting influx or efflux of ions produces an electrical change that acts as a signal to the neuron. A signal of sufficient strength to reach threshold level will initiate an action potential (the "all" of the all-or-none reaction).

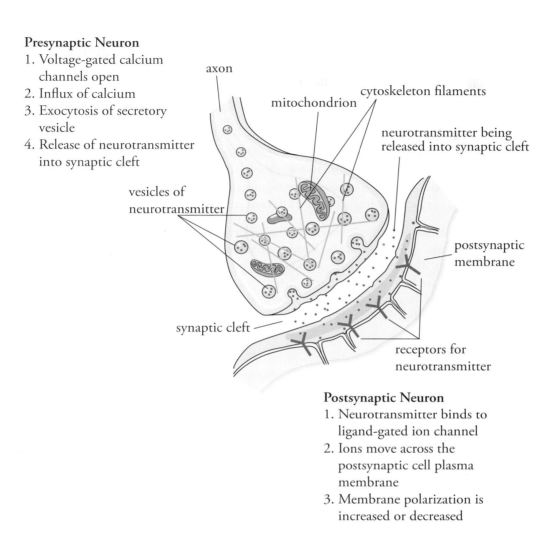

Presynaptic Neuron
1. Voltage-gated calcium channels open
2. Influx of calcium
3. Exocytosis of secretory vesicle
4. Release of neurotransmitter into synaptic cleft

axon

mitochondrion

cytoskeleton filaments

neurotransmitter being released into synaptic cleft

vesicles of neurotransmitter

postsynaptic membrane

synaptic cleft

receptors for neurotransmitter

Postsynaptic Neuron
1. Neurotransmitter binds to ligand-gated ion channel
2. Ions move across the postsynaptic cell plasma membrane
3. Membrane polarization is increased or decreased

Figure 19   A Typical Synapse

The nervous system contains more than 30 different chemicals that act as neurotransmitters; you must be familiar with two of them:

1. **Acetylcholine (ACh)** triggers skeletal muscle contraction and is degraded by the enzyme **acetylcholinesterase.** It is an important parasympathetic neurotransmitter.
2. Epinephrine (also called adrenaline) increases heart rate and blood pressure and decreases metabolic activity, such as that of the smooth muscle of the digestive system. It is an important sympathetic neurotransmitter.

Functional Organization of the Human Nervous System

The nervous system must receive information, decide what to do with it, and cause muscles or glands to act upon that decision. Receiving information is the **sensory** function of the nervous system (carried out by the peripheral nervous system, or PNS), processing the information is the **integrative** function (carried out by the central nervous system, or CNS), and acting on it is the **motor** function (also carried out by the PNS). **Motor neurons** carry information from the nervous system toward organs which can act upon that information, known as **effectors**. Notice that "motor" neurons do not lead only "to muscle." Motor neurons, which carry information away from the central nervous system and innervate effectors, are called **efferent** neurons (remember, efferents go to effectors). **Sensory neurons**, which carry information toward the central nervous system, are called **afferent** neurons.

The main anatomical division of the nervous system is between the central nervous system and the peripheral nervous system. The CNS is the brain and spinal cord. The PNS includes all other axons, dendrites, and cell bodies. The great majority of neuronal cell bodies are found within the central nervous system. Sometimes they are bunched together to form structures called **nuclei.** (Don't confuse this with the nucleic-acid-containing nuclei of cells.) Somas located outside the central nervous system are found in bunches known as **ganglia.** Finally, it is worth noting that most axons in the CNS and PNS are myelinated.

The peripheral nervous system can be subdivided into several functional divisions (Figure 20). The portion of this system concerned with conscious sensation and deliberate, voluntary movement of skeletal muscle is the **somatic** division. The portion concerned with digestion, metabolism, circulation, perspiration, and other involuntary processes is the **autonomic** division. Both the somatic and autonomic divisions include afferent and efferent functions. The efferent portion of the autonomic division is further split into two subdivisions: sympathetic and parasympathetic. When the **sympathetic** system is activated, the body is prepared for "fight or flight." When the **parasympathetic** system is activated, the body is prepared to "rest and digest."

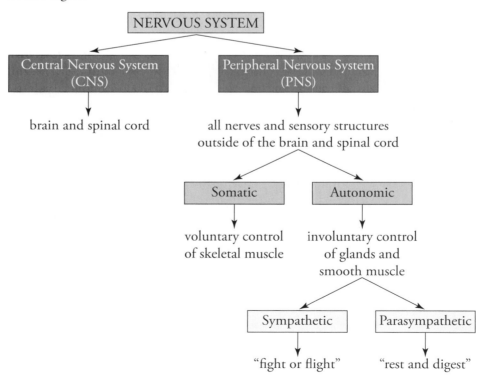

Figure 20 Overall Organization of the Nervous System

Reflexes

The simplest example of nervous system activity is the **reflex**. This is a direct motor response to sensory input which occurs without conscious thought. In fact, it usually occurs without any involvement of the brain at all. In the simplest example, a sensory neuron transmits an action potential to a synapse with a motor neuron in the spinal cord, which causes an action to occur. For example, in the **muscle stretch reflex**, a sensory neuron detects stretching of a muscle (Figure 21). The sensory neuron has a long dendrite and a long axon, which transmits an impulse to a motor neuron cell body in the spinal cord. The motor neuron's long axon synapses with the muscle that was stretched and causes it to contract. That is why the quadriceps (thigh) muscle contracts when the patellar tendon is stretched by tapping with a reflex hammer. A reflex such as this one, involving only two neurons and one synapse, is known as a **monosynaptic reflex arc**.

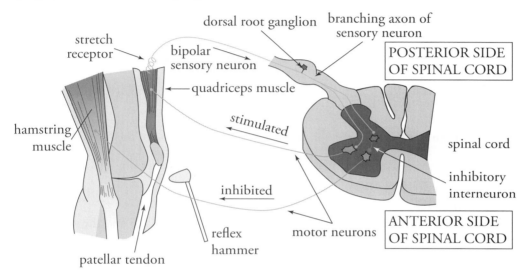

Figure 21　The Muscle Stretch Reflex

Something else also happens when a physician taps the patellar tendon. Not only does the quadriceps *contract*, but the hamstring also *relaxes*. If it did not, the leg would not be able to extend (straighten). The sensory neuron (that detects stretch) synapses not only with a motor neuron for the quadriceps, but also with an **inhibitory interneuron**. This is a short neuron which forms an inhibitory synapse with a motor neuron innervating the hamstring muscle. When the sensory nerve is stimulated by stretch, it stimulates both the quadriceps motor neuron and the inhibitory interneuron to the hamstring motor neuron. As a result, the quadriceps contracts and the hamstring relaxes. An interneuron is the simplest example of the integrative role of the nervous system. Concurrent relaxation of the hamstring and contraction of the quadriceps is an example of **reciprocal inhibition**.

CNS

The CNS includes the **spinal cord** and the brain. The brain has three subdivisions: the **hindbrain** (or the rhombencephalon), the **midbrain** (or the mesencephalon), and the **forebrain** (or the prosencephalon). These four regions of the CNS (which will be discussed individually) perform increasingly complex functions. The entire CNS (brain and spinal cord) floats in **cerebrospinal fluid** (**CSF**), a clear liquid that serves various functions such as shock absorption and exchange of nutrients and waste with the CNS.

8.5

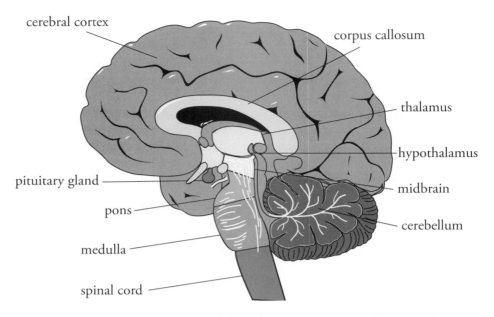

Figure 22   Organization of the CNS (Cross-Section of the Brain)

Regions of the CNS

1.   The spinal cord is connected to the brain and is protected by the CSF and the vertebral column. It is a pathway for information to and from the brain. Most sensory data is relayed to the brain for integration, but the spinal cord is also a site for information integration and processing. The spinal cord is responsible for simple spinal reflexes (like the deep tendon reflex) and is also involved in primitive processes such as walking, urination, and sex organ function.

2.   The hindbrain includes the medulla, the pons, and the cerebellum.
   •   The **medulla** (or medulla oblongata) is located below the pons and is the area of the brain that connects to the spinal cord. It regulates vital autonomic functions such as blood pressure, digestive functions (including vomiting), and respiratory rhythmicity.
   •   The **pons** is located below the midbrain and above the medulla oblongata. It is the connection point between the brain stem and the cerebellum (see Figure 22). The pons controls some autonomic functions and coordinates movement; it plays a role in balance and antigravity posture.
   •   The **cerebellum** (or "little brain") is located behind the pons and below the cerebral hemispheres. It is an integrating center where complex movements are coordinated. Both the cerebellum and the pons receive information from the vestibular apparatus in the inner ear, which monitors acceleration and position relative to gravity.

3.   The midbrain is a relay for visual and auditory information and contains much of the reticular activating system (RAS), which is responsible for arousal or wakefulness.

Another term you should be familiar with is **brainstem**. Together, the medulla, pons and midbrain constitute the brainstem, which contains important processing centers and relays information to or from the cerebellum and cerebrum.

4. The forebrain includes the **diencephalon** and the **telencephalon**.
    a) The diencephalon includes the thalamus and hypothalamus:
    *   The **thalamus** is located near the middle of the brain below the cerebral hemispheres and above the midbrain. It contains relay and processing centers for sensory information.
    *   The hypothalamus interacts directly with many parts of the brain. It contains centers for controlling emotions and autonomic functions, and has a major role in hormone production and release. It is the primary link between the nervous and the endocrine systems. By controlling the pituitary gland, the hypothalamus is the fundamental control center for the endocrine system.
    b) All parts of the CNS up to and including the diencephalon form a single symmetrical stalk, but the telencephalon consists of two separate **cerebral hemispheres**. Generally speaking, the areas of the left and right hemispheres have the same functions. However, the left hemisphere primarily controls the motor functions of the right side of the body, and the right hemisphere controls those of the left side.
    *   The cerebral hemispheres are connected by a thick bundle of axons called the **corpus callosum**. This enables communication between the two hemispheres.

The cerebrum is the largest region of the human brain and consists of large, paired cerebral hemispheres. Each hemisphere consists of the cerebral cortex, an outer layer of gray matter, plus an inner core of white matter. Gray matter is composed of trillions of somas; white matter is composed of myelinated axons.

The cerebral hemispheres are responsible for conscious thought, intellectual functions, and processing. They are divided into four lobes:

*   **Frontal lobes** initiate all voluntary movement and are involved in complex reasoning and problem solving.
*   **Parietal lobes** are involved in general sensations such as touch, temperature, and taste.
*   **Temporal lobes** process auditory and olfactory sensation and are involved in short-term memory.
*   **Occipital lobes** process visual sensation.

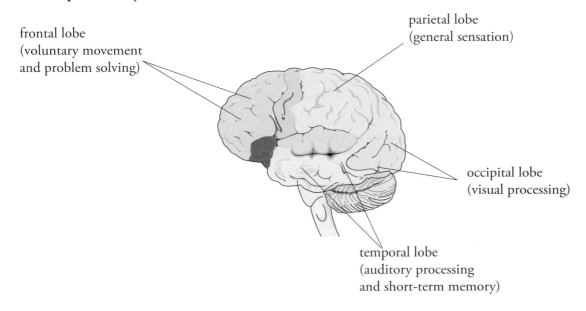

frontal lobe
(voluntary movement
and problem solving)

parietal lobe
(general sensation)

occipital lobe
(visual processing)

temporal lobe
(auditory processing
and short-term memory)

Figure 23   Principal Areas of the Cerebral Cortex

8.5

Structure	General Function	Specific Functions
Spinal cord	Simple reflexes	• controls simple stretch and tendon reflexes • controls primitive processes such as walking, urination, and sex organ function
Medulla	Involuntary functions	• controls autonomic processes such as blood pressure, blood flow, heart rate, respiratory rate, swallowing, vomiting • controls reflex reactions such as coughing or sneezing • relays sensory information to the cerebellum and the thalamus
Pons	Relay station and balance	• controls antigravity posture and balance • connects the spinal cord and medulla with upper regions of the brain • relays information to the cerebellum and thalamus
Cerebellum	Movement coordination	• integrating center • coordination of complex movement, balance and posture, muscle tone, spatial equilibrium
Midbrain	Eye movement	• integration of visual and auditory information • visual and auditory reflexes • wakefulness and consciousness • coordinates information on posture and muscle tone
Thalamus	Integrating center and relay station	• relay center for somatic (conscious) sensation • relays information between the spinal cord and the cerebral cortex
Hypothalamus	Homeostasis and behavior	• controls homeostatic functions (such as temperature regulation, fluid balance, appetite) through both neural and hormonal regulation • controls primitive emotions such as anger, rage, and sex drive • controls the pituitary gland
Basal nuclei	Movement	• regulate body movement and muscle tone • coordination of learned movement patterns • general pattern of rhythm movements (such as controlling the cycle of arm and leg movements when walking) • subconscious adjustments of conscious movements
Limbic system	Emotion, memory, and learning	• controls emotional states • links conscious and unconscious portions of the brain • helps with memory storage and retrieval
Cerebral cortex	Perception, skeletal muscle movement, integration center	• divided into four lobes (frontal, parietal, temporal, and occipital) with specialized subfunctions • conscious through processes and planning, awareness, and sensation • intellectual function (intelligence, learning, reading, communication) • abstract thought and reasoning • memory storage and retrieval • initiation and coordination of voluntary movement • complex motor patterns
Corpus callosum	Connection	• connects the left and right cerebral hemispheres

Table 6   Summary of Brain Functions

PNS

Remember, there are two divisions of the PNS: the somatic system and the autonomic nervous system (ANS). All somatic motor neurons innervate skeletal muscle cells and use acetylcholine as their neurotransmitter. They mediate voluntary control of skeletal muscle.

The ANS controls all involuntary processes that regulate and maintain our systems and processes. The ANS innervates cardiac muscle, smooth muscle, and glands:

- Cardiac muscle is found in your heart.
- Smooth muscle is found in the walls of hollow tubes (e.g., blood vessels, respiratory tract, digestive tract) and hollow organs (e.g., bladder).
- There are several types of glands controlled by the ANS; some examples are sweat glands, glands that release hormones, or glands that release digestive secretions.

The sympathetic system primarily uses the neurotransmitter norepinephrine as it drives the fight or flight response. The parasympathetic system primarily uses acetylcholine as it maintains your rest and digest state. Remember that these two branches of the ANS generally act in opposition to one another; at any given moment, one or the other is active.

The following table summarizes the main effects of the ANS.

Organ or System	Parasympathetic: rest and digest	Sympathetic: fight or flight
digestive system: glands	stimulation	inhibition
motility	stimulation (stimulates digestion)	inhibition (inhibits digestion)
sphincters	relaxation	contraction
urinary system: bladder	contraction (stimulates urination)	relaxation (inhibits urination)
urethral sphincter	relaxation (stimulates urination)	contraction (inhibits urination)
bronchial smooth muscle	constriction (closes airways)	relaxation (opens airways)
cardiovascular system		
heart rate and contractility	decreased	increased
blood flow to skeletal muscle	—	increased
skin	—	sweating and $\uparrow$ blood flow (flushing)
eye: pupil	constriction	dilation
muscles controlling lens	near vision accommodation	accommodation for far vision
adrenal medulla	—	release of epinephrine
genitals	erection / lubrication	ejaculation / orgasm

Table 7 Effects of the Autonomic Nervous System

Adrenal Medulla

The adrenal gland is named for its location: "Ad-" connotes "above," and "renal" refers to the kidney. There are two adrenal glands, one above each kidney. The adrenal has an inner portion known as the medulla and an outer portion known as the cortex. The cortex is an important endocrine gland, secreting glucocorticoids (the main one is cortisol), mineralocorticoids (the main one is aldosterone), and some sex hormones.

The adrenal medulla, however, is part of the sympathetic nervous system. It is embryologically derived from sympathetic postganglionic neurons and is directly innervated by sympathetic preganglionic neurons. Upon activation of the sympathetic system, the adrenal gland is stimulated to release epinephrine, also known as adrenaline. Epinephrine is a slightly modified version of norepinephrine, the neurotransmitter released by sympathetic postganglionic neurons. Epinephrine is a hormone because it is released into the bloodstream by a ductless gland, but in many ways it behaves like a neurotransmitter. It elicits its effects very rapidly, and the effects are quite short-lived. Epinephrine released from the adrenal medulla is what causes the sudden flushing and sweating one experiences when severely startled. In general, epinephrine's effects are those listed in Table 7 for the sympathetic system. Stimulation of the heart is an especially important effect.

Sensory Organs

Humans can respond to five types of stimuli: **tactile** (touch), **olfactory** (smell), **gustatory** (taste), **auditory** (hearing), and visual. Sensory receptors provide an organism with crucial information about its environment. Sensory receptors convey information to the organism in the form of action potentials that carry information to the central nervous system. There are several types of sensory receptors:

1. **Mechanoreceptors** respond to mechanical disturbances. These include **stretch receptors, tactile receptors, proprioceptors** (which provide cues to changes in pressure or tension in muscles), and **auditory receptors.**
2. **Chemoreceptors** respond to particular chemicals, and register taste and smell. For example, the hair-like projections of the **taste receptors**, located in the taste buds, are sensitive to molecules in the mouth. The four basic types of gustatory receptors register sourness, sweetness, saltiness, and bitterness. **Olfactory receptors** are also chemoreceptors. They are located in the olfactory epithelium of the nasal cavity and detect airborne chemicals. Olfactory receptors allow us to smell things.
3. **Thermoreceptors** are stimulated by changes in temperature.
4. **Electromagnetic receptors** are stimulated by electromagnetic waves. In humans, the only examples are **photoreceptors**: rods and cones in the eye. Rods are more sensitive to dim light and are responsible for night vision. Cones require abundant light and are responsible for color and high-acuity vision.
5. **Nociceptors** are pain receptors. They are stimulated by tissue injury.

Modality	Receptor	Receptor type	Organ	Stimulus
Vision	rods and cones	electromagnetic	retina	light
Hearing	auditory hair cells	mechanoreceptor	organ of Corti	vibration
Olfaction	olfactory nerve endings	chemoreceptor	individual neurons	airborne chemicals
Taste	taste cells	chemoreceptor	taste bud	food chemicals
Touch (a few examples)	Pacinian corpuscles free nerve endings temperature receptors	mechanoreceptor nociceptor thermoreceptor	skin	pressure pain temperature
Interoception (two examples)	aortic arch baroreceptors pH receptors	baroreceptor chemoreceptor	aortic arch aortic arch / medulla oblongata	blood pressure pH

Table 8   Summary of Sensation

Vestibular and Auditory Systems

The ear serves two distinct functions: maintenance of postural equilibrium and reception of sound. There are three basic divisions of the ear—inner, external, and middle. The **inner ear** is the location of the **vestibular apparatus**, which interprets positional information required for maintaining equilibrium. The vestibular apparatus consists of three **semicircular canals,** oriented perpendicularly to one another. Movement of the head causes movement of fluid within the canals and displacement of specialized hair cells. This sends sensory impulses via the **vestibular nerve** to centers in the cerebellum, midbrain, and cerebrum, where directional movement and position are interpreted.

The auditory system involves all three divisions of the ear. The external (or outer) ear is composed of the **pinna**, which funnels sound waves into the **ear canal**. At the middle ear, sound waves cause vibrations in the **tympanic membrane**, setting into motion the three auditory bones—the **malleus, incus,** and **stapes**. The arrangement of these bones is like that of levers, so that movement of the malleus is amplified by the incus, and movement of the incus is amplified by the stapes. Movement of the stapes is transmitted across the **oval window** into the inner ear, setting up vibrations in the fluid of the **cochlea**, which causes bending of **auditory hair cells** in the **organ of Corti**.

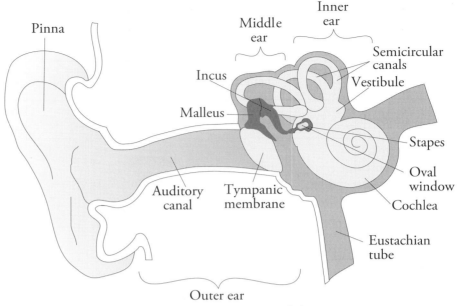

Figure 24 The Structure of the Ear

Summary: From Sound to Hearing
sound waves → auricle → external auditory canal → tympanic membrane → malleus → incus →
stapes → oval window → fluid of the cochlea → auditory hair cells → neurotransmitters stimulate
auditory neurons → brain → perception

Visual System

The eye is designed to detect visual stimuli. The structures of the eye first form an image on the retina, which detects light and converts the stimuli into action potentials to send to the brain. Light enters the eye by passing through the **cornea,** the clear portion at the front of the eye. Light is bent or refracted as it passes through the cornea, which is curved and thus acts as a lens. At its borders, the cornea is continuous with the white of the eye, the **sclera.** Beneath the sclera is a layer called the **choroid.** It contains darkly pigmented cells; this pigmentation absorbs excess light within the eye. Beneath the choroid is the **retina,** the surface upon which light is focused.

Just inside the cornea is a chamber that contains a fluid called **aqueous humor.** Behind this is a membrane called the **iris** with an opening called the **pupil.** The iris is the colored part of the eye, and muscles in the iris regulate the diameter of the pupil. Behind the iris is the **lens.** Its role is to fine-tune the angle of incoming light, so that the beams are perfectly focused upon the retina. The curvature of the lens (and thus its refractive power) is varied by the **ciliary muscle.**

Light passes through another chamber on its way from the lens to the retina. This chamber contains a thick, jelly-like fluid called **vitreous humor.** The retina is located at the back of the eye. It contains electromagnetic receptor cells (photoreceptors) known as rods and cones, which are responsible for detecting light. The rods and cones synapse with neurons that form the optic nerve.

Thus, transmission of light through the human eye follows the following pathway: light enters the cornea, traverses the aqueous humor, passes through the pupil, and proceeds through the lens and the vitreous humor until it reaches the light receptors of the retina. Electrical signals are then transmitted via the **optic nerve** to visual centers in the brain.

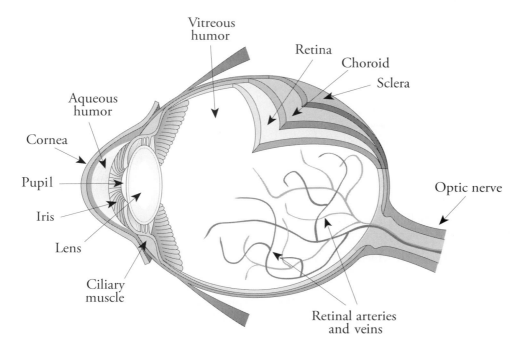

Figure 25   Structure of the Eye

The lens is a transparent structure that focuses light rays on the retina. **Myopia** (nearsightedness) occurs when the lens focuses light from a distant object in front of the retina. **Hyperopia** (farsightedness) occurs when light from a nearby object is focused behind the retina. Normal vision is called **emmetropia.**

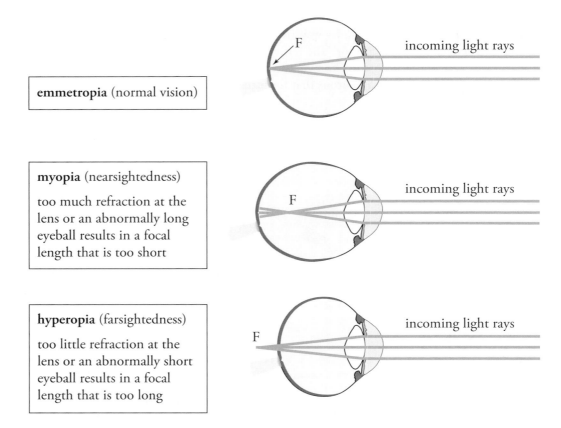

Figure 26 Defects in Visual Acuity ("F" denotes the focal point)

The retina senses light rays with two types of photoreceptors located in its outer layer: **rods**, which are specialized to register dim light, and **cones**, which are specialized to register bright light as well as color. Both rods and cones contain pigments, allowing them to absorb energy from light rays. The pigment that mediates rod reception is **rhodopsin**. Cones are subdivided into three types: red-absorbing, blue-absorbing, and green-absorbing. Light reception in cones is mediated by **opsin**, which is similar to rhodopsin.

8.6 RESPIRATORY SYSTEM

Functions of the Respiratory System

Single-cell eukaryotes that require oxygen to perform oxidative phosphorylation can acquire it by simple diffusion of oxygen from the surrounding medium. Larger organisms, such as the vertebrates, evolved a respiratory system to exchange O_2 and CO_2 between the atmosphere and the blood, and a circulatory system to transport those gases between the respiratory system and the rest of the tissues of the body.

Additional tasks performed by the respiratory system include the following:

1. pH regulation: In the blood, CO_2 is converted to carbonic acid by the RBC enzyme carbonic anhydrase. When CO_2 is exhaled by the lungs, the amount of carbonic acid in the blood is decreased, and as a result the pH of the blood increases (becomes more alkaline). Hence, minute-to-minute variations in respiration affect blood pH. **Hyperventilation** (too much breathing) causes alkalinization of the blood, known as **respiratory alkalosis**. **Hypoventilation** (too little breathing) causes acidification of the blood, or **respiratory acidosis**.
2. Thermoregulation: Breathing results in significant heat loss.
3. Protection from disease and particulate matter: The lungs provide a large moist surface where chemicals and pathogens can do harm. There are two protection mechanisms. First, specialized cells secrete mucus, which traps pathogens and inhaled particles. Other cells have cilia that constantly sweep the layer of mucus up so it is swallowed or coughed out; this is called the **mucociliary escalator.** Second, alveolar macrophages patrol alveoli and engulf foreign particles.

Anatomy of the Respiratory System

Simple movement of air into and out of the lungs is called **ventilation,** whereas the actual exchange of gases (between either lungs and blood, or blood and other tissues of the body) is called **respiration.** Inhaled air follows this pathway:

nose ➔ nasal cavity ➔ pharynx ➔ larynx ➔ trachea ➔ bronchi ➔ terminal bronchioles ➔ respiratory bronchioles ➔ alveolar ducts ➔ alveoli

Parts of the respiratory system that participate only in ventilation are referred to as the **conduction zone;** this starts at the nose and ends at the respiratory bronchioles. The parts that participate in actual gas exchange are referred to as the **respiratory zone;** this starts at respiratory bronchioles and ends at alveoli.

Conduction Zone

The **nose** is important for warming, humidifying, and filtering inhaled air; nasal hairs and sticky mucus act as filters. The **nasal cavity** is an open space within the nose. The **pharynx** is another word for the throat, a common pathway for air and food. The **larynx** has three functions:

1. It is made entirely of cartilage and thus keeps the airway open.
2. It contains the **epiglottis**, which seals the trachea during swallowing to prevent the entry of food.
3. It contains the **vocal cords**, which are folds of tissue positioned to partially block the flow of air and vibrate, thereby producing sound.

The **trachea** is a passageway which must remain open to permit air flow. Rings of cartilage prevent its collapse. The trachea branches into two **primary bronchi**, each of which supplies one lung. Each bronchus branches repeatedly to supply the entire lung. Collapse of bronchi is prevented by small plates of cartilage. Very small bronchi are called **bronchioles**. They are about 1 mm wide and contain no cartilage. Their walls are made of smooth muscle, which allows their diameters to be regulated to adjust airflow into the system. The smallest (and final) branches of the conduction zone are aptly called the **terminal bronchioles**.

The smooth muscle in the walls of terminal bronchioles is too thick to allow adequate diffusion of gases; this is why no gas exchange occurs in this region. The conduction zone is strictly for ventilation.

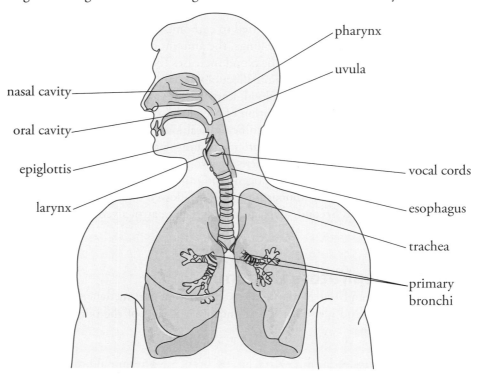

Figure 27   The Conduction Zone

Respiratory Zone

The region of the respiratory system where gas exchange occurs is the respiratory zone (Figure 28). The actual structure across which gases diffuse is called the **alveolus** (plural: **alveoli**). Alveoli are tiny sacs with very thin walls; they're so thin that they're transparent! The wall of the alveolus is only one cell thick, except where capillaries pass across its outer surface. The duct leading to the alveoli is called an **alveolar duct**, and its walls are entirely made of alveoli. The alveolar duct branches off a **respiratory bronchiole**. This is a tube made of smooth muscle, just like the terminal bronchioles, but with one important difference: the respiratory bronchiole has a few alveoli scattered in its walls. This allows it to perform gas exchange, so it is part of the respiratory zone.

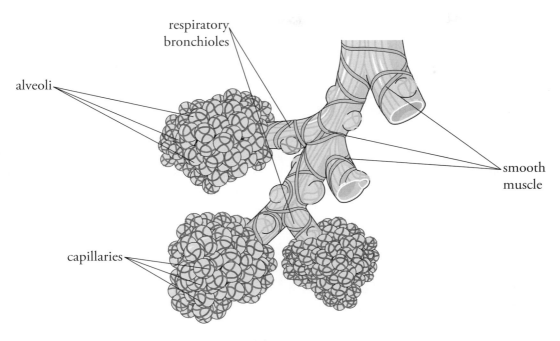

Figure 28   The Respiratory Zone

Surfactant

Imagine a beehive made of tissue paper. If you put it in a steamy bathroom, what would happen? Would all the small air spaces remain filled with air? No, the hive would collapse into a wet ball, because the mutual attraction of water molecules would overcome the flimsy support structure provided by the fine paper fibers. The tendency of water molecules to clump together creates **surface tension**, which is the force that causes wet hydrophilic surfaces (e.g., the tissue paper) to stick together in the presence of air. Think of it this way: air is hydrophobic, so hydrophilic substances in the presence of air tend to clump together. Now imagine a beehive made of thin wax paper. If you put it into a steamy room, does it collapse? No, because the wax on the surface of the paper prevents adjacent pieces of paper from being strongly attracted. In other words, the wax destroys the surface tension.

The alveoli are as fine and delicate as tissue paper, and they too tend to collapse due to surface tension. This problem is solved by a soapy substance called **surfactant** (*surf*ace *act*ive substance), which coats the alveoli. Just like the wax in our example above, surfactant reduces surface tension. Surfactant is a complex mixture of phospholipids, proteins, and ions secreted by cells in the alveolar wall.

Pulmonary Ventilation

Pulmonary ventilation is the circulation of air into and out of the lungs to continually replace the gases in the alveoli with those in the atmosphere. The drawing of air into the lungs is termed **inspiration**, and the movement of air out of the lungs is termed **expiration**. Inspiration is an active process driven by the contraction of the diaphragm, which enlarges the chest cavity (and the lungs along with the chest cavity), drawing air in. Passive expiration is driven by the elastic recoil of the lungs and does not require active muscle contraction. These processes will be described in more detail next.

Inspiration is caused by muscular expansion of the chest wall, which draws the lungs outward (expands them), and causes air to enter the system. Expansion of the chest during inspiration is driven primarily by contraction of the **diaphragm**, a large skeletal muscle that is stretched below the ribs between the abdomen and the chest cavity. The external **intercostal muscles** between the ribs also contract during inspiration, pulling the ribs upward and further expanding the chest cavity. Inspiration is an active process, requiring contraction of muscles to occur.

Resting expiration, by contrast, is a passive process (no muscle contraction required). When the diaphragm and rib muscles relax, the elastic recoil of the lungs draws the chest cavity inward, reducing the volume of the lungs and pushing air out of the system into the atmosphere. During exertion (or at other times when a more forcible exhalation is required), contraction of abdominal muscles helps the expiration process by pressing upward on the diaphragm, further shrinking the size of the lungs and forcing more air out. This is an active process called a **forced expiration**.

Volumes and Capacities

Spirometry is the measurement of the volume of air entering or exiting the lungs at the various stages of ventilation. A **spirometer** is a device used for these measurements. Data can be plotted on a **spirometric graph** (Figure 29).

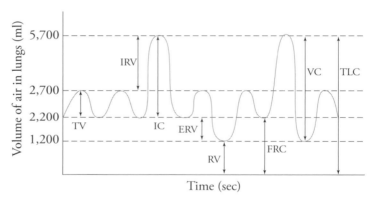

Figure 29   Lung Volumes and Capacities

- **Tidal volume (TV)** is the amount of air that moves in and out of the lungs with normal light breathing and is equal to about 10 percent of the total volume of the lungs (0.5 liters out of 5–6 liters).
- **Expiratory reserve volume (ERV)** is the volume of air that can be expired after a passive resting expiration.
- **Inspiratory reserve volume (IRV)** is the volume of air that can be inspired after a relaxed inspiration.
- **Functional residual capacity (FRC)** is the volume of air left in the lungs after a resting expiration.
- **Inspiratory capacity (IC)** is the maximal volume of air which can be inhaled after a resting expiration.
- **Residual volume (RV)** is the amount of air that remains in the lungs after the strongest possible expiration.
- **Vital capacity (VC)** is the maximum amount of air that can be forced out of the lungs after first taking the deepest possible breath.
- **Total lung capacity (TLC)** is the vital capacity plus the residual volume (TLC = VC + RV).

Gas Exchange

Pulmonary Circulation

Deoxygenated blood is carried toward the lungs by the pulmonary artery, which has left and right branches. These large arteries branch many times, eventually giving rise to a huge network of **pulmonary capillaries**, also called **alveolar capillaries**. Each alveolus is surrounded by a few tiny capillaries, which are just wide enough to permit the passage of RBCs, and have extremely thin walls to permit diffusion of gases between blood and alveolus. The capillaries drain into venules, which drain into the pulmonary veins. The lungs are supplied with lymphatic vessels as well.

The lungs are "designed" to expose a large amount of blood to a large amount of air. Hence the primary property of the lung is its enormous surface area, close to that of a tennis court. The goal is to allow O_2 from the atmosphere to diffuse into pulmonary capillaries, where it is bound by hemoglobin in RBCs. Simultaneously, CO_2 diffuses from the blood to the alveolar gas.

In the lungs, oxygen and carbon dioxide diffuse between the alveolar air and blood in the alveolar capillaries (Figure 30). The driving force for the exchange of gases in the lungs is the difference in partial pressures between the alveolar air and the blood. For diffusion to occur (from the air to the blood), gases must first pass across the alveolar epithelium, then through the interstitial liquid, and finally across the capillary endothelium. These three barriers to diffusion together form the **respiratory membrane**. Note that the pathway is reversed for diffusion from the blood to the air).

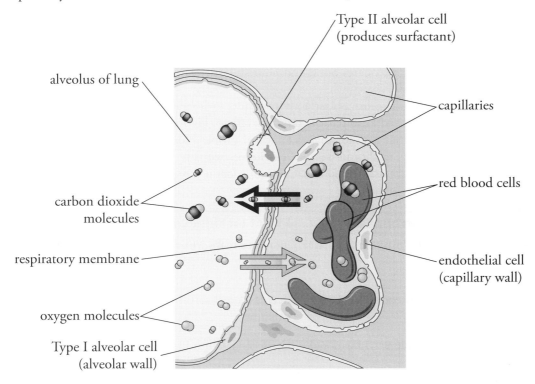

Figure 30 Diffusion of Gases Between an Alveolus and a Capillary

8.7 THE MUSCULOSKELETAL SYSTEM

The musculoskeletal system, as its name implies, is comprised of the skeleton and the muscles of the body. While the skeleton includes the cartilage and teeth, its main constituent is bone.

Overview of the Skeletal System

The skeletal system serves five roles:

1. support the body and provide our framework
2. provide an anchor for muscular contraction
3. protect vital organs such as the brain, spinal cord, heart, and lungs
4. store calcium, phosphate, and other important ions
5. synthesize formed elements of the blood (red blood cells, white blood cells, platelets). This occurs in the marrow of flat bones and is called **hematopoiesis**.

Bone is a dynamic connective tissue composed principally of matrix and cells. The matrix is made of **hydroxyapatite** (a crystalline compound of calcium and phosphorous), ions, collagen, and additional proteins. Bone contains three different cell types:

- **Osteoblasts** are located on the inner surfaces of bone tissue. They synthesize collagen and other organic components of the matrix.
- **Osteocytes** occupy minute spaces (**lacunae**) within the bony matrix and function to maintain the matrix.
- **Osteoclasts** promote ongoing breakdown, resorption, and remodeling of bone.

Overall, both osteoblasts and osteocytes build and nourish bone, while osteoclasts break bone down.

An increased ratio of osteoclast to osteoblast activity results in liberation of calcium and phosphate into the bloodstream (and a decreased ratio has the opposite effect). Hence, activity of these cells is important not only for bone structure, but also for maintenance of proper blood levels of calcium and phosphate. The hormones PTH (parathyroid hormone) and calcitonin regulate the activity of these cells and thus blood calcium levels. PTH increases blood calcium and calcitonin reduces it. The specific effects of these hormones are:

Hormone	Effect on bones	Effect on kidneys	Effect on intestines
PTH	stimulates osteoclast activity	increases reabsorption of calcium	indirectly increases intestinal calcium absorption
Calcitonin	inhibits osteoclast activity	decreases reabsorption of calcium	none

Table 9 Hormonal Control of Calcium Homeostasis

The general structure of bone may be either compact or spongy. As the names imply, **compact bone** is hard and dense, while **spongy bone** is porous. Spongy bone is always surrounded by a layer of compact bone. Spongy bone under the microscope looks like a sponge. It has a disorganized structure in which many spikes of bone surround marrow-containing cavities. The spikes of bone in spongy bone are called **spicules** or **trabeculae.**

Bone marrow is non-bony material found in the shafts of long bones and in the pores of spongy bones. **Red marrow** is found in spongy bone within flat bones and is the site of hematopoiesis. Its activity increases in response to erythropoietin, a hormone made by the kidney. **Yellow marrow,** found in the shafts of long bones, is filled with adipocytes (or fat cells) and is inactive.

8.7

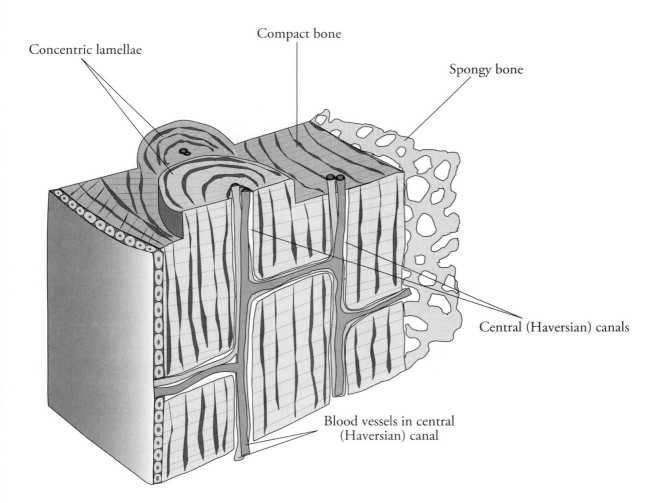

Figure 31   Compact and Spongy Bone

Compact bone has a specific organization. The basic unit of compact bone structure is the **osteon,** sometimes referred to as a **Haversian system.** In the center of the osteon is a hole called the **central (Haversian) canal,** which contains blood, lymph vessels, and nerves. Surrounding the canal are concentric rings of bone termed **lamellae** (which just means "sheets" or "layers"). Tiny channels, or **canaliculi,** branch out from the central canal to spaces called lacunae ("lakes"). In each lacuna is an osteocyte, or mature bone cell. Osteocytes have long processes which extend down the canaliculi to contact other osteocytes through gap junctions. This allows the cells to exchange nutrients and waste through an otherwise impermeable membrane. **Perforating (Volkmann's) canals** are channels that run perpendicular to central canals to connect osteons.

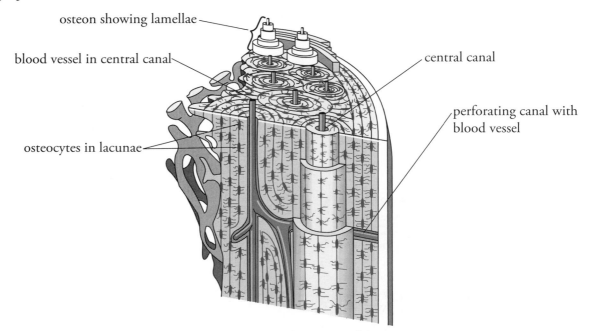

osteon showing lamellae

blood vessel in central canal

central canal

perforating canal with blood vessel

osteocytes in lacunae

Figure 32   Microscopic Structure of Compact Bone

Tissues Found at Joints

Cartilage is a strong but very flexible extracellular tissue secreted by cells called **chondrocytes.** There are three types of cartilage:

- **Hyaline cartilage** is strong and somewhat flexible. The larynx and trachea are reinforced by hyaline cartilage, and joints are lined by hyaline cartilage.
- **Elastic cartilage** is found in structures (such as the outer ear and the epiglottis) that require support and more flexibility than hyaline cartilage can provide; it contains elastin.
- **Fibrous cartilage** is very rigid and is found in places where very strong support is needed, such as the intervertebral disks of the spinal column.

Cartilage is not innervated and does not contain blood vessels; it is avascular. It receives nutrition and immune protection from surrounding fluid.

Ligaments and **tendons** are strong tissues composed of dense connective tissue.

- Ligaments connect bones to other bones.
- Tendons connect bones to muscles.

The point where one bone meets another is called a **joint.**

- Immovable joints are points where two bones are fused together. For example, the skull is formed from many fused bones.
- Slightly movable joints provide both movability and a great deal of support. The vertebral joints are an example.
- Most of the joints in the body are freely movable joints. There are several types, such as ball and socket (e.g., hip or shoulder) and hinge (e.g., knee or elbow).

All movable joints are supported by ligaments and lubricated by synovial fluid.

Overview of Muscle Tissue

8.7

There are three types of muscle which differ in cellular physiology, anatomy, and function: skeletal muscle, cardiac muscle, and smooth muscle. These three types of muscle share some characteristics and differ in others. Each will be discussed more in the sections that follow.

Skeletal Muscle

Skeletal muscle is also known as voluntary muscle, because its role is to contract in response to conscious intent. Under the microscope, skeletal muscle is striated. A skeletal muscle that traverses a joint will be responsible for bending that joint. Consider the illustration below, which shows biceps and triceps muscles traversing the elbow joint.

The biceps attaches to the upper end of the forearm and the shoulder, crossing the elbow joint. Contraction of this muscle causes the elbow joint to bend. Active straightening of the elbow joint is possible because of the action of the triceps. When muscles such as the biceps and triceps pull in opposite directions across a joint, they are said to be **antagonistic** to one another.

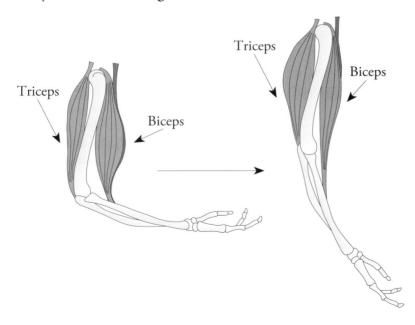

Figure 33   Flexion and Extension at the Elbow Joint

Skeletal Muscle Fiber

A skeletal muscle cell is a long, multinucleated cell in which many striations are visible. Because of their length, skeletal muscle cells are commonly referred to as muscle "fibers" or **myofibers**. A group or bundle of skeletal muscle fibers (cells) is referred to as a **fascicle**. Within each myofiber are many smaller units called **myofibrils**. The myofibril in the muscle cell is like a specialized organelle; it is responsible for the striated appearance of skeletal muscle and generates the contractile force of skeletal muscle.

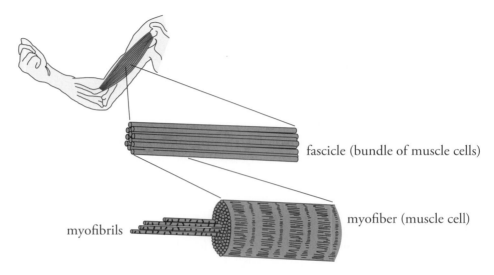

fascicle (bundle of muscle cells)

myofiber (muscle cell)

myofibrils

Figure 34   Levels of Skeletal Muscle Organization

Sarcomere

A single **sarcomere** is a segment of muscle fiber between two Z lines, as shown in Figure 35. A sarcomere is composed of a series of **thick and thin filaments** arranged parallel to each other. Each **thin filament** is anchored at one end to a Z line. The thick filaments have no connection to the Z lines. Thin and thick filaments interdigitate in a very regular manner.

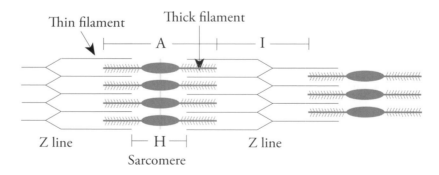

Thin filament

Thick filament

A   I

Z line   Z line

H

Sarcomere

Figure 35   Functional Unit of the Muscle Fiber

Filaments are composed of proteins. Thin filaments are composed of the protein **actin**, and thick filaments, of the protein **myosin**. Contraction of muscle is achieved by the sliding of actin and myosin filaments, each over the other, bringing the Z lines closer together.

Various sectors of the sarcomere have been named. The length of a myosin (thick) filament corresponds to the **A band**. Because the filament itself does not contract, the A band has a fixed length equal to that of the myosin strands. A given length of thin filament that does not overlap with any thick filament is called the **I band**. In the middle of the sarcomere is the **H zone**, which contains only myosin filaments with no overlapping actin filaments.

Skeletal Muscle Contraction

In order for a muscle to contract, its thin and thick filaments must physically interact. For that reason, regularly spaced **crossbridges** extend from the myosin filaments to the actin filaments. Through the physical interaction of actin and myosin, made possible by the crossbridges, contraction is thought to occur according to a **sliding filament** mechanism, in which:

1. a myosin head binds to the actin filament at a **myosin binding site**
2. myosin heads interact with the actin filaments to draw them inward
3. Z lines come closer together
4. the sarcomere shortens

The shortening of a sarcomere means that the myofiber to which it belongs shortens as well. The shortening of many sarcomeres within a myofiber means that the myofiber undergoes significant reduction in length and that amounts to contraction.

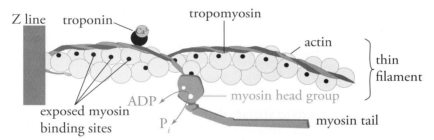

a) original position of filaments and Z line
prior to cocking of myosin head group

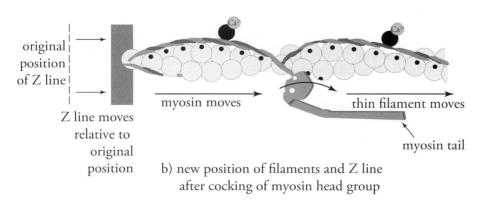

b) new position of filaments and Z line
after cocking of myosin head group

Figure 36   Filament Sliding

Troponin and Tropomyosin

Within the myofiber's sarcomeres, actin molecules are intimately associated with two regulatory proteins called **tropomyosin** and the **troponin complex**. In a resting muscle, tropomyosin molecules cover the myosin binding sites on actin. Tropomyosin and the troponin complex are intimately associated not only with actin but also with each other. Troponin has a tendency to bind calcium ions if they are present and this causes a change in its shape and position; this shifts tropomyosin off actin and exposes the myosin binding sites. In other words, calcium ions allow actin and myosin to interact and muscle contraction occurs as a consequence.

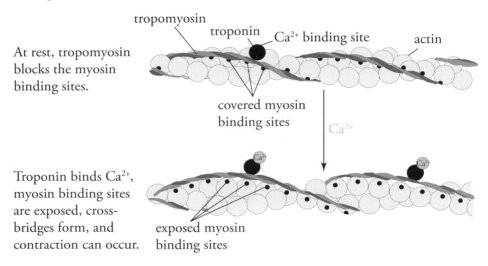

Figure 37   The Troponin/Tropomyosin Complex

Sarcolemma, Sarcoplasmic Reticulum, and Calcium

Muscle cells contain most of the typical eukaryotic organelles. However, a few of them have unique names. Within a myofiber (muscle cell), the:

- cell membrane is called the **sarcolemma**
- cytoplasm is called the **sarcoplasm**
- endoplasmic reticulum is called the **sarcoplasmic reticulum**

The sarcoplasmic reticulum is a huge, specialized smooth endoplasmic reticulum. It sequesters, stores, and releases Ca^{2+}. In order for an entire muscle fiber to contract, its action potential must be carried deep into the cell. This is accomplished by a series of invaginations in the sarcolemma called **T tubules**. As we've already seen, myofibers also contain complex and organized protein networks called sarcomeres.

Muscle contraction proceeds via the following series of events:

1. A motor neuron that innervates the myofiber undergoes an action potential, causing the motor neuron to release the neurotransmitter acetylcholine.
2. Acetylcholine binds to receptors on the sarcolemma, which is continuous with the sarcoplasmic reticulum.

8.7

3. Acetylcholine causes depolarization of both sarcolemma and sarcoplasmic reticulum.
4. The depolarization, if sufficient in magnitude, triggers an action potential, and the entire sarcolemma depolarizes.
5. The action potential causes calcium ions to move from the sarcoplasmic reticulum to the sarcoplasmic space, surrounding the fiber's actin and myosin filaments.
6. Calcium ions bind to troponin.
7. Tropomyosin undergoes a change in shape and position.
8. The sites at which actin interacts with myosin are "uncovered." Myosin heads are thus able to contact actin filaments.
9. Actin and myosin interact as "sliding filaments."

In order for a whole muscle fiber to undergo these processes synchronously, its action potential is carried deep into the fiber by a series of invaginations in the sarcolemma called T tubules. When contraction is over, calcium ions are pumped back from the sarcoplasm to the sarcoplasmic reticulum.

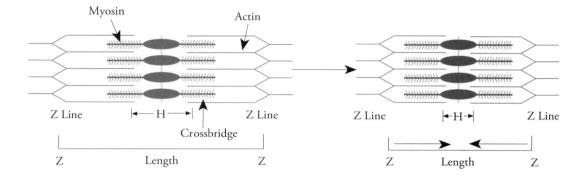

Figure 38 Shortening of Sarcomeres During Contraction

The term excitation–contraction coupling describes the rapid communication between depolarization of the skeletal muscle plasma membrane and Ca^{2+} release from the sarcoplasmic reticulum, which leads to contraction.

Energy Requirements for Muscle Contraction
Muscular function requires energy to maintain:

1. The resting potential that allows for depolarization and action potential.
2. The dynamic interaction of myosin and actin that underlies the physical shortening of the sarcomere.
3. The return of calcium ions from the sarcoplasm to the sarcoplasmic reticulum after contraction is complete.

The myofiber, like most human cells under most conditions, derives its energy most directly by dephosphorylation of ATP into ADP and inorganic phosphate. The muscle cell stores only very small amounts of ATP. In order to sustain its activity, therefore, it must somehow regenerate ATP from ADP and inorganic phosphate, and for that, it needs other energy sources.

Myofibers store (relatively small) amounts of **phosphocreatine**, which, like ATP and GTP, embodies a high-energy phosphate bond. Dephosphorylation of phosphocreatine, therefore, releases energy, which the myofiber uses to regenerate ATP from ADP and inorganic phosphate. Yet, the total amount of ATP and phosphocreatine normally stored within a muscle cell is sufficient to maintain meaningful contraction for only 5 or 10 seconds. For contractile activity that lasts longer, the cell must resort to yet another source of ATP generation.

Muscle cells store glycogen, which is readily broken down into glucose. Glucose then undergoes glycolysis to produce ATP and pyruvate, which, in the presence of an adequate oxygen supply, enters the Krebs cycle, electron transport, and oxidative phosphorylation. Where oxygen supply is inadequate to sustain the aerobic processes just mentioned, muscle cells resort to anaerobic processes alone (glycolysis and fermentation).

Cardiac Muscle

Cardiac muscle is found only in the wall of the heart. Like skeletal muscle, cardiac muscle is striated under the microscope and thus contains actin and myosin proteins arranged into sarcomeres. Muscle contraction occurs via a mechanism similar to that in skeletal muscle. Sliding filaments and excitation–contraction occur as in skeletal muscle.

Cardiac muscle is different from skeletal muscle in some important ways:

- Cardiac muscle contraction does not depend on stimulation by motor neurons.
- You have no conscious control over cardiac muscle because it is innervated by the autonomic nervous system. Cardiac muscle operates involuntarily, with the sinoatrial node acting as the initiator of its rhythmic contractions.
- Cardiac muscle cells have one nucleus per cell, but all the muscle cells of the heart are interconnected by gap junctions. This allows action potentials to propagate throughout the entire heart without allowing cells to share nuclei or cytoplasmic contents. Only small items like ions can pass through gap junctions.
- While ACh induces skeletal muscle contraction, this neurotransmitter inhibits depolarization of the SA node and thus decreases the heart rate.

Smooth Muscle

Smooth muscle is found in the walls of hollow tubes and hollow organs (such as the stomach, bladder, and uterus). It is responsible for gastrointestinal motility, constriction of blood vessels, uterine contractions, urination, and so on. You have no conscious control over smooth muscle because it is innervated by the autonomic nervous system.

Smooth muscle cells are mononucleate, elongated, and nonstriated. These cells still contain actin and myosin filaments, but they are scattered in a network instead of organized into sarcomeres. Like cardiac muscle, smooth muscle cells are connected by gap junctions so that the action potential is readily and rapidly transmitted from one cell to the next.

Smooth muscle contracts via a mechanism similar to skeletal and cardiac muscle; contraction is triggered by an action potential that releases calcium ions from the sarcoplasmic reticulum. However, smooth muscle cells do not use tropomyosin and troponin to control actin and myosin. Instead, they use a protein called **calmodulin**, which binds calcium.

8.8 EXCRETORY SYSTEM

Overview

Excretion is the disposal of waste products. "The excretory system" generally refers to the kidneys, even though the liver, large intestine, and skin are involved in excretion too. Let's begin by summarizing the excretory roles of these organs to see where the kidneys fit into the picture.

The liver is responsible for excreting many wastes by chemically modifying them and releasing them into bile. In particular, the liver deals with hydrophobic or large waste products, which cannot be filtered out by the kidney. The liver also synthesizes **urea** and releases it into the bloodstream. Urea is a carrier of excess nitrogen and is excreted in urine.

The large intestine processes wastes destined for excretion; these are molecules we ingest but do not absorb into our blood. The colon is also capable of excreting excess ions (e.g., sodium, chloride, calcium) into the feces, using active transport.

Skin produces sweat, which contains water, ions, and urea. In other words, sweat is similar to urine. In this sense, the skin is an excretory organ. However, sweating is not primarily controlled by the amount of waste that needs to be excreted, but rather by temperature and level of sympathetic nervous system activity. Therefore, the excretory role of the skin is secondary.

Most humans have two kidneys, which are responsible for several important functions:

1. excreting hydrophilic wastes
2. maintaining constant solute concentration
3. maintaining constant pH
4. maintaining constant fluid volume, which is important for blood pressure and cardiac output

Gross Anatomy of the Urinary System

Each kidney is a filtration system that removes unwanted materials from the blood and passes them to the bladder for storage and eventual elimination. Blood enters the kidney from a large **renal artery**, which is a direct branch of the lower portion of the aorta. Purified blood is returned to the circulatory system by the large **renal vein**, which empties into the inferior vena cava. Urine leaves each kidney in a **ureter**, which empties into the **urinary bladder**. The bladder is a muscular organ which stretches as it fills with urine. There are two sphincters controlling release of urine from the bladder: an **internal sphincter** made of smooth (involuntary) muscle and an **external sphincter** made of skeletal (voluntary) muscle.

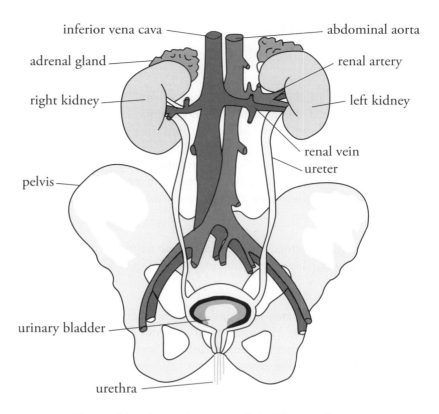

Figure 39   Gross Anatomy of the Urinary System

A frontal section (separating front from back) through the kidney demonstrates its internal anatomy. The outer region is known as the **cortex**, and the inner region is the **medulla**. It is important to note that there is an osmolarity gradient in the interstitium of the kidney: the cortex has a low osmolarity and the medulla has a high osmolarity. This will be important later because it drives reabsorption and urine concentration in the renal tubules. Let's add two nomenclature reminders here:

- **Osmolarity** is the measure of solute concentration, usually compared to the plasma. In the renal system, the main solutes are ions like Na^+, Cl^-, and K^+. Saying the cortex has a low osmolarity just means it is not very salty. Saying the renal medulla has a high osmolarity means it is quite salty.
- **Interstitium** is a generic word for "tissue." It literally means "an in-between region"; in this case it refers to the kidney tissue in between the renal tubules.

Let's return to kidney anatomy. The **medullary pyramids** are pyramid-shaped striations within the medulla. This appearance is due to the presence of many collecting ducts. Urine empties from the collecting ducts and leaves the medulla at the tip of a pyramid, known as a **papilla** (plural: **papillae**). Each papilla empties into a space called a **calyx** (plural: **calyces**). The calyces converge to form the **renal pelvis**, which is a large space where urine collects. The renal pelvis empties into the ureter.

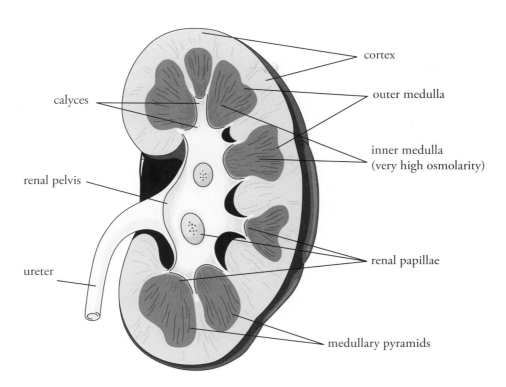

Figure 40   Internal Anatomy of the Kidney

The Nephron

The functional unit of the kidney is the nephron. It consists of two components:

1. **capsule**: a rounded region surrounding the capillaries where filtration takes place
2. **renal tubule**: a coiled tube that receives filtrate from the capillaries in the capsule at one end and empties into a **collecting duct** at the other end

Capsule and Filtration

Blood from the renal artery flows into an **afferent arteriole**, which branches into a ball of capillaries known as the **glomerulus**. Blood pressure causes fluid (essentially blood plasma) to leak out of the glomerular capillaries. The fluid passes through a filter known as the **glomerular basement membrane (GBM)** and enters **Bowman's capsule**. The lumen of Bowman's capsule is continuous with the lumen of the rest of the tubule. **Filtrate,** the fluid in the tubule, will eventually be made into urine.

The glomerular basement membrane acts like a colander. Small molecules are squeezed into the renal tubule during filtration; these molecules include water, ions, glucose, amino acids, and urea. Substances which are too large to pass through the glomerular basement membrane are not filtered; they remain in the glomerular capillary blood and drain into an **efferent arteriole**. These substances include blood cells (both RBC and WBC) and plasma proteins.

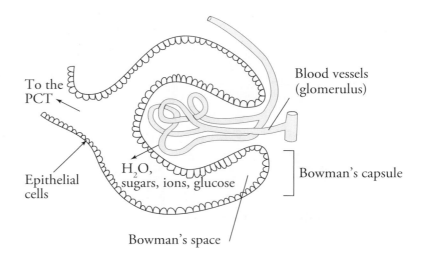

Figure 41 Filtration of Blood at the Glomerulus

Filtration occurs in the renal cortex, the outer layer of the kidney. The **glomerular filtration rate (GFR)** depends directly on blood pressure:

- Constriction of the efferent arteriole increases blood pressure in the glomerulus and increases GFR.
- Dilation of the afferent arteriole increases blood flow to the glomerulus; this increases blood pressure and GFR.

Reabsorption and Secretion

The tubule of the nephron contains five different regions. In order, they are:

1. Proximal convoluted tubule (PCT)
2. Descending loop of Henle
3. Ascending loop of Henle
4. Distal convoluted tubule (DCT)
5. Collecting duct

Coming out of Bowman's capsule, the filtrate consists of water and many useful small hydrophilic molecules; it will eventually become urine. Before this happens, some useful substances must be returned to the bloodstream and some additional waste substances will need to be added to the filtrate.

- Useful substances are extracted from the tubule, moved into the kidney interstitium, and picked up by capillaries that surround the tubule. This is a process called **reabsorption**, and it occurs throughout the nephron tubule.
- Additional waste products are moved from the kidney interstitium into the tubule filtrate. This process, called **secretion,** happens predominantly in the DCT and collecting duct; this is the primary way that many drugs and toxins are deposited in the urine. Some secretion also occurs in the PCT. Secretion adds waste substances to the filtrate so they can be eliminated in urine.

Renal Blood Vessels

Many blood vessels surround the nephron. They carry arterial blood toward the capsule for filtration, and then surround the tubule to carry filtered blood and reabsorbed substances away from the tubule:

- **Peritubular capillaries** surround the proximal and distal tubules in the cortex.
- **Vasa recta** go into the medulla to surround the loop of Henle.

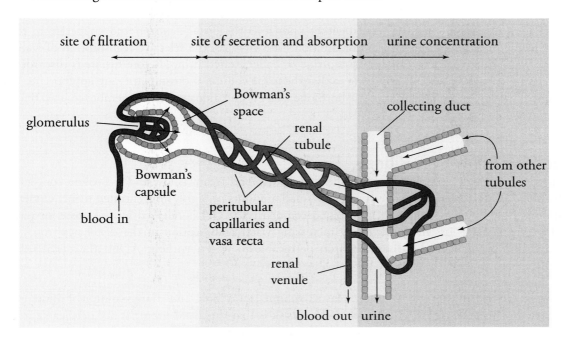

Figure 42   Blood Vessels and the Renal Tubule

These blood vessels return reabsorbed substances to the bloodstream; they drain into venules that lead to the renal vein.

Renal Tubule

Bowman's capsule empties into the first part of the tubule, the PCT. Here, most of the reabsorption occurs. All solute movement in the PCT is accompanied by water movement, so a lot of water reabsorption occurs in this region also; roughly 70 percent of the volume of the filtrate is reabsorbed in the PCT. For useful substances, the PCT reabsorbs as much as possible. Like Bowman's capsule, the PCT is located in the renal cortex, the outer layer of the kidney.

The PCT empties into the next region of the nephron, the loop of Henle. This is a long loop that dips down into the renal medulla. The loop of Henle has two parts:

- The descending loop of Henle starts in the cortex and goes down into the renal medulla. It is permeable to water, but not to ions. Because the renal interstitium has a high osmolarity, water is reabsorbed. This makes the filtrate more concentrated.
- The ascending loop of Henle starts in the medulla and heads back up toward the cortex. It is permeable to ions but not water. Because the filtrate is highly concentrated at the bottom of the loop of Henle, ions are reabsorbed as the filtrate moves up. These ions (mostly Na^+ and Cl^-) make the medullary interstitium salty.

As we continue through the tubule, the loop of Henle becomes the DCT, which is located in the renal cortex. The filtrate composition is optimized and fine-tuned in the DCT. Reabsorption here is more regulated than in the PCT, usually via hormones. Some secretion also happens here. The DCT dumps into a collecting duct and by the end of the collecting duct, whatever remains in the renal tubule gets excreted as urine. Many collecting ducts merge to form larger tributaries which empty into renal calyces and then the renal pelvis. Urine is sent to the bladder for storage, via the ureter.

The DCT and the collecting duct are together known as the distal nephron and cooperate in the last step of urine formation: concentration or dilution. This involves the selective reabsorption of water and is where we decide whether to make dilute urine or concentrated urine. Before filtrate is discarded into the ureter as urine, adjustments are made so that the urine volume and osmolarity are appropriate. This is controlled by two hormones: antidiuretic hormone (ADH) and aldosterone. Remember that ADH is also known as vasopressin.

Endocrine Role of the Kidney

When you are dehydrated, the volume of fluid in your bloodstream is low and the solute concentration in the blood is high. Hence, you need to make small amounts of highly concentrated urine. Under these conditions (low blood volume and high blood osmolarity), ADH is released by the posterior pituitary. ADH prevents water loss in the urine by increasing water reabsorption in the distal nephron. This is accomplished by making the distal nephron permeable to water; without ADH, the distal tubule is impermeable to water.

In contrast, after drinking a lot of water, plasma volume is too high, and a large volume of dilute urine is necessary. In this case, no ADH is secreted. The result is that the distal tubule is not permeable to water. This means that any water in the filtrate remains in the tubule and is lost in the urine. The reason that drinking alcohol causes many bathroom runs is that it inhibits ADH secretion by the posterior pituitary.

When blood pressure is low, aldosterone is released by the adrenal cortex. It increases reabsorption of Na^+ by the distal nephron. The result is increased plasma osmolarity, which leads to increased thirst and water retention, which raises the blood pressure. When the blood pressure is high, aldosterone is not released. As a result, sodium is lost in the urine; plasma osmolarity (and eventually blood pressure) fall.

ADH and aldosterone work together to increase blood pressure. First, aldosterone causes sodium reabsorption, which results in increased plasma osmolarity. This causes ADH to be secreted, which results in increased water reabsorption and thus increased plasma volume.

There are a few other hormones that affect the kidney, and the kidney makes one as well. All are peptides except aldosterone, which is a steroid. You should know the basic role and source of each of the following hormones:

Hormone	Source	Target and effect
Aldosterone	Adrenal cortex	Increases sodium reabsorption and potassium secretion in the distal nephron; this increases blood volume through the action of ADH and thus increases blood pressure
Antidiuretic hormone (ADH) or vasopressin	Posterior pituitary	Increases water reabsorption in the distal nephron, to increase urine concentration, dilute the blood, increase plasma volume, and increase systemic blood pressure
Calcitonin	Thyroid	Decreases serum $[Ca^{2+}]$ by deposition in bone, reduced absorption in the gut, and excretion in urine
Parathyroid hormone (PTH)	Parathyroid	Increases serum $[Ca^{2+}]$ by breaking down bone, increased absorption in the gut, and reabsorption from the filtrate
Erythropoietin (EPO)	Kidney	Increases synthesis of red blood cells in the bone marrow

Table 10 Hormones Affecting or Secreted by the Kidney

Countercurrent Multiplier

A system called the **countercurrent multiplier** allows the kidney to reabsorb 99% of the filtrate in the tubule and to produce urine that has a much higher osmolarity than plasma. The basis of this system is a series of tubes running in opposite directions through the interstitial space of the kidney, and a combination of active and passage transport across the tubule wall:

- The descending loop of Henle runs down, from the cortex into the medulla. It is permeable to water, but not to ions, so water is reabsorbed.
- Like the loop of Henle, vasa recta blood vessels form a loop; the ascending portions of the vasa recta are near the descending limb of the loop of Henle and carry off water that leaves the descending limb.
- The ascending loop of Henle runs up, from the medulla to the cortex of the kidney. It is permeable to ions but not water, so ions are reabsorbed. These ions contribute to the high osmolarity in the medulla.
- The collecting duct runs down, from the cortex to the medulla. The high osmolarity of the interstitium sucks water out of the collecting duct in the presence of ADH.

The countercurrent multiplier makes the medulla very salty, and this facilitates water reabsorption from the descending loop of Henle and the collecting duct. This is how the kidney is capable of making urine with a much higher osmolarity than plasma.

8.8

Now that we have looked at all aspects of renal physiology, let's look at a full labelled diagram of the nephron:

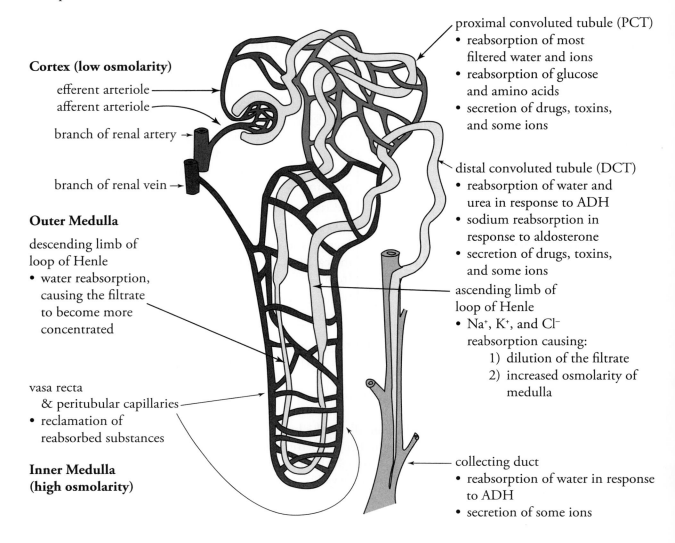

proximal convoluted tubule (PCT)
- reabsorption of most filtered water and ions
- reabsorption of glucose and amino acids
- secretion of drugs, toxins, and some ions

Cortex (low osmolarity)
- efferent arteriole
- afferent arteriole
- branch of renal artery →
- branch of renal vein →

distal convoluted tubule (DCT)
- reabsorption of water and urea in response to ADH
- sodium reabsorption in response to aldosterone
- secretion of drugs, toxins, and some ions

Outer Medulla

descending limb of loop of Henle
- water reabsorption, causing the filtrate to become more concentrated

ascending limb of loop of Henle
- Na^+, K^+, and Cl^- reabsorption causing:
  1) dilution of the filtrate
  2) increased osmolarity of medulla

vasa recta
  & peritubular capillaries
- reclamation of reabsorbed substances

Inner Medulla (high osmolarity)

collecting duct
- reabsorption of water in response to ADH
- secretion of some ions

Figure 43 Regions and Functions of the Nephron

Renal Regulation of Blood Pressure

Since GFR depends directly on pressure, the kidney has built-in mechanisms to help regulate systemic and local (glomerular) blood pressure. The **juxtaglomerular apparatus (JGA)** contains baroreceptors that monitor systemic blood pressure. When there is a decrease in blood pressure, juxtaglomerular (JG) cells secrete an enzyme called **renin** into the bloodstream. Renin catalyzes the conversion of **angiotensinogen** (a plasma protein made by the liver) into **angiotensin I**, which is further converted to **angiotensin II** by **angiotensin-converting enzyme (ACE)** in the lungs. Angiotensin II is a powerful vasoconstrictor that immediately raises the blood pressure. It also stimulates the release of aldosterone; see Figure 44.

The cells of the **macula densa** are chemoreceptors that monitor filtrate osmolarity in the distal tubule. A low filtrate osmolarity indicates a low filtration rate; the macula densa stimulates the JG cells to release renin. The macula densa also increases blood flow to the glomerulus, which increases filtration.

Let's look at a summary of how these two processes work together to increase systemic blood pressure:

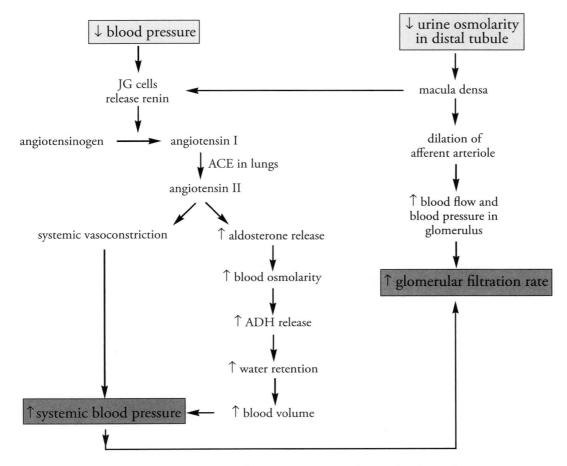

Figure 44   Regulation of Blood Pressure and GFR by the Kidney

Renal Regulation of pH

The kidney is essential for maintaining constant blood pH. It accomplishes this by a direct mechanism:

- When plasma pH is too high, HCO_3^- is excreted in the urine.
- When the plasma pH is too low, H^+ is excreted in the urine.

These modifications affect the CO_2 equilibrium reaction we saw earlier in this chapter:

$$CO_2 + H_2O \rightleftharpoons H_2CO_3 \rightleftharpoons HCO_3^- + H^+$$

By excreting molecules in the urine, they are lost from the body and the equilibrium shifts to compensate for the change. This impacts pH but takes a while to have an effect. This is why the respiratory system (which controls CO_2 levels) is used for short-term or quick adjustments to physiological pH.

8.9 DIGESTIVE SYSTEM

The digestive system includes the **alimentary canal** (also called the **gastrointestinal tract** or **GI tract**) and four **accessory organs**. The alimentary canal is a continuous tube from mouth to anus and each portion is seen as a separate organ. It includes the following:

1. mouth or oral cavity
2. throat or pharynx
3. esophagus
4. stomach
5. small intestine
6. large intestine

We will review each of these in turn. Later in this chapter, we will review the accessory organs.

Macronutrients (which are found in both liquid and solid foods) can be grouped into three types: **carbohydrate, protein,** and **fat**. In order to be of use to the body, these foods must be broken down into smaller particles that can be absorbed from the lumen of the digestive tract into the blood stream. Digestion is of two types: **mechanical** and **chemical**. Mechanical digestion begins with the shredding and grinding of food into small pieces by chewing (**mastication**). It continues with vigorous churning in the stomach. Chemical digestion occurs by means of enzymes produced by several different organs associated with the alimentary canal. Enzymes break down food into absorbable molecules. Here are the organs of the digestive system that we will be reviewing in this chapter:

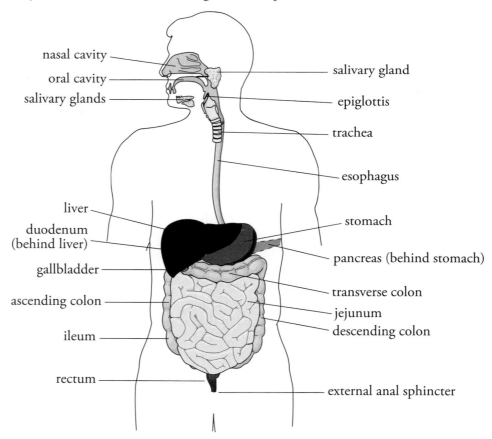

Figure 45 Organs of the Digestive System

Alimentary Canal

Mouth

As food is chewed, it mixes with saliva, which contains the digestive enzyme **salivary amylase**. Salivary amylase initiates (but does not complete) the digestion of starch (a carbohydrate), hydrolyzing glycosidic bonds to produce component sugars. Saliva also lubricates the food and contains lysozyme, an enzyme that degrades the bacterial cell wall; this is an important part of innate immune protection. Chewing is a type of mechanical digestion. By the time the food is ready to be swallowed, it is called a **bolus.**

Esophagus

The esophagus has no enzymatic function but serves as a conduit for food from the mouth to the stomach. It is a muscular structure with separate sets of muscle fibers arranged circumferentially and longitudinally. Transit through the esophagus results from a highly coordinated series of contractions, involving both circular and longitudinal muscles, known as **peristalsis**. This process squeezes a bolus of chewed food downward to the stomach. Peristalsis continues throughout the gastrointestinal tract.

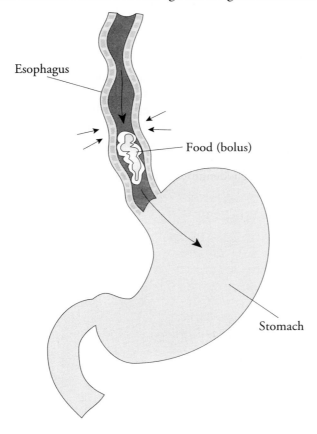

Figure 46   Peristalsis

Stomach

The **cardiac sphincter** (so named because it is found near the heart) is at the end of the esophagus, or the entrance to the stomach. It prevents reflux from the stomach into the esophagus.

The stomach is a large hollow muscular organ that serves three purposes:

1. storage and regulated release of chyme into the small intestine
2. partial digestion of food, especially proteins
3. destruction of microorganisms

Among the stomach's most striking features is its relatively low pH. Specialized cells, called **parietal cells**, in the lining of the stomach secrete **hydrochloric acid** (**HCl**) into the stomach's lumen. The acidity of the stomach is part of innate immunity, as it kills microorganisms in the food we eat. It is also essential to the functioning of the gastric enzyme **pepsin**. Secreted by **chief cells** in the stomach wall, pepsin initiates the chemical breakdown of proteins. Once food has been churned and digested by pepsin, it passes through the **pyloric sphincter** into the first section of the small intestine, the **duodenum**. One way to think about this is that the pyloric sphincter releases chyme (from the stomach) a squirt at a time.

Small Intestine and Pancreas

The small intestine is a tube about an inch wide and 10 feet long. It is divided into three segments: the duodenum, **jejunum,** and **ileum.** Digestion begins in the mouth, continues in the stomach, and is completed in the duodenum and jejunum. Absorption begins in the duodenum and continues throughout the small intestine. In the small intestine, the liquid food mixture, or **chyme,** is processed by enzymes that act on protein, carbohydrate, and fat. Unlike pepsin, which is produced by the organ into which it is released, the enzymes of the small intestine are synthesized in a separate organ—the pancreas. Pancreatic enzymes are delivered directly to the duodenum via the **pancreatic duct.**

8.9

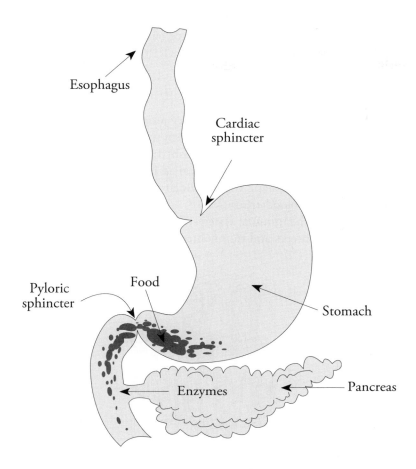

Figure 47   Release of the Pancreatic Enzymes

Some pancreatic enzymes are secreted into the small intestine in an inactive form. These inactive precursors are called **zymogens**. To be activated, zymogens normally must be cleaved by an enzyme. For example, **trypsinogen** is one of the zymogens released into the duodenum. It is activated by an enzyme in the duodenum called **enterokinase** (also called **enteropeptidase**). The activation process produces **trypsin**, an active protein-degrading enzyme. Trypsin cleaves a number of other zymogens into their active forms.

You should be familiar with the names and targets of a few other pancreatic enzymes. **Pancreatic amylase**, chemically identical to salivary amylase, continues the digestion of carbohydrates, which was initiated in the mouth. **Pancreatic lipase** serves in the enzymatic breakdown of fats (lipids). Trypsin and **chymotrypsin** are the two most important proteolytic, or protein-digesting, enzymes in the gastrointestinal tract. These two enzymes break peptide bonds, reducing large proteins into small chains composed of only a few amino acids.

Food particles are broken down by digestive enzymes into smaller subunits, which enter the blood stream by being absorbed across the wall of the small intestine into regional capillaries. From the small intestine, blood travels directly to the liver, where further processing occurs.

The key feature that allows the small intestine to accomplish absorption is its large surface area; this results from 1) length, 2) villi, and 3) microvilli. **Villi** (singular: **villus**) are macroscopic (multicellular) projections in the wall of the small intestine. **Microvilli** are microscopic foldings of the cell membranes of individual intestinal epithelial cells. The luminal surface of the small intestine is known as the **brush border** due to the brush-like appearance of microvilli.

The intestinal villus is a finger-like projection of the wall of the gut into the lumen. It has three very important structures:

1. The villus contains capillaries, which absorb dietary monosaccharides and amino acids. The capillaries merge to form veins, which merge to form the large **hepatic portal vein**, which transports blood containing amino acid and carbohydrate nutrients from the gut to the liver.
2. The villus also contains small lymphatic vessels called **lacteals**, which absorb dietary fats. The lacteals merge to form large lymphatic vessels, which transport dietary fats to the thoracic duct, which empties into the bloodstream.
3. **Peyer's patches** are part of the immune system. They are collections of lymphocytes dotting the villi that monitor GI contents and thus confer immunity to gut pathogens and toxins.

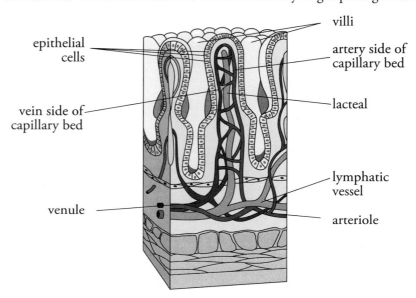

Figure 48   An Intestinal Villus

Some duodenal epithelial cells secrete enzymes. As we saw earlier, duodenal **enterokinase** activates the pancreatic zymogen trypsinogen. Other duodenal enzymes are peculiar in that they are not truly secreted, but rather do their work inside or on the surface of the brush border epithelial cell. These duodenal enzymes are called **brush border enzymes.** Their role is to hydrolyze the smallest carbohydrates and proteins (like disaccharides and dipeptides) into monosaccharides and amino acids. Lactose, sucrose, and maltose are all degraded into monosaccharides in this way.

Other duodenal epithelial cells secrete hormones. One important duodenal hormone is **cholecystokinin (CCK),** which is secreted in response to fats in the duodenum. It causes the pancreas to secrete digestive enzymes, stimulates gallbladder contraction (bile release), and decreases gastric motility.

Substances not absorbed in the duodenum must be absorbed in these lower segments of the small intestine, the jejunum and the ileum. A valve called the **ileocecal valve** separates the ileum from the cecum, which is the first part of the large intestine.

Large Intestine

The large intestine is the last part of the alimentary canal. The sections are:

- cecum and appendix
- ascending colon
- transverse colon
- descending colon
- sigmoid colon
- rectum
- anus

The colon is the largest portion of the large intestine. Like the rest of the intestine, the large intestine is a muscular tube. It is 3 or 4 feet long and several inches wide. Its role is to absorb water and minerals, and to form and store feces until the time of **defecation**. Abnormalities of colon function result in poor fluid absorption and diarrhea, which can cause dehydration and death.

The first part of the colon is the **cecum**. Entrance of chyme into the cecum is controlled by the ileocecal valve. The **appendix** is a finger-like appendage of the cecum. It is composed primarily of lymphatic tissue.

The colon contains billions of bacteria of various species. Many are facultative or obligate anaerobes. Undigested materials are metabolized by colonic bacteria. This often results in gas, which is given off as a waste product of bacterial metabolism. **Colonic bacteria** are important for two reasons:

1. The presence of large numbers of normal bacteria helps keep dangerous bacteria from proliferating, due to competition for space and nutrients.
2. Colonic bacteria supply us with **vitamin K,** which is essential for blood clotting.

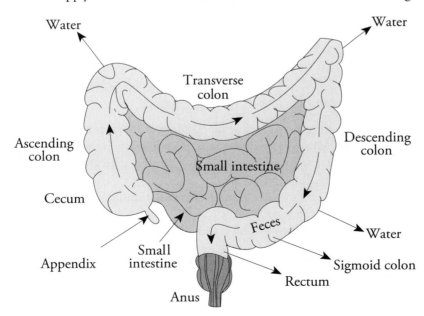

Figure 49   Large Intestine

The last portion of the colon is called the **rectum**. Exit of feces (defecation) from the rectum occurs through the **anus**. Defecation is controlled by the **anal sphincter**, which has an internal portion and an external portion. The internal anal sphincter consists of smooth muscle, which is under autonomic control. The external anal sphincter consists of skeletal muscle and is under voluntary control. (Note that this is the same arrangement as seen in the urinary sphincters.) Most of the wastes from a meal are defecated about a day after it is eaten. However, the wastes from a meal are first present in stool after just a few hours and some residue of a meal is typically still present in the colon after several days.

Digestive Accessory Organs

There are four digestive accessory organs that play a role in digestion but are not actually part of the alimentary canal. They are:

1. salivary glands
2. pancreas
3. liver
4. gallbladder

8.9

Salivary glands make and release saliva, which we have already discussed. The pancreas and liver are essential for GI function; the gallbladder is not essential.

Pancreas

We have already talked about how the pancreas makes and releases many enzymes that are essential for chemical digestion. The pancreas also makes and secretes bicarbonate into the duodenum. This neutralizes the low pH of chyme once it moves into the small intestine; the stomach has structural characteristics that protect it from the low pH of the chyme, but the small intestine does not.

The pancreas also has endocrine function via cells in small regions called the islets of Langerhans. By way of review, there are three types of cells in the islets, and each secretes a particular hormone into the bloodstream:

1. α cells secrete glucagon in response to low blood sugar. Glucagon mobilizes stored fuels by stimulating the liver to hydrolyze glycogen and release glucose into the bloodstream, and by stimulating adipocytes (fat cells) to release fats into the bloodstream.
2. β cells secrete insulin in response to elevated blood sugar (e.g., after a meal). Its effects are opposite (or antagonistic) to those of glucagon; insulin stimulates the removal of glucose from the blood for storage as glycogen or fat.
3. δ cells secrete somatostatin, which inhibits many digestive processes such as gastric secretions and motility.

Liver and Gallbladder

Also active in the duodenum is **bile**, which is produced in the liver and stored in the **gallbladder**. Bile is also concentrated in the gallbladder and is released when a fatty meal is eaten. Bile is a complex mixture of water, electrolytes, cholesterol, bilirubin, steroid hormones, and several other substances. Unlike pancreatic secretions, bile contains no enzymes, but instead acts as an **emulsifier**, helping to separate large globules of fat molecules into smaller globules in order to increase the surface area available for the action of lipase. Bile enters the midsection of the duodenum via the **common bile duct.**

Bile production is only one of the important functions of the liver. The liver also plays a significant role in carbohydrate metabolism (for example, converting glucose to a storage form, glycogen), converts amino acids to **keto acids** and urea, and processes toxins. Another of its functions is the degradation of senescent (aged) erythrocytes.

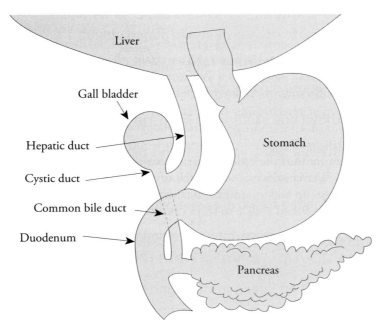

Figure 50　Pancreas, Gallbladder, and Duodenum

8.10   REPRODUCTIVE SYSTEMS

Male Reproductive System

Anatomy

The principal male reproductive structures that are visible on the outside of the body are the scrotum and the penis. The scrotum is essentially a bag of skin containing the male gonads, which are known as **testes** (testicles). The testes have two roles:

1. synthesis of sperm (**spermatogenesis**)
2. secretion of male sex hormones (androgens, e.g., testosterone) into the bloodstream

Let's start by tracing the path of a sperm from its origination to its final destination. The sites of spermatogenesis within the testes are the **seminiferous tubules**. Walls of the seminiferous tubules are formed by cells called **Sertoli cells**. Sertoli cells protect and nurture the developing sperm, both physically and chemically; their role will be discussed in more detail below. The tissue between the seminiferous tubules is simply referred to as testicular interstitium. Important cells found in the testicular interstitium are the **Leydig cells**. They are responsible for androgen (testosterone) synthesis.

The seminiferous tubules empty into the **epididymis**, a long coiled tube located on the posterior (back) of each testicle (Figure 51). The epididymis from each testicle empties into a **vas deferens** (also called **ductus deferens**), which circles up and around the bladder. Near the back of the urinary bladder, the **vas deferens** joins the duct of the seminal vesicle to form the **ejaculatory duct.**

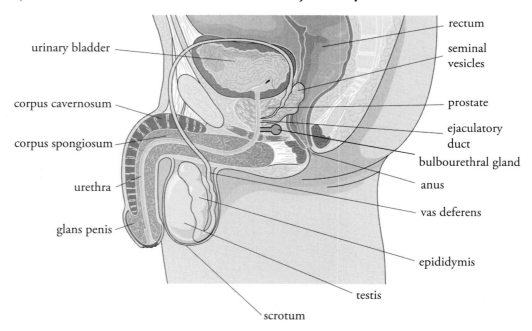

Figure 51   The Male Reproductive System

A pair of glands known as **seminal vesicles** is located on the posterior surface of the bladder. They secrete about 60 percent of the total volume of the **semen** into the ejaculatory duct. Semen, a highly nourishing fluid for sperm, is produced by three separate glands: the seminal vesicles, the **prostate**, and the **bulbo-urethral glands**. These are collectively referred to as the **accessory glands** (see Table 11). The ejaculatory duct empties into the **urethra** as it passes through the prostate gland. One final set of glands, the bulbo-urethral glands, contributes to the semen near the beginning of the urethra.

Gland	Secretions	Function of secretions	% of total ejaculate volume
Seminal vesicles	Mostly fructose	Nourishment of sperm	60%
Prostate gland	Fructose and a coagulant	Nourishment, allows semen to coagulate after ejaculation	35%
Bulbourethral glands	Thick, alkaline mucus	Lubricate urethra, neutralize acids in male urethra and in female vagina	3%
Testes	Sperm	Male gamete	2%

Table 11 Accessory Glands

The urethra exits the body via the penis. Penile erection facilitates deposition of semen near the opening of the uterus during intercourse. Specialized **erectile tissue** in the penis allows erection. It is composed of modified veins and capillaries surrounded by a connective tissue sheath. Erection occurs when blood accumulates at high pressure in the erectile tissue. Three compartments contain erectile tissue: the **corpora cavernosa** (there are two of these) and the **corpus spongiosum** (only one).

8.10

Spermatogenesis

What processes in a human being involve meiosis? Only one: **gametogenesis**. This is the process whereby diploid germ cells undergo **meiotic division** to produce **haploid gametes**. Meiotic cell division fosters genetic diversity in the population (by independent assortment of genes and by recombination). The gametes produced by the male are known as **spermatozoa**, or sperm; females produce **ova**, or eggs. The role of the sperm is to swim through the female genital tract to reach the egg and fuse with it. This fusion, known as **syngamy**, results in a **zygote**. The gametes produced by males and females differ dramatically in structure but contribute equally to the genome of the zygote (except in the special case of the two different sex chromosomes, X and Y, given to male offspring). Although both gametes contribute equally to the genome, the egg provides every other part of the zygote, since the only part of the sperm that enters the egg is a haploid genome. The term for this is **maternal inheritance**. For instance, mitochondria are inherited maternally.

Sperm synthesis is called spermatogenesis (Figure 52). It begins at puberty and occurs in the testes throughout adult life. The seminiferous tubule is the site of spermatogenesis. The entire process of spermatogenesis occurs with the aid of the specialized Sertoli cells found in the wall of the seminiferous tubule. Immature sperm precursors are found near the outer wall of the tubule, and nearly-mature spermatozoa are deposited into the lumen; from there they are transported to the epididymis. The cells that give rise to spermatogonia (and to their female counterparts, oogonia) are known as **germ cells**; under the right conditions, they *germ*inate, and give rise to a complete organism.

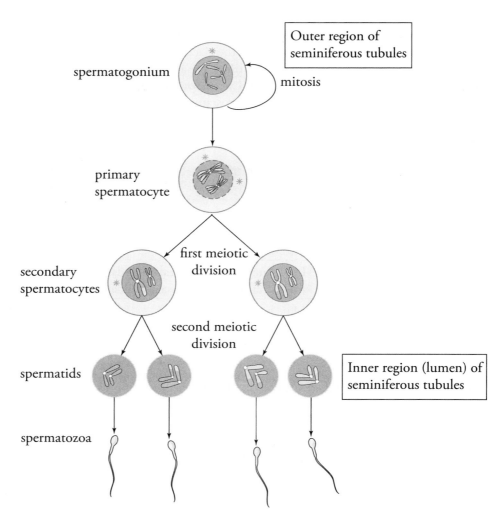

spermatogonium

Outer region of
seminiferous tubules

mitosis

primary
spermatocyte

first meiotic
division

secondary
spermatocytes

second meiotic
division

spermatids

Inner region (lumen) of
seminiferous tubules

spermatozoa

Figure 52   Spermatogenesis

8.10

The table below gives the names of the sperm precursors, along with the meiotic role of each stage, and some mnemonic comments.

Stage	Jobs	Mnemonic
Spermatogonium	1. Mitotically reproduce prior to meiosis 2. Replicate DNA in S phase of meiosis	The spermatoGONium is GONNA become a sperm.
Primary spermatocyte	Meiosis I	Any gamete precursor (male or female) with "cyte" undergoes a meiotic division.
Secondary spermatocyte	Meiosis II	The *secondary* spermatoCYTE undergoes the *second* meiotic division.
Spermatid	Turn into a spermatozoan	The spermatid's a kid, almost mature.
Spermatozoan	Finish maturing in: 1. seminiferous tubule 2. epididymis	Remember that a mature sperm is called a spermatozoan.

Table 12   Gametogenesis

8.10

Spermatids develop into spermatozoa in the seminiferous tubules with the aid of Sertoli cells. DNA condenses, the cytoplasm shrinks, and the cell changes shape so there is a head, containing the haploid nucleus and an **acrosome,** and a flagellum, which forms the tail. The acrosome is a lysosome-like compartment in the head of the sperm that contains hydrolytic enzymes required to penetrate the ovum. Spermatozoa contain many mitochondria to power motility. The final stages of sperm maturation occur in the epididymis, where spermatozoa gain motility.

Androgens and Estrogens

All hormones involved in the development and maintenance of male characteristics are termed **androgens**, while those involved in development and maintenance of female characteristics are termed **estrogens**. The primary androgen produced in the testes is testosterone. It is converted into dihydrotestosterone within the cells of target tissues. The primary estrogen produced in the ovaries is estradiol.

Testosterone is required in the testes for spermatogenesis. Testosterone levels start to increase at puberty and remain high for the remainder of adult life. Elevated levels of testosterone are responsible for the development and maintenance of male secondary sexual characteristics, which include maturation of the genitalia, male distribution of facial and body hair, deepening of the voice, and increased muscle mass.

The role of estrogen in the female is analogous to the role of testosterone in the male. Beginning at puberty, estrogen is required to regulate the menstrual cycle and for the development and maintenance of female secondary sexual characteristics (maturation of the genitalia, breast development, wider hips, and pubic hair).

During puberty and adult life, sex steroid production is controlled by the hypothalamus and the anterior pituitary. **Gonadotropin releasing hormone (GnRH)** from the hypothalamus stimulates the pituitary to release the gonadotropins: follicle-stimulating hormone (FSH) and luteinizing hormone (LH). In men, LH acts on Leydig cells to stimulate testosterone production, and FSH stimulates the Sertoli cells. In women FSH stimulates the granulosa cells to secrete estrogen, and LH simulates the formation of the corpus luteum and progesterone secretion. Feedback inhibition by the steroids inhibits the production of GnRH and LH and FSH. Inhibin, produced by Sertoli cells and the granulosa cells, provides further feedback regulation of FSH production (Figure 53).

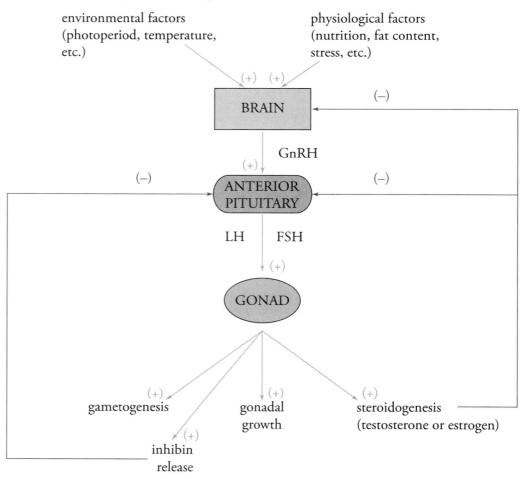

Figure 53   Regulation of Sex Steroid Production

Female Reproductive System

Anatomy

Female external genitalia include the **labium majus**, **labium minus**, and **glans clitoris**. The opening of the vagina is found between the labia minora. Female internal genitalia include:

- **Vagina**: site of sperm deposition during intercourse and also the birth canal a baby passes through during childbirth.
- **Cervix**: the lower and narrow end of the uterus. It is usually covered in mucus and contains an opening that connects the uterus and the vagina.
- **Uterus**: site of implantation, where an embryo/fetus develops and grows, contracts during labor and delivery. Uterine walls contain an **endometrium**, which (in the absence of pregnancy) is shed each month to produce menstrual bleeding, and the **myometrium**, which is a thick layer of smooth muscle.
- **Fallopian tubes**, also called **uterine tubes**: tubes that connect each ovary to the uterus. Each fallopian tube ends in finger-like structures called **fimbriae;** these brush up against the ovary.
- **Ovaries**: female gonads. Ovaries contain follicles and are the site of estrogen and progesterone synthesis, as well as oogenesis.

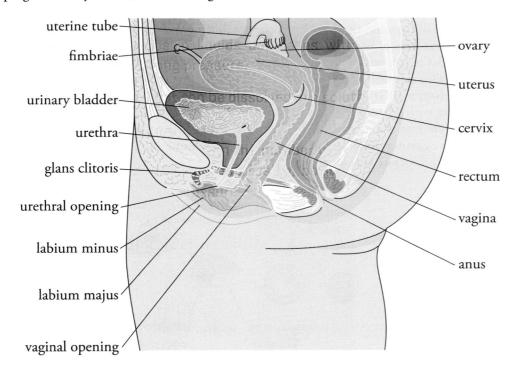

Figure 54   The Female Reproductive System

Oogenesis and Ovulation

Oogenesis begins prenatally. In the ovary of a female embryo, germ cells divide mitotically to produce large numbers of **oogonia**. Oogonia not only undergo mitosis in utero, but they also enter the first phase of meiosis and are arrested in prophase I (as primary oocytes). These cells remain frozen in prophase I of meiosis for decades, until they reenter the meiotic cycle. Beginning at puberty and continuing on a monthly basis, hormonal changes stimulate completion of the first meiotic division and ovulation. This meiotic division yields a large secondary oocyte (containing all of the cytoplasm and organelles) and a small **polar body** (containing half the DNA, but no cytoplasm or organelles). The polar body disintegrates. The second meiotic division (i.e., completion of oogenesis) occurs only if the secondary oocyte is fertilized by a sperm; this division is also unequal, producing a large ovum and the second polar body. Note that if fertilization does occur, the nuclei from the sperm and egg do not fuse immediately. They must wait for the secondary oocyte to release the second polar body and finish maturing to an ootid and then an ovum. Finally, the two nuclei fuse, and a diploid ($2n$) zygote is formed.

Before we move on to a discussion of the menstrual cycle, you will need more background information on oogenesis. The primary oocyte is not an isolated cell. It is found in a clump of supporting cells called **granulosa cells**, and the entire structure (oocyte plus granulosa cells) is known as a **follicle**. The granulosa cells assist in maturation. An immature primary oocyte is surrounded by a single layer of granulosa cells, forming a **primordial follicle**.

As the primordial follicle matures, the granulosa cells proliferate to form several layers around the oocyte, and the oocyte itself forms a protective layer of mucopolysaccharides termed the **zona pellucida**. There may be several follicles in the ovary; they are surrounded and separated by **thecal cells**. Of the several maturing follicles, only one progresses to the point of ovulation each month; all others degenerate. The mature follicle is known as a **Graafian follicle**. During ovulation, the Graafian follicle bursts, releasing the secondary oocyte with its zona pellucida and protective granulosa cells into the abdomen. The fimbriae sweep the oocyte into the uterine tube. At this point the layer of granulosa cells surrounding the ovum is known as the **corona radiata**. The follicular cells remaining in the ovary after ovulation form a new structure called the **corpus luteum** (Figure 55).

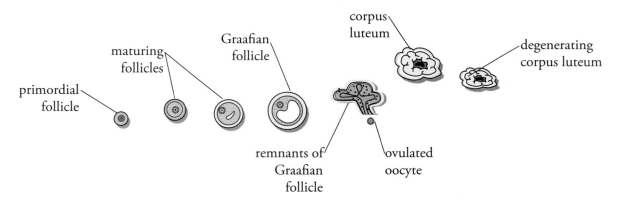

Figure 55   The Fate of a Follicle

Estrogen is made and secreted by the granulosa cells (with help from the thecal cells) during the first half of the menstrual cycle. Both estrogen and progesterone are secreted by the corpus luteum during the second half of the cycle. Estrogen is a steroid hormone that plays an important role in the development of female secondary sexual characteristics, in the menstrual cycle, and during pregnancy. Progesterone is also a steroid hormone involved in the hormonal regulation of the menstrual cycle and pregnancy, but with different effects than estrogen.

Menstrual Cycle

The menstrual cycle is (on average) a 28-day cycle that includes events occurring in the ovary (discussed above and referred to as the **ovarian cycle**), as well as events occurring in the uterus (the shedding of the old endometrium and preparation of a new endometrium for potential pregnancy), referred to as the **uterine cycle**.

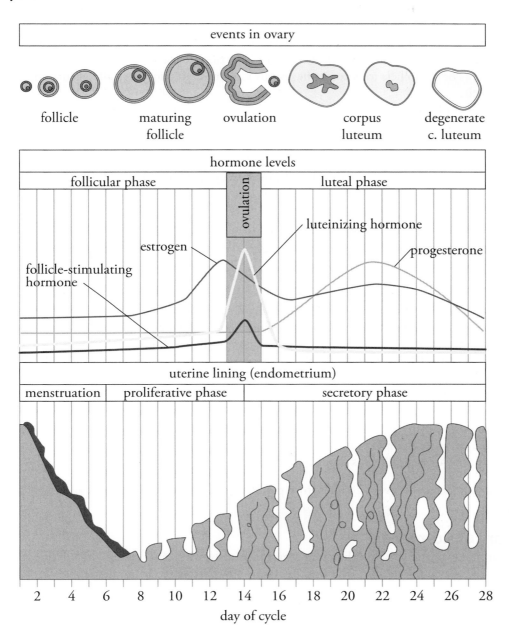

Figure 56   Menstrual Cycle

8.10

Ovarian Cycle

The ovarian cycle can be subdivided into three phases (Figure 56):

1. During the **follicular phase**, a primary follicle matures and secretes estrogen. Rising estrogen levels have a positive feedback effect on granulosa cells, encouraging them to make even more estrogen. Maturation of the follicle is under the control of follicle stimulating hormone (FSH) from the anterior pituitary. The follicular phase lasts about 13 days.
2. In the **ovulatory phase**, a secondary oocyte is released from the ovary. This is triggered by a surge of luteinizing hormone (LH) from the anterior pituitary. The surge also causes the remnants of the follicle to become the corpus luteum. Ovulation typically occurs on day 14 of the cycle.
3. The **luteal phase** begins with full formation of the corpus luteum in the ovary. This structure secretes both estrogen and progesterone, and has a life span of about two weeks. The average length of the luteal phase is about 14 days.

The hormones secreted from the ovary during the ovarian cycle direct the uterine cycle.

Uterine Cycle

The uterine cycle covers the same 28 days that were discussed above, but the focus is on the preparation of the endometrium for potential implantation of a fertilized egg. The uterine cycle can also be subdivided into three phases (Figure 56):

1. The first phase is **menstruation**, triggered by the degeneration of the corpus luteum and subsequent drop in estrogen and progesterone levels. The sharp decrease in these hormones causes the previous cycle's endometrial lining to slough out of the uterus, producing the bleeding associated with this time period. Menstruation typically lasts about 5 days.
2. During the **proliferative phase** of the menstrual cycle, estrogen produced by the follicle induces the proliferation of a new endometrium. This phase lasts about 9 days.
3. After ovulation the **secretory phase** occurs. Here, estrogen and progesterone produced by the corpus luteum further increase development of the endometrium, including secretion of glycogen, lipids, and other material. If pregnancy does not occur, death of the corpus luteum and decline in the secretion of estrogen and progesterone trigger menstruation once again. The secretory phase typically lasts about 14 days.

The menstrual cycle repeats every 28 days from puberty until menopause (at about age 50–60).

Summary of Hormones

The anterior pituitary and the hypothalamus play a role in the menstrual cycle by regulating the secretion of estrogen and progesterone from the ovary (Figure 56). Estrogen and progesterone then regulate the events in the uterus. The following is a summary:

- GnRH from the hypothalamus stimulates the release of FSH and LH from the anterior pituitary.

- Under the influence of FSH, granulosa and thecal cells develop during the follicular phase and secrete estrogen. Secretion of GnRH, FSH, and LH is initially inhibited by estrogen; however, estrogen, which increases throughout the follicular stage, reaches a threshold near the end of this phase and has a positive effect on LH secretion.

- This sudden surge in LH causes ovulation.

8.10

- After ovulation, LH induces the follicle to become the corpus luteum and to secrete estrogen and progesterone (this marks the beginning of the secretory phase).

- If pregnancy does not occur, the combined high levels of estrogen and progesterone provide feedback to strongly inhibit secretion of GnRH, FSH, and LH. When LH secretion drops, the corpus luteum regresses, no longer secretes estrogen or progesterone, and menstruation occurs.

8.11   DEVELOPMENT AND EMBRYOLOGY

Hormonal Changes During Pregnancy

There are still a couple of points we have not made completely clear: How can pregnancy occur if the uterine lining is lost each month, and why does the body discard the endometrium?

Recall that the physiological reason for endometrial shedding is a decrease in estrogen and progesterone levels, which occurs as the corpus luteum degenerates. Why does the corpus luteum degenerate? Due to a decrease in luteinizing hormone. Why does LH decrease? Due to feedback inhibition from the high levels of estrogen and progesterone secreted by the corpus luteum.

Let's begin with why LH levels decrease. During pregnancy, ovulation should be prevented. The way ovulation is prevented is for the constant high levels of estrogen and progesterone seen during pregnancy to inhibit secretion of LH by the pituitary—no LH surge, no ovulation. Constant high levels of estrogen inhibit LH release. The result is pregnancy without continued ovulation. The secondary result is the one we were trying to explain: when the corpus luteum secretes a lot of estrogen and progesterone during the menstrual cycle, LH levels drop, causing the corpus luteum to degenerate. The point is that the corpus luteum degenerates unless fertilization has occurred.

So how can pregnancy occur? If pregnancy is to occur, the endometrium must be maintained, because it is the site of gestation (i.e., where the **embryo** lives and is nourished). If fertilization takes place, within a few days a developing embryo becomes implanted in the endometrium, and a **placenta** begins to develop. The **chorion** is the portion of the placenta that is derived from the zygote. It secretes **human chorionic gonadotropin**, or **hCG,** which can take the place of LH in maintaining the corpus luteum. In the presence of hCG, the corpus luteum does not degenerate, estrogen and progesterone levels stay elevated, and menstruation does not occur. hCG is the hormone tested for in pregnancy tests because its presence absolutely confirms the presence of an embryo.

Fertilization

As we saw in the previous section, every month, a secondary oocyte is ovulated and enters the uterine tube. It is surrounded by the corona radiata (a protective layer of granulosa cells) and the zona pellucida (located just outside the egg cell membrane). The oocyte will remain fertile for about a day. If intercourse occurs, sperm are deposited near the cervix, and will survive for two or three days. They swim through the uterus toward the secondary oocyte.

Fertilization is the fusion of a spermatozoan with the secondary oocyte (Figure 57). It normally occurs in a fallopian tube. In order for fertilization to occur, a sperm must penetrate the corona radiata and bind to and penetrate the zona pellucida. It accomplishes this using the **acrosome reaction**. The acrosome is

8.11

a large vesicle in the sperm head containing hydrolytic enzymes which are released by exocytosis. After the corona radiata has been penetrated, an **acrosomal process** containing actin elongates toward the zona pellucida. The acrosomal process has **bindin**, a species-specific protein which binds to receptors in the zona pellucida. Finally, the sperm and egg plasma membranes fuse, and the sperm nucleus enters the secondary oocyte. In about 20 minutes, the secondary oocyte completes meiosis II, giving rise to an ootid and the second polar body. The ootid matures rapidly, becoming an **ovum**. Then the sperm and egg nuclei fuse, and the new diploid cell is known as a **zygote**.

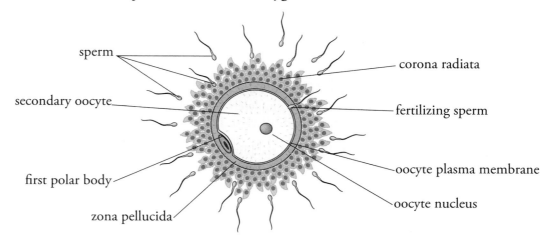

Figure 57   Fertilization

8.11

Penetration of an ovum by more than one sperm is known as **polyspermy**. It is normally prevented by the **fast block** to polyspermy and the **slow block** to polyspermy, which occur upon penetration of the egg by a spermatozoan. The fast block consists of a depolarization of the egg plasma membrane. This depolarization prevents other spermatozoa from fusing with the egg cell membrane. The slow block results from a Ca^{2+} influx caused by the initial depolarization. The slow block is also known as the **cortical reaction**. It has two components: swelling of the space between the zona pellucida and the plasma membrane, and hardening of the zona pellucida. The Ca^{2+} influx has one other noteworthy effect. It causes increased metabolism and protein synthesis, referred to as **egg activation**.

Cleavage

The process of **embryogenesis** begins within hours of fertilization, but proceeds slowly in humans. The first stage is **cleavage**, in which the zygote undergoes many cell divisions to produce a ball of cells known as the **morula**. The first cell division occurs about 36 hours after fertilization.

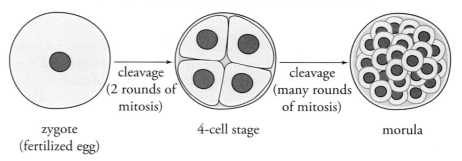

Figure 58   Cleavage

As cell divisions continue, the morula is transformed into a **blastocyst** (Figure 59). This process is known as **blastulation**. The blastocyst consists of a ring of cells called the **trophoblast** surrounding a cavity, and an **inner cell mass** adhering to the inside of the trophoblast at one end of the cavity. The trophoblast will give rise to the chorion (the zygote's contribution to the placenta). The inner cell mass will become the embryo.

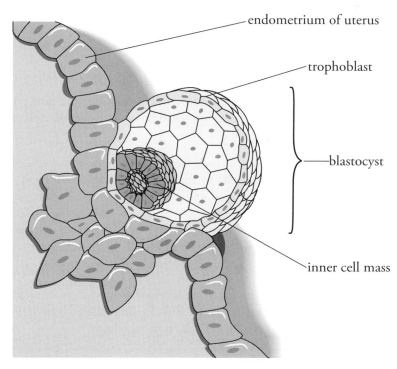

Figure 59 The Blastocyst at the Beginning of Implantation

Implantation and the Placenta

The developing blastocyst reaches the uterus and burrows into the endometrium, or **implants**, about a week after fertilization (Figure 59). The trophoblast secretes proteases that lyse endometrial cells. The blastocyst then sinks into the endometrium and is surrounded by it, absorbing nutrients through the trophoblast into the inner cell mass. The embryo receives a large part of its nutrition in this manner for the first few weeks of pregnancy. This is why the secretory phase of the endometrial cycle occurs: endometrial cells store glycogen, lipids, and other nutrients so that the early embryo may derive nourishment directly from the endometrium. Later, an organ develops which is specialized to facilitate exchange of nutrients, gases, and even antibodies between the maternal and embryonic bloodstreams: the placenta. Because it takes about three months for the placenta to develop, it is during the first trimester (three months) of pregnancy that hCG is essential for maintenance of the endometrium. During the last six months of pregnancy, the corpus luteum is no longer needed because the placenta itself secretes sufficient estrogen and progesterone for maintenance of the endometrium.

Development of the placenta involves formation of **placental villi**. These are chorionic projections extending into the endometrium, into which fetal capillaries will grow. Surrounding the villi are sinuses (open spaces) filled with maternal blood.

8.11

The embryo is not the only important structure derived from the inner cell mass. There are three others: amnion, yolk sac, and allantois. The **amnion** surrounds a fluid-filled cavity which contains the developing embryo. Amniotic fluid is the "water" that "breaks" (is expelled) before birth. The **yolk sac** is important in reptiles and birds because it contains the nourishing yolk. Mammals do not store yolk. Our yolk sac is important because it is the first site of red blood cell synthesis in the embryo. Finally, the **allantois** develops from the embryonic gut and forms the blood vessels of the umbilical cord, which transport blood between embryo and placenta.

Post-Implantation Development

We have examined embryogenesis from fertilization through blastulation. The next phase is **gastrulation**. During gastrulation, the three **primary germ layers (ectoderm, mesoderm, and endoderm)** become distinct.

In primitive organisms, the **blastula** (equivalent to blastocyst) is a hollow ball of cells, and gastrulation involves **invagination** (involution) of these cells to form layers. Imagine pushing your fist into a big soft round balloon to create an inner layer (contacting your fist) and an outer layer (contacting the air). The inner layer is the endoderm, and the outer layer is the ectoderm. The mesoderm (middle layer) develops from the endoderm. The cavity (where your fist is) is primitive gut, or **archenteron**. The opening (where your wrist is) is the **blastopore**, and will give rise to the anus. The whole structure is the **gastrula**. (Don't be confused: The *gastr*ula has a *blast*opore; the *blast*ula has no opening.)

In humans, things are a little different. The gastrula develops from a double layer of cells called the **embryonic disk**, instead of from a spherical blastula. But the end result is the same: three layers. You need to know what parts of the human body are derived from each layer.

Ectoderm	Mesoderm	Endoderm
• Entire nervous system • Pituitary gland (both lobes), adrenal medulla • Cornea and lens • Epidermis of skin and derivatives (hair, nails, sweat glands, sensory receptors) • Nasal, oral, anal epithelium	• All muscle, bone, and connective tissue • Entire cardiovascular and lymphatic system, including blood • Urogenital organs (kidneys, ureters, gonads, reproductive ducts) • Dermis of skin	• GI tract epithelium (except mouth and anus) • GI glands (liver, pancreas, etc.) • Respiratory epithelium • Epithelial lining of urogenital organs and ducts • Urinary bladder

Table 13 Fates of the Primary Germ Layers

One key thing to note is that **ectoderm** and epithelium are not synonymous. Epithelium outside the body (epidermis) is derived from ectoderm, but epithelium inside the body (gut lining) comes from endoderm.

The next step after gastrulation is **neurulation**, the formation of the nervous system. It proceeds by the invagination and pinching off of a layer of ectoderm along the dorsum (back) of the embryo to form the **dorsal neural groove**. This gives rise to the **neural tube**, which gives rise to the brain and spinal cord. The formation of the neural tube is induced by instructions from the underlying notochord, which is mesodermal in origin. It gives rise to the vertebral column. Other ectodermal cells migrate through the body to form peripheral nervous system ganglia.

Neurulation is one component of **organogenesis**, the development of organ systems. By the eighth week of gestation, all major organ systems are present, and the embryo is now called a **fetus**. Even though the developmental process has attained staggering complexity, by the end of the first trimester the fetus is still only 5 cm long. During the second and third trimesters, the fetus grows substantially. The organ systems that were initially formed in the first trimester undergo further development and maturation.

Birth and Lactation

The technical term for birth is **parturition**. It is dependent on uterine wall muscle contraction. The very high levels of progesterone secreted throughout pregnancy repress contractions in uterine muscle, but near the end of pregnancy uterine excitability increases. This increased excitability likely results from several factors, including a change in the ratio of estrogen to progesterone, the presence of the hormone oxytocin secreted by the posterior pituitary, and mechanical stretching of the uterus and cervix.

Weak contractions of the uterus occur throughout pregnancy. As pregnancy reaches full term, however, rhythmic **labor contractions** begin. This is likely the result of a positive feedback reflex: increased pressure on the cervix crosses a threshold that causes the posterior pituitary to increase secretion of oxytocin. Oxytocin causes uterine contractions to increase in intensity, creating greater pressure on the cervix that stimulates still more oxytocin release and even stronger contractions.

The first stage of labor is dilation of the cervix. The second stage is the actual birth, involving movement of the baby through the cervix and birth canal, pushed by contraction of uterine (smooth) and abdominal (skeletal) muscle. The third stage is expulsion of the placenta, after it separates from the wall of the uterus. Contractions of the uterus after birth help to minimize blood loss.

During pregnancy, milk production and secretion would be a waste of energy, but after parturition it is necessary. During puberty, estrogen stimulates development of breasts in women. Increased levels of estrogen and progesterone secreted by the placenta during pregnancy cause the further development of glandular and adipose breast tissue. However, while these hormones stimulate breast development, they inhibit the release of prolactin and thus the production of milk. After parturition, levels of estrogen and progesterone fall and milk production begins. Every time suckling occurs, the pituitary gland is stimulated by the hypothalamus to release a large surge of prolactin, prolonging the ability of breasts to secrete milk. If the mother stops breast-feeding the infant, prolactin levels fall and milk secretion ceases. The converse is also true: milk secretion can continue for years, as long as nursing continues. Breasts do not leak large amounts of milk when the infant is not nursing. This is because the posterior pituitary hormone oxytocin is necessary for **milk letdown** (release). Oxytocin is also released when suckling occurs.

8.12   CELLS, TISSUES, ORGANS

Organization in living things exists in a hierarchical structure. Arranged from the simplest to most complex, they are: atoms, molecules, organelles, cells, tissues, organs, organ systems, organisms, populations, communities, ecosystem, biome, and biosphere. In other words, cells make up tissues, tissues make up organs, organs make up organ systems, organ systems make up an organism, and so on.

The human body consists of approximately 100 trillion cells, of which there are about 220 different types. Cells are generally grouped together to form **tissues**, groups of cells that function together as a unit and usually have similar structures. The space between cells is filled by a nonliving material, called the extracellular matrix, intercellular matrix, or interstitium.

There are four major types of tissues in the human body: epithelial tissue, muscle tissue, nervous tissue, and connective tissue. **Epithelial tissue** is located at the body's surface and where the body meets the external environment, such as the lining of the digestive tract. There are three common shapes of epithelial cells: **squamous** (flat), **columnar** (tall and thin), and **cuboidal** (shaped like a cube). Here are some examples of each:

- Epithelial tissue of the skin is made of many layers of (or stratified) squamous cells lying on a basement membrane.
- **Endothelial cells** are squamous epithelial cells that make up blood vessels.
- Alveoli of the lung are made of many squamous epithelial cells and a smaller number of cuboidal cells that make and secrete surfactant.
- Columnar cells line most of the digestive tract.
- Ciliated columnar cells make up the upper respiratory tract, such as the trachea and bronchi.
- Cuboidal cells make up the epithelia of kidney tubules and many glands.

Not all cells in your body are these shapes. For example, hepatocytes (liver cells) are polygonal in shape, the acinar cells of the pancreas are shaped like pyramids.

There are three types of **muscle tissue**. Skeletal muscle allows gross motor movement and is made of myofibers. Cardiac muscle tissue is found in the heart and smooth muscle tissue lines hollow organs and tubes. Cardiac and smooth muscle cells are both called myocytes.

Nerve tissue is made of neurons (or nerve cells) and glial cells, both of which were discussed earlier in this chapter.

There are six types of **connective tissue**:

1. cartilage, made of chondrocytes
2. bone tissue, containing osteoblasts, osteoclasts, and osteocytes
3. tendons
4. ligaments
5. fat (adipose), made of adipocytes
6. blood, containing red blood cells (erythrocytes) and white blood cells (leukocytes)

All together there are 78 main organs within the human body, many of which we've explored in this chapter. Of the 78 organs, only five organs are vital for survival: the heart, brain, kidneys, liver, and lungs. If you think about what each of these organs do for us, you will appreciate why they are important enough to make this list. Organs coordinate and work together in organ systems, and organ systems also work together. This coordination and cooperation are essential to maintain homeostasis and facilitate survival of the organism.

8.12

CHAPTER 8 KEY TERMS

A band
ABO blood group
absolute refractory period
accessory glands
accessory organs
acetylcholine (ACh)
acetylcholinesterase
acrosomal process
acrosome
acrosome reaction
actin
action potential
adenohypophysis
adrenal cortex
adrenal gland
adrenaline
adrenal medulla
adrenocorticotropic hormone (ACTH)
afferent
afferent arteriole
albumin
aldosterone
alimentary canal
allantois
alveolar capillaries
alveolar duct
alveoli
alveolus
amnion
anal sphincter
androgens
angiotensin-converting enzyme (ACE)
angiotensin I
angiotensin II
angiotensinogen
antagonistic
anterior pituitary
antidiuretic hormone (ADH)
anus
aorta
aortic semilunar valves
appendix
aqueous humor
archenteron
arteries
arterioles
atria
atrioventricular (AV) node
atrioventricular (AV) valve

auditory
auditory hair cells
auditory receptors
autonomic
AV bundle (bundle of His)
axon
bicarbonate
bicuspid (or mitral) valve
bile
bindin
blastocyst
blastopore
blastula
blastulation
bolus
bone marrow
Bowman's capsule
brainstem
bronchioles
brush border
brush border enzymes
bulbourethral glands
calcitonin
calmodulin
calyces
calyx
canaliculi
capillaries
capsule
carbohydrate
carbonic acid
carbonic anhydrase
cardiac output (CO)
cardiac sphincter
cartilage
catecholamines
cecum
central nervous system (CNS)
central (or Haversian) canal
cerebellum
cerebral cortex
cerebral hemispheres
cerebrospinal fluid (CSF)
ceruminous (wax) glands
cervix
chemical
chemoreceptors
chief cells
cholecystokinin (CCK)

chondrocytes
chorion
choroid
chyme
chymotrypsin
ciliary muscle
cleavage
cochlea
collecting duct
colonic bacteria
columnar
common bile duct
compact bone
conduction zone
cones
connective tissue
contractility
cooperatively
cornea
corona radiata
coronary arteries
coronary veins
corpora cavernosa
corpus callosum
corpus luteum
corpus spongiosum
cortex
cortical reaction
cortisol
countercurrent multiplier
cretinism
crossbridges
cuboidal
cutaneous vasoconstriction
cutaneous vasodilation
defecation
dendrites
depolarized
dermis
diaphragm
diastole
diencephalon
dorsal neural groove
ductus deferens
duodenum
ear canal
ectoderm
effectors
efferent
efferent arteriole
egg activation
ejaculatory duct
elastic cartilage

electromagnetic receptors
embryo
embryogenesis
embryonic disk
emmetropia
emulsifier
endocrine glands
endoderm
endometrium
endothelial cells
enterokinase
enteropeptidase
epidermis
epididymis
epiglottis
epinephrine
epithelial tissue
erectile tissue
erythroblastosis fetalis
erythropoietin
estrogens
exocrine organs
expiration
expiratory reserve volume (ERV)
external sphincter
fallopian tubes
fascicle
fast block
fat
feedback inhibition
fertilization
fetus
fibrin
fibrinogen
fibrous cartilage
filtrate
fimbriae
follicle
follicle stimulating hormone (FSH)
follicular phase
forced expiration
forebrain
formed elements
frontal lobes
functional residual capacity (FRC)
functional syncytium
gallbladder
gametogenesis
ganglia
gastrointestinal tract or GI tract
gastrula
gastrulation
germ cells

glans clitoris
glomerular basement membrane (GBM)
glomerular filtration rate (GFR)
glomerulus
glucagon
glucocorticoids
gluconeogenesis
glycogen
glycogenesis
glycogenolysis
goiter
gonadotropin releasing hormone (GnRH)
Graafian follicle
granulosa cells
growth hormone (GH)
gustatory
hair follicles
haploid gametes
Haversian system
heart
heart rate
hematocrit
hematopoiesis
heme
hemoglobin
hemolytic disease of the newborn
hemophilia
hemostasis
hepatic portal vein
hindbrain
homeostasis
homeotherms
human chorionic gonadotropin, or hCG
hyaline cartilage
hydrochloric acid (HCl)
hydroxyapatite
hyperglycemia
hyperopia
hyperpolarized
hyperventilation
hypodermis
hypoglycemia
hypothalamic-pituitary control axis
hypothalamic-pituitary portal system
hypothalamus
hypothyroidism
hypoventilation
hypoxia
H zone
I band
ileocecal valve
ileum
implants

incus
inferior vena cava
inhibitory interneuron
inner cell mass
inner ear
inspiration
inspiratory capacity (IC)
inspiratory reserve volume (IRV)
insulin
integrative
intercostal muscles
internal sphincter
internodal tract
interstitium
invagination
iris
ischemia
islets of Langerhans
jejunum
joint
juxtaglomerular apparatus (JGA)
keratin
keratinized
keto acids
labium majus
labium minus
labor contractions
lacteals
lacunae
lamellae
larynx
lens
leukocytes
Leydig cells
ligaments
ligand-gated ion channels
limbic systems
lipolysis
luteal phase
luteinizing hormone (LH)
lymph
lymph nodes
macronutrients
macula densa
malleus
mastication
maternal inheritance
mechanical
mechanoreceptors
medulla
medullary pyramids
megakaryocytes
meiotic division

melanin
melanocytes
menstruation
mesoderm
microvilli
midbrain
milk letdown
mineralocorticoids
monosynaptic reflex arc
morula
motor
motor neurons
mucociliary escalator
muscle stretch reflex
muscle tissue
myelination
myelin sheaths
myocytes
myofibers
myofibrils
myometrium
myopia
myosin
myosin binding site
nasal cavity
negative feedback
nerve tissue
neural tube
neuroendocrine cells
neurohypophysis
neurons
neurotransmitters
neurulation
nociceptors
nodes of Ranvier
nose
nuclei
occipital lobes
olfactory
olfactory receptors
oligodendrocytes
oogonia
opsin
optic nerve
organ of Corti
organogenesis
osmolarity
osteoblasts
osteoclasts
osteocytes
osteon
ova
oval window

ovarian cycle
ovaries
ovulatory phase
ovum
oxytocin
pacemaker of the heart
pancreas
pancreatic amylase
pancreatic duct
pancreatic lipase
papilla
papillae
parafollicular cells
parasympathetic
parathormone
parathyroid hormone
parietal cells
parietal lobes
parturition
pepsin
perforating (or Volkmann's) canals
perfusion
peripheral nervous system (PNS)
peristalsis
peritubular capillaries
Peyer's patches
pharynx
phosphocreatine
photoreceptors
pinna
placenta
placental villi
plasma
platelet plug
polar body
polyspermy
pons
portal systems
positive feedback
posterior pituitary
potassium leak channels
presynaptic neuron
primary bronchi
primary germ layers
primordial follicle
prolactin
proliferative phase
proprioceptors
prostate
protein
pulmonary
pulmonary capillaries
pulmonary circulation

pulse
pupil
Purkinje fibers
pyloric sphincter
reabsorption
reciprocal inhibition
rectum
red marrow
reflex
relative refractory period
releasing and inhibiting factors
releasing and inhibiting hormones
renal artery
renal pelvis
renal tubule
renal vein
renin
repolarized
residual volume (RV)
respiration
respiratory acidosis
respiratory alkalosis
respiratory bronchiole
respiratory membrane
respiratory zone
resting membrane potential (RMP)
retina
Rh blood group
rhodopsin
right and left bundle branches
rods
salivary amylase
saltatory conduction
sarcolemma
sarcomere
sarcoplasm
sarcoplasmic reticulum
Schwann cells
sclera
sebaceous (oil) glands
secretion
secretory phase
semen
semicircular canals
seminal vesicles
seminiferous tubules
sensory
sensory neurons
sensory receptors
Sertoli cells
serum
sex hormones
sinoatrial (SA) node

sliding filament
slow block
somatic
somatostatin
somatotropin (STH)
spermatogenesis
spermatozoa
spicules
spinal cord
spirometer
spirometric graph
spirometry
spongy bone
squamous
stapes
stratum basale
stretch receptors
stroke volume (SV)
subcutaneous tissue
sudoriferous (sweat) glands
superior vena cava
surface tension
surfactant
sympathetic
synapse
synaptic cleft
synaptic terminals
synaptic vesicles
syngamy
systemic circulation
systole
tactile
tactile receptors
taste receptors
telencephalon
temporal lobes
tendons
terminal bronchioles
testes
thalamus
thecal cells
thermoreceptors
thick and thin filaments
thin filament
thoracic duct
threshold
thrombin
thrombus
thyroid
thyroid-stimulating hormone (TSH)
thyroxine (T4)
tidal volume (TV)
tissues

total lung capacity (TLC)
trabeculae
trachea
transfusion reaction
tricuspid valve
triiodothyronine (T3)
trophoblast
tropic hormones
tropomyosin
troponin complex
trypsin
trypsinogen
T tubules
tympanic membrane
urea
ureter
urethra
urinary bladder
uterine cycle
uterine tubes
uterus
vagina
vasa recta

vas deferens
vasopressin
veins
ventilation
ventricles
venules
vestibular apparatus
vestibular nerve
villi
vital capacity (VC)
vitamin K
vitreous humor
vocal cords
voltage-gated calcium channels
voltage-gated potassium channels
voltage-gated sodium channels
yellow marrow
yolk sac
zona pellucida
zygote
zymogens

ANATOMY AND PHYSIOLOGY DRILL

1. Which of the following is true?

   A. The SA node is the pacemaker of the heart.
   B. Arteries always carry oxygenated blood.
   C. The aorta leaves the right ventricle of the heart.
   D. Large veins are elastic and contain valves.

2. Which of the following cells secretes glucagon in the pancreas?

   A. Alpha cells
   B. Beta cells
   C. Delta cells
   D. Hepatocytes

3. Which organ is responsible for release of epinephrine into the bloodstream?

   A. Adrenal cortex
   B. Spinal cord
   C. Adrenal medulla
   D. Liver

4. Which of the following could trigger an action potential in a neuron?

   A. An efflux of potassium ions
   B. A large number of negatively charged proteins in the cell
   C. Stimulus from another cell causing sodium ion channels in the membrane to open
   D. Allowing potassium ions, but not sodium ions, to diffuse down their gradient

5. Which statement best supports the fact that oxygen concentration is different across the alveoli and the capillary?

   A. The alveoli and the capillary are both thin walled.
   B. Hemoglobin in the blood has a very high affinity for oxygen.
   C. Oxygen transport between alveoli and capillaries occurs through diffusion.
   D. Alveolar air pressure and capillary blood pressure are slightly different.

6. The functional unit of respiration in the human body is the:

   A. bronchiole.
   B. alveolus.
   C. lung.
   D. capillary.

7. Which of the following molecules serves as an extra energy supply for muscles?

   A. ATP
   B. Phosphocreatine
   C. GTP
   D. Ca^{2+}

8. During the contraction of a skeletal muscle, the actin filaments:

   A. get attached to the binding sites on the myosin filaments.
   B. are pulled closer when the myosin heads rotate.
   C. require ATP while attaching themselves to the myosin filaments.
   D. become thinner than the myosin filaments.

9. In the adult human, where are the majority of blood cells produced?

A. Spleen
B. Kidney
C. All bones in the body
D. Bones in the axial skeleton

10. Glomerular filtration is the process by which blood plasma and other constituents are transferred to the Bowman's capsule. Which of the following factors has the least effect on the regulation of glomerular filtration?

A. Diameter of the glomerular efferent arteriole
B. Hormones present in blood plasma
C. Blood pressure in the glomerular afferent arteriole
D. Diameter of the glomerular afferent arteriole

11. How does the structure below help in the process of digestion?

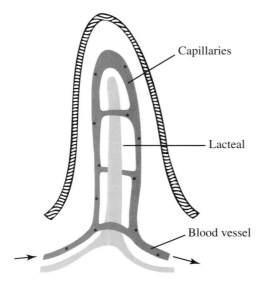

A. Increase the rate of absorption of nutrients by means of a thick-walled outer membrane
B. Provide more surface area for the absorption of nutrients
C. Increase the rate of absorption of nutrients by the means of thick-walled capillaries
D. Have the ability to move, so they can easily remove toxins from food

12. Which of the following correctly lists where the oocyte is released from at ovulation, where fertilization occurs, and where the blastocyst implants, respectively?

A. Ovary, fallopian tube, uterus
B. Ovary, uterus, abdominal cavity
C. Fallopian tube, fallopian tube, uterus
D. Ovary, uterus, uterus

13. Which of the following cell types is responsible for the nourishment of the developing sperm cells?

A. Sertoli cells, which respond to FSH
B. Nurse cells, which respond to FSH
C. Bartoli cells, which respond to LH
D. Leydig cells, which respond to LH

Want More Practice?
Register your book online for more drill questions!

Answers and Explanations

1. **A**   The sinoatrial node is the pacemaker of the heart (choice A is correct). Arteries carry oxygenated blood in systemic blood vessels, but not in the pulmonary circulatory system (eliminate option B). The aorta leaves the left ventricle of the heart (eliminate choice C). Arteries are elastic and large veins contain valves (eliminate choice D).

2. **A**   Alpha cells secrete glucagon in the pancreas (choice A is correct). Beta cells make and release insulin (eliminate choice B), delta cells release somatostatin (eliminate choice C), and hepatocytes are liver cells and do not make or release hormones (eliminate choice D).

3. **C**   The adrenal cortex produces various hormones including cortisol and aldosterone (eliminate choice A). The spinal cord does not release substances into the bloodstream (eliminate choice B). The adrenal medulla produces epinephrine (also known as adrenaline, choice (C) is correct). The liver produces many blood proteins but does not make or release hormones (eliminate choice D).

4. **C**   Potassium ions leaving the cell cause repolarization or hyperpolarization but will not get a neuron to threshold (eliminate choices A and D). The presence of a large number of negatively charged proteins is a reason why the RMP is negative, but this is not relevant to initiating an action potential (eliminate choice B). Stimulus from another cell causing sodium ion channels in the membrane to open would allow sodium ions to flow across the concentration gradient. This could get a neuron to threshold (choice C is correct).

5. **C**   While thin-walled capillaries facilitate gas diffusion, they do not explain the difference in oxygen concentration across the alveoli and capillary (eliminate choice A). Diffusion occurs only when there is a concentration gradient across a membrane. In the lungs, oxygen diffuses across the alveoli membrane and is picked up by red blood cells in the capillaries (choice C is correct). The presence of oxygen-bound hemoglobin in the capillary does not explain why the oxygen concentration is different across the alveoli and capillary (eliminate choice B). Partial pressure difference of oxygen in alveolar air and capillary blood is responsible for oxygen diffusion from the alveoli to the capillary. Total air pressure and blood pressure are not relevant (eliminate choice D).

6. **B**   Bronchioles do not participate in gas exchange (eliminate choice A). The functional unit of any organ is the smallest part of the organ that carries out the organ's function. For example, in the kidney, the smallest part that filters blood to produce urine is the nephron, so the nephron is the functional unit of the kidney. In the respiratory system, the alveolus is the smallest part that actually participates in gas exchange, so it is the functional unit of respiration (choice B is correct). The lungs are too large to be considered the functional unit (eliminate choice C). Capillaries do not belong solely to the respiratory system (eliminate choice D).

7. **B**   First muscle cells rely on ATP for energy (eliminate choice A). Phosphocreatine acts as a secondary energy source for muscles; it can be dephosphorylated to create ATP out of ADP and P_i when muscle ATP is low (choice B is correct). GTP and Ca^{2+} are not important energy sources in muscle cells (eliminate choices C and D).

8. **B** The actin filament has a binding site at which the myosin filament attaches itself (eliminate choice A). Myosin heads rotate to pull actin filaments closer which makes the sarcomere shorter (choice B is correct). Myosin filaments need ATP while detaching themselves from the actin filaments (eliminate choice C). Actin filaments are naturally thin protein filaments; their thickness does not change during muscle contraction (eliminate choice D).

9. **D** The spleen produces blood cells during fetal development (eliminate choice A). While the kidney plays a role in blood-cell development through secretion of erythropoietin, it does not directly produce blood cells (eliminate choice B). In an adult, most blood cell production occurs in the red bone marrow of the ribs, vertebrae, sternum, and pelvis. Together with the skull, these bones make up the axial skeleton of the body. Most bone marrow is a fatty, dormant tissue not involved in blood cell production (choice D is correct; eliminate option C).

10. **B** Glomerular filtration does not depend on blood-borne hormones (choice B is correct). Glomerular filtration rate (GFR) depends directly on blood pressure (eliminate choice C); constriction of the efferent arteriole increases blood pressure in the glomerulus and increases GFR (eliminate choice A). Dilation of the afferent arteriole increases blood flow to the glomerulus; this increases blood pressure and GFR (eliminate choice D).

11. **B** Villi of the small intestine are finger-like projections. Their shape increases the surface area for the absorption of nutrients (choice B is correct). The other answer choices are not relevant.

12. **A** At ovulation, an oocyte is released from the ovary (eliminate choice C). It is swept into a fallopian tube, where fertilization occurs (eliminate choices B and D). The blastocyst implants into the uterine wall and this is where the embryo develops (choice A is correct).

13. **A** Sertoli cells are also known as supporting cells or sustentacular cells, because they help nurture the developing sperm. They respond to FSH from the anterior pituitary gland (choice A is correct). Nurse and Bartoli cells are not cell types associated with the male reproductive system (eliminate choices B and C). Leydig cells are found outside the seminiferous tubules; they respond to LH and secrete testosterone (eliminate choice D).

Quick Review

Circulatory and Lymphatic Systems

- Circulatory and lymphatic systems transport materials (e.g., O_2, CO_2, nutrients, wastes, hormones, etc.) around the body.

- The lymphatic system helps filter and return tissue fluid (lymph) to the circulatory system.

- Deoxygenated blood returning from the body enters the heart at the right atrium and is pumped to the lungs by the right ventricle.

- Oxygenated blood returns to the heart at the left atrium and is pumped to the body by the left ventricle.

- AV valves (tricuspid on the right and bicuspid, or mitral, on the left) separate atria and ventricles.

- Semilunar valves (pulmonary on the right and aortic on the left) separate ventricles and arteries.

- Veins always return blood to the heart. Most veins carry deoxygenated blood; an exception are the pulmonary veins, which return blood from the lungs to the heart.

- Arteries always carry blood away from the heart. Most arteries carry oxygenated blood; an exception are the pulmonary arteries, which carry blood from the heart to the lungs.

- Cardiac muscle is a functional syncytium; cells are connected by intercalated disks, which contain gap junctions. These gap junctions are electrical synapses that easily allow the transmission of the action potential, and thus contraction, to spread from cell to cell.

- The SA node is the pacemaker of the heart. It generates 120 beats per minute and is continuously controlled by the autonomic nervous system.

- Cardiac output is directly proportional to stroke volume and heart rate.

- Blood is approximately 55% plasma, 45% percent erythrocytes (red blood cells), and 1% leukocytes (white blood cells) and platelets.

- ABO and Rh antigens on the surface of erythrocytes determine blood type:

Blood Type	Genotype	Can Receive from	Can Donate to
A	$I^A I^A$ or $I^A i$	A or O	A or AB
B	$I^B I^B$ or $I^B i$	B or O	B or AB
O	ii	O only	O, A, B, or AB (universal donor)
AB	$I^A I^B$	O, A, B, or AB (universal recipient)	AB only

- Oxygen is transported in the blood bound to hemoglobin, a protein in red blood cells.

- Carbon dioxide is transported in the blood primarily as bicarbonate ion; some also binds to hemoglobin.

Endocrine System

- The endocrine system controls our overall physiology and homeostasis by hormones that travel through the bloodstream.

- Hormones are released from endocrine glands, travel to distant target tissues via the blood, bind to receptors on target tissues, and exert effects on target cells.

- Peptide hormones are made from amino acids, bind to receptors on the cell surface, and typically affect target cells via second messenger pathways. Effects tend to be rapid and temporary.

- Steroid hormones are derived from cholesterol, bind to receptors in the cytoplasm or nucleus, and alter transcription. Effects tend to occur more slowly and are more permanent.

- Anterior pituitary hormones are made and released from the anterior pituitary. They are all peptide hormones and include FSH, LH, ACTH, TSH, prolactin, and GH.

- Oxytocin and vasopressin (ADH) are peptide hormones; they are made by the hypothalamus but released from the posterior pituitary gland.

- Calcium homeostasis is controlled by PTH (parathyroids) and calcitonin (thyroid).

- Blood pressure is controlled by aldosterone (adrenal cortex) and ADH (posterior pituitary).

- Blood sugar levels are controlled by insulin and glucagon, both released from the pancreas.

- Sex steroids include testosterone, estrogen, and progesterone. They are released from the adrenal cortex and gonads.

- Stress hormones are cortisol (long term; from adrenal cortex) and epinephrine (or adrenalin; short term; from adrenal medulla).

Integumentary System

- Skin is made of three main layers: epidermis (epithelial tissue), dermis (connective tissue), and hypodermis (adipose tissue).

- Epidermis provides a barrier to infection and water loss.

- Dermis is where sweat glands, nerves, blood vessels, and sensory receptors are found.

- Hypodermis is a layer of fat for protection and insulation.

- Thermoregulation is primarily a function of the dermis.

- When temperatures rise, blood vessels in the dermis dilate to release heat and sweat glands are activated.

- When temperature falls, blood vessels constrict to retain heat. Also, involuntary skeletal muscle contractions occur (shivering) to produce heat.

Nervous System

- The neuron is the basic structural and functional unit of the nervous system. It has several specialized structures that allow it to transmit action potentials.

- Neurons receive incoming information via dendrites. Signals are summed by the axon hillock, and if the signal is greater than the threshold (–50 mV), an action potential is initiated and fired down the axon.

- An action potential is an all-or-none signal that includes depolarization (via voltage-gated sodium channels) and repolarization (via voltage-gated potassium channels); it begins and ends at the cell's resting potential of –70 mV.

- A second action potential cannot fire during the absolute refractory period because voltage-gated sodium channels are resetting.

- A second action potential can fire during the relative refractory period but more stimulatory signal is required to reach threshold.

- Glial cells are specialized, non-neuronal cells that provide structural and metabolic support to neurons; Schwann cells (PNS) and oligodendrocytes (CNS) are examples.

- Saltatory conduction is mediated by the myelin sheath; this accelerates action potential transmission.

- Neurons communicate with other neurons, organs, and glands at synapses.

- Most synapses are chemical in nature: an action potential causes the release of a neurotransmitter into the synaptic cleft; binding of the neurotransmitter to receptors on the postsynaptic cell triggers a change, either stimulatory or inhibitory, in the postsynaptic cell.

- The central nervous system includes the spinal cord and brain; specialized areas control specific aspects of human behavior, movement, intelligence, emotion, and reflexes.

- Important regions of the brain include the medulla, pons, cerebellum, midbrain, brainstem, thalamus hypothalamus, corpus callosum, and cerebral hemispheres.

- Four lobes of the cerebral hemispheres are frontal, parietal, temporal, and occipital lobes.

- The peripheral nervous system includes somatic (voluntary) and autonomic (involuntary) subdivisions.
    - The sympathetic branch of the autonomic system controls our fight-or-flight response; norepinephrine is the primary neurotransmitter and is augmented by epinephrine from the adrenal medulla.
    - The parasympathetic branch of the autonomic system controls our rest-and-digest state; acetylcholine is the primary neurotransmitter.

- Humans have several types of receptors (mechanoreceptors, chemoreceptors, nociceptors, thermoreceptors, electromagnetic receptors, and proprioceptors) that allow us to detect a variety of stimuli.

- From sound to hearing: sound waves → auricle → external auditory canal → tympanic membrane → malleus → incus → stapes → oval window → fluid of the cochlea → auditory hair cells → neurotransmitters stimulate auditory neurons → brain → perception.

- From light to vision: light → cornea → aqueous humor → pupil → lens → vitreous humor → light receptors (rods and cones) of the retina → electrical signals → optic nerve → brain → perception.

Respiratory System

- Primary functions of the respiratory system are gas exchange, thermoregulation, and pH regulation; pH regulation by the respiratory system is very fast.

- Organs of the respiratory system are divided into the conduction zone and respiratory zone.

- The conduction zone is for ventilation only and includes the nose, nasal cavity, pharynx, larynx, trachea, and respiratory tree from primary bronchi to terminal bronchioles.

- Larynx is made entirely of cartilage and includes the epiglottis (which separates food and air) and vocal cords (for sound production).

- Respiratory zone is for gas exchange and includes respiratory bronchioles, alveolar ducts, and alveoli.

- Surfactant reduces surface tension inside alveoli and helps them stay inflated.

- Inspiration is an active process and requires contraction of the diaphragm to expand the chest cavity; an increase in the size of the chest cavity (and lungs) reduces their pressure, and air flows in.

- Pathway of inhaled air: nose → nasal cavity → pharynx → larynx → trachea → bronchi → terminal bronchioles → respiratory bronchioles → alveolar ducts → alveoli.

- Expiration is primarily a passive process; the diaphragm relaxes and lung elastic recoil helps return them to their resting state. Reduction in the size of the chest cavity increases pressure and pushes air out.

- Forced expiration requires contraction of abdominal muscles to forcibly reduce the size of the chest cavity.

- Ventilation rate is determined primarily by CO_2 levels and the need to regulate pH, according to the following equilibrium: $CO_2 + H_2O \rightleftharpoons H_2CO_3 \rightleftharpoons H^+ + HCO_3^-$.

- As CO_2 levels increase, pH falls and ventilation rate increases; the reverse is also true.

Musculoskeletal System

- Bone is a dense connective tissue that functions in body support, protection, and mineral storage.

- Resorption and deposition of bone is regulated by parathyroid hormone and calcitonin, respectively, to regulate blood calcium levels.

- Osteoblasts build bone, osteoclasts collapse bone, and osteocytes are mature (retired) osteoblasts.

- Compact bone is organized into osteons—long cylinders of hard, dense bone; compact bone forms the outer shell of all bones and the shaft (diaphysis) of long bones.

- Spongy bone contains more space than compact bone and is filled with red bone marrow; this is where blood cell formation takes place. Spongy bone forms the core of flat bones and is found at the ends (epiphyses) of long bones.

- Cartilage is made by chondrocytes.

- Three types of cartilage are hyaline (e.g., trachea), elastic (e.g., outer ear), fibrous (e.g., intervertebral disks).

- Ligaments connect bones to other bones.

- Tendons connect bones to muscles.

- There are three types of muscle tissue: skeletal, cardiac, and smooth.

- Skeletal muscles are voluntary, striated, multinucleated, and attached to bones. They are individually innervated.

- Skeletal muscles are bundled into fascicles of many myofibers (cells), which contain myofibrils (strings of sarcomeres).

- Actin and myosin are organized into sarcomeres, which are contractile units of the skeletal muscle cell.

- The arrangement of actin and myosin produces a characteristic banding pattern (striations):
  - A band is the length of the thick/myosin filament.
  - I band is where only the thin/actin filament is present.
  - H zone is where only myosin is present.

- Increased overlap of actin and myosin during the Sliding Filament Theory produces sarcomere shortening. I band and H zone get shorter and Z lines move closer together.

- The four steps of the Sliding Filament Theory are binding of myosin to actin (cross-bridge formation), pulling of actin toward the center of the sarcomere (power stroke), release of actin from myosin (via ATP binding), and resetting myosin to a high-energy conformation (ATP hydrolysis).

- Muscle contraction starts with depolarization of the muscle cell; this triggers release of calcium into the cytosol from the sarcoplasmic reticulum. Calcium binds troponin and changes shape, pulling tropomyosin off actin. This exposes myosin binding sites on actin and allows contraction to occur. This process is known as excitation–contraction coupling.

- Cardiac muscle is also striated, meaning that it, too, is organized into sarcomeres. Sliding filaments and excitation–contraction occur as in skeletal muscle. However, cardiac muscle is involuntary and autorhythmic. The cells are uninuclear and connected by gap junctions to form a functional syncytium.

- Smooth muscles are involuntary and lack striations and sarcomeres; actin and myosin filaments are dispersed in the cytoplasm and controlled by calmodulin. Calcium is still needed for contraction.

Excretory System

- Organs of the excretory system include the kidneys, liver, large intestine, and skin.

- Kidneys filter blood to remove hydrophilic wastes; they also play a major role in homeostasis by regulating blood pressure, pH, ion balance, and water balance.

- Urine is produced by first filtering the blood, then by modifying the filtrate via reabsorption (moving substances from the filtrate to the blood) and secretion (moving substances from the blood to the filtrate), and finally by concentrating the filtrate to conserve body water.

- Filtration occurs at the glomerulus, most reabsorption and secretion occur in the PCT, selective reabsorption and secretion occur in the DCT, and concentration occurs in the collecting duct.

- The Loop of Henle establishes a concentration gradient in the medulla; this gradient is critical for the reabsorption of water and the creation of concentrated urine.

- ADH increases water permeability of the distal tubule (DCT and collecting duct) to allow reabsorption of water. Aldosterone increases Na^+ reabsorption at the distal tubule. Both hormones work together to help regulate blood pressure.

- When systemic blood pressure falls, kidneys release renin.

- Renin is an enzyme that converts the blood protein angiotensinogen into angiotensin I, which is further converted to angiotensin II.

- Angiotensin II is a potent vasoconstrictor and also increases the release of aldosterone; the ultimate goal is to increase blood pressure.

Digestive System

- Digestive system organs are divided into two categories: alimentary canal and accessory organs.

- The alimentary canal is the long muscular tube consisting of the mouth, esophagus, stomach, small intestine, and large intestine.

- Peristalsis moves food through the alimentary canal.

- Accessory organs have a digestive role but are not part of the tube; they include salivary glands, liver, gallbladder, and pancreas.

- The mouth breaks down food mechanically by chewing and also begins starch digestion via salivary amylase.

- The stomach is primarily a storage tank for food. Mechanical digestion occurs through churning of the food, chemical digestion occurs by acid hydrolysis, and protein digestion begins via pepsin.

- Almost all chemical digestion and nutrient absorption take place in the small intestine (duodenum, jejunum, and ileum).

- The large intestine (cecum, colon, rectum, and anus) primarily reabsorbs water and stores feces; no digestion takes place in the large intestine.

- The liver produces bile (secreted into the small intestine), which emulsifies fat to increase the efficiency of fat digestion. The gallbladder stores and concentrates bile.

- The pancreas secretes the majority of the digestive enzymes used in the small intestine, along with bicarbonate to help neutralize the acid entering the small intestine from the stomach.

- The pancreas is also a major endocrine organ, secreting insulin and glucagon to regulate blood glucose.

Reproductive System

- Primary sex organs (testes in males, ovaries in females) produce gametes and sex hormones.

- Spermatogenesis takes place in seminiferous tubules and results in four haploid sperm from a single spermatogonium. It begins at puberty and continues on a daily basis throughout the life of the male. FSH stimulates spermatogenesis and LH stimulates testosterone production.

- GnRH from the hypothalamus controls release of FSH and LH from the anterior pituitary.

- Sperm travel from the seminiferous tubules to the epididymis, then to the vas deferens, and then to the urethra.

- Semen is a supportive fluid for sperm, produced by the seminal vesicles, prostate, and bulbourethral glands.

- Oogenesis begins prenatally, producing primary oocytes. It occurs again on a monthly basis, beginning at puberty and ending at menopause; this produces one secondary oocyte (which is ovulated) and the first polar body.

- Oogenesis is completed only if the secondary oocyte is fertilized, in which case an ovum and the second polar body will be produced.

- FSH stimulates follicle development and estrogen secretion during the first half of the menstrual cycle.

- LH stimulates ovulation and the formation of the corpus luteum, as well as progesterone and estrogen secretion, during the second half of the menstrual cycle.

- Estrogen stimulates growth of the endometrium during the first half of the menstrual cycle; progesterone and estrogen maintain and enhance the endometrium during the second half of the menstrual cycle.

- If fertilization does not take place, estrogen and progesterone levels fall, and the endometrium is sloughed off via menstruation.

Development and Embryology

- Fertilization takes place in the fallopian tubes via sperm and ovum fusion.

- The nuclear genome is 50% maternal and 50% paternal, but the mitochondrial genome is inherited from the ovum.

- The zygote becomes a morula via cleavage, the morula becomes a blastula via blastulation, and the blastula implants in the endometrium of the uterus about a week after fertilization.

- The blastula (or blastocyst) contains an inner cell mass and an outer trophoblast.

- The trophoblast becomes the placenta and the inner cell mass becomes the embryo.

- The first eight weeks of development are the embryonic stage, during which gastrulation (formation of the three primary germ layers), neurulation (formation of the nervous system), and organogenesis (formation of the major organ systems) occur.

- The fetal stage begins at the eighth week of development and ends at the birth of the baby.

- Labor is a positive feedback cycle triggered by mild (initially) uterine contractions that push the baby's head on the cervix. This stimulates the release of oxytocin, which causes a stronger uterine contraction, and a bigger stretch of the cervix. This positive feedback loop will continue until the birth of the baby.

- Prolactin stimulates milk production and oxytocin stimulates milk ejection in a baby-driven cycle.

Cells, Tissues, Organs

- Levels of organization of living things: atoms, molecules, organelles, cells, tissues, organs, organ systems, organisms, populations, communities, ecosystem, biome, biosphere.

- Humans have 220 types of cells, four major types of tissues, 78 main organs, and 11 organ systems.

- Four major types of tissues are epithelial tissue, muscle tissue, nervous tissue, and connective tissue.

- Five organs (heart, brain, kidneys, liver, and lungs) are vital for survival.

- Organ systems are as follows: circulatory, lymphatic, endocrine, integumentary, nervous, respiratory, muscular, skeletal, excretory, digestive, and reproductive systems.

Chapter 9

General Chemistry

9.1 GENERAL CHEMISTRY FUNDAMENTALS

Metric Units

To express measurements of physical quantities, scientists use the *Système International d'Unitès* (the International System of Units), abbreviated SI. Six of the seven **base units** of SI are given below:

SI Base Unit	Abbreviation	Measures
meter	m	length
kilogram	kg	mass
second	s	time
mole	mol	amount of substance
kelvin	K	temperature
ampere	A	electric current

Table 1

The units of any physical quantity can be written in terms of the SI base units. For example, the SI unit of speed is meters per second (m/s), the SI unit of energy (the joule) is kilograms times meters² per second² ($kg \cdot m^2/s^2$), and so forth.

Multiples of the base units that are powers of 10 are often abbreviated and precede the symbol for the unit. For example, m is the symbol for milli-, which means 10^{-3} (one thousandth). So, one thousandth of a second, 1 millisecond, would be written as 1 ms. Some of the most common power-of-10 prefixes are given in the list below:

Prefix	Symbol	Multiple
nano-	n	10^{-9}
micro-	μ	10^{-6}
milli-	m	10^{-3}
centi	c	10^{-2}
kilo-	k	10^{3}
mega-	M	10^{6}

Table 2

Two other units, ones that are common in chemistry, are the liter and the angstrom. The liter (abbreviated L) is a unit of volume equal to 1/1,000 of a cubic meter. The cubic meter is the SI unit for volume:

$$1L = 10^{-3} \ m^3$$

From the relationship above, we see that one cubic meter is equal to one thousand liters. $1 \text{ m}^3 = 1{,}000 \text{ L}$

One milliliter is the same volume as one cubic centimeter. The relationship between milliliters, cubic centimeters, and liters is the following:

$$1 \text{ mL} = 1 \text{ cm}^3 = 1 \text{ cc}$$

$$1{,}000 \text{ mL} = 1{,}000 \text{ cm}^3 = 1 \text{ L}$$

The most common way of expressing solution concentrations is molarity (M), which is defined as moles of solute per liter of solution (moles/L). Ordinarily, the liter is used to express the volumes of liquids and gases, but not solids.

The **angstrom**, abbreviated Å, is a unit of length equal to 10^{-10} m. Atomic radii and bond lengths are typically around 1 to 3 Å.

Density

The **density** of a substance is its mass per volume:

$$\text{Density: } \rho = \frac{\text{mass}}{\text{volume}} = \frac{m}{V}$$

In SI units, density is expressed in kilograms per cubic meter (kg/m^3). However, in chemistry, densities of liquids and solids are more often expressed in grams per cubic centimeter (g/cm^3), whereas densities of gases are expressed in grams per liter (g/L). Most liquids and solids have a density of around 1 to 20 g/cm^3. Here is the conversion between density units:

$$\text{g/cm}^3 \rightarrow \text{multiply by } 1{,}000 \rightarrow \text{kg/m}^3$$

$$\text{g/cm}^3 \leftarrow \text{divide by } 1{,}000 \leftarrow \text{kg/m}^3$$

Molecular Formulas

When two or more atoms form a *covalent bond*, in which electrons are shared between two atoms, they create a **molecule**. For example, the H_2O molecule is formed from two O-H bonds. A compound's **molecular formula** gives the identities and numbers of the atoms in the molecule. The formula $C_4H_4N_2$, for example, tells us that this molecule contains 4 carbon atoms, 4 hydrogen atoms, and 2 nitrogen atoms.

Formula and Molecular Weight

Each element has an associated atomic weight, which is the common term for atomic mass. The unit for atomic weight is the **atomic mass unit**, abbreviated **amu**. By definition, one atomic mass unit is equal to exactly 1/12 the mass of an atom of carbon-12, the most abundant naturally occurring form of carbon. The masses of all other atoms are determined from this standard. The periodic table lists the mass of each element; it is a weighted average of the atomic masses of all its naturally occurring forms. For example, the atomic mass of hydrogen is listed as 1.0 (amu), and nitrogen as 14.0 (amu).

If we know the chemical formula, we can calculate the **formula weight**, which is the sum of the atomic weights of all the atoms in the molecule. The formula weight for the $C_4H_4N_2$ molecule is the sum of the weights of four carbon atoms, four hydrogen atoms, and two nitrogen atoms. Its weight is

$$4(12) + 4(1) + 2(14) = 80$$

(The unit *amu* is often not explicitly included.) When a compound exists as discrete molecules, the term **molecular weight** (**MW**) is usually used instead of formula weight. The term formula weight is commonly used for ionic compounds, such as NaCl, that are held together by strong attractive forces between oppositely charged species. For example, the molecular weight of water, H_2O, is $2(1) + 16 = 18$. The formula weight of NaCl is $23.0 + 35.5 = 58.5$.

The Mole

A **mole** is a unit of measure that contains 6.02×10^{23} entities. A mole of atoms is a collection of 6.02×10^{23} atoms; a mole of molecules contains 6.02×10^{23} molecules, and so on. This number, 6.02×10^{23}, is called **Avogadro's number**, denoted by N_A (or N_0). It is the number of atoms contained in exactly 12 grams of carbon-12. This link between the number of atoms and mass means that a mole of any chemical substance has a mass denoted by its atomic mass units. For example, sodium has a mass of 23 atomic mass units, so 1 mole of sodium atoms has a mass of 23 grams. The relationship among moles, grams, and molecular weight is shown in the following formula:

$$\# \text{ moles} = \frac{\text{mass in grams}}{\text{molecular weight (MW)}}$$

Oxidation Numbers

The **oxidation number**, or oxidation state, of an atom indicates the number of electrons gained or lost from the neutral atom. *Positive* oxidation numbers indicate a *loss* of electrons. *Negative* oxidation numbers indicate a *gain* of electrons. Neutral species have an oxidation number of zero. For a neutral molecule, the sum of all oxidation numbers must add up to zero. If they do not, the result is a charged species called an **ion**.

Most atoms have more than one possible oxidation number. For the transition metals (Groups 3–12 in the periodic table), oxidation numbers are easiest to determine from the oxidation numbers of the other elements to which the transition metal is bound. Fortunately, certain elements have only one oxidation number, which indicates their tendency to gain or lose electrons. For the PCAT you should know the common oxidation numbers, which are these:

- All group 1 elements have an oxidation number of +1.
- All group 2 elements have an oxidation number of +2.
- All group 3 elements have an oxidation number of +3.
- Fluorine always has an oxidation number of –1.
- Oxygen almost always has an oxidation number of –2 (oxygen has a –1 oxidation state in peroxides, which contain an O-O bond such as in H_2O_2).
- Hydrogen has an oxidation number of either +1 or –1. Use this rule of thumb: +1 when bonded to nonmetals, –1 when bonded to metals. (See Section 9.2, Table 4, to distinguish between metals and nonmetals.)

Consider $K_2Cr_2O_7$. Since we know that oxygen has an oxidation number of –2 and potassium, a Group 1 element, has an oxidation number of +1, we can solve for the oxidation number of chromium:

K	2	×	+1	=	+2	
O	7	×	–2	=	–14	
Cr	2	×	__	=	+12	(since the sum must be zero)

The oxidation state of each chromium in $K_2Cr_2O_7$ is +6. Similarly, the oxidation state of manganese in MnO_4^- is +7: the total for oxygen is $4 \times -2 = -8$, so Mn must be +7 for an overall charge of –1.

9.2 ATOMIC STRUCTURE

Subatomic Particles

An **atom** is the smallest unit of any element that has all of the chemical and physical properties of that element. All atoms have a central **nucleus**, which contains **protons** and **neutrons**, known collectively as **nucleons**. Each proton has an electric charge of +1 elementary unit, the magnitude of electric charge associated with a single electron, whereas neutrons are electrically neutral. **Electrons** occupy regions of space outside of the nucleus, and each has an elementary charge of –1. There is an electrostatic attraction between the positively charged nucleus and the negatively charged electrons. In every neutral atom the number of electrons is equal to the number of protons.

The number of protons in the nucleus of an atom is called its **atomic number, Z**. The atomic number of an atom is unique and determines an element's identity, and Z may be shown explicitly by a subscript before the symbol of the element. For example, every beryllium atom contains four protons, indicted as $_4$Be.

A proton and a neutron each have a mass slightly more than one atomic mass unit (1 amu = 1.66×10^{-27} kg), whereas an electron has a mass that is only about 0.05 percent the mass of either a proton or a neutron. This means that virtually all of the mass of an atom is due to the mass of the nucleons. The number of protons plus the number of neutrons in the nucleus of an atom gives the atom's **mass number, A**. If we let N stand for the number of neutrons, then $A = Z + N$.

In designating a particular atom of an element, we refer to its mass number. For example, a beryllium atom has 4 protons. If it contains 5 neutrons, then its mass number is $4 + 5 = 9$, and we would write this as $_4^9$Be or simply as ^{9}Be. We can also write the mass number after the name of the elements with a hyphen; ^{9}Be is beryllium-9.

When representing an element by its one- or two-letter symbol, we can also include information about its numbers of electrons, neutrons, and protons. Notice that the number of protons, Z, identifies the element in the periodic table.

$$_Z^A X$$

where A = number of neutrons + protons, Z = number of protons, and X is an element's one- or two-letter symbol.

Isotopes

If two atoms of the same element differ in their numbers of neutrons, then they are called **isotopes**. Beryllium, for example, has an isotope with 3 neutrons, ^{7}Be (or beryllium-7). It also has an isotope with 5 neutrons, which is ^{9}Be (beryllium-9).

Notice that these atoms—like all isotopes of a given element—*have the same atomic number but different mass numbers.*

Atomic Weight

Elements exist naturally as a collection of their isotopes. The **atomic weight of an element** is the weighted average of the masses of its naturally occurring isotopes. For example, boron has two naturally occurring isotopes: boron-10, with an atomic mass of 10.013 amu, and boron-11, with an atomic mass of 11.009 amu. Since boron-10 accounts for 20 percent of all naturally occurring boron, and boron-11 accounts for the other 80 percent, the atomic weight of boron is

$$(20\%)(10.013 \text{ amu}) + (80\%)(11.009 \text{ amu}) = 10.810 \text{ amu}$$

This is the value listed in the periodic table. (Recall that the atomic mass unit is defined so that the most abundant isotope of carbon, carbon-12, has a mass of precisely 12 amu.)

Ions

An **ion** is a charged species that has gained or lost one or more electrons. A negatively charged ion is called an **anion**, while a positively charged ion is called a **cation**.

We designate how many electrons an atom has gained or lost by placing this number as a superscript after the chemical symbol for the element. For example, if a lithium atom loses 1 electron, it becomes the lithium cation Li^{1+}, or simply Li^+. It has an oxidation number, or *state*, of +1. If a phosphorus atom gains 3 electrons, it becomes the phosphorus anion P^{3-}, and has an oxidation state of −3.

The Bohr Model of the Atom

In 1913 the Danish physicist Niels Bohr realized that the model of atomic structure of his time was inconsistent with experimental data. Bohr described a new model of the atom. In this model that would later take his name, he proposed that the electrons in an atom orbited the nucleus in circular paths, much as the planets orbit the Sun in the Solar System. Distance from the nucleus was related to the energy of the electrons; electrons with greater amounts of potential energy orbited the nucleus at greater distances. However, the electrons in the atom cannot assume any arbitrary energy, but have *quantized* energy states, and thereby orbit only at certain allowed distances from the nucleus.

If an electron absorbs energy that's exactly equal to the difference in energy between its current level and that of an available higher lever, it "jumps," or is *promoted*, to that higher level. The electron can then "drop," or *decay*, to a lower energy level, emitting a *photon* whose energy is exactly equal to the difference in energy between the levels. This model predicted that elements would have line spectra with positions in the electromagnetic spectrum corresponding to the energy of its photons, rather than having the continuous spectrum that would result if transitions between all possible energies could occur. An electron could gain or lose only very specific amounts of energy due to the quantized nature of the energy levels. Therefore, only photons with certain energies are observed, and those specific energies correspond to very specific wavelengths of energy *emitted* that appear as bright lines in the **emission line spectrum**. The **absorption line spectrum** contains dark lines corresponding to the wavelength of energy *absorbed*.

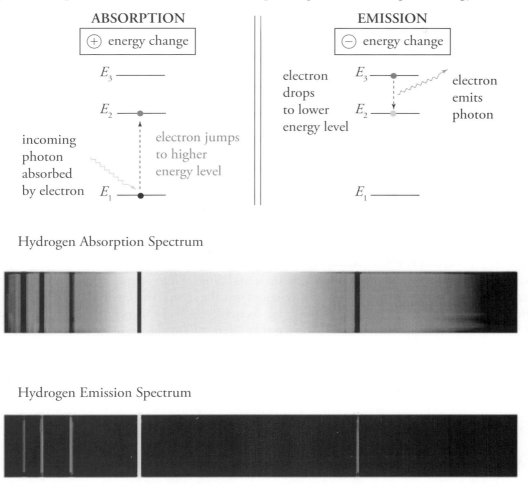

Hydrogen Absorption Spectrum

Hydrogen Emission Spectrum

Figure 1

In the transition depicted in Figure 2 on the next page, an electron is initially in its **ground state** ($n = 1$), its lowest possible energy level. When this electron absorbs a photon, it jumps to a higher energy level, known as an **excited state** (in this case $n = 3$). Electrons excited to high energy don't always relax to the ground state in large jumps; rather they can relax in a series of smaller jumps, gradually coming back to the ground state. From the $n = 3$ excited state the electron can relax in one of two ways, either dropping into the $n = 2$ level, or directly back to the $n = 1$ ground state. In the first scenario, we can expect to detect a photon with energy corresponding to the difference between $n = 3$ and $n = 2$. In the latter case, we'd detect a more energetic photon of energy corresponding to the difference between $n = 3$ and $n = 1$.

Note: Distances between energy levels are not drawn to scale.

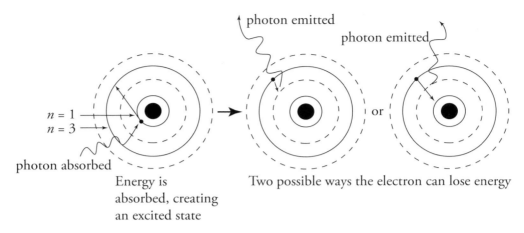

$n = 1$
$n = 3$

photon absorbed

Energy is
absorbed, creating
an excited state

Two possible ways the electron can lose energy

Figure 2

Not all electron transitions produce photons we can see with the naked eye, but all transitions in an atom will produce photons either in the ultraviolet, visible, or infrared region of the electromagnetic spectrum.

The Atom in Modern Perspective

With the advent of **quantum mechanics**, our understanding of the atom changed dramatically. An important precursor to the field of quantum mechanics was the atomic theory of Max Planck. According to Planck, electrons are able to exist only at discrete energy levels. In fact, energy itself can occur only in discrete amounts called **quanta**. Planck theorized that electrons are able to move from one energy level to the next only when they are given enough energy to jump to that level; an electron cannot absorb an excess of energy that is not sufficient for a transition to a higher energy level. Based on the work of Planck, Louis de Broglie hypothesized that electrons and other particles can behave like waves. That is, they have both energy and momentum. This is summarized by the equation

$$\Delta E = hf$$

where ΔE is the difference in energy between two allowed energy levels for an electron, h is Planck's constant, which has a value of 6.63×10^{-34} J • s, and f is the frequency of the electromagnetic radiation used to increase the energy of the electron. Each allowable energy level is therefore separated by a quantum of energy, hf. Since (wavelength)(frequency) = velocity, and electromagnetic radiation travels at the speed of light (c), we can arrive at the equation $c = \lambda f$, where λ is the wavelength of the electromagnetic radiation.

Substituting for f, the quantum equation becomes

$$\Delta E = h\frac{c}{\lambda}$$

Werner Heisenberg determined that it is impossible to simultaneously determine both the position and the momentum of an electron. Heisenberg showed that an electron's location in space at any given time may be determined with certainty only at the expense of the determination of its momentum at that instant. Since it is theoretically impossible to determine both of these variables simultaneously, we cannot assume that electrons travel in only spherical orbits.

Electron Quantum Numbers

Quantum mechanics was a new theory of the electronic structure of atoms that was consistent with observable facts. It stated that electrons held by an atom can exist only at discrete energy levels; that is, electron energy levels are **quantized**. This quantization is described by a unique "address" for each electron, consisting of four quantum numbers designating the shell, subshell, orbital, and spin.

The First Quantum Number

The first, or **principal**, quantum number is the **shell number**, n. It's related to the size and energy of an orbital. Loosely speaking, an **orbital** describes a three-dimensional region around the nucleus in which the electron is most likely to be found, and corresponds to Bohr's orbits. The value of n can be any whole number starting with 1; the greater the value of n, the greater the electron's energy and average distance from the nucleus.

The Second Quantum Number

An electron's second quantum number, the **subshell number**, is denoted by the letter l. It describes the *shape* (and energy) of an electron's orbital. The possible values for l depend on the value of n as follows: $l = 0, 1, 2, \ldots, n - 1$. For example, if the principal quantum number is $n = 3$, then l could be 0, 1, or 2. Letters are assigned to the values of l: the $l = 0$ subshell is called the **s subshell**, $l = 1$ is the **p subshell**, $l = 2$ is the **d subshell**, and $l = 3$ is the **f subshell**. The PCAT primarily uses this spectroscopic notation—that is, s, p, d, and f—for the subshells.

The Third Quantum Number

An electron's third quantum number, the **orbital number**, is denoted by m_l. It describes the three-dimensional *orientation* of an orbital. The possible values of m_l depend on the value of l as follows: $m_l = -l$, $-(l-1)$, $\ldots$, -1, 0, $\ldots$, $(l-1)$, l. For example, if $l = 2$, then m_l could be $-2, -1, 0, 1,$ or 2. We use the possible values of the orbital quantum number to tell us how many orbitals are in each subshell.

- If $l = 0$, then m_l can only be equal to 0 (one possibility), so each s subshell has just 1 orbital.
- If $l = 1$, then m_l can equal $-1, 0, 1$ (three possibilities), so each p subshell has 3 orbitals.
- If $l = 2$, then $m_l = -2, -1, 0, 1,$ or 2 (five possibilities), so each d subshell has 5 orbitals.
- If $l = 3$, then there are seven possible values for m_l, so the f subshell contains 7 orbitals.

You should be able to recognize the shapes of the orbitals in the s and p subshells. Each s subshell has just one spherically symmetric orbital, and is pictured as a 3-dimensional sphere.

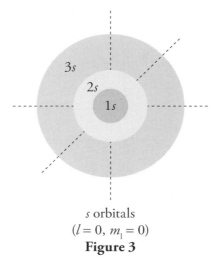

s orbitals
($l = 0$, $m_l = 0$)
Figure 3

Each p subshell has three orbitals, each depicted as a dumbbell, with different spatial orientations, p_x, p_y, and p_z.

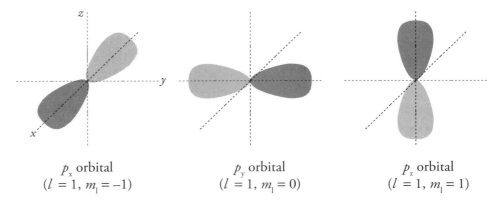

p_x orbital
$(l = 1, m_1 = -1)$

p_y orbital
$(l = 1, m_1 = 0)$

p_z orbital
$(l = 1, m_1 = 1)$

Figure 4

The Fourth Quantum Number

An electron's fourth quantum number is the **spin number**, m_s, which designates the electron's intrinsic magnetism. Regardless of the values of the n, l, or m_1, the value of m_s can be either +½ (**spin up**) or −½ (**spin down**). Every orbital can accommodate 2 electrons, one spin up and one spin down. If an orbital is full, we say that the electrons it contains are "spin-paired."

Tabular Summary of Quantum Numbers

Symbol and Name	Definitions	Possible Values	Related Quantities
n shell	size and energy of orbital	{positive integers}	principal shell
l subshell	shape and energy of orbital	$\{0, 1, 2, ..., n - 1\}$	n subshells per shell
m_1 orbital	orientation of orbital	$\{-l, ..., 0, ..., + l\}$	$2l + 1$ orbitals per subshell, n^2 orbitals per shell
m_s electron spin	spin of electron in orbital	$\{+\frac{1}{2}, -\frac{1}{2}\}$	2 electrons per orbital, $4l + 2$ electrons per subshell, $2n^2$ electrons per shell

Table 3

Diamagnetic and Paramagnetic Atoms

An atom that has all of its electrons spin-paired is **diamagnetic**. The individual magnetic fields that it creates cancel, leaving no net magnetic field. Helium, beryllium, and neon, for example, are diamagnetic. Atoms such as these will be *repelled* by an externally produced magnetic field.

If an atom's electrons are not all spin-paired, it is **paramagnetic**. Paramagnetic atoms, such as iron (Fe), are *attracted* into externally produced magnetic fields.

Excited State Versus Ground State

Electron configurations describe the *most probable* location of electrons. The electron configuration corresponding to the lowest energy is the **ground state configuration**. If an electron absorbs sufficient energy, it is promoted from its ground state to an excited state.

Emission Spectra

When an electric current is passed through a glass tube filled with a small sample of an element in gaseous form, the gas begins to glow with a color characteristic of that particular element. If this light emitted by the gas is then passed through a prism, thereby separating the light into its component wavelengths, the result is the element's characteristic emission spectrum.

An atom's emission spectrum gives an energetic "fingerprint" of that element because it consists of a unique sequence of bright lines that correspond to specific wavelengths and energies based on its electron configuration (see Figure 1).

The Pauli Exclusion Principle and Hund's Rule

Electrons will always be added to the lowest available energy level (as defined by the four quantum numbers). According to the **Pauli Exclusion Principle**, no electron in any one atom may have all four quantum numbers identical to another electron in the same atom. While it is possible to have two electrons with the same n, l, and m_ℓ, these two electrons must differ in m_s. Two electrons that differ only in spin quantum number are spin paired, and share an orbital within a subshell of a particular shell in the same atom.

Hund's Rule states that no two electrons will become spin paired unless there are no empty orbitals at the energy level of the orbitals that are presently being filled. To illustrate this, consider the three $2p$ orbitals of carbon. Each of these orbitals has the same energy as the other two orbitals. When orbitals have identical energies, they are **degenerate**. Applying Hund's Rule, one electron enters each of the three p orbitals; it is not until a fourth electron is placed into a p orbital that spin pairing occurs, with one spin up and one spin down.

The Aufbau Principle and Electron Configuration

The **Aufbau Principle** describes the order in which orbitals are filled. Electrons are placed into orbitals from the lowest energy orbital available to the highest energy orbital available.

As indicated in Figure 5, orbitals are filled in the order 1s, 2s, 2p, 3s, 3p, 4s, 3d, 4p, 5s, 4d, 5p, 6s, 4f, 5d, 6p, 7s, 5f, 6d. To determine the lowest possible electron configuration for an atom, first determine the number of electrons to be placed into orbitals (equal to the atomic number for neutral atoms), and use Figure 5.

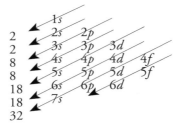

Figure 5

Consider vanadium ($Z = 23$). The number of electrons in subshells is indicated as superscripts, so vanadium's electron configuration is $1s^2 2s^2 2p^6 3s^2 3p^6 4s^2 3d^3$. Notice that the sum of the superscripts gives the total number of electrons for the atom. The electron configuration just determined for vanadium is its ground state. Any other configuration for vanadium that contains 23 electrons and does not violate the Pauli Exclusion Principle or Hund's Rule is an excited state. It is often an excited state configuration that is asked for when electron configuration questions are given on the PCAT.

The Periodic Table and Electron Configurations

Mendeleev's Periodic Table

The first version of the periodic table of the elements was proposed in 1869 by the Russian scientist Dmitri Mendeleev. A contemporary version of the periodic table is presented in Table 4. For PCAT purposes, only the elements set forth on the classic periodic table are relevant.

PERIODIC TABLE OF THE ELEMENTS

1																	18
1 **H** 1.008	**2**											**13**	**14**	**15**	**16**	**17**	**2** **He** 4.00
3 **Li** 6.94	**4** **Be** 9.01											**5** **B** 10.81	**6** **C** 12.01	**7** **N** 14.01	**8** **O** 16.00	**9** **F** 19.00	**10** **Ne** 20.18
11 **Na** 22.99	**12** **Mg** 24.30	**3**	**4**	**5**	**6**	**7**	**8**	**9**	**10**	**11**	**12**	**13** **Al** 26.98	**11** **Si** 28.09	**15** **P** 30.97	**16** **S** 32.06	**17** **Cl** 35.45	**18** **Ar** 39.95
19 **K** 39.10	**20** **Ca** 40.08	**21** **Sc** 44.96	**22** **Ti** 47.87	**23** **V** 50.94	**24** **Cr** 52.00	**25** **Mn** 54.94	**26** **Fe** 55.85	**27** **Co** 58.93	**28** **Ni** 58.69	**29** **Cu** 63.55	**30** **Zn** 65.38	**31** **Ga** 69.72	**32** **Ge** 72.63	**33** **As** 74.92	**34** **Se** 78.97	**35** **Br** 79.90	**36** **Kr** 83.80
37 **Rb** 85.47	**38** **Sr** 87.62	**39** **Y** 88.91	**40** **Zr** 91.22	**41** **Nb** 92.91	**42** **Mo** 95.95	**43** **Tc**	**44** **Ru** 101.07	**45** **Rh** 102.91	**46** **Pd** 106.42	**47** **Ag** 107.87	**48** **Cd** 112.41	**49** **In** 114.82	**50** **Sn** 118.71	**51** **Sb** 121.76	**52** **Te** 127.60	**53** **I** 126.90	**54** **Xe** 131.29
35 **Cs** 132.91	**56** **Ba** 137.33	57–71 *	**72** **Hf** 178.49	**73** **Ta** 180.95	**74** **W** 183.84	**75** **Re** 186.21	**76** **Os** 190.23	**77** **Ir** 192.22	**78** **Pt** 195.08	**79** **Au** 196.97	**80** **Hg** 200.59	**81** **Tl** 204.38	**82** **Pb** 207.2	**83** **Bi** 208.98	**84** **Po**	**85** **At**	**86** **Rn**
87 **Fr**	**88** **Ra**	89–103 †	**104** **Rf**	**105** **Db**	**106** **Sg**	**107** **Bh**	**108** **Hs**	**109** **Mt**	**110** **Ds**	**111** **Rg**	**112** **Cn**	**113** **Nh**	**114** **Fl**	**115** **Mc**	**116** **Lv**	**117** **Ts**	**118** **Og**

*Lanthanides	**57** **La** 138.91	**58** **Ce** 140.12	**59** **Pr** 140.91	**60** **Nd** 144.24	**61** **Pm**	**62** **Sm** 150.36	**63** **Eu** 151.97	**64** **Gd** 157.25	**65** **Tb** 158.93	**66** **Dy** 162.50	**67** **Ho** 164.93	**68** **Er** 167.26	**69** **Tm** 168.93	**70** **Yb** 173.05	**71** **Lu** 174.97
†Actinides	**89** **Ac**	**9** **Th** 232.04	**91** **Pa** 231.04	**92** **U** 238.03	**93** **Np**	**94** **Pu**	**95** **Am**	**96** **Cm**	**97** **Bk**	**98** **Cf**	**99** **Es**	**100** **Fm**	**101** **Md**	**102** **No**	**103** **Lr**

Table 4

Each element is represented by its one- or two-letter chemical symbol. Above each chemical symbol is the atomic number (number of protons) for that element. Below each chemical symbol is that element's atomic weight. Elements to the left of those shaded are metals, and elements to the right, including H, are nonmetals. The shaded elements are the semimetals. There is no need for you to memorize the periodic table for the exam, but you should be familiar with the location of the more popular elements: H, Li, C, N, O, F, Na, Mg, P, S, Cl, K, Ca, Fe, Cu, Br, Ag, and I.

Periods and Groups

The outermost electrons of every atom in a period, or row, have the same principal quantum number, n. Potassium (K), for example, is in period 4, so $n = 4$. Each vertical column in the periodic table is called a **group**. The *alkali metals* form Group I, the *alkaline earths* Group 2, the *chalcogens* Group 16, the *halogens* Group 17, and the *noble gases* Group 18. Every member of a group has the same number of valence, or outermost, electrons and may be expected to have similar chemical properties to other members of the group. In addition to the designation of groups, we can designate blocks of the periodic table. The blocks are identified by the letter that corresponds to the subshell presently being filled. The two rows farthest to the left (and He) are called the *s* block, the next 10 rows the *d* block, the six rows farthest to the right are called the *p* block, and the actinides and lanthanides are the *f* block.

9.2

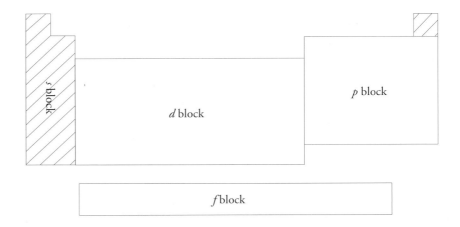

Figure 6

Blocks in the Periodic Table

Blocks (*s, p, d,* or *f*) indicate the highest-energy subshell containing electrons in the ground-state of an atom that falls within that block. For example, carbon is in the *p* block, and its electron configuration is $1s^2 2s^2 2p^2$ (it has 6 protons, and therefore 6 electrons in its neutral state). For any element in the *p* block, the *p* subshell is filling, first with electrons spin up, and then spin-paired.

We can illustrate how to use this block diagram to write electron configurations using chlorine ($Z = 17$). At $n = 1$, two electrons fill the $1s$ orbital, giving us $1s^2$. At $n = 2$, the next two electrons fill the $2s$ orbital giving $2s^2$. Moving to the *p* block, six electrons fill the $2p$ orbitals, giving us $2p^6$. At $n = 3$, two electrons fill the $3s$ orbital, giving us $3s^2$. With five electrons remaining, we move to the *p* block and complete the electron configuration with $3p^5$. The electron configuration is therefore $1s^2 2s^2 2p^6 3s^2 3p^5$, which is the correct ground state electron configuration for chlorine.

Elements in Group 18 are called the noble gases. Their subshells are completely filled (they have a closed shell electron configuration), with all electrons spin-paired. This makes them largely unreactive.

To find the **valence electron configuration**, we find the closest noble gas whose atomic number is less than that of the atom whose configuration we are after. In the case of chlorine ($Z = 17$), the closest noble gas with a smaller atomic number is neon ($Z = 10$). Starting with neon's closed shell, we have 7 additional electrons to assign. To get to $Z = 17$, we see that the electron configuration of chlorine is the same as that of neon plus $3s^2 3p^5$, which we can write as [Ne] $3s^2 3p^5$. Notice that according to the Aufbau Principle, the *d* block fills as $(n - 1)d$. For example, the electron configuration for scandium (Sc, atomic number 21) is [Ar]$4s^2 3d^1$. The *f* block fills as $(n - 2)f$.

In summary, the blocks in the table tells us in which subshell the outermost (valence) electrons of the atom will be. The period (row) gives the valence shell, *n*. Electrons for an atom in the *d* block of Period *n* fill the $(n - 1)d$ subshell, and those in the *f* block fill the $(n - 2)f$ subshell.

Electron Configurations

Now that we've described the electron quantum numbers, let's see how we assign them to each electron in an atom. There are three basic rules:

1) *Electrons occupy the lowest energy orbitals available.* (This is the Aufbau Principle.) Electron subshells are filled in order of increasing energy. The periodic table is logically constructed, so it is easy to determine electron configurations based on where atoms appear in the table.

2) *Electrons in the same subshell occupy available orbitals singly, before pairing up.* (This is Hund's Rule.)

3) *No two electrons in the same atom can have the same set of four quantum numbers.* (This is the Pauli Exclusion Principle.)

For example, let's find the quantum numbers for all the electrons in an oxygen atom, $(Z = 8)$. Oxygen is $1s^2 2s^2 2p^4$, but do the p electrons fill the orbitals spin up or spin down? Designating the $2p$ orbitals as $2p_x 2p_y 2p_z$, the electrons can fill either as $2p_x^2 2p_y^2$ or as $2p_x^2 2p_y^1 2p_z^1$. Which is correct? According to Hund's Rule, the second option is correct. The electrons enter each $2p$ orbital singly, and then spin pair. The complete electron configuration for oxygen can now be written like this:

$$\text{Oxygen} = 1s^2 2s^2 2p^4$$

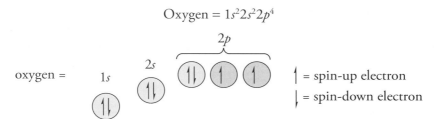

Figure 7

Here are the electron configurations for the first ten elements:

Z			$1s$	$2s$	$2p$		
1	Hydrogen	$1s^1$	↑				
2	Helium	$1s^2$	↑↓				
3	Lithium	$1s^2 2s^1$	↑↓	↑			
4	Beryllium	$1s^2 2s^2$	↑↓	↑↓			
5	Boron	$1s^2 2s^2 2p^1$	↑↓	↑↓	↑	●	●
6	Carbon	$1s^2 2s^2 2p^2$	↑↓	↑↓	↑	↑	●
7	Nitrogen	$1s^2 2s^2 2p^3$	↑↓	↑↓	↑	↑	↑
8	Oxygen	$1s^2 2s^2 2p^4$	↑↓	↑↓	↑↓	↑	↑
9	Fluorine	$1s^2 2s^2 2p^5$	↑↓	↑↓	↑↓	↑↓	↑
10	Neon	$1s^2 2s^2 2p^6$	↑↓	↑↓	↑↓	↑↓	↑↓

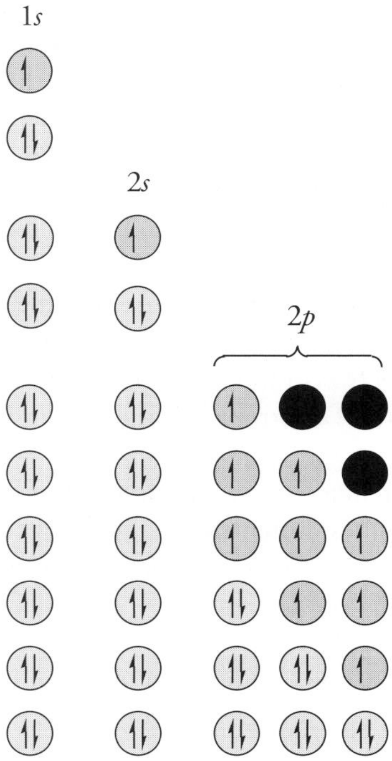

Figure 8

From Figure 9, we see that the electron configuration for argon is

$$Ar = 1s^2 2s^2 2p^6 3s^2 3p^6$$

Notice that $3s$ and $3p$ subshells have their full complement of electrons. In fact, the noble gases (those elements in Group 18) all have their outer 8 electrons in filled subshells: 2 in the ns subshell and 6 in the np. (The lone exception, of course, is helium; but its only subshell, the $1s$, is filled—with 2 electrons.) Because their 8 valence electrons are in filled subshells, we say that these atoms—Ne, Ar, Kr, Xe, and Rn—have a complete **octet**.

Some Anomalous Electron Configurations

Anomalies occur among atoms when the anticipated electron configuration is not the actual configuration observed. For these atoms, there are other considerations that affect their electron configurations, such as the added stability gained *by having a filled, or half-filled, subshell*. For example, consider chromium (Cr, $Z = 24$). We would expect its electron configuration to be $[Ar] 4s^2 3d^4$. Recalling that a d subshell can hold a maximum of 10 electrons, chromium achieves a more stable state by promoting one of its $4s$ electrons to the $3d$ subshell, giving it two half-filled subshells and an electron configuration of $[Ar]4s^1 3d^5$. As another example, copper (Cu, $Z = 29$) has an expected electron configuration of $[Ar] 4s^2 3d^9$. However, a copper atom obtains a more stable, lower-energy state by promoting one of its $4s$ electrons into the $3d$ subshell, yielding $[Ar] 4s^1 3d^{10}$ to give a *filled d* subshell.

Other atoms that display the same type of behavior include molybdenum (Mo, $Z = 42$, in the same family, or group, as chromium), as well as silver and gold (Ag and Au, $Z = 47$ and $Z = 79$, respectively, which are in the same family as copper).

Electron Configurations of Ions

Recall that an ion is a charged species. Atoms that gain electrons (anions) accommodate them in the first available orbital with the lowest available energy. For example, fluorine (F, $Z = 9$) has the electron configuration $1s^2 2s^2 2p^5$. When a fluorine atom gains an electron to become the fluoride ion, F^-, the additional electron goes into the $2p$ subshell, giving the electron configuration $1s^2 2s^2 2p^6$, which is the same as the configuration of neon. For this reason, F^- and Ne are said to be **isoelectronic**.

If an atom gains one or more electrons to become an anion, we find its isoelectronic atom by moving to the *right* in the periodic table by a number of elements equal to the number of electrons gained. Conversely, if an atom loses electrons to become a cation, we move to the *left* in the table by a number of elements equal to the number of electrons lost in order to find its isoelectronic atom.

Electrons that are removed (*ionized*) from an atom always come from the valence shell, which is usually the one with the highest potential energy, or the least stable orbital. For example, lithium (Li) can lose its $2s^1$ electron to obtain the noble gas electron configuration of He ($1s^2$). For **transition metals** (the elements in the d block), *the valence s electrons are always lost before the d electrons*. Valence electrons from the highest n level are ALWAYS lost first. For example, the electron configuration for titanium (Ti, $Z = 22$) is $[Ar] 4s^2 3d^2$. The electron configuration of Ti^{2+} is not $[Ar] 4s^2$—it's actually $[Ar] 3d^2$.

9.3 STOICHIOMETRY

The Formation of Molecules

Nitrogen will form bonds with three or four hydrogens (NH_3 and NH_4^+), while fluorine will form a bond with one hydrogen atom (HF). The subscript is known as a **stoichiometric number**. The stoichiometric number 3 on the H in the NH_3 molecule indicates that there are three hydrogens for each nitrogen in this molecule. While there are three hydrogens **bonded** to each nitrogen, the subscript 3 gives only the **ratios** between constituent atoms, *not* information on bonding.

The molecular formula of glucose, for example, is $C_6H_{12}O_6$, which tells us that there are 6 carbons, 12 hydrogens, and 6 oxygens in a molecule of glucose. It also tells us that there are 2 hydrogen atoms and 1 oxygen atom for every carbon atom in a molecule of glucose. The molecular formula, however, tells us nothing about how these elements are bonded together.

Empirical Formulas

The $C_4H_4N_2$ molecule contains 4 atoms of carbon, 4 atoms of hydrogen, and 2 nitrogen atoms. Their CHN ratio is 4:4:2. The smallest whole number ratio in this molecule is 2:2:1. If we use *these* numbers, we get the molecule's **empirical formula**: C_2H_2N. In general, to reduce a molecular formula to the empirical formula, divide all the subscripts by their greatest common factor. Here are a few more examples:

Molecular Formula	Empirical Formula
$C_6H_{12}O_6$	CH_2O
$K_2S_2O_8$	KSO_4
$Fe_4Na_8O_{35}P_{10}$	$Fe_4Na_8O_{35}P_{10}$
$C_{30}H_{27}N_3O_{15}$	$C_{10}H_9NO_5$

Table 5

Percentage Composition by Mass

The molecular or empirical formula can be used to determine a percent mass composition. For example, we can find the mass composition of carbon, hydrogen, and nitrogen in $C_4H_4N_2$. Using the compound's empirical formula, C_2H_2N, the empirical formula weight is $2(12) + 2(1) + 14 = 40$, so each element's contribution to the total mass is

$$\%C = \frac{2(12)}{40} = \frac{12}{20} = \frac{60}{100} = 60\%, \quad \%H = \frac{2(1)}{40} = \frac{1}{20} = \frac{5}{100} = 5\%, \quad \%N = \frac{14}{40} = \frac{7}{20} = \frac{35}{100} = 35\%$$

We can also use information about the percentage composition to determine a compound's empirical formula. Suppose a substance is analyzed and found to consist, by mass, of 70 percent iron and 30 percent oxygen. Because we are given percentages, to find the empirical formula for this compound, we base our calculations on 100 grams of the substance. One hundred grams would then contain 70g of Fe and 30g of O. We now have to convert grams to moles in order to get molar ratios.

$$\text{\# moles of Fe} = \frac{70 \text{ g}}{55.8 \text{ g/mol}} \approx \frac{70}{56} = \frac{5}{4} \quad \text{and} \quad \text{\# moles of O} = \frac{30 \text{ g}}{16 \text{ g/mol}} = \frac{15}{8}$$

To obtain the empirical formula, we find the ratio of Fe to O as small whole numbers:

$$\text{Ratio of Fe to O} = \frac{5/4 \text{ mol}}{15/8 \text{ mol}} = \frac{5}{4} \cdot \frac{8}{15} = \frac{2}{3}$$

Since the ratio of Fe to O is 2:3, the empirical formula of the substance is Fe_2O_3.

Chemical Equations and Stoichiometric Coefficients

The equation

$$2Al + 6HCl \rightarrow 2AlCl_3 + 3H_2$$

describes the reaction of aluminum metal (Al) with hydrochloric acid (HCl) to produce aluminum chloride ($AlCl_3$) and hydrogen gas (H_2). The **reactants** are on the left side of the arrow, and the **products** are on the right side. A chemical equation is **balanced** if, for every element represented, the number of atoms on the left side is equal to the number of atoms on the right side. This illustrates the **Law of Conservation of Mass** (or of **Matter**), which says that the amount of matter (and thus mass) does not change in a chemical reaction. For a *balanced* reaction such as the one above, the coefficients (2, 6, 2, and 3) that precede each compound are known as **stoichiometric coefficients**. They tell us in what proportion the reactants react and in what proportion the products are formed. For this reaction, 2 atoms of Al react with 6 molecules of HCl to form 2 molecules of $AlCl_3$ and 3 molecules of H_2. The equation also means that 2 *moles* of Al react with 6 *moles* of HCl to form 2 *moles* of $AlCl_3$ and 3 *moles* of H_2. The stoichiometric coefficients give the ratios of the number of molecules (or moles) that apply to the combination of reactants and the formation of products. They do *not* give the ratios by mass.

Balancing Equations

When balancing a chemical equation, start with the most complex species in the reaction and leave the simplest for last. For the reaction above:

$$Al + HCl \rightarrow AlCl_3 + H_2 \text{ (unbalanced)}$$

The most complex species is $AlCl_3$. To get 3 atoms of Cl on the product side, we need to have 3 atoms of Cl on the reactant side. We therefore put a 3 in front of the HCl:

$$Al + 3HCl \rightarrow AlCl_3 + H_2 \text{ (unbalanced)}$$

The Cl's are balanced, but the H's are still unbalanced. Because we have 3 H's on the left, we need 3 H's on the right, so we put a coefficient of 3/2 in front of the H_2:

$$Al + 3HCl \rightarrow AlCl_3 + \frac{3}{2}H_2$$

All the atoms are now balanced. Because it is customary to write stoichiometric coefficients as whole numbers, we multiply through by 2 and obtain

$$2Al + 6HCl \rightarrow 2AlCl_3 + 3H_2$$

Stoichiometric Relationships in Balanced Reactions

Once the equation for a chemical reaction is balanced, the stoichiometric coefficients tell us the relative amounts of the reactant species that combine and the relative amounts of the product species that are formed. For example, recall that the reaction

$$2Al + 6HCl \rightarrow 2AlCl_3 + 3H_2$$

tells us that 2 moles of Al react with 6 moles of HCl to form 2 moles of $AlCl_3$ and 3 moles of H_2. We can convert from moles to mass by multiplying the coefficient by the atomic or molecular weight. Thus, 2 mol Al × (26.98 g/mol) = 53.96 g Al, which reacts with 6 mol HCl × (36.46 g/mol) = 218.8 g HCl, producing 2 mol $AlCl_3$ × (133.33 g/mol) = 266.66 g $AlCl_3$ and 3 mol H_2 × (2.02 g/mol) = 6.05 g H_2. Notice that mass is conserved: within error, 272.8 g of reactant produces 272.8 g of product.

The Limiting Reactant

Let's look again at the reaction of aluminum with hydrochloric acid. Suppose we have 4 moles of Al and 18 moles of HCl. We have enough HCl to make 6 moles of $AlCl_3$ and 9 moles of H_2, but there is only enough Al to make 4 moles of $AlCl_3$ and 6 moles of H_2. There isn't enough aluminum metal (Al) to make use of all the available HCl. As the reaction proceeds, we'll run out of aluminum. This means that aluminum is the **limiting reactant**, because it limits how much product the reaction can produce.

Now suppose that the reaction begins with 4 moles of Al and 9 moles of HCl. There's enough Al metal to produce 4 moles of $AlCl_3$ and 6 moles of H_2, but there is only enough HCl to make 3 moles of $AlCl_3$ and 4.5 moles of H_2. There isn't enough HCl to react with all of the aluminum metal. Here HCl is the limiting reactant.

9.4 PERIODIC TRENDS AND BONDING

Periodic Trends

There are five periodic trends that are governed by electron configuration: **electronegativity, atomic radius, ionization energy, electron affinity,** and **acidity**. Here is a mnemonic device that should help you remember this. Those trends that contain a word beginning with the letter "e" increase from left to right across the periodic table and from bottom to top. This is illustrated in Figure 10.

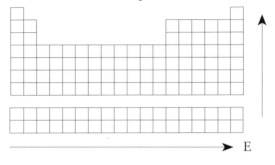

Figure 9

Electronegativity

Electronegativity (EN) is the affinity of a particular atom for electrons when that atom is engaged in a chemical bond. It is not a directly measurable quantity. A **nonpolar covalent bond** occurs between atoms that have differences in electronegativity less than or equal to 0.5. In a polar covalent bond, the electrons forming the bond are more attracted to the atom with the greater electronegativity.

Atomic Radius

Atomic radius decreases from left to right within a period. Because the number of protons increases from left to right, as do the number of electrons in the neutral atoms, the electrostatic attractive forces increase and the atomic radii decrease. Down a group, as n increases, the atomic radius becomes larger.

Ionization Energy

Because there is an electrostatic attraction between the positively charged nucleus and the electrons in the atom, it takes energy to remove an electron. The amount of energy necessary to remove an electron from an isolated, gaseous atom in its ground state is called the **ionization energy** (often abbreviated **IE**). Removing the least tightly bound electron has an associated IE_1. As we move from left to right across a period, or up a group, the ionization energy *increases* since the valence electrons are more tightly bound.

The ionization energy of any atom with a noble gas configuration will always be very large because of the added stability associated with a closed valence shell. For example, the ionization energy of neon is 4 times greater than that of lithium. Valence shells that are half filled also have higher ionization energies because of their additional stability.

The second ionization energy (IE_2) of an atom, X, is the energy required to remove the next least tightly bound electron from the cation X^+. Note that IE_2 will always be greater than IE_1, because an electron is being removed from a positively charged species.

Electron Affinity

The energy associated with the addition of an electron to an isolated atom is known as the atom's **electron affinity** (often abbreviated **EA**). If energy is released when an electron is added, the electron affinity is negative. If adding an electron requires energy, then EA is positive.

The halogens (Group 17) have large negative electron affinities, because adding an electron gives them a closed valence shell, which is especially stable. Therefore, they readily form an anion and energy is released. The noble gases (Group 18) and alkaline earth metals (Group 2) have positive electron affinities because they have closed valence shells. Electron affinities generally become more negative as we move from left to right in the periodic table, or up a group, but valence shell electron configurations produce anomalies because of the additional stability associated with filled and half-filled subshells.

Acidity

Acidity is a measure of how well a compound donates protons, accepts electrons, or lowers pH in a chemical system. A binary acid has the structure HX, and can dissociate in water in the following manner: $HX \rightarrow H^+ + X^-$. Stronger acids lose a proton because they form stable X^- anions. When moving across a row, the more electronegative the element, the more stable the anion. Acidity therefore increases from left to right across a period. The vertical trend, however, is driven by orbital overlap and the size of the anion. The larger the anion, the poorer the orbital overlap with the proton ($n = 1$) and the weaker the bond. Also, repulsive interactions among electrons are reduced as n increases, so the anion becomes more stable. Therefore, acidity increases down a group in the periodic table. This means that HI, for example, is a much stronger acid than HCl.

Atomic and Molecular Interactions: Bonding

A chemical bond is an electrostatic interaction between atoms, ions, or molecules that results in the formation of a chemical compound. If electrons are shared between atoms, those electrons are electrostatically attracted to two nuclei and form a covalent bond. If there is a transfer of one or more electrons from one atom to another, then the resulting ions form an ionic bond. How atoms interact with each other will depend largely on their electron configurations and periodic trends.

Lewis Dot Structures and the Octet Rule

Lewis dot structures provide a way to predict how atoms will bond together to form a molecule, or how electrons will transfer to form an ionic compound. Fluorine has a valence shell that is $2s^2 2p^5$, so there are $2 + 5 = 7$ valence electrons. Representing each valence electron by a dot, we place the dots around the symbol for the element. One dot is placed on each of four sides, and additional electrons are added by pairing them with the first ones. For fluorine we have

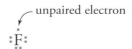

(*Note*: In Lewis structures, electrons in *d* and *f* subshells are not counted among valence electrons.)

We can also use Lewis dot structures to show multiple bonds. Here are examples:

$$:\ddot{O}\cdot \quad \cdot \ddot{O}: \quad \longrightarrow \quad :\ddot{O}\,\,\ddot{O}: \quad \longrightarrow \quad :O::O: \quad \longrightarrow \quad \ddot{O}=\ddot{O}$$

$$H\cdot \quad \cdot\dot{C}\cdot \quad \cdot\ddot{N}: \quad \longrightarrow \quad H:C\,\,N: \quad \longrightarrow \quad H:C::N: $$

$$\Downarrow$$

$$H\!-\!C\!\equiv\!N:$$

The Lewis dot structures for the second period elements are

$$Li\bullet \quad \bullet Be\bullet \quad \bullet \dot{B}\bullet \quad \bullet \dot{C}\bullet \quad \cdot\dot{\ddot{N}}\cdot \quad :\dot{\ddot{O}}\cdot \quad :\dot{\ddot{F}}\bullet \quad :\ddot{Ne}:$$

The octet rule states that atoms prefer to have a noble gas valence shell configuration. An octet may be achieved in the three ways outlined below:

1. A metal may lose electrons to form a cation that is isoelectronic with the previous noble gas. An example of this is the Mg^{2+} cation, which is isoelectronic with neon (Ne). The formation of this ion is given by the equation

$$\bullet Mg\bullet \quad \longrightarrow \quad Mg^{2+} + 2e^-$$

2. A nonmetal may gain electrons to form an anion that is isoelectronic to the next noble gas, with anions shown in brackets. An example of this is the F^- anion, which is isoelectronic with neon. The formation of this anion is given by the equation

$$:\ddot{F}\bullet \;+\; e^- \quad \longrightarrow \quad \left[:\ddot{\ddot{F}}:\right]$$

3. Both HF and NH_3 molecules illustrate how Lewis dot structures depict covalent bonds. Fluorine would like to gain a single electron, while nitrogen would like to gain three electrons. As a result, the Lewis dot structures are the following, where an "x" indicates an electron from H:

$$H\overset{x}{\bullet}\ddot{F}: \qquad H\overset{x}{\bullet}\ddot{N}\overset{x}{\bullet}H$$
$$\overset{x\ \bullet}{H}$$

Notice that by sharing electrons, H and F now have filled valence shells.

Formal Charge

A proposed Lewis dot structure for a molecule consisting of 1 atom each of hydrogen, carbon, and nitrogen is drawn below with N as the central atom:

$$H\cdot \quad \cdot\ddot{N}: \quad \cdot\ddot{C}\cdot \quad \Longrightarrow \quad H:N::C: \quad \Longrightarrow \quad H\!-\!N\!\!=\!\!C: \quad (?)$$

This, though, does not give the correct structure for this molecule. One way to evaluate a proposed Lewis structure is to calculate the **formal charge** of each atom in the molecule. The formal charges won't give the actual charges on the atoms; rather they will tell us which option is predicted to be the most stable. The formula for calculating the formal charge of an atom in a covalent compound is

$$\text{Formal charge (FC)} = V - \left[\frac{B}{2} + L \right]$$

where V is the number of valence electrons, B is the number of bonding electrons, and L is the number of lone-paired (non-bonding) electrons. For the Lewis structures shown above, the formal charges are these:

Formal charges

$$\underset{\text{H}}{\textcircled{0}} \; \underset{\text{C}}{\textcircled{0}} \; \underset{\text{N}}{\textcircled{0}} \qquad\qquad \underset{\text{H}}{\textcircled{0}} \; \underset{\text{N}}{\textcircled{+1}} \; \underset{\text{C}}{\textcircled{-1}}$$

$$\text{H} : \text{C} :: \text{N} : \qquad\qquad \text{H} : \text{N} :: \text{C} :$$

Formal charge on H = $1 - \frac{1}{2}(2) - 0 = 0$ Formal charge on H = $1 - \frac{1}{2}(2) - 0 = 0$

Formal charge on C = $4 - \frac{1}{2}(8) - 0 = 0$ Formal charge on N = $5 - \frac{1}{2}(8) - 0 = +1$

Formal charge on N = $5 - \frac{1}{2}(6) - 2 = 0$ Formal charge on C = $4 - \frac{1}{2}(6) - 2 = -1$

The most stable structure is predicted to be the one that has a formal charge of zero on all the atoms. (If this isn't possible, then the best structure is the one that *minimizes* the magnitudes of the formal charges.) The HCN structure has formal charges of zero for all the atoms, but the HNC structure does not. Thus, the HCN structure is the better choice.

Electron Group Geometry (VSEPR) and Molecular Geometry

Lewis dot structures give information about bonding, but they give no information about the geometric shape of the molecule. The **Valence Shell Electron Pair Repulsion (VSEPR)** theory is used to predict *electron group* geometry. VSEPR states that electrons occupy regions of space that minimize repulsions. Electrons form *groups*, that can consist of a single bond, multiple bonds, a lone pair of electrons, or a single electron, *but an empty orbital does not form a group*. Groups are arranged around a central atom in such a way that repulsions among groups are minimized. There are three separate repulsive forces: **lone pair–lone pair**, **lone pair–bonding pair**, and **bonding pair–bonding pair**. Lone pair–lone pair interactions create the strongest repulsive force, while bonding pair–bonding pair repulsions create the weakest repulsions. Only bonding pairs are used to determine **molecular geometry**—lone pairs cause deviations from the ideal geometry because of their strong repulsive forces. The variety of geometric shapes available to molecules with a single central atom are summarized in Table 6.

9.4

Number of Electron Groups	Electron-Group Geometry	Bonding Pairs	Nonbonding Pairs	Molecular Geometry	Example
2	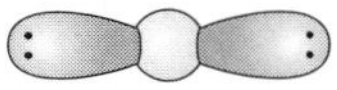	2	0	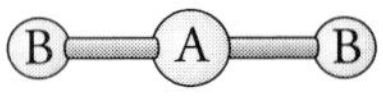 Linear	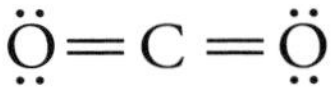 $\ddot{O}=C=\ddot{O}$
3	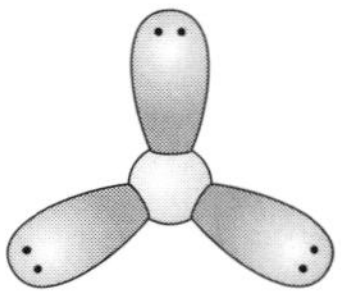	3	0	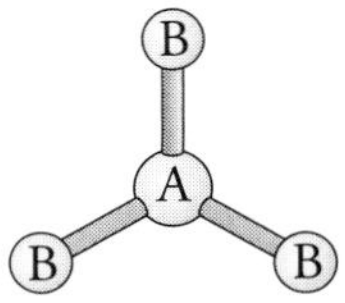 Trigonal planar	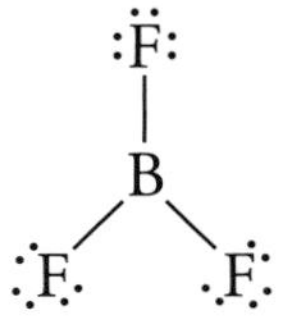 $\ddot{F}$—B—$\ddot{F}$ $\ddot{F}$
		2	1	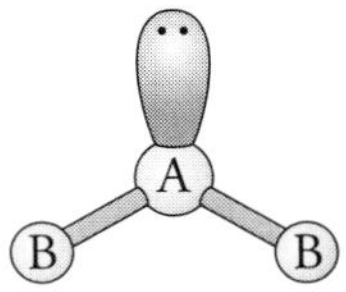 Bent (V-shaped)	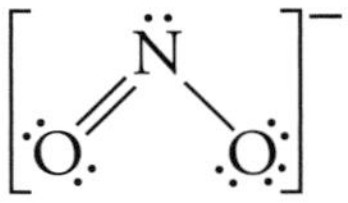 $[\ddot{O}-\dot{N}-\ddot{O}]^{-}$
4	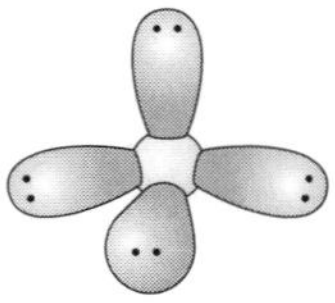	4	0	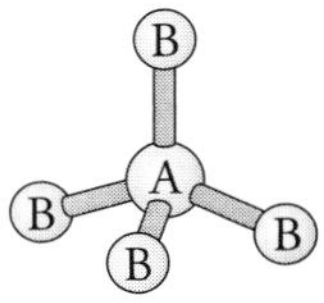 Tetrahedral	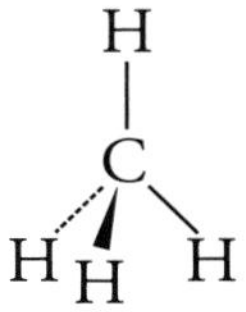 H—C—H H H
		3	1	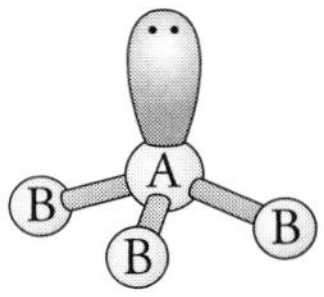 Trigonal pyramidal	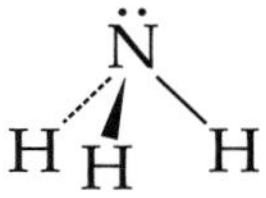 $\ddot{N}$ H H H
		2	2	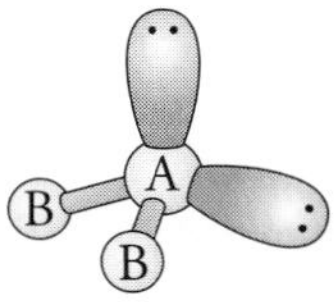 Bent (V-shaped)	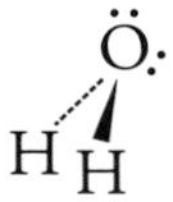 $\ddot{O}$ H H

Table 6

Number of Electron Groups	Electron-Group Geometry	Bonding Pairs	Nonbonding Pairs	Molecular Geometry	Example
5		5	0	Trigonal bipyramidal	PCl_5
		4	1	Seesaw	SF_4
		3	2	T-shaped	ClF_3
		2	3	Linear	XeF_2
6		6	0	Octahedral	SF_6
		5	1	Square pyramidal	BrF_5
		4	2	Square planar	XeF_4

Table 6 (continued)

Intramolecular Interactions: Ionic, Covalent, and Polar Covalent Compounds

In an **ionic bond**, one or more electrons are transferred from one atom to another. One atom forms a cation and the other forms an anion. Together they form an ionic bond that has strong electrostatic forces holding it together. An example of an ionic bond is the one between Na and Cl to form sodium chloride:

$$Na\cdot \ + \ \cdot\ddot{\underset{\cdot\cdot}{Cl}}\cdot \longrightarrow Na^+ \quad \left[:\ddot{\underset{\cdot\cdot}{Cl}}: \right]^-$$

Contrast this to a covalent bond, in which an electron pair is shared between two atoms.

The electronegativity of an atom determines whether a bond will be ionic or covalent. If two atoms have a difference in electronegativity that is less than 0.5, they form a nonpolar covalent bond. The electrons involved in bonding are equally attracted to two atomic nuclei. If the difference in electronegativities is greater than approximately 1.5, however, the atoms form an ionic bond through the complete transfer of one or more electrons. Between these two extremes atoms form **polar covalent bonds**.

The electrons forming the polar covalent bond are more associated with the more electronegative atom. This asymmetric charge distribution forms a **dipole**. The symbol for a dipole is an arrow with a perpendicular line through its tail. The head of the arrow is pointed in the direction of the more electronegative atom, which indicates the direction of electron flow. For HCl, the dipole is shown as

$$\overset{\longrightarrow}{H\ Cl}$$

This may also be represented two other ways:

$$\overset{\delta^+ \ \ \delta^-}{H-Cl}$$

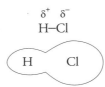

In the upper representation, δ+ denotes a partial positive charge on the hydrogen atom, and δ− is a partial negative charge on the chlorine atom. In the lower representation, the outline represents the shape of the electron cloud that is formed by the asymmetric charge distribution.

The H_2O molecule has a strong dipole because oxygen has two lone pairs of electrons that are nonbonding. Oxygen carries two partial negative charges and each hydrogen a partial positive charge.

$$\underset{\text{H}}{\overset{\text{H}}{:\ddot{\underset{\cdot\cdot}{O}}:\text{H}}} \Longrightarrow \ \ \overset{\delta^+}{\underset{\delta^-}{\overset{\text{H}}{\delta^-:\overset{|}{O}-\text{H}}}} \ \overset{\delta^+}{}$$

lone-pairs = nonbonding electrons
(unshared pairs of valence electrons)

Coordinate Covalent Bonds

Sometimes, both of the electrons in a bond come from the same atom, forming a **coordinate covalent bond**. For example, the nitrogen atom in NH_3 donates both electrons in its lone pair to boron in BF_3 to produce the coordinate covalent compound F_3BNH_3, shown here:

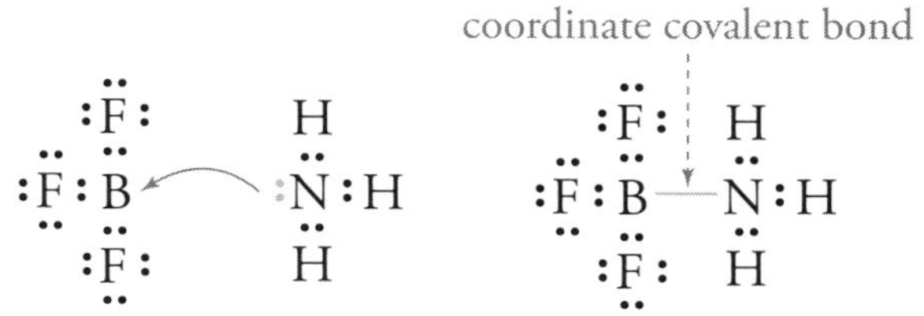

coordinate covalent bond

Since the NH_3 molecule donates a pair of electrons, it is a **ligand**, an ion or molecule that binds to a central atom. When a coordinate covalent bond breaks, the electrons that come from the ligand will leave *with* that ligand.

Intermolecular Forces

Intermolecular forces describe interactions that take place between neutral molecules. These forces are substantially weaker than the electrostatic attractive forces characteristic of ionic compounds.

Polar molecules are attracted to ions, producing **ion-dipole** forces. **Dipole-dipole forces** are the attractions between the positive dipole on one molecule and the negative dipole on another molecule. A hydrogen bond is a specialized dipole-dipole force that forms when hydrogen is bonded to a very electronegative element, such as O, N, or F. This is a comparatively strong dipole-dipole bond that is indicated by dotted lines from hydrogen to the electronegative atom.

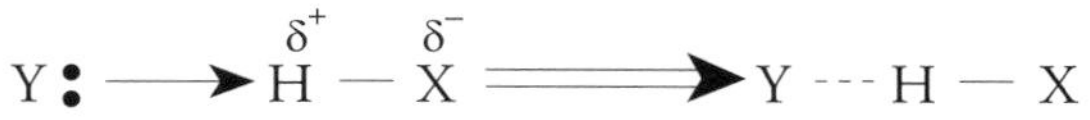

Water, for example, can form multiple hydrogen bonds that require a significant input of energy to break. If a molecule has a net dipole moment, it can induce a dipole in a neighboring nonpolar molecule, producing a momentary **dipole-induced dipole force**. Finally, an instantaneous dipole in a nonpolar molecule, arising from electron motions, may induce a dipole in a neighboring nonpolar molecule. The resulting momentary attraction is known as a **London dispersion force**. London dispersion forces are very weak and transient interactions between the instantaneous dipoles in nonpolar molecules. They are the weakest of all intermolecular interactions. For nonpolar molecules, London dispersion forces are the only intermolecular forces present. Low molecular weight hydrocarbons whose molecules experience only London dispersion forces are gases at room temperature. The intermolecular forces described are shown in Figure 11.

Dipole forces, hydrogen bonding, and London dispersion forces are *all* collectively known as **van der Waals forces**. However, the term "van der Waals forces" is often used to mean only London dispersion forces.

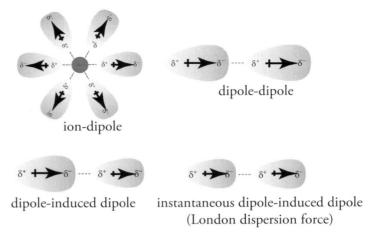

Figure 10

Despite being weak, intermolecular forces can have a profound impact on the physical properties of a particular molecule. Substances with stronger intermolecular forces will exhibit greater melting points, greater boiling points, greater viscosities, and lower vapor pressures than similar compounds with weaker intermolecular forces. This is particularly true for hydrogen bonding. The degree of hydrogen bonding that occurs within a given substance requires an input of energy to overcome the attractive forces and produce a physical separation of the molecules.

Multiple Bonds

When two atoms share a single pair of electrons, they form a *single bond*. When sharing two pairs of electrons, they form a *double bond*. A *triple bond* is formed when the atoms share three pairs of electrons. The term **bond order** is used to describe the number of bonds between two atoms: a single bond has a bond order of 1, a double bond a bond order of 2, and a triple bond a bond order of 3.

Examples of double and triple bonds are:

$$\begin{array}{c} \text{H} \\ \diagdown \\ \text{C}=\text{C} \\ \diagup \quad \diagup \\ \text{H} \end{array} \qquad :\text{N} \equiv \text{N}:$$

The bond order affects the bond *length* and bond *strength*. A triple bond is shorter and stronger than a double bond, and a double bond is shorter and stronger than a single bond. Among the three kinds of bonds, a single bond is the longest and weakest. This does not mean, however, that it is the most reactive.

Resonance

Resonance occurs through the *p* orbital framework of adjacent atoms in a molecule. The single depiction of the polyatomic nitrate ion (NO_3^-) shown below is not entirely accurate. All three of the ion's oxygen atoms are equivalent, so there is no reason for the ion to choose to locate its double bond at one particular oxygen, leaving the other two oxygens with single bonds. The nitrate ion exists as an intermediate among three separate structures in which the double bond between the nitrogen (N) and oxygen (O) atoms is *delocalized*. Thus, NO_3^- has a structure that is an intermediate or average among these three:

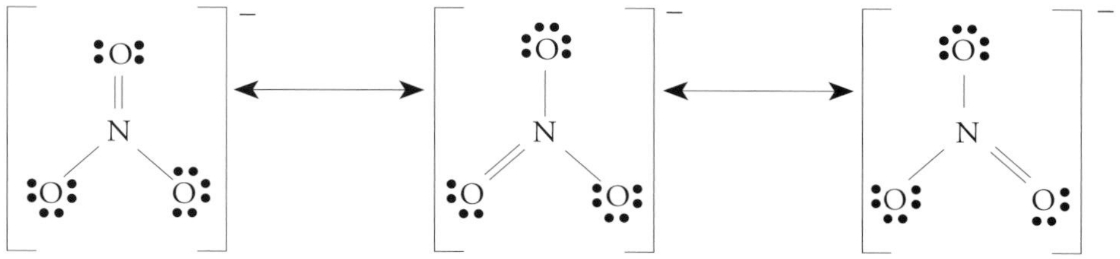

These structures are called **resonance forms**. The NO_3^- ion represents a **resonance structure** for which there are three resonance forms, indicated with double-headed arrows. The average structure, which shows the partial double bond character of the N—O bonds, is this:

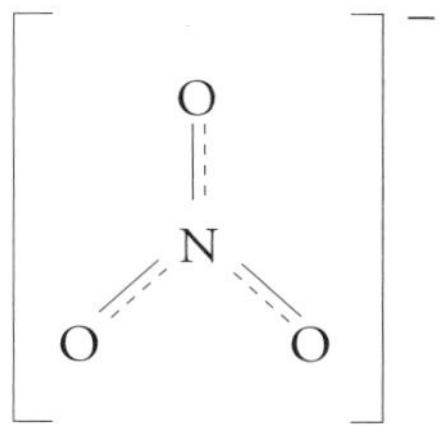

Each N—O bond has a bond order of $1\frac{1}{3}$, so each is shorter than a single bond but longer than a double bond.

Chemical Reaction Classes

In broad terms, there are 6 types of chemical reactions:

- synthesis (combination)
- decomposition
- single displacement
- double displacement (ion exchange, metathesis)
- oxidation-reduction (redox)
- combustion

Oxidation-reduction, or redox reactions may take the form of any of the six other classes. They are addressed later in this chapter; the other types of reactions are discussed next.

Synthesis

A **synthesis reaction** is the direct combination of two or more compounds, or elements, to form a new chemical compound. The general form of a synthesis reaction is

$$A + B \rightarrow AB$$

Examples of synthesis reactions include the reaction between hydrogen and oxygen gases to form water (also a redox reaction). The physical state of each species (solid, liquid, gas, or aqueous) is indicated in parentheses.

$$2H_2(g) + O_2(g) \rightarrow 2H_2O(l)$$

A synthesis reaction also occurs between barium oxide and water to form barium hydroxide:

$$BaO(s) + H_2O(l) \rightarrow Ba(OH)_2(aq)$$

Decomposition

A **decomposition reaction** is the opposite of a synthesis reaction. In a decomposition, two or more compounds, or elements, are formed from a single chemical compound. The general form of a decomposition reaction is

$$AB \rightarrow A + B$$

Examples of decomposition reactions include the electrolysis of water to form hydrogen and oxygen gases:

$$2H_2O(l) \rightarrow 2H_2(g) + O_2(g)$$

and the decomposition of aluminum trichloride to form aluminum metal and chlorine gas:

$$2AlCl_3(s) \rightarrow 2Al(s) + 3Cl_2(g)$$

Single Displacement

In a **single displacement reaction**, an element reacts with a compound to form a new compound and an element. The general form of a single displacement reaction is

$$A + BX \rightarrow AX + B$$

Examples include the reaction between copper metal and sulfuric acid to form hydrogen gas and copper(II) sulfate:

$$Cu(s) + H_2SO_4(aq) \rightarrow CuSO_4(aq) + H_2(g)$$

and the displacement of bromine by chlorine in sodium bromide:

$$2NaBr(aq) + Cl_2(g) \rightarrow 2NaCl(aq) + Br_2(l)$$

(All of the single displacement reactions just described also represent oxidation reduction reactions.)

Double Displacement

In a **double displacement reaction**, two compounds exchange ions with one another. The result is the formation of two new chemical compounds. The general form of a double displacement reaction is

$$AX + BY \rightarrow AY + BX$$

Examples include the neutralization reaction between sodium hydroxide and hydrochloric acid:

$$NaOH(aq) + HCl(aq) \rightarrow NaCl(aq) + H_2O(l)$$

This particular reaction also represents an acid–base reaction. Another example is the reaction between silver nitrate and sodium chloride to form silver chloride and sodium nitrate:

$$AgNO_3(aq) + NaCl(aq) \rightarrow NaNO_3(aq) + AgCl(s)$$

Oxidation–Reduction

An oxidation reaction cannot happen without a concomitant reduction reaction occurring. In this regard, we may consider an **oxidation–reduction** reaction (**redox**) as consisting of two half reactions: the oxidation half and the reduction half.

Oxidation is a loss of electrons. Reduction is a gain of electrons. You can remember this using the mnemonic OIL RIG (oxidation is loss, reduction is gain).

An oxidation half reaction takes the form:

$$M^c \rightarrow M^{(c+n)} + ne^-$$

For example:

$$Fe^{2+} \rightarrow Fe^{3+} + e^-$$

A reduction half reaction takes the form:

$$M^c + ne^- \rightarrow M^{(c-n)}$$

For example:

$$Al^{3+} + 3e^- \rightarrow Al^0$$

An **oxidizing agent**, or **oxidant**, is a species that causes an oxidation to occur. An oxidizing agent oxidizes another species by accepting electrons from that species. By accepting these electrons, the oxidizing agent is reduced.

A **reducing agent**, or **reductant**, is a species that causes a reduction to occur. A reducing agent reduces another species by giving up electrons to that species. By giving up these electrons, the reducing agent is oxidized.

Combustion Reaction

A combustion reaction, which is a type of redox reaction, occurs when a compound and an oxidant react to form heat and a new product. For example,

$$2C_2H_6(g) + 7O_2(g) \rightarrow 4CO_2(g) + 6H_2O(g) + \text{heat}$$

The oxidant in this reaction is oxygen gas. Notice that oxygen is reduced from 0 to –2, and carbon is oxidized from –3 to +4.

9.5 PHASE CHANGES AND PHASES (SOLIDS AND GASES)

Phase Transitions

Kinetic energy is the energy of motion. Temperature is a measure of the average kinetic energy of the molecules in an object or a system. The temperature of a substance directly affects its **state** or **phase**: that is, whether it is a **solid** (*s*), **liquid** (*l*), or **gas** (*g*). Kinetic energy is also related to the degree of disorder, or **entropy**. In general, the higher the average kinetic energy of a substance's molecules, the greater the entropy.

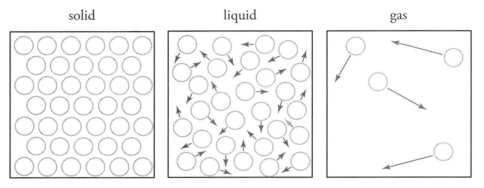

solid   liquid   gas

Figure 11

If we increase the temperature at a given pressure, a solid typically undergoes a phase change from a liquid and then into a gas. Phase changes are the result of breaking (or forming) intermolecular interactions.

In the solid phase, matter is held together by intermolecular interactions in an orderly array. There isn't enough kinetic energy to overcome the intermolecular forces. As a solid is heated, the average kinetic energy of the molecules increases. The solid melts and becomes liquid. At the molecular level, the molecules in a liquid are still in contact and interact with each other, but they are not locked into fixed positions. Liquids have more internal kinetic energy and greater entropy than solids. When the liquid is heated, the kinetic energy increases until the molecules have enough energy to overcome intermolecular forces and vaporize into the gas phase. Molecules in the gas phase move freely and experience few, if any, intermolecular forces.

We can illustrate these transitions with H_2O. Ice is composed of highly organized H_2O molecules held rigidly together by hydrogen bonds. The molecules have limited motion. If we increase the temperature of the ice, the molecules will eventually absorb enough energy to disrupt the organized structure of the solid. The fixed hydrogen bonds are replaced with hydrogen bonds in which the molecules are *not* in fixed positions. This is the transition from solid to liquid. If we continue to increase the temperature, the kinetic energy of the molecules eventually becomes great enough for the individual molecules to overcome the intermolecular attractive forces and move freely. This is the transition from liquid to vapor. At this point the H_2O molecules are free to move randomly, forming a high-entropy, chaotic swarm.

Phases and Temperature and Pressure Dependence

Within a system, all matter that has a particular set of properties is said to be in a single phase. In certain cases, a pure substance may adopt more than one crystalline structure in the solid phase. Diamond and graphite, for example, are two different solid phases of carbon. For the PCAT:

- A gas takes the shape of the container that holds it and expands to fill the available volume.
- A liquid conforms to the shape of the container that holds it, but it does not expand to fill the available volume.
- A solid neither conforms to the shape of the container that holds it nor expands to fill the available volume.

Whether a substance is a solid, liquid, or gas depends primarily on temperature and pressure. As the temperature is increased under constant pressure, a substance will transition from the solid phase to the liquid phase. As temperature increases, the substance will then transition from the liquid phase to the gas phase. As the pressure of a gas is increased at constant temperature, the molecules are forced into closer proximity and intermolecular interactions occur, forming a liquid. If the pressure of a liquid is decreased at constant temperature, more molecules on the liquid surface can escape into the vapor phase until all of the liquid forms a gas.

The Available Phase Changes

Figure 13 illustrates the various phase changes that occur, and the associated terms for those changes. **Fusion** occurs when a solid becomes a liquid. The opposite of fusion is **crystallization**.

Vaporization occurs when a liquid becomes a gas. The opposite of vaporization is **condensation**.

Some solids skip the liquid phase altogether, such as solid CO_2 (dry ice). The direct conversion of a solid to a gas is called **sublimation**. The opposite of sublimation is **deposition**.

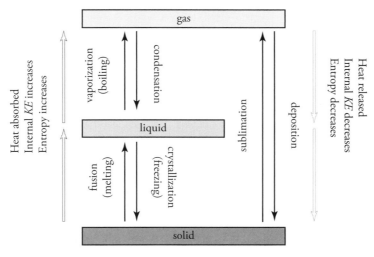

Figure 12

The Thermodynamics of Phase Changes

Melting, vaporization, and sublimation involve a change from a lower energy state to a higher energy state (entropy and kinetic energy increase). Deposition, condensation, and freezing involve a change from a higher energy state to a lower energy state (entropy and kinetic energy decrease).

Because energy is always conserved, the transition from a phase or state that contains more energy to one that contains less energy must involve the release of energy. That is, it must be **exothermic**. Deposition, condensation, and freezing are all exothermic processes.

Conversely, a transition from a phase or state that contains less energy to one that contains more energy requires an energy input. Such a process is **endothermic**. Melting, vaporization, and sublimation are endothermic processes.

Calorimetry

When a sample undergoes a phase change, it absorbs or releases energy *without* a change in temperature. The energy is used to overcome intermolecular interactions.

> When a substance absorbs or releases heat, one of two things can happen: either its temperature changes, *or* it will undergo a phase change, *but not both at the same time.*

The amount of heat absorbed or released by a sample is proportional to its change in temperature. The constant of proportionality is called the substance's **heat capacity, C**, which is the product of its **specific heat**, c, and its mass, m; that is, $C = mc$. The heat capacity is also related to the amount of heat added to or released by a substance, q, and its change in temperature: $q = C\Delta T$. From these two equations, we derive the relationship

$$q = mc\Delta T$$

where

q = heat added to (or released by) a sample
m = mass of the sample
c = specific heat of the substance
ΔT = temperature change

A substance's specific heat is an *intrinsic* property of that substance and tells us how resistant it is to changing its temperature and is measured in $J/(g\bullet°C)$. For example, the specific heat of liquid water is 4.184 J per gram•°C. (A **calorie** is the amount of heat required to raise the temperature of 1 gram of water by 1°C and is equal to 4.184 J exactly.) The specific heat of copper, however, is much less;

only 0.385 J/g•°C, or 0.09 cal/g•°C. If we had 1 g of water and 1 g of copper and each absorbed 10 calories of heat, the resulting changes in their temperatures would be

$$\Delta T_{water} = \frac{q}{mc_{water}} \qquad \Delta T_{copper} = \frac{q}{mc_{copper}}$$

$$= \frac{10 \text{ cal}}{(1 \text{ g})(1\frac{\text{cal}}{\text{g}\bullet°\text{C}})} \qquad = \frac{10 \text{ cal}}{(1 \text{ g})(0.09\frac{\text{cal}}{\text{g}\bullet°\text{C}})}$$

$$= 10°\text{C} \qquad = 111°\text{C}$$

Thus, while the temperature change is proportional to the heat absorbed, it's *inversely* proportional to the substance's heat capacity. A substance like water, with a relatively high specific heat, will undergo a smaller change in temperature than a substance (like copper) with a lower specific heat. Keep in mind that the specific heat of a substance also depends on its phase. For example, the specific heat of ice is different from that of liquid water.

Notice that the *change* in temperature can be expressed in either degrees Celsius or Kelvin. Because the magnitude of the change is the same using either scale, no conversion is needed.

Heats of Phase Changes

When matter undergoes a phase transition, energy is either absorbed or released. The amount of energy required to complete a transition is called the **change in enthalpy,** symbolized ΔH *where H has units of kJ/mol.* For example, the amount of heat that must be absorbed to change a solid into liquid is called the **heat of fusion** (ΔH_{fus}), and the energy absorbed when a liquid changes to gas is the **heat of vaporization** (ΔH_{vap}). The magnitude of ΔH is directly related to the strength and number of the substance's intermolecular forces.

The amount of heat required to cause a change of phase depends on both the identity and amount of substance. For example, the heat of fusion of H_2O is 6.0 kJ/mol. To melt a 2 mol sample of ice (at 0°C), 12 kJ of heat would be needed. The heat of vaporization of H_2O is about 41 kJ/mol, so vaporizing a 2 mol sample of liquid water (at 100°C) would require 82 kJ of heat. If the 2 mol sample of steam (at 100°C) condensed back to liquid, 82 kJ of heat would be released. In general, the amount of heat, q, accompanying a phase transition is given by

$$q = n \times \Delta H_{\text{phase change}}$$

where n is the number of moles of the substance. If ΔH and q are positive, heat is absorbed; if ΔH and q are negative, heat is released.

Heating Curves

A **heating curve** (or a **phase change diagram**) is a graphical representation of the phase changes a substance undergoes as a function of q and T. One such representation is shown in Figure 14.

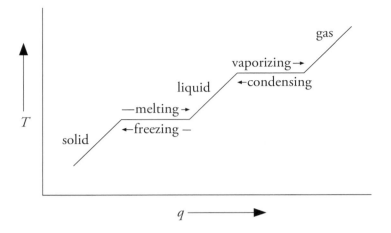

Figure 13

The horizontal lines denote the amount of heat energy that is added or released during a phase change. Notice that the temperature does not change during these transitions. Horizontal components of the graph are given by the formula:

$$q = n\Delta H$$

The length of a horizontal line divided by the number of moles gives a value for ΔH.

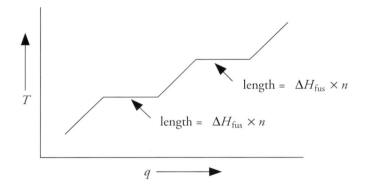

Figure 14

Lines that are not horizontal represent the thermodynamics of a system that is not undergoing a phase change. Relationships here are given by the equation:

$$q = mc\Delta T$$

Therefore, for a heating curve, we can calculate the heat capacity of each phase.

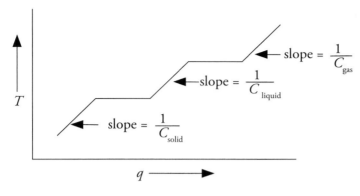

Figure 15

Notice that the heating curve is obtained at constant pressure. If pressure is changed, the phase change diagram must also be changed.

Phase Diagrams

The phase of a substance doesn't depend just on the temperature, it also depends on the pressure. For example, even at high temperatures, a substance can enter the liquid phase if the pressure is high enough, and at low temperature, a substance can become a gas if that pressure is low enough. A substance's **phase diagram** shows how its phases are determined by temperature and pressure. The following figure is an example of a phase diagram.

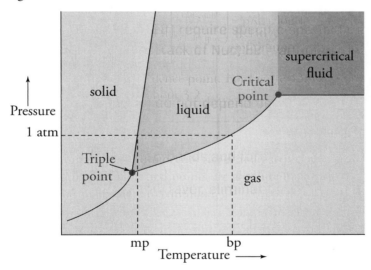

Figure 16

The boundary lines between phases represent points at which the two phases exist simultaneously. For example, a glass of liquid water at 0°C containing ice cubes is a two-phase system, and if its temperature and pressure were plotted in a phase diagram, it would be on the solid-liquid boundary line. Crossing a boundary line implies a phase transition. Notice that the solid phase is favored at low temperatures and high pressures, while the gas phase is favored at high temperatures and low pressures.

The temperature at the point where the horizontal line extends from 1 atm and crosses the solid-liquid boundary is the substance's **normal melting point**. The temperature where the line crosses the liquid-gas boundary is the **normal boiling point**.

The **triple point** is the temperature and pressure at which all three phases exist simultaneously in equilibrium. In a perfectly insulated thermos, for example, the gas, liquid, and solid phases of ice water would be in equilibrium.

At the **critical point** the substance displays properties of both a liquid (such as high density) and a gas (such as low *viscosity*, a resistance to flow). A substance in which the liquid and gas phases are no longer distinct is called a **supercritical fluid**. No amount of increased pressure can force the substance back into its liquid phase.

The Phase Diagrams for Water and CO₂

Water is the most common of a handful of substances that are denser in the liquid phase than in the solid phase. As a result, the solid-liquid boundary line in the phase diagram for water has a slightly *negative* slope, as opposed to the usual positive slope for most other substances. Compare these diagrams:

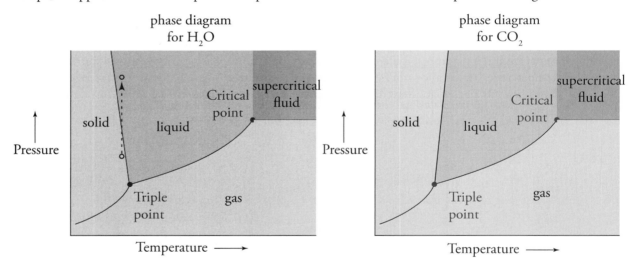

Figure 17

For H_2O, an increase in pressure at constant temperature can favor the *liquid* phase, not the solid phase, as would be the case for most other substances, such as CO_2. The density of ice is lower than that of water, because the H_2O molecules move apart to maximize hydrogen bonding interactions in the solid. Consequently, the solid/liquid line has a negative slope rather than the more typical positive slope shown in the CO_2 diagram. For H_2O the liquid phase is favored with increasing pressure as the water molecules are forced into closer proximity. This is why glaciers move and why ice floats on its liquid.

Types of Solids

Ionic Solids

An **ionic solid** is held together by the electrostatic attraction between cations and anions in a lattice structure. The bonds that hold all the ions together in the crystal lattice are the same as the bonds that hold each pair of ions together. Ionic bonds are strong, so most ionic substances (like NaCl and other salts) are solid at room temperature. The strength of the bonds is primarily dependent on the magnitudes of the charges and the size of the ions. The greater the charge, the stronger the attractive force between the ions. The smaller the distance between nuclei, the stronger the electrostatic attraction. This relationship is described by Coulomb's Law: $E = k(q_1)(q_2)/r^2$, where q_1 and q_2 are the charges on the cation and anion, r is the internuclear distance, and k is a proportionality constant.

The ionic structure of sodium chloride is shown below. Each corner ion is shared by eight cells, each ion on an edge is shared by 4 cells, an ion on a face is shared by two cells, and an ion in the center is not shared. For sodium the unit cell has $(12 \times \frac{1}{4}) + (1 \times 1) = 4$ ions, and chloride has $(6 \times \frac{1}{2}) + (8 \times \frac{1}{8}) = 4$ ions. The ratio of Na^+ to Cl^- is 4:4 or 1:1, which gives the ionic formula NaCl.

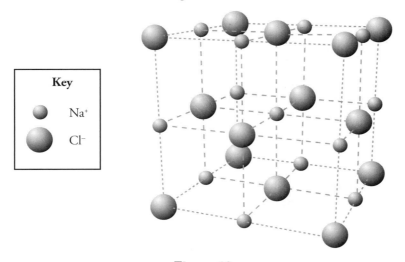

Key

● Na^+

● Cl^-

Figure 18

Network Solids

In a **network solid**, atoms form an interconnected **lattice** of covalent bonds. Just like an ionic solid, in a network solid the *inter*molecular forces are identical to the *intra*molecular forces. A network solid behaves like one large molecule. It is very strong and tends to be very hard solid at room temperature. Diamond (a form of carbon) and quartz (a form of silica, SiO_2) are examples of network solids.

Metallic Solids

A metallic solid is held together by a high density of shared, delocalized valence electrons that are no longer exclusively associated with a single atom. **Metallic bonding** is often referred to as an *electron sea*. The delocalized electrons are called **conduction electrons**. As a result of their metallic bonding, metals are excellent conductors of electricity and heat, and are *malleable* (hammered or pressed without cracking) and *ductile* (able to be drawn into a thin wire). Metallic bonds vary widely in strength, but almost all metals are solids at room temperature.

Molecular Solids

Molecular solids are held together by one of three types of *inter*molecular interactions—hydrogen bonds, dipole-dipole forces, or London dispersion forces. Since these forces are *significantly* weaker than ionic, network, or metallic bonds, molecular compounds typically have much lower melting and boiling points than the other types of solids mentioned. Molecular solids are often liquids or gases at room temperature, and are more likely to be solids as the strength of their intermolecular forces increases.

Gases

Temperature

As the average kinetic energy of a system increases, the temperature increases. Conversely, as the average kinetic energy of a system decreases, the temperature decreases. A temperature scale may be either **absolute** or **relative**. The absolute temperature scale is the **Kelvin (K).** The **Celsius** (°C) and the **Fahrenheit** (°F) scales are examples of relative scales, in which two points of known energy are selected and fixed with chosen values. The freezing point of water at 1 atm on the Celsius scale is 0°C, and the boiling point temperature of water at 1 atm is 100°C. The Fahrenheit scale sets the temperature of the freezing point of water at 1 atm at 32°F, and the boiling point at 1 atm at 212°F.

Absolute zero (0 K) is defined as the temperature at which virtually all motion has ceased. The Kelvin temperature scale is related to the Celsius scale in that one degree Kelvin is equal in magnitude to one degree Celsius. Absolute zero on the Celsius scale is –273.15°C, so the conversion from Celsius to Kelvin is given by

$$K = °C + 273.15$$

Notice that while a temperature in K and °C does not have the same value, a *difference* in temperature (ΔT) in K and °C does. As with all problems on the PCAT, *watch your units*!

Pressure

Pressure is a measure of the **force per unit area**. For a gas, this is the force that moving gas particles have with the walls of their container:

$$P = \frac{F}{A}$$

The pressure of a gas depends on the number of collisions with the walls, the velocity of the colliding gas molecules, and their mass. As each of these factors increases, the pressure increases. The number of collisions with the walls will increase if the number of molecules increases or the volume decreases. The velocity of the colliding gas molecules will increase as the temperature (the average kinetic energy) increases.

Pressure is measured in the SI units of **pascals (Pa)**.

$$P = \frac{F}{A} = \frac{N}{m^2} = \text{Pa}$$

Pressure may also be measured in **atmospheres (atm)**, **millimeters of mercury (mmHg)**, or **torr.**

$$1 \text{ atm} = 760 \text{ mmHg} = 760 \text{ torr} = 1.013 \times 10^5 \text{ Pa}$$

STP

Standard temperature and pressure (STP) is defined as 0°C and 760 torr. This is a reference point for the comparison of one gas to another. One mole of an ideal gas at STP occupies a volume of 22.4 liters (or 0.0224 cubic meters in SI units). It should be noted that gas STP differs from the standard state for thermodynamic functions such as enthalpy. The temperature at STP for a gas is 0°C (273 K); the temperature of the standard thermodynamic state is 25°C (298 K). Both are defined at a pressure of 760 torr, or 1 atm.

Kinetic Molecular Theory

The **kinetic molecular theory** assumes that gases behave in an ideal way. There are five basic premises:

1. Gases are composed of molecules, or particles, which are in rapid, random translational motion (straight-line motion). Because these particles have mass and velocity, they possess kinetic energy given by $KE = \frac{1}{2}mv^2$.
2. The particles undergo collisions with the walls of their container and with one another. These collisions are perfectly elastic; there is no loss of kinetic energy during any collision.
3. At any instant in time, the particles are separated by a distance much greater than the size of the particles themselves. Thus, the space occupied by the particles is negligible with regard to the size of the container.
4. There are no attractive or repulsive forces between the particles.
5. The average kinetic energy of the particles is directly proportional to the absolute temperature of the particles.

The first statement says that any particle that possesses both mass and velocity will have a kinetic energy given by $KE = \frac{1}{2}mv^2$.

The second states that all collisions are elastic. In practice, perfectly elastic collisions are extremely rare.

The third states that there is no excluded volume. That is, none of the volume of the container is excluded from use by any one gas molecule at any moment in time. This, of course, is not true. The only way this could be true is if only one gas molecule was present in a given volume or if the gas particles were truly point masses.

The fourth states that gas particles do not influence each other except in collisions. However, as we have seen, all molecules will exert either repulsive or attractive forces upon one another, such as London dispersion forces.

The fifth states that at a given temperature all gases have the same average kinetic energy. Their velocities, however, are mass dependent. Higher masses have lower velocities; that is, heavy particles move more slowly.

Deviations from Ideality

Deviations in Pressure

As the temperature of a gas is decreased, the kinetic energy of individual gas particles decreases. As a result, the velocity of the particles decreases, which leads to a higher probability of inelastic collisions (violation of premise 2). Molecules that are moving at a slower velocity are also more likely to experience the attractive or repulsive forces of other gas molecules in the container (violation of premise 4). Any of these factors will lead to an actual pressure that is less than the ideal pressure. *The actual pressure exerted by a gas is always less than or equal to the pressure calculated by the ideal gas law.*

Deviations in Volume

As the pressure of a gas is increased, the volume occupied by the individual gas particles themselves becomes more important. As pressure goes up, the volume in which gas particles move goes down. Therefore, the average separation between any two gas molecules must also decrease (violation of premise 3). Individual gas molecules now occupy a more significant amount of the total volume. Thus, there is an *excluded volume,* which is the volume occupied by the gas molecules themselves. The actual volume of the gas is equal to the volume of the container plus the excluded volume. *The actual volume occupied by a gas is always greater than or equal to the volume calculated based on ideal behavior.*

Approaching Ideal-Gas Behavior

The actual pressure and volume of a real gas are less than those obtained assuming ideal behavior. In particular, *high pressures, low temperatures, and higher masses cause real gases to deviate the most from ideal-gas behavior.* That is, $P_{real} < P_{ideal}$ because the real gases *do* experience intermolecular forces, which reduces the force of the collisions with the walls of the container. Moreover, $V_{real} < V_{ideal}$ because molecules of real gases *do* have volumes that reduce the effective empty volume of the container. Gases with a higher mass deviate the most from ideal behavior because they take up more volume, as do those with weak intermolecular forces. You can remember pressure and volume relationships between ideal gases and real gases using this phrase: *the ideal world is greater than the real world.*

The Gas Laws

Boyle's Law

Boyle's Law states that under conditions of constant temperature and with a constant number of moles of gas, the product of pressure and volume is a constant:

$$PV = \text{constant}$$

If the pressure or volume changes for a given system, then:

$$P_1 V_1 = P_2 V_2$$

Notice that pressure and volume are inversely proportional:

$$P \propto \frac{1}{V}$$

$$V \propto \frac{1}{P}$$

Charles's Law

Charles's Law establishes the relationship between volume and temperature in degrees K where a constant number of moles of gas is at a constant pressure:

$$\frac{V}{T} = \text{constant}$$

or

$$V = (\text{constant})(T)$$

$$\frac{V_1}{T_1} = \frac{V_2}{T_2}$$

or

$$V_1 T_2 = V_2 T_1$$

That is, temperature and volume for a given system are directly proportional:

$$V \propto T$$
$$T \propto V$$

Gay-Lussac's Law

Gay-Lussac's Law includes Charles's Law and the relationship between pressure and temperature under conditions of constant volume and a constant number of moles of gas:

$$\frac{P}{T} = \text{constant}$$

or

$$P = (\text{constant})(T)$$

If pressure or temperature change for a given system, then

$$\frac{P_1}{T_1} = \frac{P_2}{T_2}$$

or

$$P_1 T_2 = P_2 T_1$$

This means that temperature is directly proportional to pressure and that pressure is, therefore, also directly proportional to temperature:

$$P \propto T$$
$$T \propto P$$

The Combined Gas Law

The **Combined Gas Law** unites the relationships found in Boyle's Law, Charles's Law, and Gay-Lussac's Law, for conditions in which the number of moles of gas is constant:

$$\frac{PV}{T} = \text{constant}$$

or

$$PV = (\text{constant})(T)$$

If pressure, volume, or temperature change for a given system, then

$$\frac{P_1 V_1}{T_1} = \frac{P_2 V_2}{T_2}$$

or

$$P_1 V_1 T_2 = P_2 V_2 T_1$$

Avogadro's Hypothesis

Avogadro's Hypothesis establishes the relationship between the number of moles (n) of gas and its volume when the pressure and temperature are constant:

$$\frac{V}{n} = \text{constant}$$

or

$$V = (\text{constant})(n)$$

If the volume or number of moles changes for a given system, then

$$\frac{V_1}{n_1} = \frac{V_2}{n_2}$$

or

$$V_1 n_2 = V_2 n_1$$

The volume of a gas is directly proportional to its number of moles:

$$V \propto n$$
$$n \propto V$$

This hypothesis also asserts that under conditions in which the temperature and pressure are identical, the volume of one mole of a gas is equal to the volume of one mole of any other gas.

The Ideal Gas Law and the Gas Constant

Avogadro's Hypothesis may be incorporated into the combined gas law to give the following relationship:

$$\frac{PV}{nT} = \text{constant}$$

Since it holds for any ideal gas, the constant is called the **universal gas constant** and is symbolized by R. Thus,

$$\frac{PV}{nT} = R$$

or

$$PV = nRT$$

We can summarize the laws like this:

In a system with constant n:

At constant P : $\dfrac{V_1}{T_1} = \dfrac{V_2}{T_2}$

At constant T : $P_1V_1 = P_2V_2$

At constant V : $\dfrac{P_1}{T_1} = \dfrac{P_2}{T_2}$

The Ideal Gas Law

The volume, temperature, and pressure of an ideal gas are related by a simple equation called the **Ideal Gas Law**. Most real gases under ordinary conditions act very much like ideal gases, so the ideal gas law applies to most gas behavior:

Ideal Gas Law

$$PV = nRT$$

where

P = the pressure of the gas in atmospheres
V = the volume of the container in liters
n = the number of moles of the gas
R = the universal gas constant, 0.0821 L-atm•K-mol
T = the absolute temperature of the gas (that is, T in kelvins)

PCAT questions on gas behavior typically take one of two forms. The first type of question simply gives you some facts, in which you use $PV = nRT$ to determine a missing variable. In the second type "before" and "after" scenarios are presented, in which you determine the effect of changing the volume, temperature, or pressure. In this case, you use the relationships that apply to changing conditions. We'll solve a typical example of each type of question.

9.5

1. If two moles of helium at 27°C fill a 3 L balloon, what is the pressure?

We use the ideal gas law, check our units and convert where necessary, and solve for P:

$$PV = nRT$$
$$P = \frac{nRT}{V}$$
$$P = \frac{(2 \text{ mol})(0.082 \text{ L-atm/K-mol})(300 \text{ K})}{3 \text{ L}}$$
$$P = 16 \text{ atm}$$

2. Argon, at a pressure of 2 atm, fills a 100 mL vial at a temperature of 0°C. What would the pressure of the argon be if we increase the volume to 500 mL, and the temperature is 100°C?

The number of moles of argon in the vial has not changed. Since R is a constant, the ratio of PV/T, which is equal to nR, remains constant. Again, after checking units and converting where necessary.

$$\frac{P_1V_1}{T_1} = \frac{P_2V_2}{T_2} \quad \Rightarrow \quad P_2 = P_1\frac{V_1}{V_2}\frac{T_2}{T_1}$$
$$P_2 = (2 \text{ atm})\left(\frac{0.1 \text{ L}}{0.5 \text{ L}}\right)\left(\frac{373 \text{ K}}{273 \text{ K}}\right)$$
$$P_2 = 0.55 \text{ atm}$$

Mixtures of Gases

Dalton's Law

Vapor Pressure is the pressure created over a liquid by the molecules of that liquid that have enough kinetic energy to escape to the vapor phase. The higher the temperature, the greater the kinetic energy and the higher the vapor pressure. **Dalton's Law of Partial Pressures** states that the pressure exerted by a mixture of gases that behaves ideally is equal to the sum of the pressures exerted by the individual gases at the same temperature and volume:

$$P_T = P_A + P_B$$

where P_T is the total pressure exerted by a mixture of gases A and B, and P_A and P_B are the pressures that gases A and B would exert alone under the same set of conditions. Substituting this relationship into the ideal gas law gives

$$P_T = \frac{(n_A + n_B)RT}{V}$$

where n_A and n_B are the number of moles of gases A and B, respectively. We can alternatively state that the partial pressure exerted by gas A is equal to the product of the total pressure exerted by the mixture and the mole fraction of gas A that is present:

$$P_A = P_T X_A$$

where X_A is the mole fraction of gas A, which is given by

$$X_A = \frac{n_A}{n_T} = \frac{n_A}{n_A + n_B}$$

Raoult's Law

Raoult's Law describes a relationship similar to Dalton's Law, but pertains to certain **ideal solutions**. Raoult's Law asserts that the vapor pressure exerted by a component of a liquid mixture is equal to the product of the vapor pressure of the pure component and the mole fraction of that component in the *liquid* phase:

$$P_A = X_{A(\ell)} P^*_A$$

where P_A is the vapor pressure exerted by liquid component A, $X_{A(\ell)}$ is the mole fraction of A in the liquid phase, and P^*_A is the vapor pressure of pure A. In the case of a nonvolatile solute dissolved in a solvent, the vapor pressure of the solution can be calculated from

$$P_{soln} = X_{solv} P^*_{solv}$$

where

P_{soln} = vapor pressure of the solution

X_{soln} = mol fraction of the solvent

P^*_{solv} = vapor pressure of the pure solvent

Graham's Law of Effusion

Gaseous particles move constantly in random motions. **Diffusion** occurs when they disperse in a container. **Effusion** occurs when a particle passes through an opening. The rates of diffusion and effusion depend on the velocities of the gas particles, and therefore are mass and temperature dependent.

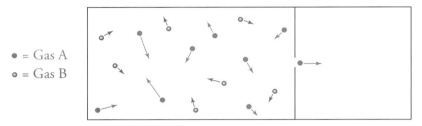

Figure 19

If Gas A and Gas B have different molar masses, the heavier molecules will move, on average, slower than the lighter ones. The average kinetic energies of Gas A and Gas B are the same at a given temperature. The average kinetic energy of a molecule of Gas A is $\frac{1}{2}m_A(v_A^2)_{avg}$, and the average kinetic energy of a molecule of Gas B is $\frac{1}{2}m_B(v_B^2)_{avg}$. Setting these equal to each other, we get

$$\frac{1}{2}m_A(v_A^2)_{avg} = \frac{1}{2}m_B(v_B^2)_{avg} \quad\Rightarrow\quad \frac{(v_A^2)_{avg}}{(v_B^2)_{avg}} = \frac{m_B}{m_A} \quad\Rightarrow\quad \frac{rms\ v_A}{rms\ v_B} = \sqrt{\frac{m_B}{m_A}}$$

The abbreviation **rms** stands for *root-mean-square*; it's the square root of the mean [average] of the square of speed. Therefore, rms v is a measure of the average speed of the molecules. For example, if Gas A is hydrogen gas (H_2, molecular weight = 2) and Gas B is oxygen gas (O_2, molecular weight = 32), the hydrogen molecules will move, on average, four times faster than oxygen molecules:

$$\sqrt{\frac{m_B}{m_A}} = \sqrt{\frac{32}{2}} = \sqrt{16} = 4$$

This result gives rise to **Graham's Law of Effusion**:

Graham's Law of Effusion

$$\frac{\text{rate of effusion of Gas A}}{\text{rate of effusion of Gas B}} = \sqrt{\frac{\text{molar mass of Gas B}}{\text{molar mass of Gas A}}}$$

The distinction between the relationships of temperature to the kinetic energy and to the speed of the gas is an important one. The molecules of two different gases at the same temperature have the same average kinetic energy, but the molecules of two different gases at the same temperature don't have the same average *speed*. Lighter molecules travel faster, because the kinetic energy depends on both the mass and the speed of the molecules.

Also, it's important to remember that not all the molecules of the gas in a container—even if there's only one type of molecule—travel at the same speed. Their speeds cover a wide range. As the temperature of the sample is increased, only the *average* speed increases. In fact, since $KE \propto T$, the root-mean-square speed is proportional to $\sqrt{T}$. The figure below shows the distribution of molecular speeds for a gas at three different temperatures. Notice that the rms speeds increase, and the shape under the peaks broaden, as the temperature is increased.

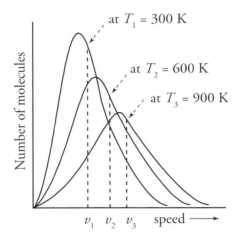

Figure 20

9.6 REACTION KINETICS: RATE, RATE LAWS, AND CATALYSIS

Kinetics

Kinetics is the study of the rates of chemical reactions and their pathways. It focuses on both the speed and the mechanism by which it occurs. Kinetics answers *how* a reaction proceeds from reactants to products.

Thermodynamics, in contrast, is concerned with the interrelationships among heat, work, and energy, and the stability of the system. It answers *whether or not* a reaction will occur. Thermodynamics is pathway independent.

Reaction Mechanisms

Breaking a chemical bond in a chemical reaction requires an input of energy, while the formation of a chemical bond involves the release of energy. A **reaction mechanism** is the pathway by which reactants are converted to products. Each reaction may have different available pathways that have different steps, different rates, and different combinations of possible products. The particular mechanism that predominates, since often a reaction will proceed simultaneously along competitive pathways, depends on the reaction conditions. These include reactant concentrations, pressure, temperature, and the absence or presence of a catalyst.

Each mechanism is comprised of a series of elementary steps. Consider the overall reaction:

$$2AB + C \rightleftharpoons A_2C + B_2$$

One possible mechanism for this reaction is

Step 1:	$AB \rightarrow A + B$
Step 2:	$A + C \rightarrow AC$
Step 3:	$AC + A \rightarrow A_2C$
Step 4:	$B + B \rightarrow B_2$

Another possible mechanism for this reaction is

Step 1:	$AB + C \rightleftharpoons ABC$
Step 2:	$ABC \rightleftharpoons AC + B$
Step 3:	$AB \rightarrow A + B$
Step 4:	$AC + A \rightarrow A_2C$
Step 5:	$B + B \rightarrow B_2$

Elementary steps are distinguished by the number of reactant molecules involved in that particular step. A step involving only one reactant molecule, such as step 1 in the first mechanism or step 2 or 3 in the second mechanism, is called a **unimolecular process**. A step involving two reactant molecules, such as step 2, 3, or 4 in the first mechanism or step 1, 4, or 5 in the second mechanism, is called a **bimolecular process**. Elementary steps involving more than two reactant molecules are rare: therefore, most mechanistic steps are either unimolecular or bimolecular.

For each elementary step in a mechanism, there is an energy barrier that must be overcome in order for that step to proceed. This energy barrier is termed the **activation energy (E_a)** for that step. The higher the energy of activation, the less likely that step is to occur. For any mechanism, the step with the highest activation energy is the slowest step. The slowest step in a series of steps will limit the overall progression from reactants to products, so this step is termed the **rate-determining step**. Because steps are dependent on reaction conditions, the rate-determining step under a given set of reaction conditions may change as reaction conditions change.

Another important feature of elementary steps is **microscopic reversibility**. While an overall chemical reaction may not be considered to be reversible, *all* elementary steps are reversible. Thus, for every forward process, the reverse process also occurs in *exactly* the reverse manner.

If $AB \rightarrow A + B$, then $A + B \rightarrow AB$ by reversing the path.

If a substance is formed and later consumed, such as we see for the product *ABC* of step 1 of the second mechanism above, it is called an **intermediate**. An intermediate is a detectable substance that is neither reactant nor product. It is formed and then consumed within a mechanistic pathway. The detection of such intermediates is often crucial in determining the mechanism of a reaction.

An intermediate should not be confused with a **transition state**. The latter is a high-energy species found at the peak of the reaction curve. Intermediates are found in the troughs of reaction curves. This is discussed in greater detail when reaction diagrams are presented.

Reaction Rates

A **reaction rate** can be expressed either as the amount of product formed or as the amount of reactant consumed in a given amount of time.

Consider the general reaction:

$$aA + bB \rightarrow cC + dD$$

The rate at which the reaction proceeds can be measured as the rate at which reactant A or reactant B is consumed (a negative sign), or as the rate at which either reactant C or reactant D is formed (a positive sign):

$$\text{Rate of Reaction} = \frac{-\Delta[A]}{a\Delta t} = \frac{-\Delta[B]}{b\Delta t} = \frac{\Delta[C]}{c\Delta t} = \frac{\Delta[D]}{d\Delta t}$$

Consider the following example:

$$N_2O_4(g) \rightarrow 2NO_2(g)$$

The rate of this reaction is given by

$$\text{Rate of Reaction} = \frac{-\Delta[N_2O_4]}{\Delta t} = \frac{\Delta[NO_2]}{2\Delta t}$$

We can see that for every 1 mole of N_2O_4 consumed, 2 moles of NO_2 are produced.

The Effect of Concentration: The Rate Law

Concentration has a marked effect on the rate of reaction. In general, a reaction will slow as time passes because reactants are being consumed. As the concentration of reactants decreases, there are fewer collisions between reactant molecules. Thus, the reaction rate is proportional to reactant concentration. Considering the general reaction:

$$aA + bB \rightarrow cC + dD$$

the **Rate Law** is given by

$$\text{Rate} = k[A]^x[B]^y$$

where k is the rate constant and $[A]$ and $[B]$ are the concentrations of A and B, respectively. The value of x is the *order of the reaction with respect to A* and the value of y is the *order of the reaction with respect to B*. The **overall order** of this reaction is given by the sum of x and y, whose values must be experimentally determined. The values of x and y bear no relationship to the stoichiometric numbers a and b.

For instance, it has been experimentally determined that the rate law expression for

$$NO_2(g) + CO(g) \rightarrow NO(g) + CO_2(g)$$

is given by

$$\text{Rate} = k[NO_2]^2$$

This reaction is second order in $[NO_2]$.

The elementary steps for this reaction are

$$2NO_2(g) \xrightarrow{slow} NO(g) + NO_3(g)$$
$$NO_3(g) + CO(g) \xrightarrow{fast} NO_2(g) + CO_2(g)$$
$$\overline{NO_2(g) + CO(g) \longrightarrow NO(g) + CO_2(g)}$$

The sum of the elementary steps gives the overall reaction. Notice that the slowest elementary step gives the experimentally determined rate law for the overall reaction, which makes sense. The reaction can proceed only as fast as the slowest step.

While a rate law can be directly written from an elementary step, the rate law for an overall reaction must be determined experimentally.

The rate has units of molarity/second (M/s) unless another unit of time is specified. This means that the units of k change with the reaction order. In this example, the units of k are $M^{-1}s^{-1}$, but if the reaction had been first order in $[NO_2]$, k would have units of s^{-1} in order to obtain a rate in M/s. If the temperature of the reaction is changed, a new rate constant must be calculated.

The following are the important points to remember about a rate constant:

- The value of k is unique to each reaction at a given temperature.
- The value of k will change if the temperature is changed.
- The value of k does *not* change with time.
- The value of k is not dependent on the concentrations of either reactants or products.
- The value of k *must* be determined experimentally.
- The units of k depend on the overall order of the reaction.

The value of k does not change with time; therefore, its value will be the same at any point of the reaction if all other conditions remain the same.

The Effect of Catalysts

Catalysts are substances that are added to reaction systems to lower the energy of activation. Catalysts have no effect on the equilibrium concentrations of reactants and products. While catalysts are usually thought of as speeding up a reaction, they may also *slow down* a reaction. A catalyst that's used to slow down a reaction is called an **inhibitory catalyst,** or **inhibitor.** The following discussion focuses on catalysts that speed up reactions. You should be aware that an inhibitor will have the reverse effect on a reaction process.

A catalyst provides an alternative pathway that lowers the overall activation energy of the reaction system. It does not appear in the balanced equation for the reaction, and is neither consumed nor produced during the course of a reaction.

Catalysts may be classified into two categories: **homogeneous catalysts** and **heterogeneous catalysts.** A homogeneous catalyst is in the same phase as the reactants. An example is an acid or a base added catalytically to an organic reaction. **Enzymes** are proteins that act as homogeneous catalysts for specific biochemical reactions.

A heterogeneous catalyst is in a different phase than that of the reactants. Heterogeneous catalysts are usually solids that supply a surface upon which the reaction may occur. An example is "poisoned palladium" (palladium with added graphite), which is often used as a hydrogenation catalyst in organic chemistry.

The Effect of Temperature: The Arrhenius Equation

A change in the temperature of a reaction will lead to a change in the value of the rate constant. The average kinetic energy of the molecules in a reaction system is proportional to the temperature (in Kelvin) of the system, because for a reaction to occur collisions must occur. There also must be sufficient energy during the collision to overcome the activation energy.

From experimental evidence, Svante Arrhenius was able to develop the mathematical relationship between activation energy, absolute temperature (Kelvin), and the rate constant at that temperature. The result is the **Arrhenius equation:**

$$k = Ae^{-\frac{E_a}{RT}}$$

which, in terms of log, base 10, may be written

$$\log k = \log A - \frac{E_a}{2.303 \, RT}$$

The following equation is used to determine the rate constant, k_2, at a temperature, T_2, when the rate constant, k_1, is known at temperature T_1. In this case, the Arrhenius equation becomes

$$\log \frac{k_2}{k_1} = \frac{E_a}{2.303 \, R} \left(\frac{T_2 - T_1}{T_1 T_2} \right)$$

Notice that the rate constant of a reaction is different for different temperatures, and that the magnitude of the change in the rate constant is directly proportional to the activation energy of the reaction—the larger the activation energy, the greater the change in rate constant for the same temperature change. Also notice that the rate constant is independent of concentration.

9.7 CHEMICAL EQUILIBRIUM

Equilibrium Dynamics

In a reversible reaction, **chemical equilibrium** is a state that is reached when there is no net change in the concentrations of products or reactants. At equilibrium, the rate of formation of products is equal to that of reactants. In an equilibrium state, reactants and products continue to be formed, but their overall concentrations do not change. Thus, equilibrium is a *dynamic condition*—forward and reverse reactions occur simultaneously and at the same rate. It is also *independent of the path taken to reach equilibrium*—the ratio of products to reactants will not change as long as temperature and, in some cases, pressure and volume do not change.

The Equilibrium Constants (K_{eq}, K_c, K_p)

The equilibrium constant, K_{eq}, is the ratio of the concentrations of products to the concentrations of reactants at equilibrium. For the general reaction:

$$a\text{A} + b\text{B} \rightleftharpoons c\text{C} + d\text{D}$$

the equilibrium constant is given by

$$K_{eq} = \frac{[\text{C}]^c [\text{D}]^d}{[\text{A}]^a [\text{B}]^b}$$

The concentrations are the equilibrium concentrations (not the initial concentrations), and they are usually measured in molarity (M), defined as moles/liter (mol/L). Pure liquids and pure solids do not appear in the equilibrium equation. If all reactants and products are gases, the partial pressures of the gases can be used in place of molarity, and the equilibrium constant is expressed as K_p. We can convert between K_{eq} and K_p using this equation:

$$K_p = K_{eq}(\text{RT})^{\Delta n}$$

where Δn is the total number of moles of gas in the products – the total number of moles of gas in the reactants. If they are equal, then Δn is zero and $K_p = K_{eq}$. K_c is used to indicate gases expressed as molar concentrations.

The magnitude of K_{eq} is independent of the amounts of reactants and products, but it is *not independent* of changes in temperature and, in some cases, pressure or volume. A change in one of these factors does not *necessarily* correspond to the change in K_{eq}, however. For example, some reactions will have a *decrease* in K_{eq} with an *increase* in temperature.

When the system is at equilibrium, the value of the equilibrium constant tells us the relative amounts of reactants and products. If K_{eq} is large, then the ratio of products to reactants is high. If K_{eq} is close to 1, the relative concentrations of products and reactants are similar. And, if K_{eq} is small, then the ratio of products to reactants is low.

Use these values as a guide:

- If $K_{eq} > 10^3$, then products are favored over reactants.
- If K_{eq} is between 10^{-3} and 10^3, then neither reactants nor products is favored.
- If $K_{eq} < 10^{-3}$, then reactants are favored over products.

The Reaction Quotient

The reaction quotient, Q, is related to the equilibrium constant, K_{eq}. While K_{eq} gives the ratio of products to reactants at equilibrium, the reaction quotient gives the same ratio of concentrations that are not necessarily at equilibrium. At equilibrium $Q = K_{eq}$. If the equation for the reaction is

$$a\text{A} + b\text{B} \rightleftharpoons c\text{C} + d\text{D}$$

Then the equation for the reaction quotient is

$$Q = \frac{(\text{C})^c\,(\text{D})^d}{(\text{A})^a\,(\text{B})^b}$$

Parentheses are used instead of brackets to designate concentrations other than equilibrium concentrations.

The reaction quotient can be calculated for any concentrations of reactants and products. As shown in Table 7, for example, if $Q > K_{eq}$, then the numerator of Q is greater than the numerator of K_{eq}. The numerator corresponds to the concentrations of products, so the reaction must proceed toward reactants to reduce product concentrations

Relationship	Interpretation	Change as Reaction Approaches Equilibrium
$Q > K_{eq}$	Products in excess	Decrease in products, increase in reactants. Reaction shifts toward reactants.
$Q = K_{eq}$	At equilibrium	No change
$Q < K_{eq}$	Reactants in excess	Decrease in reactants, increase in products. Reaction shifts toward products.

Table 7

9.7

Le Châtelier's Principle

Shifts in Equilibrium

Once a reaction is at equilibrium, a variety of factors may cause a shift away from equilibrium. The addition or removal of either a reactant or a product will affect the concentration of that substance, but it will not affect the value of K_{eq}. Therefore, when a product or reactant is added or removed, the system will seek ways in which to reestablish the equilibrium condition. The tendency of a system to return to a condition of chemical equilibrium is described by **Le Châtelier's principle**:

- When a system at equilibrium is subjected to a stress, the equilibrium will shift in a direction that tends to alleviate the effect of that stress.

Changes in pH

For an aqueous solution, an increase in pH means lowering the H^+ concentration and raising the OH^- concentration. Conversely, a decrease in the pH of an aqueous solution means a higher H^+ concentration and a lower OH^- concentration.

Consider the general acid dissociation reaction:

$$HA \rightleftharpoons H^+ + A^-$$

By increasing the concentration of H^+, $Q > K_{eq}$ and the reaction is driven to the left, which means that [HA] increases, [A^-] decreases, and the pH of the solution is lowered:

$$\uparrow HA \rightleftharpoons \uparrow H^+ + \downarrow A^-$$

If [H^+] is decreased, then $Q > K_{eq}$ and the reaction is driven to the right. This means that [HA] decreases, [A^-] increases, and the pH is raised:

$$\downarrow HA \rightleftharpoons \downarrow H^+ + \uparrow A^-$$

Effects of Changes in Pressure and Volume

Le Châtelier's principle states that the pressure of a gas at equilibrium is directly proportional to the number of moles of gas and inversely proportional to its volume.

To predict changes in equilibrium resulting from pressure changes due to a change in volume, Le Châtelier's principle can be used as follows:

- If volume is decreased, then pressure is increased. The reaction will be pushed in the direction in which there are fewer moles of gas.
- If volume is increased, then pressure is decreased, and the reaction will shift in the direction with more moles of gas.

If both sides of a reaction contain an equal number of gaseous moles, then there is no change in equilibrium when the pressure is changed. However, if they are not equal, then the system will act to relieve the stress resulting from the increased pressure: equilibrium will shift to the side with fewer moles of gas.

The Effect of Changes in Temperature

To determine the effects of temperature, we first determine whether a reaction is endothermic or exothermic. An endothermic reaction *consumes* heat and an exothermic reaction *gives off* heat. Stating this in Le Châtelier terms: heat is a reactant in an endothermic reaction and heat is a product in an exothermic reaction.

> If we add heat to an endothermic reaction, the reaction will be driven toward products, but if we add heat to an exothermic reaction, the reaction will be driven toward reactants.

9.8   SOLUTIONS

Solutions in Qualitative Terms

Basic Definitions

A **solution**—a homogeneous mixture of two or more substances—may exist in any phase (gas, liquid, or solid).

A **solute** dissolves in a **solvent**. If it is not clear which is the solvent, the solvent is the compound that is present in the largest quantity, and all other compounds present are considered solutes. Exceptions occur in the health sciences, in which a 75% ethanol solution is 75% ethanol in water. Water is the solvent, but it has the lower concentration.

For a solute to dissolve in a liquid, it must have similar intermolecular forces. This gives rise to the saying, "like dissolves like." For example, nonpolar molecules dissolve in nonpolar solvents, and polar molecules dissolve in polar solvents. Ionic compounds with very strong electrostatic attractive forces between cations and anions as described by Coulomb's Law, such as $Mg(OH)_2$, have limited solubility in a polar solvent such as water. The affinity for water is simply not strong enough to completely overcome the strong electrostatic interaction of the ions.

When a solute is added to a solvent, the solvent molecules surround the solute molecules in a process called **solvation**. Solvation depends on the intermolecular forces present between the solvent and the solute.

Hydration describes the solvation process when the solvent is water. Substances that are water soluble have a significant electrostatic energy, form hydrogen bonds, or have a large dipole moment.

Thermodynamics of Solutions

Solvation is controlled by two different thermodynamic properties: the tendency of a system to seek a minimum energy state and to maximize entropy. **Heat of solution** is the enthalpy change that occurs when a solute dissolves in a solvent. It may be either positive (energy absorbed) or negative (energy released). As with other thermodynamic systems, a **positive heat of solution** indicates an **endothermic solvation,** and a **negative heat of solution** indicates an **exothermic solvation**.

An exothermic solvation results from the dissolution of a solute that has a greater affinity for solvent molecules than for other solute molecules. Conversely, an endothermic solvation results from the dissolution of a solute that has a lower affinity for solvent molecules than for other solute molecules. A solution that has a negative heat of solution is lower in enthalpy than the pure solute and the pure solvent. Conversely, a positive heat of solution indicates that the solution has a higher enthalpy than the solute and the solvent.

Relative Concentrations

A solution is **saturated** when no more solute molecules will dissolve in the quantity of solvent available. A solution may become **supersaturated** under certain conditions, however. A supersaturated solution is an unstable system in which more solute molecules have been dissolved than would be possible under normal conditions. A solution may become supersaturated if prepared at a higher temperature and then slowly cooled. The solution will eventually stabilize through precipitation of the excess dissolved solute molecules.

A **concentrated solution** is one in which there is a relative abundance of solute molecules, whereas a **dilute solution** is one in which there are relatively few solute molecules. The terms "concentrated" and "dilute" can qualitatively describe the amount of solute in a solution. There are other quantitative expressions for solution concentration such as molarity, molality, and mole fraction, described below.

Qualitative Solubility

Solubility is the ability of a solute to dissolve in a solvent. The solubility of gases in a liquid solvent is determined using **Henry's Law,** where C is solubility, k is the Henry's Law constant for the gas under consideration, and P is the gas pressure, or **partial pressure** of the particular gaseous solute over the solution.

$$C = kP_{gas}$$

Notice that the solubility of a gas is directly proportional to the pressure of that gas above the solution: as pressure is increased, solubility is also increased.

The heat of solution for gases in liquid solvents is almost always negative. As temperature is increased, gas solubility decreases. For example, when a pot of water is heated, dissolved gases such as CO_2 are released at a lower temperature than the boiling point of water. They are seen as small bubbles at the bottom of the pot well before the water begins to boil.

Liquids are said to be **miscible** in other liquids when they are soluble in all proportions. Liquids that do not dissolve in one another are **immiscible**.

Some general solubility rules for aqueous solutions can be stated as follows:

- All alkali and ammonium (NH_4^+) compounds are soluble. The alkali metals are included in Group 1 (Li^+, Na^+, K^+, Rb^+, Cs^+).
- All acetates (CH_3COO^-), chlorates (ClO_3^-), nitrates (NO_3^-), and perchlorates (ClO_4^-) are soluble.
- Pb^{2+}, Hg^{2+}, and Ag^+ salts are insoluble, *unless* they are paired with one of the anions from the previous rules.

Solubility: pH and Temperature

The solubility of a substance is affected by several factors, including temperature, the presence of common ions, and pH.

For a system with an endothermic heat of solution, solubility will generally increase with increasing temperature and decrease with decreasing temperature. For a system with an exothermic heat of solution, solubility will typically decrease with increasing temperature and increase with decreasing temperature.

If a basic or acidic ion is produced in a dissolution process, a change in pH will affect the solubility of the solute. A solute that dissociates into an acidic ion will have enhanced solubility in a solution with a high pH (basic), and diminished solubility in a solution with a low pH (acidic). Conversely, a solute that dissociates into a basic ion will be more soluble in a solution with a low pH (acidic) and less soluble in a solution with a high pH (basic).

Solutions in Quantitative Terms: Concentration

Concentration Measurements

There are various ways in which concentration may be expressed. Recall that solution concentrations are expressed as moles of solute per liter of solution, or molarity (M):

$$\text{Molarity } (M) = \frac{\text{moles of solute}}{\text{liters of solution}}$$

Concentration is denoted by enclosing the solute in brackets. For instance, "$[Na^+] = 1.0\ M$" indicates a solution whose concentration is 1 mole of sodium ions per liter of solution.

Molality

Molality is expressed in terms of mass (moles/kilogram of solvent) and is symbolized as m. For dilute aqueous solutions, however, molality and molarity are nearly identical, as the density of water is approximately 1 kilogram per liter.

Mole Fraction

The **mole fraction** of a solution is usually of interest only in problems involving gases, or problems concerned with vapor pressure. Mole fraction (X_s, where s is the substance under consideration) is defined as

$$X_s = \frac{\text{moles of solute (s)}}{\text{total moles of solution}}$$

Parts per Million and Parts per Thousand

Parts per million (**ppm**) and **parts per thousand** (**ppt**) are often used in the health sciences. These units denote a very low concentration of solute in a solution. One ppm is the equivalent of 1 mg/L and one ppt is equal to 1 g/L:

$$1\ \text{ppm} = 1\text{mg/L}$$

$$1\ \text{ppt} = 1\text{g/L}$$

Solubility and Saturation: K_{sp}

The **solubility product constant**, K_{sp} is the equilibrium constant that results when a solid is in equilibrium with its solution:

$$A_aB_b(s) \rightleftharpoons aA^{+n}(aq) + bB^{-m}(aq)$$

Recall that pure liquids and pure solids do not appear in equilibrium expressions. Since A_aB_b is a pure solid, it does not affect the equilibrium constant, which then reduces to

$$K_{sp} = [A^{+n}]^a[B^{-m}]^b$$

K_{sp} is the solubility product constant for a substance; it is *not* the solubility of that substance. Solubility is the amount of substance (expressed in grams) that may be dissolved in a unit volume of solution. Solubility may be calculated from a known value of K_{sp}, or vice versa.

For example, assume that it is known that the solubility of A_2B is 1×10^{-2} moles per liter of solution. We may now calculate K_{sp}.

From the equilibrium expression:

$$A_2B(s) \rightleftharpoons 2A^+(aq) + B^{2-}(aq)$$

we see that for every one A_2B that is dissolved, two A^+ and one B^{2-} go into solution.

$$A_2B(s) \rightleftharpoons 2A^+(aq) + B^{2-}(aq)$$
$$1-x \qquad 2x \qquad x$$

Knowing that solubility, x, is 1×10^{-2} M, and employing the equilibrium expression for this reaction:

$$K_{sp} = [A^+]^2[B^{2-}] = [2x]^2[x] = [4x^2][x] = 4x^3 = (4)(1 \times 10^{-2})^3 = 4 \times 10^{-6}$$

Similarly, if K_{sp} is known, solubility may be determined.

Temperature and pressure also affect solubility:

Phase Solubility Rules
1. The solubility of solids in liquids tends to increase with increasing temperature.
2. The solubility of gases in liquids tends to decrease with increasing temperature.
3. The solubility of gases in liquids tends to increase with increasing pressure.

Colligative Properties

When a substance is solvated, it can either enter the solution through solvation or dissociation.

Many covalently bonded molecules that have dipoles or that can hydrogen bond are solvated by water. Examples include methanol, ethanol, glucose, and fructose. The greater the alkyl portion of the molecule, the less soluble it is in water. Examples here include octanol $C_8H_{17}OH$, (0.3 g/L) and dodecanoic acid $C_{11}H_{23}COOH$, (0.15 g/L).

Ionic compounds dissociate in water. Solutes that dissociate into constituent ions are **electrolytes**. **Strong electrolytes** dissociate completely or nearly completely, while **weak electrolytes** dissociate only slightly. Examples of strong electrolytes include salts of the alkali metals (Group 1) and of ammonium, some salts of the alkaline earth metals, all nitrates, chlorates, perchlorates, and acetates. Examples of weak electrolytes include weak acids and bases, such as carbonic acid, phosphoric acid, acetic acid, and ammonia.

A **colligative property** is a property that depends only on the number of particles present in solution and **not** on the identity of those particles. Colligative properties are valid only for aqueous solutions when the total concentration of particles (molality) is equal to or less than 0.5 m. The four most important colligative properties for the PCAT are discussed in the following sections. These include vapor-pressure depression, boiling-point elevation, freezing-point depression, and osmotic pressure.

9.8

Vapor-Pressure Depression

Vapor pressure is the pressure exerted by the gaseous phase of a liquid that evaporated from the exposed surface of the liquid. The weaker a substance's intermolecular forces, the higher its vapor pressure and the more easily it evaporates. For example, if we compare diethyl ether, $H_5C_2OC_2H_5$, and water, we notice that while water undergoes hydrogen bonding, diethyl ether does not, so despite its greater molecular mass, diethyl ether will vaporize more easily and have a higher vapor pressure than water. Easily vaporized liquids—liquids with *high* vapor pressure like diethyl ether—are said to be **volatile.**

When a solvent contains a dissolved solute, the solute occupies part of the surface area of the solution and prevents solvent molecules from escaping the surface. The vapor pressure of the solution is lowered, which means that more energy must be added for the solution to reach its *normal boiling point* at 1 atmosphere. Thus, the solution will boil at a higher temperature. For example, salted water (say, for cooking spaghetti) boils at a higher temperature than unsalted water.

If we have a solution of two liquids, A and B, then Dalton's Law states that the total vapor pressure is equal to the partial vapor pressure of A plus the partial vapor pressure of B. That is, $P = P_A + P_B$. **Raoult's Law** says that the partial vapor pressure of A (or B) is proportional to its mole fraction in the solution:

$$P_A = X_A P°_A$$

The presence of B causes X_A to be less than 1, which results in a **vapor-pressure depression**. In fact, because $X_A = 1 - X_B$, we can write the formula for vapor-pressure depression in terms of B like this:

Vapor-Pressure Depression
$$\Delta P_A = -X_B P^\circ_A$$

Most solutions deviate from Raoult's Law because of intermolecular attractive forces and the volatility of the solvent. Despite these deviations, Raoult's Law works very well for the solvent in dilute solutions.

Boiling-Point Elevation

Because the surface of a solution contains solute molecules, heat must be added to the solution for its vapor pressure to reach a normal boiling point. The difference in temperature between the normal boiling point and the temperature associated with the increased boiling point is the **boiling point elevation**.

Boiling-Point Elevation
$$\Delta T_b = k_b i m$$

In this equation, k_b is the solvent's boiling-point elevation constant, i is the solute's **van't Hoff factor**, which is a solute's tabulated dissociation factor, and m is the molal concentration of the solution. The van't Hoff factor for NaCl, for example, is 2, because for each formula unit of NaCl, there are two ions in solution: Na^+ and Cl^-. In contrast, ethanol has a van't Hoff factor of 1. For water, $k_b \approx 0.5°C \,/\, m$.

Freezing-Point Depression

During freezing, the molecules in a liquid will assemble into an orderly, tightly packed array. However, the presence of solute particles will interfere with the efficient arrangement of the solvent molecules into a solid lattice. As a result, a liquid will be less able to achieve a solid state when a solute is present, and the freezing point of the solution will decrease. This gives rise to a **freezing point depression**. (Or, equivalently, the melting point of a solid containing a solute is decreased.) It is the opposite of the boiling point elevation, so the equation for freezing-point *depression* has a *minus* sign whereas the equation for boiling-point *elevation* has a *plus* sign.

Freezing-Point Depression
$$\Delta T_f = -k_f i m$$

Osmotic Pressure

Osmosis describes the net movement of water across a semipermeable membrane from a region of low solute concentration to a region of higher solute concentration. The semipermeable membrane prohibits the transfer of solutes, but allows water to transverse through it. In the following figure, the net movement of water will be to the right where the solute concentration is highest:

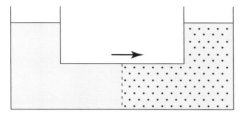

Figure 21

Osmotic pressure (Π) can be defined as the pressure it would take to *stop* osmosis from occurring. If a pressure gauge were added to the same system, osmotic pressure could be measured.

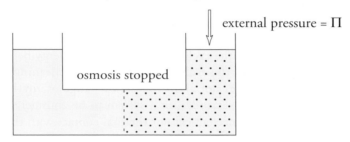

Figure 22

The osmotic pressure of a solution is given by the **van't Hoff equation**:

$$\Pi = MiRT$$

where Π is osmotic pressure in atm, M is the molarity of the solution, i is the tabulated van't Hoff factor, R is the universal gas constant (0.0821 L-atm•K-mol), and T is the temperature in kelvins.

Again, changes in osmotic pressure are affected only by the number of particles in solution (taking into account the van't Hoff factor), not by the identity of those particles.

Hints on Colligative Properties Questions

Colligative properties questions will, in general, come in two forms: (1) questions dealing with *equimolar* solutions, and (2) questions dealing with solutions in which *equal masses* of solute are utilized. Depending on which type of question it is, it's possible to simplify answer choices based on which factor of the colligative properties questions you're being asked to examine.

Questions about equimolar solutions are asking for the comparison of van't Hoff factors. Equimolar, aqueous solutions have identical molalities, so the solute with the largest i will produce the largest colligative change.

Questions in which equal masses of solute are utilized are often more concerned with the calculation of m. Small, low MW salts will have the greater number of moles in a given mass, and hence have a larger value of m and a larger colligative change. In general, when equal masses of solute are added to a solution, the lightest one gives the largest colligative change.

9.9 THERMOCHEMISTRY/THERMODYNAMICS

Basic Definitions and Concepts of Thermodynamics

Thermodynamics is the study of heat and its interconversions with other energy forms. The **system (sys)** is the object under investigation. The **surroundings (surr)** are everything outside the system. The **universe (univ)** is the sum of the system and the surroundings.

An **open** system is a system that allows for the exchange of matter and energy between the surroundings and the system. A **closed** system allows for the exchange of energy only, meaning that mass is conserved within the system. An **isolated** system does not allow for the exchange of anything (matter or energy) between the system and the surroundings. In order for a system to be considered an isolated system, it must be a closed system that is in neither mechanical nor thermal contact with the surroundings. While thermodynamics usually focuses on the system, changes in the thermodynamic properties of the surroundings must also be considered.

A variety of functions is used to determine the thermodynamic characteristics of a system. A **state function** is determined only by the current state of the system, not by the path taken to achieve this state. Common thermodynamic state functions are pressure, temperature, volume, internal energy, enthalpy, entropy, and free energy. Neither work nor heat is a state function.

The **path** that a system takes to reach a given state may be given by a single step or by multiple steps. If a path is reversible, it may be reversed at any point to restore the original values. An **irreversible path** is characterized by an inability to reverse the direction of the path.

The **energy** of a system is a state function that may take many different forms: **kinetic, potential, heat, electrical, light, sound, magnetic, chemical**, and others.

There are two principal ways by which a system can gain or lose energy: by heat transfer or by work (the two common thermodynamic nonstate functions). Heat transfer occurs only when there is a temperature difference, or gradient, between the two objects. (In chemical thermodynamics, these two items are typically the system and the surroundings, but they could be two items within the system itself.) In the case of a system with a temperature higher than its surroundings, energy in the form of heat is transferred from the system to the surroundings ($-Q$). In the case of a system with a temperature lower than the surroundings, heat is transferred from the surroundings into the system ($+Q$).

Thermodynamic work principally takes the form of mechanical work (as when lifting an object) or of electrical work (as in a car battery). Work done by the system is negative (less energy is available to the system). Work done by the surroundings upon the system is positive (more energy is available to the system). There are many types of work, but we will focus here on the mechanical work done by expanding gases (work done by the system on the surroundings), which may be represented by the equation:

$$W = -P\Delta V \qquad \text{Work done by the system}$$

where W is work, P is the pressure of the system, and ΔV is the internal volume change undergone by the system. Work performed by a reversible process is always greater than the work performed by an irreversible process.

Entropy

Entropy is a measure of the number of microstates in a system, but is usually described as the disorder of a system. As disorder increases, so does entropy. Entropy increases in transitioning from a solid to a liquid to a gas. Here are other situations in which entropy increases:

- Entropy increases as temperature increases.
- Entropy increases in a reaction if that reaction produces more product molecules than it contained reactant molecules.
- Entropy increases when pure liquids and/or pure solids form solutions.
- The entropy of the universe, S_{univ}, always increases.

Heats of Formation, Heats of Reaction, and Hess's Law

Recall that enthalpy (H) is a measure of the heat released when pressure is held constant, and has units of kJ/mol. The **heat of formation** (ΔH_f) of a substance is the enthalpy required for the formation of one mole of that substance from its elements. The standard heat of formation (ΔH_f^0) is the change in enthalpy for such a process under standard conditions, which are defined as a temperature of 298.15 Kelvin (25°C) at a pressure of 1 atm. This should not be confused with STP (standard temperature and pressure), where temperature is defined as 273.15 Kelvin (0°C). The (ΔH_f^0) of all elements in their naturally occurring state is defined as zero.

The **heat of reaction** (ΔH^0) is given by the sum of the heats of formation of the products minus the sum of the heats of formation of the reactants. Recall that

- An **endothermic** reaction has a positive ΔH^0.
- An **exothermic** reaction has a negative ΔH^0.

Consider the following reaction:

$$H_2(g) + \frac{1}{2} O_2(g) \rightarrow H_2O(g) \qquad \Delta H^0 = -241.8 \text{ kJ}$$

The heat of formation is taken, by definition, to be zero for both H_2 and O_2, since these are the natural elemental forms of the elements H and O under standard conditions, respectively. Therefore, since the heat of reaction is equal to the heats of formation of the products minus the heats of formation of the reactants, we can say that the heat of formation of $H_2O(g)$ is equal to −241.8 kilojoules per mole.

Note that the heat of formation of *liquid* water is not the same as the heat of formation of *gaseous* water:

$$H_2(g) + \frac{1}{2}O_2(g) \rightarrow H_2O(g) \rightarrow H_2O(\ell) \quad \Delta H^0 = -285.8 \text{ kJ}$$

The extra 44 kilojoules of enthalpy given off is the result of a transition from the more energetic gaseous form to the less energetic liquid form.

Heats of reaction for complex reactions are determined via the use of **Hess's Law**. Consider the following reaction:

$$CO_2(g) + 4\,H_2(g) \rightarrow CH_4(g) + 2H_2O(\ell)$$

One method to determine the heat of reaction involves the heats of formation of each reactant and of each product.

For reactants:

- The heat of formation of H_2 is, by definition, zero.
- The heat of formation of $CO_2(g)$ is

$$C(s) + O_2(g) \rightarrow CO_2(g) \quad \Delta H_f^0 = -393.5 \text{ kJ/mol}$$

- Therefore, the heat of formation of the reactants is −393.5 kilojoules.

For products:

- The heat of formation of $CH_4(g)$ is

$$C(s) + 2H_2(g) \rightarrow CH_4(g) \quad \Delta H_f^0 = -74.85 \text{ kJ/mol}$$

- The heat of formation of $H_2O(\ell)$ is −285.8 kJ/mol, as given above.
- Therefore, the heat of formation of the products is

$$-74.85 + 2(-285.8) = -646.45 \text{ kJ}$$

- Thus, the heat of reaction is

$$-646.45 - (-393.5) = -252.95 \text{ kJ}$$

Gibbs Free-Energy and Reaction Spontaneity

The **free energy** of a system (or **Gibbs free-energy, G**) at constant temperature is given by the equation

$$\Delta G = \Delta H - T\Delta S$$

where all thermodynamic quantities refer to the system, and T is given in kelvin. Under standard conditions, both ΔG and ΔH are at 298 K and have units of kJ/mol, however, ΔS is at 273 K and has units of J/mol. As always, watch your units!

Gibbs free-energy is a measure of the energy available to the system for the performance of useful work. The value of ΔG may be either positive or negative depending upon the signs and magnitudes of ΔH and ΔS. *Only ΔG can determine the spontaneity of a reaction.*

- When ΔG of a reaction is negative, the reaction is spontaneous in the forward direction.
- When ΔG of a reaction is positive, the reaction is nonspontaneous in the forward direction (it is spontaneous in the reverse direction).
- When ΔG of a reaction is equal to zero, the reaction is at equilibrium.

A reaction with a positive ΔG is termed an **endergonic** reaction. A reaction with a negative ΔG is termed an **exergonic** reaction. All of the possible relationships between ΔG and ΔH, T, and ΔS are shown in Table 8.

ΔH	$-$	T	ΔS	ΔG
+		low	+	+
+		high	+	−
+		low	−	+
+		high	−	+
−		low	+	−
−		high	+	−
−		low	−	−
−		high	−	+

Free-energy Changes

Table 8

From these observations it is clear, for example, that only those endothermic reactions that occur at a high temperature with an increase in entropy will occur spontaneously. The probability of obtaining a negative entropy at high temperature is not large (recall that a gas possesses more entropy than a liquid and a liquid possesses more entropy than a solid).

Reactions at Equilibrium

A reaction may be characterized by its equilibrium constant, K_{eq}. For a reaction, the change in Gibbs free-energy (ΔG) is

$$\Delta G = \Delta G^\circ + RT\ln K_{eq}$$

where ΔG is the change in Gibbs free-energy of the reaction at a constant temperature and a constant pressure. ΔG° is the standard free energy change of the reaction at 298 K and 1 atm. At equilibrium $\Delta G = 0$.

The Three Laws of Thermodynamics

There are three laws of thermodynamics. The **First Law of Thermodynamics** states that for any isolated system energy is constant. This law is simply a restatement of the general **principle of conservation of energy**, and means energy is neither created nor destroyed.

The **Second Law of Thermodynamics** introduces the concept of entropy. This law states that no process may exist in which a system is cycled from its point of origin to other points and back to its point of origin, with the heat produced being converted entirely to useful work. In other words, the entropy of the universe is constantly increasing.

The **Third Law of Thermodynamics** is perhaps the least useful thermodynamic law for the PCAT. This law, in effect, states that absolute zero is unattainable.

Reaction Diagrams, ΔH, ΔG, and Activation Energy

Reaction diagrams depict the relationship between the energy of the reaction system (energy coordinate) and the progress of the reaction (reaction coordinate). The energy coordinate may represent enthalpy (ΔH) or Gibbs free-energy (ΔG).

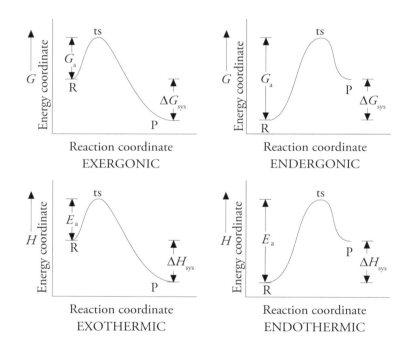

Figure 23

In the graph of free energy versus reaction coordinate, the vertical distance is a measure of the **free energy of activation**, or how much free energy is required to activate, or start, the reaction. In the graph of enthalpy versus reaction coordinate, the vertical distance is a measure of the **enthalpy of activation**, or how much heat is required to activate the reaction. For the PCAT, enthalpy of activation is the activation energy, E_a.

The **transition state** (**ts**) of a system is the highest energy state that the system achieves during the course of its reaction. At this state, some of the bonds of the reactants are partially broken, and some of the new bonds that will be in the products have begun to form.

For a reversible reaction, the reaction diagram for the reverse reaction is the mirror image of the reaction diagram for the forward reaction.

For the PCAT, you should also be familiar with reaction diagrams of multistep processes. Represented below are typical reaction diagrams for exothermic one-step and two-step reactions.

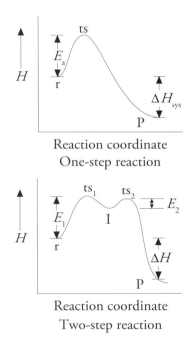

Figure 24

The two-step diagram has two separate activation energies, labeled E_1 and E_2. An intermediate in a reaction pathway is an unstable species that has a relatively short lifetime in the reaction mixture compared to the products and the reactants. In terms of a reaction diagram, a trough in the pathway is indicative of an intermediate, I.

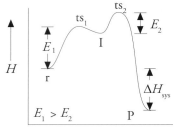

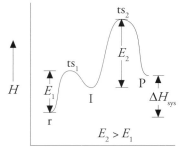

Figure 25

The slowest step in a multistep reaction is the **rate-determining step**, which is the step in the reaction diagram that has the greatest *individual* activation energy. The rate-determining step is *not* determined by the step with the highest-energy transition state. In the top diagram of Figure 25, you will notice that the second step has the highest-energy transition state, but that the first step has the highest activation energy ($E_1 > E_2$). For this system, the rate-determining step is the first step. In the bottom diagram of Figure 26, the rate-determining step is the second step.

Kinetics and Thermodynamic Reaction Energetics

A catalyst reduces the activation energy of a reaction (or a step in a multistep reaction). Therefore, catalysts affect E_a, but they do not affect the ultimate changes in state functions between reactants and products (e.g., ΔH, ΔG). In the reaction diagram depicted in Figure 27, the solid line represents the uncatalyzed reaction pathway, while the dashed line represents the pathway with the catalyst present. When competing reactions occur in solution, be aware that a catalyst may lower the activation energy of one reaction over another. This may mean that the less desired product is the more energetically preferred product.

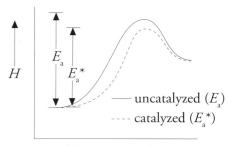

Figure 26

9.10   ACIDS AND BASES

Definitions and Concepts

Arrhenius Acids and Bases

Arrhenius gave us the most straightforward definitions of acids and bases:

>*Acids ionize in water to produce hydrogen (H^+) ions.*
>*Bases ionize in water to produce hydroxide (OH^-) ions.*

For example, HCl is an acid,

$$HCl(aq) \rightarrow H^+(aq) + Cl^-(aq)$$

and NaOH is a base:

$$NaOH(aq) \rightarrow Na^+(aq) + OH^-(aq)$$

It's important to remember that H^+ does not exist by itself. Rather, it will protonate a molecule of water to give H_3O^+. However, for purposes of the PCAT, it doesn't matter which of the two you use: H^+ or H_3O^+.

9.10

Brønsted-Lowry Definitions of Acid and Base

According to the **Brønsted-Lowry** definitions, an acid is a **proton donor** and a base is a **proton acceptor.** Consider this reaction:

$$HCl(g) + H_2O(l) \rightarrow H_3O^+(aq) + Cl^-(aq)$$

In Brønsted-Lowry terms, the HCl molecule is an acid because it *donates a proton* to the H_2O molecule. The H_2O molecule is a base because it *accepts a proton from* the HCl molecule.

Consider in Brønsted-Lowry terms the reaction between ammonia (NH_3) and water:

$$NH_3(aq) + H_2O(l) \rightarrow NH_4^+(aq) + OH^-(aq)$$

In Brønsted-Lowry terms, the NH_3 molecule is a base because it accepts a proton from the H_2O molecule. The H_2O molecule is an acid because it *donates a proton* to the NH_3 molecule. Note that in Arrhenius terms, water is neither an acid nor a base. In Brønsted-Lowry terms, it might be either an acid *or* a base. That is, it is **amphoteric.**

Conjugate Acids and Bases

When a Brønsted-Lowry acid donates an H^+, the remaining structure is called the **conjugate base** of the acid. Likewise, when a Brønsted-Lowry base bonds with an H^+ in solution, this new species is called the **conjugate acid** of the base. To illustrate these definitions, consider this reaction:

acid–base conjugate pair

$$NH_3 + H_2O \rightleftharpoons NH_4^+ + OH^-$$

acid–base conjugate pair

Considering only the forward direction, NH_3 is the base and H_2O is the acid. The products are the conjugate acid and base of the reactants: NH_4^+ is the conjugate acid of NH_3, and OH^- is the conjugate base of H_2O:

acid $\cdots\cdots\cdots\rightarrow$ conjugate base

$$NH_3 + H_2O \rightleftharpoons NH_4^+ + OH^-$$

base $\cdots\cdots\cdots\rightarrow$ conjugate acid

Now consider the reverse reaction in which NH_4^+ is the acid and OH^- is the base. The conjugates are the same as for the forward reaction: NH_3 is the conjugate base of NH_4^+, and H_2O is the conjugate acid of OH^-:

conjugate base $\leftarrow\cdots\cdots\cdots$ acid

$$NH_3 + H_2O \rightleftharpoons NH_4^+ + OH^-$$

conjugate acid $\leftarrow\cdots\cdots\cdots$ base

Notice that the acid and base in an acid-base conjugate pair differ by one proton, and that there are two acid-base conjugate pairs in an acid-base reaction.

forming conjugates:

$$\text{acid} \underset{+ H^+}{\overset{- H^+}{\rightleftharpoons}} \text{base}$$

The Relative Strengths of Conjugate Acid-Base Pairs

Let's once again look at the dissociation of HCl in water:

$$HCl(aq) + H_2O(l) \rightarrow H_3O^+(aq) + Cl^-(aq)$$

no basic properties in water

The chloride ion (Cl^-) is the conjugate base of HCl. Since this reaction goes to completion, there must be no reverse reaction. Therefore, Cl^- has no tendency to accept a proton and thus does not act as a base. The conjugate base of a strong acid has no basic properties in water.

On the other hand, hydrofluoric acid, HF, is a moderately weak acid since its dissociation is not complete:

$$HF(aq) + H_2O(l) \rightleftharpoons H_3O^+(aq) + F^-(aq)$$

Since the reverse reaction does take place to a significant extent, the conjugate base of HF, the fluoride ion, F^-, *does* have some tendency to accept a proton, and so behaves as a moderately weak base. The conjugate base of a moderately weak acid is a moderately weak base.

In fact, the weaker the acid, the more the reverse reaction is favored, and the stronger its conjugate base. To summarize, a strong acid forms a weak conjugate base, and a weak acid forms a strong conjugate base.

The same ideas can be applied to bases:

1) The conjugate acid of a strong base has no acidic properties in water. For example, the conjugate acid of LiOH is Li^+, which does not act as an acid in water. A strong base has a weak conjugate acid.
2) A weak base has a strong conjugate acid. For example, the conjugate acid of Cl^- is the strong acid HCl.

Amphoteric Substances

Take a look at the dissociation of carbonic acid (H_2CO_3), a weak acid:

$$H_2CO_3(aq) + H_2O(l) \rightleftharpoons H_3O^+(aq) + HCO_3^-(aq)$$

The conjugate base of carbonic acid is HCO_3^-, which also has an ionizable proton. Carbonic acid is said to be **polyprotic**, because it has more than one proton to donate.

Let's look at how the conjugate base of carbonic acid dissociates:

$$HCO_3^-(aq) + H_2O(l) \rightleftharpoons H_3O^+(aq) + CO_3^{2-}(aq)$$

In the first reaction, HCO_3^- acts as a base, but in the second reaction, it acts as an acid. Recall that when a substance can act as either an acid or a base, it is amphoteric. The conjugate base of a weak polyprotic acid is always amphoteric, because it can either donate or accept another proton. We expect HCO_3^- to be a weaker acid than H_2CO_3; in general, every time a polyprotic acid donates a proton, the resulting species will be a weaker acid than its predecessor, because removing a proton from a negatively charged species is less favorable.

Lewis Definition of Acid and Base

The **Lewis definitions** of acid and base describe an acid as an electron pair acceptor and a base as an electron pair donor. This is broader than the Brønsted-Lowry definition. Any substance that qualifies as an acid or a base in the Brønsted-Lowry sense qualifies also in the Lewis sense. Yet, there are some substances that qualify as Lewis acids and bases that do not qualify as Brønsted-Lowry acids and bases.

Amines and phosphines, with their lone pairs, are frequently used on the PCAT as prototypical Lewis bases. Trivalent boron or aluminum compounds are frequently used as Lewis acids because of their vacant *p*-orbital, as shown below. The amine donates an electron pair to an electron deficient borane.

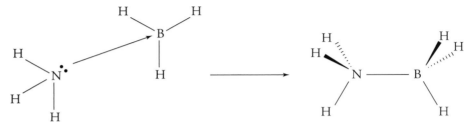

Figure 27

Lewis bases are sometimes referred to as "ligands" when used in conjunction with transition metals, because they donate electron pairs to form bonds.

If we consider the reversible reaction below:

$$AlCl_3 + H_2O \rightleftharpoons (AlCl_3OH)^- + H^+$$

then according to the Lewis definition, $AlCl_3$ and H^+ are acids because they accept electron pairs; H_2O and $(AlCl_3OH)^-$ are bases because they donate electron pairs. Lewis acid/base reactions frequently result in the formation of coordinate **covalent bonds**, in which both shared electrons come from the same species (here, the lone pair of electrons on oxygen). For example, in the reaction above, water acts as a Lewis base since it donates both of the electrons involved in the coordinate covalent bond between OH^- and $AlCl_3$. $AlCl_3$ acts as a Lewis acid, since it accepts the electrons involved in this bond.

Strong and Weak Acids and Bases

Whether an acid is strong or weak depends on how completely it ionizes in water. If we use HA to denote a generic acid, its dissociation in water has the form

$$HA(aq) + H_2O(l) \rightleftharpoons H_3O^+(aq) + A^-(aq)$$

The strength of the acid is directly related to how much the products are favored over the reactants. Disregarding pure solids and liquids, the equilibrium expression for this reaction is

$$K_a = \frac{[H_3O^+][A^-]}{[HA]}$$

This is written as K_a, rather than K_{eq}, to emphasize that this is the equilibrium expression for an acid-dissociation reaction. In fact, K_a is known as the **acid-ionization** (or **acid-dissociation**) **constant** of the acid (HA). If $K_a > 1$, then the numerator is greater than the denominator and the products are favored, and we say the acid is strong; if $K_a < 1$, then the reactants are favored and the acid is weak. We can also rank the relative strengths of acids by comparing their K_a values: the larger the K_a value, the stronger the acid; the smaller the K_a value, the weaker the acid.

The acids for which $K_a > 1$—the strong acids—are so few that you should memorize them for the PCAT:

Common Strong Acids	
Hydroiodic acid	HI
Hydrobromic acid	HBr
Hydrochloric acid	HCl
Perchloric acid	$HClO_4$
Sulfuric acid	H_2SO_4
Nitric acid	HNO_3

Table 9

The values of K_a for these acids are so large that most tables of acid ionization constants don't even list them. On the PCAT, you may assume that any acid that's not in this list is a weak acid. (Other acids that fit the definition of *strong* are so uncommon that it's very unlikely they'd appear on the test. For example, $HClO_3$ has a pK_a of −1, and could be considered strong, but it is definitely one of the weaker strong acids and is not likely to appear on the PCAT.)

For the ionization of a base in water, the equilibrium is

$$B(aq) + H_2O(l) \rightarrow HB^+(aq) + OH^-(aq)$$

Once again, since water does not appear in the equilibrium expression, the equilibrium constant may be expressed as K_b:

$$K_b = \frac{[HB^+][OH^-]}{[B]}$$

In fact, K_b is known as the **base-ionization** (or **base-dissociation**) **constant**. We can rank the relative strengths of bases by comparing their K_b values: the larger the K_b value, the stronger the base; the smaller the K_b value, the weaker the base.

For the PCAT, you should know the following strong bases that may be used in aqueous solutions:

Common Strong Bases
Group 1 hydroxides (Example: NaOH)
Group 1 oxides (Example: Li_2O)
Some group 2 hydroxides ($Ba(OH)_2$, $Sr(OH)_2$, $Ca(OH)_2$)
Metal amides (Example: $NaNH_2$)

Table 10

Weak bases include ammonia (NH_3) and amines, as well as the conjugate bases of many weak acids.

Ionization of Water, pH, and pOH

Water is subject to the ionizing equilibrium:

$$H_2O(l) \rightleftharpoons H^+(aq) + OH^-(aq)$$

This is called the **autoionization of water**. Omitting the pure liquid, the equilibrium expression is

$$K_w = [H^+][OH^-] = 1 \times 10^{-14}$$

From this expression and the equilibrium equation, we can see that, in the absence of outside influences, the concentration of hydrogen ions must be equal to the concentration of hydroxide ions. Therefore, $[H^+] = [OH^-] = 1 \times 10^{-7}$ M. Although the ion product constant for water, K_w, was obtained for pure water, it is valid for any aqueous solutions at 25°C.

This is one of the most important relationships in all of acid/base chemistry, since it establishes the inverse relationship between $[H^+]$ and $[OH^-]$ for all dilute (< 1 M) aqueous solutions.

The pH Scale

The pH scale measures the concentration of H^+ (or H_3O^+) ions in a solution. Because the molarity of H^+ tends to be quite small and can vary over many orders of magnitude, the pH scale is logarithmic:

$$pH = -\log[H^+]$$

This formula establishes the relationship $[H^+] = 10^{-pH}$. Since $[H^+] = 10^{-7}$ M in pure water, the pH of water is $-(-7) = 7$. At 25°C, this defines a pH neutral solution. If $[H^+]$ is greater than 10^{-7} M, then the pH will be less than 7, and the solution is said to be acidic. If $[H^+]$ is less than 10^{-7} M, the pH will be greater than 7, and the solution is basic (or alkaline). Notice that a *low* pH means a *high* $[H^+]$ and the solution is *acidic*; a *high* pH means a *low* $[H^+]$ and the solution is basic.

pH > 7	basic solution
pH = 7	neutral solution
pH < 7	acidic solution

Relationships Between pH and pOH

When attacking questions about the relationship between [H$^+$] and pH, or [OH$^-$] and pOH, it is important to remember the following: *logs are exponents!*

In order to determine, for example, the pH of a system in which [H$^+$] = 1 × 10^{-2}, we must look to the exponent. Since logs are exponents, log [10^{-2}] = –2, and the –log of 10^{-2} is 2. If [H$^+$] = 1 × 10^{-10}, then we know that pH = 10. The same is true for determining pOH from [OH$^-$].

Acidity and basicity refer to the hydrogen ion concentration of an aqueous solution. An acid is a substance that when added to water *increases its hydrogen ion concentration* (decreases its pH). A base is a substance that when added to water *decreases its hydrogen ion concentration* (increases its pH).

The range of the pH scale for most solutions falls between 0 and 14, but some strong acids and bases extend the scale past this range. For example, a 10 M solution of HCl will fully dissociate into H$^+$ and Cl$^-$. Therefore, the [H$^+$] = 10 M, and the pH = –1.

Because aqueous solutions maintain an equilibrium characterized by K_w = [H$^+$][OH$^-$] = 1 × 10^{-14}, it is also true that when added to water (a) an acid decreases the hydroxide ion concentration (increases pOH), and (b) a base increases the hydroxide ion concentration (decreases pOH). Thus, an alternate measurement expresses the acidity or basicity in terms of the hydroxide ion concentration, [OH$^-$], by using pOH. The same formula applies for hydroxide ions as for hydrogen ions.

$$pOH = -\log[OH^-]$$

This formula implies that [OH$^-$] = 10^{-pOH}.

Acids and bases are inversely related: the greater the concentration of H$^+$ ions, the lower the concentration of OH$^-$ ions, and vice versa. Since [H$^+$][OH$^-$] = 10^{-14} at 25°C, the values of pH and pOH have the following relationship at 25°C:

$$pH + pOH = 14$$

This means that if you know the pOH of a solution, you can find the pH, and vice versa. For example, if the pH of a solution is 5, then the pOH must be 9. If the pOH of a solution is 2, then the pH must be 12.

The scenario is slightly more complicated when the concentrations of [H$^+$] and [OH$^-$] have pre-exponential factors other than 1, but these situations can be handled by trying to put boundaries on the possible values of pH. If [H$^+$] = 6.7 × 10^{-8}, we can no longer say that pH = 8. However, since 6.7 × 10^{-8} is *between* 10^{-8} and 10^{-7}, we know that the pH must fall somewhere between 8 and 7. Since (6.7 × 10^{-8}) > 10^{-8}, we know there is more H$^+$ in solution than at pH = 8, and hence a lower pH value. On the PCAT, narrowing the answer down to between two integers, as we just did, will allow you to unequivocally choose the correct answer of the four choices.

Rather than reporting acid or base strengths in exponents, strengths are generally given as pK_a or pK_b. As the similarity in nomenclature to pH might suggest, these values are simply –log K_a and –log K_b, respectively. As is the case with [H$^+$] and pH, pK_a and pK_b have an inverse relationship with K_a and K_b. The following relations can then be summarized:

- Strong acids and bases have small values of pK_a and pK_b.
- Weak acids and bases have large values of pK_a and pK_b.

Relationships Between Conjugate Pairs

pK_a and pK_b Because H^+ concentrations are generally very small and can vary over such a wide range, the pH scale gives us more convenient numbers to work with. The same is true for pK_a and pK_b. Remember that the larger the K_a value, the stronger the acid, and the *lower* the pK_a value, the stronger the acid. For example, acetic acid (CH_3COOH) has a K_a of 1.75×10^{-5}, and hypochlorous acid ($HClO$) has a K_a of 2.9×10^{-8}. Since the K_a of acetic acid is larger than that of hypochlorous acid, we know this means that more molecules of acetic acid than hypochlorous acid will dissociate into ions in aqueous solution. In other words, acetic acid is a stronger acid than hypochlorous acid. In fact, the pK_a of acetic acid is 4.8, and the pK_a of hypochlorous acid is 7.5. The acid with the lower pK_a value is the stronger acid. The same pattern applies to pK_b: the lower the pK_b value, the stronger the base.

Let's now look at the relationship between the K_a and the K_b for an acid-base conjugate pair by working through an example question. Let K_a be the acid-dissociation constant for formic acid ($HCOOH$) and K_b the base-dissociation constant of its conjugate base (the formate ion, $HCOO^-$). If K_a is equal to 5.6×10^{-11}, what is $K_a \times K_b$?

The equilibrium for the dissociation of $HCOOH$ is

$$HCOOH(aq) + H_2O(l) \rightleftharpoons H_3O^+(aq) + HCOO^-(aq)$$

so

9.10

$$K_a = \frac{[H_3O^+][HCOO^-]}{[HCOOH]}$$

The equilibrium for the dissociation of $HCOO^-$ is

$$HCOO^-(aq) + H_2O(l) \rightleftharpoons HCOOH(aq) + OH^-(aq)$$

so

$$K_b = \frac{[HCOOH][OH^-]}{[HCOO^-]}$$

Therefore,

$$K_a K_b = \frac{[H_3O^+][HCOO^-]}{[HCOOH]} \times \frac{[HCOOH][OH^-]}{[HCOO^-]} = [H_3O^+][OH^-]$$

This is K_w, the ion-product constant of water, whose value (at 25°C) is 1×10^{-14}.

In fact, for any acid-base conjugate pair,

$$K_a K_b = K_w = 1 \times 10^{-14}$$

This gives us a way to quantitatively relate the strength of an acid and its conjugate base. For example, the value of K_a for HF is about 7×10^{-4}; therefore, the value of K_b for its conjugate base, F⁻, is about 1.4×10^{-9}. For HCN, $K_a \approx 5 \times 10^{-10}$, so K_b for CN⁻ $\approx 2 \times 10^{-5}$.

It also follows from our definitions that for an acid-base conjugate pair at 25°C, we'll have

$$pK_a + pK_b = 14$$

If the introduction of an acid increases the concentration of H_3O^+ ions, then the equilibrium is disturbed, and the reverse reaction is favored, thereby decreasing the concentration of OH⁻ ions. Similarly, if the introduction of a base increases the concentration of OH⁻ ions, then the equilibrium is again disturbed; the reverse reaction is favored, decreasing the concentration of H_3O^+ ions. However, in either case, the product of $[H_3O^+]$ and $[OH^-]$ will remain equal to K_w.

For example, suppose we add 0.002 moles of HCl to water to create a 1-liter solution. Since the dissociation of HCl goes to completion (it's a strong acid), it will create 0.002 moles of H_3O^+ ions, so $[H_3O^+]$ = 0.002 M. Since H_3O^+ concentration has been increased, we expect the OH⁻ concentration to decrease, which it does:

$$[OH^-] = \frac{K_w}{[H_3O^+]} = \frac{1 \times 10^{-14}}{2 \times 10^{-3}} = 5 \times 10^{-12} M$$

9.10

pH Calculations

For Strong Acids
Strong acids dissociate completely in water, so as noted above, the hydrogen ion concentration will be the same as the concentration of the acid. That means that you can calculate the pH directly from the molarity of the solution. For example, a 0.01 M aqueous solution of HCl will have $[H^+]$ = 0.01 M and pH = 2.

For Weak Acids
Weak acids equilibrate with their dissociated ions. In fact, for a weak acid at equilibrium, the concentration of undissociated acid will be much greater than the concentration of hydrogen ion. To get the pH of a weak acid solution, you need to use the equilibrium expression.

As an example, if 0.2 mol of HCN (hydrocyanic acid, a weak acid) is added to water to create a 1-liter solution, how do we find the pH? Initially, [HCN] = 0.2 M, and none of it has dissociated. If x moles of HCN are dissociated at equilibrium, then the equilibrium concentration of HCN is $0.2 - x$. Each molecule of HCN dissociates into one H⁺ ion and one CN⁻ ion, so if x moles of HCN have dissociated, there will be x moles of H⁺ and x moles of CN⁻:

	HCN	⇌	H⁺	+	CN⁻
initial:	0.2 M		0 M		0 M
at equilibrium:	$(0.2 - x)$ M		x M		x M

(Actually, the initial concentration of H^+ in water is 10^{-7} M, but its contribution is so small that it can be neglected for this calculation.) By finding x, we know $[H^+]$, and therefore the pH. So, we use the equilibrium expression:

$$K_a = \frac{[H^+][CN^-]}{[HCN]} = \frac{x^2}{0.2 - x}$$

The K_a for HCN is 4.9×10^{-10}. Because the K_a is so small, not much of the HCN dissociates. We can therefore substitute 0.2 for $(0.2 - x)$, and solve the equation above for x:

$$\frac{x^2}{0.2} \approx 4.9 \times 10^{-10}$$
$$x^2 \approx 1 \times 10^{-10}$$
$$\therefore x \approx 1 \times 10^{-5}$$

Since $[H^+]$ is approximately 1×10^{-5} M, the pH is about 5.

We simplified the computation by assuming that the concentration of hydrogen ion $[H^+]$ was insignificant compared to the concentration of undissociated acid $[HCN]$. It turned out that $[H^+] \approx 10^{-5}$ M, which is much less than $[HCN] = 0.2$ M, our assumption was valid. On the PCAT, you should always simplify the math wherever possible.

Neutralization Reactions

An acid and a base react to form a **neutralization reaction**. Oftentimes this reaction, which is exothermic, will produce a salt and water. Here is an example:

$$HCl(aq) \quad + \quad NaOH(aq) \quad \rightarrow \quad NaCl(aq) \quad + \quad H_2O(l)$$

$$\text{acid} \qquad\qquad \text{base} \qquad\qquad\quad \text{salt} \qquad\qquad \text{water}$$

This class of reaction takes place when you take an antacid to relieve excess stomach acid. The antacid is a weak base, usually carbonate, that reacts in the stomach to neutralize the acid.

If a strong acid and strong base react (as in the example above), the resulting solution will have a pH = 7. Neutralization reactions involving a weak acid or weak base generally will not be pH neutral.

No matter how weak an acid or base is, when mixed with an equimolar amount of a strong base or acid, we can expect complete neutralization and an exothermic reaction.

To determine just how much base (B) to add to an acidic solution for complete neutralization (or how much acid (A) to add to a basic solution), we use the following formula:

$$a \times [A] \times V_A = b \times [B] \times V_B$$

where a is the number of acidic hydrogens per formula unit and b is a constant that tells us how many H_3O^+ ions the base can accept. The product $a[A] \times V_A$ gives the number of moles of A: (mol/L) × L. It requires bB moles of B for complete neutralization to occur.

For example, let's calculate how much 0.1 M NaOH solution is needed to neutralize 40 mL of a 0.3 M HCl solution:

$$V_B = \frac{a[A]V_A}{b[B]} = \frac{1(0.3\,M)(0.040\,L)}{1(0.1\,M)} = 0.1\,L$$

Hydrolysis of Salts

A **salt** is an ionic compound consisting of a cation and an anion. In water, the salt dissociates into ions. Depending on how these ions react with water, the resulting solution will be either acidic, basic, or neutral. To predict the outcome, there are essentially two possibilities for both the cation and the anion:

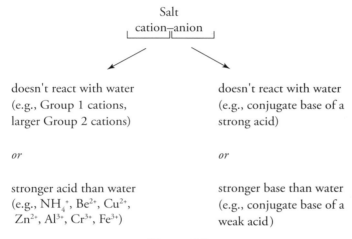

Figure 28

Whether the solution will be acidic, basic, or neutral depends on which combination of possibilities applies. Recall that the reaction of a substance with water—such as a salt or an ion—is called a hydrolysis reaction.

If we dissolve NaCl in water, for example, Na^+ and Cl^- ions become hydrated. Therefore, the solution will be pH neutral.

In water, NH_4Cl will form NH_4^+ and Cl^- ions. The ammonium ion is a stronger acid than water (it is the conjugate acid of NH_3, a weak base). As a result, a solution of this salt will be acidic and have a pH less than 7. Thus, NH_4Cl is an acidic salt.

Sodium acetate, CH_3COONa in water forms Na^+ and CH_3COO^-. The CH_3COO^- ion is a moderately strong base: it is the conjugate base of acetic acid (CH_3COOH), a moderately weak acid. Therefore, a solution of the salt will be basic and have a pH greater than 7. This makes CH_3COONa a basic salt.

Finally, let's consider NH_4CN. In solution it will form NH_4^+ and CN^-. The NH_4^+ ion is a moderately strong acid, and CN^- is a strong base (it is the conjugate base of HCN, a weak acid). In a case like this, we need to compare K_a and K_b values to identify the reaction that occurs:

$$NH_4^+(aq) + H_2O(l) \rightleftharpoons NH_3(aq) + H_3O^+(aq) \quad (K_a = 6.3 \times 10^{-10})$$

$$CN^-(aq) + H_2O(l) \rightleftharpoons HCN(aq) + OH^-(aq) \quad (K_b = 1.6 \times 10^{-5})$$

The K_b of $CN^- > K_a$ of NH_4^+, so more OH^- will form than H_3O^+ and the solution will be basic.

Henderson-Hasselbalch Equation

By taking the log of both sides of the equation for pK_a (below) and rearranging the terms, we derive the Henderson-Hasselbalch (HH) equation:

$$K_a = \frac{[H^+][A^-]}{[HA]}$$

$$pH = pK_a + \log\frac{[A^-]}{[HA]}$$

Or, similarly, for basic systems:

$$pOH = pK_b + \log\frac{[BH^+]}{[B]}$$

The HH equation is useful in that it allows us to gauge ratios of acid and conjugate base concentrations of a system depending on the pH.

Buffers

A **buffer** is composed of a weak acid and its conjugate base, or a weak base and its conjugate acid. A buffer is designed to resist a change in pH when an external acid or base is added to the solution. The acid component of a buffer system neutralizes added base, while the base component of a buffer system neutralizes added acid. Problems involving buffers can generally be solved using the Henderson-Hasselbalch equation.

Buffers are usually made by mixing equal parts of a weak acid (or base) and its conjugate. For example, an acetic acid/acetate buffer would likely be comprised of equal moles of acetic acid and sodium acetate. Since the acid [HA] and the conjugate base [A−] are equimolar in solution, we know from the Henderson-Hasselbalch equation that the pH of the solution will be the pK_a of acetic acid (4.75) because log(1) = 0. The acetic acid equilibrium reaction causes the solution to resist a change in pH because of the existence of both acetic acid and acetate:

$$CH_3COOH(aq) + H_2O(l) \rightleftharpoons CH_3COO^-(aq) + H_3O^+(aq)$$

If a small amount of a strong acid is added, it will protonate the acetate causing the reaction to adjust to maintain the pK_a. If, for example, we had 1 L of a 1 M acetate buffer solution (1 mol CH_3COOH/ 1 mol CH_3COO^-), and we added 0.01 moles HCl, what would be the resulting pH?

In this scenario, 0.01 moles of acetate ion will be protonated, forming 0.01 moles of acetic acid. Solving for pH:

$$pH = 4.75 + \log\frac{0.99}{1.01}$$

The pH is now 4.74. In contrast, if 0.01 moles of HCl were added to 1 L of water, the pH of the solution would be $-\log 10^{-2} = 2$. The presence of a buffer has prevented the large change in pH from occurring.

Adding large amounts of acid or base would overwhelm the buffering capacity of the solution. Therefore, a buffer is more effective at resisting changes in pH near its pK_a. When choosing a buffer:

- The more concentrated the buffer, the more effective it will be.
- The pK_a of the buffer should be chosen to approximate the pH that is desired.

Acid-Base Titrations

An **acid-base titration** is a laboratory technique used to determine the identity of an unknown acid or base. We can use this technique to determine a pK_a or pK_b. The procedure consists of adding a strong acid or base of *known* identity and concentration—the **titrant**—to a solution containing the unknown base or acid. The titrant is added in measurable amounts, and the pH of the solution is recorded using a pH meter or by conductance. The conductivity of the solution will decrease as neutralization proceeds, it will be zero when complete neutralization occurs, and it will rise when excess titrant is added and those ions are in solution.

9.10

A titration curve is a plot of pH vs. volume of titrant added. The titration curve of HF (a moderately weak acid) with NaOH (a strong base) is shown in Figure 29.

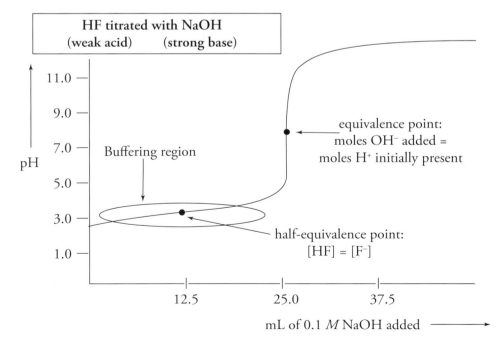

Figure 29

When the amount of titrant added is 0, the pH is the pH of the original solution of HF. As NaOH is added, an equivalent amount of HF will be neutralized according to the reaction

$$NaOH(aq) + HF(aq) \rightarrow Na^+(aq) + F^-(aq) + H_2O(l)$$

As HF is neutralized, the pH will increase. The pH does not increase rapidly because the solution is behaving as a buffer: [HF] is in equilibrium with [F$^-$], and the solution contains a weak acid and its conjugate base. This equilibrium position is called the **midpoint**, or **half-equivalence point**), where pH = pK_a.

Once the buffering capacity is exceeded, the pH increases dramatically.

When there is just enough NaOH added to completely neutralize all the HF, we have reached the **acid-base equivalence point** or **endpoint**, and [$^-$OH] = [H$^+$]. At this point, we have Na$^+$ ions and F$^-$ ions in solution. Notice that the pH of this solution is basic at its equivalence point. In fact, we can generalize trends as follows:

- For a weak acid (titrated with a strong base), the equivalence point will occur at a pH > 7.
- For a weak base (titrated with a strong acid), the equivalence point will occur at a pH < 7.
- For a strong acid (titrated with a strong base) or for a strong base (titrated with a strong acid), the equivalence point will occur at pH = 7.

9.10

Therefore, the pH at the equivalence point of our titration tells us whether the acid (or base) we were titrating was weak or strong, as shown in Figures 30 and 31.

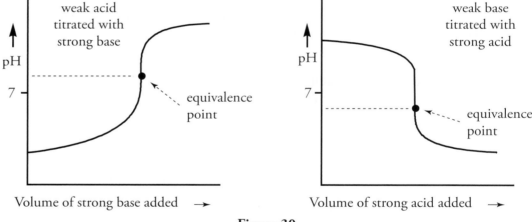

Figure 30

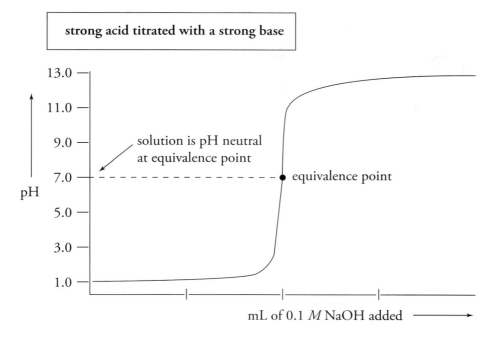

Figure 31

We can determine the pK_a (or pK_b) of the unknown weak acid or weak base. The Henderson-Hasselbalch equation then tells us that

$$pH_{\text{at half-equiv}} = pK_a + \log\left(\frac{[\text{F}^-]_{\text{at half-equiv}}}{[\text{HF}]_{\text{at half-equiv}}}\right) = pK_a + \log 1 = pK_a + 0$$

The pK_a of HF equals the pH at the half-equivalence point. For Figure 32, we see that this occurs around pH 3.2, so we conclude that the pK_a of HF is about 3.2.

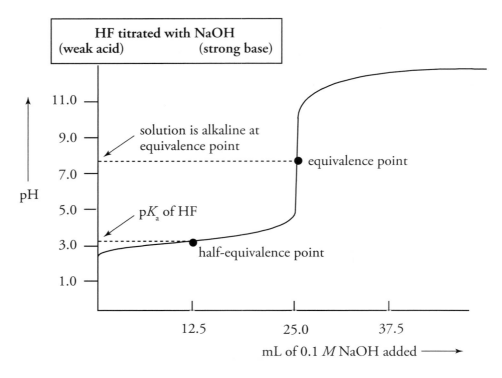

Figure 32

The titration curve of a polyprotic acid (like H_2SO_4 or H_3PO_4) will have more than one equivalence point. The number of equivalence points is equal to the number of ionizable hydrogens the acid can donate.

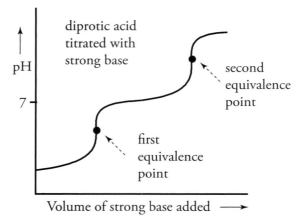

Figure 33

Indicators and the End Point

An **indicator** is a substance that will change color at the end point of a titration curve. It does so because of color differences between its protonated and deprotonated form at the indicated pH. Phenolphthalein is a weakly acidic molecule that is often used as an indicator because its protonated, neutral form is colorless, while its deprotonated, anionic form is pink. The equilibrium is shown below with the protonated form on the left and deprotonated on the right. Notice that when [Phn(H)] = [Phn⁻], we are at the pK_a of phenolphthalein.

$$Phn(H) + B^- \rightleftharpoons Phn^- + BH$$
$$\text{clear} \qquad\qquad \text{pink}$$

For maximum accuracy, an indicator should be chosen that changes color within +/– 1 pH range of the endpoint.

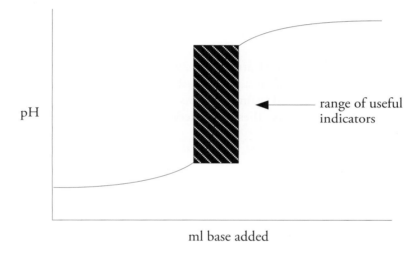

Figure 34

9.10

9.11 ELECTROCHEMISTRY

Redox Reactions

In an electrochemical process, electrons flow from one chemical substance to another and are driven by an **oxidation-reduction**, or **redox**, reaction. Electrons are transferred from a substance that is oxidized to one that is reduced. You may find the pneumonic OIL RIG to be useful in remembering that Oxidation Is Loss, Reduction Is Gain.

A **reductant**, or **reducing agent**, donates electrons and in the process is oxidized. The **oxidant**, or **oxidizing agent**, accepts electrons and in the process is reduced. Notice that the terms reductant and oxidant indicate what is happening to the *other* species.

Consider the following redox reaction:

$$Cu(NO_3)_2(aq) + Zn(s) \rightarrow Zn(NO_3)_2(aq) + Cu(s)$$

Any element in its pure, free state at STP (1 atm, 1 M, 298 K) has an oxidation state of 0. In this reaction, copper undergoes a change in oxidation state from +2 to 0, while the oxidation state of zinc changes from 0 to +2. Therefore, copper is reduced (gains electrons) and zinc is oxidized (loses electrons). For this reaction, we can write two **half reactions**. These are reactions that represent either the oxidation half or reduction half of a redox reaction.

The half reaction for the reduction of copper is

$$Cu^{2+} + 2e^- \rightarrow Cu^0$$

and the half reaction for the oxidation of zinc is

$$Zn^0 \rightarrow Zn^{2+} + 2e^-$$

In this case, two electrons are transferred in each half reaction:

$$Cu^{2+} + Zn^0 + 2e^- \rightarrow Cu^0 + Zn^{2+} + 2e^-$$

or

$$Cu^{2+} + Zn^0 \rightarrow Cu^0 + Zn^{2+}$$

The reaction is balanced as written. In a balanced redox reaction, *the number of electrons lost by the reductant is equal to the number of electrons gained by the oxidant.*

Redox Couples

Consider the half reaction:

$$Cu^{2+} + 2e^- \rightarrow Cu^0$$

If zinc metal is coupled with Cu^{2+}, the zinc metal is oxidized, and the copper^{2+} ion is reduced. This is because Zn is a weaker oxidizing agent than Cu^{2+}:

$$Zn^0 + Cu^{2+} \rightarrow Zn^{2+} + Cu^0$$

However, Fe^{3+} is a stronger oxidizing agent than Cu. When copper metal is placed in a solution of Fe^{3+}, the copper metal is oxidized, and Fe^{3+} is reduced:

$$2Fe^{3+} + Cu^0 \rightarrow 2Fe^{2+} + Cu^{2+}$$

In each of these reactions there is a **redox couple**, which consists of an oxidized form and a reduced form of a given species. The three redox couples in these reactions are Cu^{2+}/Cu, Zn^{2+}/Zn, and Fe^{3+}/Fe^{2+}. Notice that redox couples are written in oxidized form/reduced form.

Electrochemical Potential

Reduction Potentials

The potential of a redox process, symbolized as E_{cell}, is the difference in electrical potential between two half reactions, which together constitute an electrochemical cell. It is a measure of the driving force for the reaction against some standard, and is measured in volts. The standard cell potential, $E°_{cell}$, is the potential of a redox process measured under standard conditions. More specifically, these conditions are 1 M for solutions, 1 atm for gases, pure solids and pure liquids for other substances, and 298 K. The cell potential depends strongly on concentrations and temperature.

By convention, *half-reaction potentials are tabulated as reduction potentials*. The more negative the reduction potential the stronger the reductant. Elements with low electronegativity, such as the Group 1 elements, are strong reductants (they are the most easily oxidized) and have large negative potentials. Those with positive potentials are strong oxidants (they are the most easily reduced).

9.11

Reduction	$E°$ (volts)
$Li^+ + e^- \longrightarrow Li(s)$	−3.05
$Al^{3+} + 3e^- \longrightarrow Al(s)$	−1.66
$Fe^{3+} + e^- \longrightarrow Fe^{2+}$	+0.77
$MnO_4^- + 8H^+ + 5e^- \longrightarrow Mn^{2+} + 4H_2O$	+1.49

Table 11

Reduction potentials are always listed from the most negative $E°$ to the most positive. To obtain an oxidation potential, simply reverse the tabulated reaction and reverse the sign of $E°$.

The Electromotive Force

The **standard half cell** is the **hydrogen electrode**:

$$2H^+(aq, 1\ M) + 2e^- \rightarrow H_2(g, 1\ atm)$$

The electromotive force (**emf**) is represented by $E°$. By definition, the electromotive force of the hydrogen half cell is 0 V.

Since electromotive force will be altered by changes in **concentration** (for solutes), **pressure** (for gases), and **temperature**, all electromotive forces recorded at nonstandard conditions are represented by E. For electromotive forces at nonstandard conditions, the temperature and concentration (or pressure) must also be given.

The electromotive forces of half reactions may be summed to produce a **cell emf.**

$$Pb^{2+} + 2e^- \rightarrow Pb(s) \qquad E° = -0.13V$$
$$2I^- \rightarrow I_2 + 2e^- \qquad E° = -0.54V$$
$$\overline{\qquad\qquad\qquad\qquad\qquad\qquad\qquad}$$
$$Pb^{2+} + 2I^- \rightarrow Pb(s) + I_2 \qquad E°_{cell} = -0.67V$$

Notice that $E°$ values are independent of stoichiometric coefficients for the half reaction. Electromotive forces are independent of the total amount of material present and depend only on concentration. The most common error made on the PCAT is multiplying half-reaction electromotive forces by stoichiometric coefficients.

For example, consider the following balanced redox reaction:

$$14H^+ + Cr_2O_7^{2-} + 6Fe^{2+} \rightarrow 2Cr^{3+} + 6Fe^{3+} + 7H_2O$$

This reaction comes from the half reactions:

$$Cr_2O_7^{2-} + 14H^+ + 6e^- \rightarrow 2Cr^{3+} + 7H_2O \quad E° = +1.33V$$

and

$$Fe^{2+} \rightarrow Fe^{3+} + e^- \qquad\qquad E° = -0.77V$$

The total electromotive force for this reaction is $E° = 1.33$ V + (-0.77) V = 0.56 V, not 1.33 V + 6(−0.77) V = −3.26 V. By incorrectly using stoichiometric coefficients in this example, you would predict the wrong numerical answer and sign for this redox equation.

Galvanic Cells

An electrochemical cell generates electricity from a spontaneous redox reaction, or uses electricity to drive a nonspontaneous redox reaction. A **galvanic**, or **voltaic**, cell uses the energy released during a spontaneous redox reaction to generate electricity. Because the process is spontaneous, $\Delta G < 0$. In contrast, an electrolytic cell consumes electrical energy from an external source to drive a nonspontaneous redox reaction ($\Delta G > 0$). Consider the reaction of dichromate with iodine:

$$14H^+ + Cr_2O_7^{2-} + 6I^- \rightarrow 2Cr^{3+} + 3I_2 + 7H_2O$$

Initially, an acidic solution containing the dichromate ion will be orange. After the reduction to chromate, the solution will be green. Likewise, a solution containing iodide (I^-) will be colorless; however, a solution containing I_2 will be yellow-brown.

Suppose that instead of mixing our two solutions, we connect them via a platinum wire connected to a **galvanometer** (to detect current), as shown below. Platinum is chosen because it will not react with either of our initial solutions. The galvanometer will indicate a flow of electrons from one solution to the other.

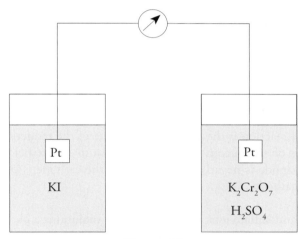

Figure 35

Initially, in the solution containing the iodide, electrons flow from the iodide ions to the platinum wire, thus forming iodine:

$$2I^- \rightarrow I_2 + 2e^-$$

These electrons are then transferred through the wire to the solution containing the dichromate ion. The dichromate ions are reduced to chromate ions:

$$Cr_2O_7^{2-} + 14H^+ + 6e^- \rightarrow 2Cr^{3+} + 7H_2O$$

However, this process cannot continue. A consumption of the iodide ions in the oxidation vessel will leave an excess of positively charged potassium ions in this vessel. This buildup of positive charge will prevent the further release of electrons from the remaining iodide ions. Eliminating this excess positive charge is accomplished by using a salt bridge.

9.11

A **salt bridge** is a link between the oxidation and reduction vessels that allows for the transfer of ions, thereby ensuring electrical neutrality. To be effective, the counter ions must not be reactive under the conditions of either half reaction, they must not form a precipitate or complex, and they should be highly soluble in the solution medium. A complete galvanic cell for the redox reaction of iodide and dichromate is depicted below.

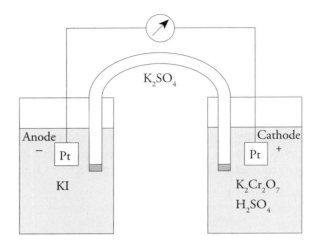

Figure 36

The site of the oxidation half reaction is the **anode**, and the site of the reduction half reaction is the **cathode**. The salt bridge consists of an aqueous solution of potassium sulfate held into a U-tube by plugs of glass wool. Notice that the anode is negatively charged and the cathode is positively charged: electrons flow from the anode to the cathode.

The flow of potassium ions and sulfate ions in the salt bridge maintains a charge balance in the reaction vessels and allows the redox reactions to proceed, thereby producing a measurable current in the galvanometer.

We can represent this same process in a **cell diagram**, where the anode is written on the left and the cathode on the right. Vertical lines indicate a phase boundary. Here is the cell diagram for this reaction:

$$(Pt) \mid I^-, I_2 \parallel Cr_2O_7^{2-}, H^+, Cr^{3+} \mid (Pt)$$

Because the Pt electrodes are inert, they are shown in parentheses. The double vertical line symbolizes the salt bridge, which has a phase boundary in each solution. Thus, the reaction at the anode is the oxidation of iodide to iodine, and the reaction at the cathode is the reduction of Cr^{6+} to Cr^{3+}. A galvanic cell produces a current (which results from the voltage) for the performance of useful work.

9.11

To summarize, in a galvanic cell:

- the redox reaction is spontaneous
- the cell creates an electron flow
- oxidation occurs at the anode
- reduction occurs at the cathode
- the cathode is the positive electrode
- the anode is the negative electrode
- electrons flow from the anode to the cathode

Electrolytic Cells

In an electrochemical cell, we drive a nonspontaneous redox reaction by supplying an electrical current.

Electroplating is an important application of electrolysis. This technique is often employed to improve the appearance and durability of metal objects. For example, a thin film of chromium is applied over steel automobile bumpers to improve their appearance and to retard corrosion of the underlying steel. Silver plating is common on eating utensils. The typical apparatus for electroplating a fork is shown below:

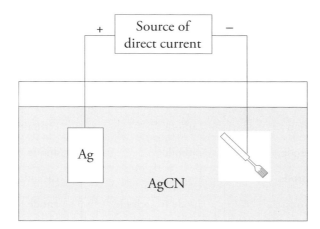

Figure 37

In this example, a direct current is supplied to the system from an external source. The silver bar is the anode, the site of oxidation, and the fork is the cathode, the site of reduction. At the anode, the silver is oxidized to furnish Ag^+ ions to the solution. At the cathode, the Ag^+ ions in solution are reduced to silver metal, which adheres to the surface of the fork. The half reactions are

Anode:	$Ag(s) \rightarrow Ag^+ + e^-$
Cathode:	$Ag^+ + e^- \rightarrow Ag(s)$

Current flows in a direction opposite to that of the electron flow. The purpose of the **external current source** is to supply electrons to the cathode for the reduction process. As time passes, silver metal from the anode is transferred to the cathode. You should note that electron flow in an electrolytic cell is confined to the wires attaching the anode and cathode to the external current source. Electrons do not flow through the electrolytic medium itself. Also notice that in an electrolytic cell, the anode is positively charged and the cathode is negatively charged. However, for both a galvanic and an electrolytic cell, by definition *oxidation occurs at the anode, and reduction occurs at the cathode.*

9.11

In an electrolytic cell:

- the redox reaction is nonspontaneous*
- the cell requires an electron flow*
- oxidation occurs at the anode
- reduction occurs at the cathode
- the anode is the positive electrode*
- the cathode is the negative electrode*
- electrons flow from the anode to the cathode
- current flows from the cathode to the anode

Items marked with asterisks differ from the case of a galvanic cell.

A Comparison of Galvanic and Electrolytic Cells

Table 12 summarizes the similarities and differences between galvanic and electrolytic cells:

	Galvanic	Electrolytic
type of redox reaction	spontaneous	nonspontaneous
electron flow	created	supplied
site of oxidation	anode	anode
site of reduction	cathode	cathode
positive electrode	cathode	anode
negative electrode	anode	cathode
flow of electrons	anode to cathode	anode to cathode
flow of current	cathode to anode	cathode to anode

Table 12

Concentration Cells

A **concentration cell** is a galvanic cell in which the cathodic half reaction and the anodic half reaction are identical except for the concentration of each reactant. It is possible to sustain such a cell by differing the concentrations between the two electrode vessels. Figure 38 is an example of a concentration cell containing different concentrations of silver(I) with silver electrodes:

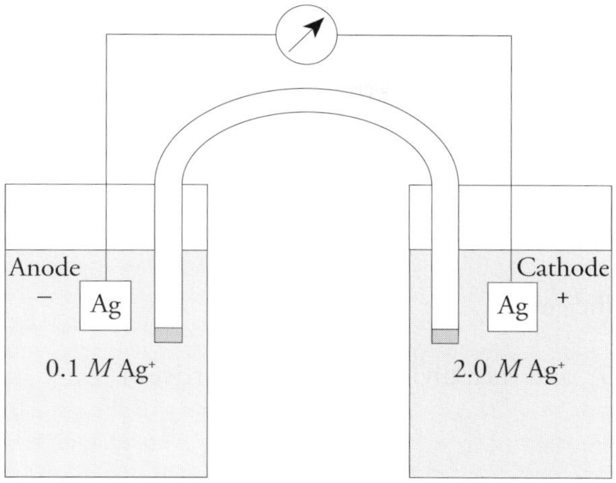

Figure 38

In this cell, the redox couple in each case is Ag^+/Ag. Since this is an example of a galvanic cell, we see that the half reaction for the right vessel will be

$$Ag^+ + e^- \rightarrow Ag(s)$$

and the half reaction for the left vessel (anode) will be

$$Ag(s) \rightarrow Ag^+ + e^-$$

The Ag^+ concentration of the more dilute solution increases, while it decreases in the more concentrated solution. The cell diagram for this cell is given by

$$Ag(s) \mid Ag^+ (aq, 0.1\ M) \parallel Ag^+ (aq, 2.0\ M) \mid Ag(s)$$

Effect of Concentration on Potentials: The Nernst Equation

The relationship between $E°$ values and $\Delta G°$ values is given by

$$\Delta G° = -nFE°$$

Notice that in a spontaneous reaction ($\Delta G° < 0$), $E°$ has a positive value.

The SI unit for the amount of electric charge is coulombs (C). We can relate the charge to moles using these relationships:

n = moles of electrons

F = Faraday's constant = 96,485 C/mole

For nonstandard conditions

$$\Delta G = -nFE$$

ΔG is given by

$$\Delta G = \Delta G^\circ + RTlnQ$$

where Q is the reaction coefficient.

Substituting for ΔG and ΔG°, and then dividing by $-nF$ we arrive at

$$E = E^\circ - \frac{RT}{nF}\ln Q$$

Using the relationship between natural log (ln) and log base 10 (log), with $R = 8.314$ and $F = 96{,}485$:

$$E = E^\circ - 2.303\frac{RT}{nF}\log Q \sim E^\circ - (2\times10^{-4})\frac{T}{n}\log Q$$

This is the **Nernst equation.**

The Nernst equation is used to calculate E under nonstandard conditions, since R and F are constants, and Q, T, and n can be determined.

The Nernst equation can also be used to calculate the equilibrium constant, K_{eq}, for electrochemical systems at equilibrium under standard conditions. For a system under standard conditions, T is 298 K, and by definition, $E = 0$ at equilibrium. Therefore, the Nernst equation reduces to

$$E^\circ = (2.303)\frac{RT}{nF}\log K_{eq} = \frac{(2.303)(8.314)(298)}{n(96{,}485)}\log K_{eq} = \frac{0.0592}{n}\log K_{eq}$$

For the concentration cell described above containing different concentrations of silver$^+$ with silver electrodes, $E = \dfrac{E^\circ - 0.0592}{1}\log\dfrac{0.10}{2.0} \sim 0 - 0.06\log 0.05 = 0.078\,\text{V}$. Since E is positive the reaction is spontaneous. That is, the concentration of the more dilute solution spontaneously increases while that of the more concentrated solution decreases.

9.12 NUCLEAR CHEMISTRY

Nuclear Stability and Radioactivity

The protons and neutrons in a nucleus are held together by a force called the **strong nuclear force**. It's stronger than the electrical force between charged particles, since for all atoms besides hydrogen, the strong nuclear force must overcome the electrical repulsion between the protons. In fact, of the four fundamental forces of nature, the strong nuclear force is the most powerful.

Atoms seek to have a balance between protons and neutrons in their nuclei. For relatively light nuclei, a neutron-to-proton ratio of one to one will tend to be stable. For heavier nuclei, a neutron-to-proton ratio as high as 1.5 to 1 may be needed to confer ideal stability. If an isotope has too many neutrons relative to protons, it may seek either to shed some of those neutrons or to convert some of those neutrons to protons. Likewise, if an isotope has too many protons, it may seek either to shed protons or convert protons to neutrons. These and related processes are collectively known as **radioactive decay**, and we'll look at three types: alpha, beta and gamma. The nucleus that undergoes radioactive decay is known as the parent, and the resulting more stable nucleus is known as the daughter.

Alpha Decay

When a large nucleus becomes more stable by reducing the number of protons and neutrons, it emits an **alpha particle**, denoted by α, that consists of 2 protons and 2 neutrons:

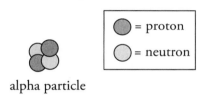

alpha particle

Figure 39

This is equivalent to a helium-4 nucleus with a +2 charge, so an alpha particle is also denoted by He^{2+}. Alpha decay reduces the parent's atomic number by 2 and the mass number by 4. For example, polonium-210 is an α-emitter. It undergoes alpha decay to form the stable nucleus lead-206:

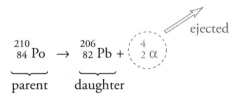

Notice that the equation is balanced: 210 = 206 + 4, and 84 = 82 + 2. Although alpha particles are emitted with high energy from the parent nucleus, this energy is quickly lost as the particle travels through matter or air. As a result, these relatively heavy particles do not typically travel far, and can be stopped by the outer layers of human skin or a piece of paper.

Beta Decay

There are actually three types of beta decay: β^-, β^+, and electron capture. Each type of beta decay involves the transmutation of a neutron into a proton, or vice versa, through the action of a force between elementary particles called the weak nuclear force.

Beta particles are more dangerous than alpha particles since they are significantly less massive. They therefore have more energy and a greater penetrating ability. However, they can be stopped by aluminum foil or a centimeter of plastic or glass.

β⁻ Decay

When an unstable nucleus contains too many neutrons, it may emit a β⁻ **particle,** a high-energy, high-speed electron. The atomic number of the resulting daughter nucleus is 1 greater than the radioactive parent nucleus, but the mass number remains the same. The isotope carbon-14, whose decay is the basis of radiocarbon dating of archaeological artifacts, is an example of a radioactive nucleus that undergoes β⁻ decay:

$$^{14}_{6}\text{C} \rightarrow {}^{14}_{7}\text{N} + {}^{0}_{-1}e^{-} \quad \text{ejected}$$

β⁻ decay is the most common type of beta decay, and when the PCAT mentions "beta decay" without any further qualification, it means β⁻ decay.

β⁺ Decay

When an unstable nucleus contains too few neutrons, it undergoes β⁺ **decay**. The **positron** is the electron's *antiparticle*; it's identical to an electron except its charge is positive. The atomic number of the resulting daughter nucleus is 1 less than the radioactive parent nucleus, but the mass number remains the same. The isotope fluorine-18, which can be used in medical diagnostic bone scans in the form Na^{18}F, is an example of a positron emitter:

$$^{18}_{9}\text{F} \rightarrow {}^{18}_{8}\text{O} + {}^{0}_{+1}e^{+} \quad \text{ejected}$$

Electron Capture

Another way for an unstable nucleus to increase the number of neutrons is to convert a proton into a neutron. Just like positron emission, **electron capture** (EC) causes the atomic number to be reduced by 1 while the mass number remains the same. The nucleus chromium-51 is an example of a radioactive nucleus that undergoes electron capture, becoming the stable nucleus vanadium-51:

$$^{51}_{24}\text{Cr} + {}^{0}_{-1}e^{-} \rightarrow {}^{51}_{23}\text{V}$$

Gamma Decay

A nucleus in an excited energy state—which is usually the case after a nucleus has undergone alpha or any type of beta decay—can "relax" to its ground state by emitting energy in the form of one or more photons of electromagnetic radiation. These photons are called **gamma photons** (symbolized by γ) and have a very high frequency and energy. Gamma photons (or gamma rays) have neither mass nor charge, and can therefore penetrate matter most effectively. They are emitted during nuclear explosions. A few inches of lead or about three meters of concrete will stop most gamma rays. Their ejection from a radioactive atom changes neither the atomic number nor the mass number of the nucleus. For example, after silicon-31 undergoes β^- decay, the resulting daughter nucleus then undergoes gamma decay:

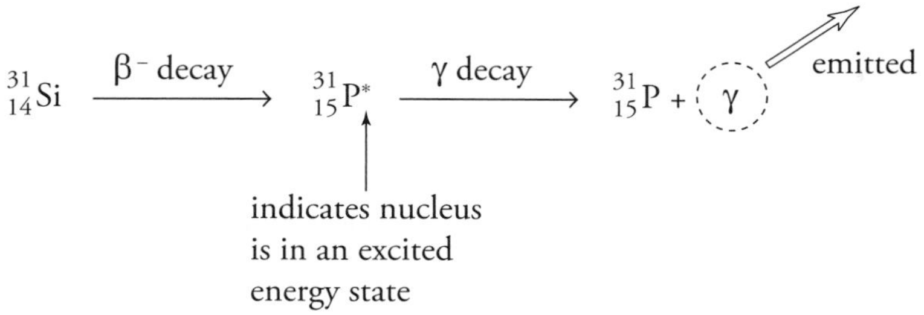

$$^{31}_{14}Si \xrightarrow{\beta^- \text{ decay}} {}^{31}_{15}P^* \xrightarrow{\gamma \text{ decay}} {}^{31}_{15}P + \gamma \quad \text{emitted}$$

indicates nucleus
is in an excited
energy state

Notice that alpha and beta decay change the identity of the nucleus, but gamma decay does not. Gamma decay is simply an expulsion of energy.

Summary of Radioactive Decay

$\boxed{N\downarrow \quad Z\downarrow}$	α Decay	Decreases the number of neutrons *and* protons in large nucleus
		    Subtracts 4 from the mass number
		    Subtracts 2 from the atomic number
		$^{A}_{Z}X \xrightarrow{\alpha} {}^{A-4}_{Z-2}Y + {}^{4}_{2}\alpha$

$\boxed{N\downarrow \quad Z\uparrow}$	β^- Decay	Decreases the number of neutrons, increases the number of protons Adds 1 to the atomic number $^{A}_{Z}X \xrightarrow{\beta^-} {}^{A}_{Z+1}Y + {}^{0}_{-1}e^-$
$\boxed{N\uparrow \quad Z\downarrow}$	β^+ Decay	Increases the number of neutrons, decreases the number of protons Subtracts 1 from the atomic number $^{A}_{Z}X \xrightarrow{\beta^+} {}^{A}_{Z-1}Y + {}^{0}_{+1}e^+$
$\boxed{N\uparrow \quad Z\downarrow}$	EC	Increases the number of neutrons, decreases the number of protons Subtracts 1 from the atomic number $^{A}_{Z}X + {}^{0}_{-1}e^- \xrightarrow{EC} {}^{A}_{Z-1}Y$
	γ Decay	Brings an excited nucleus to a lower energy state Doesn't change mass number or atomic number $^{A}_{Z}X^* \xrightarrow{\gamma} {}^{A}_{Z}X + \gamma$

9.12

Figure 40

Nuclear Binding Energy

Every nucleus that contains protons *and* neutrons has a **nuclear binding energy**. This is the energy that was released when the individual nucleons (protons and neutrons) were bound together by the strong force to form the nucleus. It's also equal to the energy that would be required to break up the intact nucleus into its individual nucleons. The greater the binding energy per nucleon, the more stable the nucleus.

When nucleons bind together to form a nucleus, some mass is converted to energy, so the mass of the combined nucleus is *less* than the sum of the masses of all its nucleons individually. The difference, Δm, is called the **mass defect**, and its energy equivalent *is* the nuclear binding energy. For a stable nucleus, the mass defect will always be positive.

$$\Delta m = \text{(total mass of separate nucleons)} - \text{(mass of nucleus)}$$

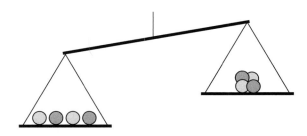

Figure 41

The nuclear binding energy, E_B, can be found from the mass defect using **Einstein's equations for mass-energy equivalence**: $E_B = (\Delta m)c^2$, where c is the speed of light (3×10^8 m/s). In the nuclear domain, masses are often expressed in atomic mass units (1 amu $\approx 1.66 \times 10^{-27}$ kg), and energy is expressed in **electronvolts** (1 eV $\approx 1.6 \times 10^{-19}$ J). In terms of these units, E_B (in eV) = [Δm(in amu)] $\times$ 931.5 MeV.

$$E = mc^2$$

E = energy (J)

m = mass (kg)

c = the speed of light, 3×10^8 m/sec

You can see that because c^2 is such a large number, a very small change in mass results in a very large change in energy. This is the source of energy characteristic of nuclear explosions.

Half-Life

The **half-life** of a radioactive substance (denoted by $t_{1/2}$) is the time it takes for half of the substance to decay; it is a first order reaction. Most half-life problems can be solved by using a simple chart.

Time	Sample
0	100%
1 half-life	50%
2 half-lives	25%
3 half-lives	12.5%

So a sample with a mass of 120 grams and a half-life of 3 years will decay as follows:

(Don't forget that the chart should start with the time at zero.)

Time (yr)	Sample (g)
0	120
3	60
6	30
9	15

Different radioactive nuclei decay at different rates; the shorter the half-life, the faster the decay. As illustrated in the following graph, the amount of a radioactive substance decreases exponentially with time, as is characteristic of a first-order reaction.

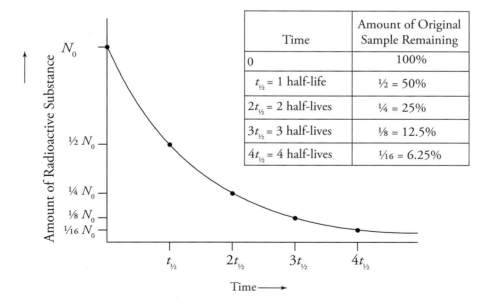

Time	Amount of Original Sample Remaining
0	100%
$t_{1/2}$ = 1 half-life	½ = 50%
$2t_{1/2}$ = 2 half-lives	¼ = 25%
$3t_{1/2}$ = 3 half-lives	⅛ = 12.5%
$4t_{1/2}$ = 4 half-lives	1/16 = 6.25%

Figure 42

As you can see, the amount of substance remaining is $\dfrac{1}{2}^n$, where n is the number of half-lives.

The equation for the exponential decay curve shown above is often written as

$$N = N_0(1/2)^{t/t_{1/2}}$$

where $t_{1/2}$ is the half-life and $\dfrac{t}{t_{1/2}}$ is the number of half-lives. For example, when $t = 3t_{1/2}$, the number of radioactive nuclei remaining, N, is $N_0(1/2)^3 = 1/8\, N_0$, just what we expect. We can also use the equation $0.693 = kt_{1/2}$, where k is the **decay constant**. Notice that the shorter the half-life, the greater the decay constant, and the more rapidly the sample decays.

9.12

CHAPTER 9 KEY TERMS

β^+ decay
β^- decay
β^- particle
absolute zero
absorption line spectrum
acid-base equivalence point or endpoint
acid-base titration
acid-ionization (or acid-dissociation) constant
acidity
activation energy (E_a)
alpha particle
amphoteric
amu
angstrom
anion
anode
Arrhenius equation
atmospheres (atm)
atom
atomic mass unit
atomic number
atomic radius
atomic weight of an element
Aufbau Principle
autoionization of water
Avogadro's Hypothesis
Avogadro's number
base-ionization (or base-dissociation) constant
bimolecular process
boiling point elevation
bond order
Boyle's Law
Brønsted-Lowry
buffer
calorie
cathode
cation
cell diagram
cell emf
Celsius (°C)
Charles's Law
chemical equilibrium
colligative property
concentration
concentration cell
condensation
conduction electrons
conjugate acid
conjugate base

coordinate covalent bond
covalent bonds
critical point
crystallization
Dalton's Law of Partial Pressures
decomposition reaction
degenerate
density
deposition
diamagnetic
diffusion
dilute solution
dipole-dipole forces
dipole-induced dipole force
double displacement reaction
d subshell
effusion
Einstein's equations for mass-energy equivalence
electrolytes
electron affinity
electron capture
electrons
electronvolts
electroplating
emf
empirical formula
endergonic
endothermic
energy
enthalpy
enthalpy of activation
entropy
enzymes
excited state
exergonic
exothermic
Fahrenheit (°F)
First Law of Thermodynamics
formal charge
formula weight
free energy
freezing
freezing point depression
f subshell
galvanic, or voltaic
galvanometer
gamma photons
gas
Gay-Lussac's Law

Gibbs free-energy
Graham's Law of Effusion
ground state configuration
group
half-life
half reactions
heat capacity
heating curve
heat of formation
heat of fusion
heat of reaction
heat of solution
heat of vaporization
Henry's Law
Hess's Law
heterogeneous catalysts
homogeneous catalysts
Hund's Rule
hydration
hydrogen electrode
ideal gas law
immiscible
indicator
inhibitor
inhibitory catalyst
intermediate
intermolecular forces
ion
ion-dipole
ionic bond
ionic solid
ionization energy
isoelectronic
isotopes
Kelvin (K)
kinetic molecular theory
kinetics
lattice
Law of Conservation of Mass (or of Matter)
Le Châtelier's principle
Lewis definitions
ligand
limiting reactant
liquid
London dispersion force
lone pair–bonding pair
lone pair–lone pair
magnetic
mass defect
mass number
metallic bonding
metallic character
microscopic reversibility

midpoint, or half-equivalence point
millimeters of mercury (mmHg)
miscible
molality
molarity
mole
molecular formula
molecular geometry
molecular solids
molecular weight (MW)
molecule
mole fraction
negative heat of solution
Nernst equation
network solid
neutralization reaction
neutrons
nonpolar covalent bond
normal boiling point
normal melting point
nuclear binding energy
nucleons
nucleus
octet
orbital
orbital number
osmosis
osmotic pressure
oxidant
oxidation number
oxidation-reduction, or redox
oxidizing agent
paramagnetic
partial pressure
parts per million (ppm)
parts per thousand (ppt)
pascals
Pauli Exclusion Principle
phase
phase change diagram
polar covalent bonds
polyprotic
positron
potential
pressure
principle of conservation of energy
proton acceptor
proton donor
protons
p subshell
quantized
quantum mechanics
radioactive decay

Raoult's Law
rate-determining step
Rate Law
reactants
reaction mechanism
redox
redox couple
reducing agent
reductant
resonance
resonance forms
rms
salt
salt bridge
saturated
Second Law of Thermodynamics
single displacement reaction
solid
solubility
solubility product constant
solute
solution
solvation
solvent
specific heat
spin down
spin number
spin up
s subshell

standard half cell
standard temperature and pressure (STP)
state function
stoichiometric coefficients
strong electrolytes
strong nuclear force
sublimation
supercritical fluid
supersaturated
synthesis reaction
temperature
thermodynamics
Third Law of Thermodynamics
titrant
torr
transition metals
transition state
triple point
unimolecular process
universal gas constant
valence electron configuration
valence shell electron pair repulsion (VSEPR)
van der Waals forces
van't Hoff equation
van't Hoff factor
vapor pressure
vapor-pressure depression
volatile

GENERAL CHEMISTRY DRILL

1. Predict which element has the ionization energies shown:

	Ionization Energy (kJ/mol)
I_1	577.5
I_2	1816.7
I_3	2744.8
I_4	11,577.5

 A. Na
 B. Si
 C. Al
 D. Mg

2. What is the valence electron configuration of Ag^+?

 A. $[Kr]4d^95s^1$
 B. $[Kr]4d^95s^2$
 C. $[Kr]4d^{10}5s^1$
 D. $[Kr]4d^{10}$

3. Order these intermolecular forces by increasing bond strength: ionic, covalent, dipole-dipole, H-bonding.

 A. Covalent < H-bonding < dipole-dipole < ionic
 B. Dipole-dipole < H-bonding < covalent < ionic
 C. Ionic < covalent < H-bonding < dipole-dipole
 D. Dipole-dipole < H-bonding < ionic < covalent

4. Which anion has a formula mass of 95 g/mol?

 A. Sulfate
 B. Nitrate
 C. Phosphate
 D. Dichromate

5. What is the mass of carbon in one gram of the artificial sweetener aspartame? The molecular formula is $C_{14}H_{18}N_2O_5$.

 A. 0.095 g
 B. 0.27 g
 C. 0.57 g
 D. 0.79 g

6. Ammonia and oxygen react to form dinitrogen monoxide and water. Given 25.0 g of ammonia and 21.5 g of oxygen, how much dinitrogen monoxide will be produced?

 A. 46.5 g
 B. 0.33 mol
 C. 0.75 mol
 D. 29.5 g

7. What is the oxidation state of chromium in dichromate?

 A. +7
 B. –3
 C. +5
 D. +6

8. A 4.25 L gas cylinder containing Cl_2 has a pressure of 28 atm at 25°C. What is the pressure inside the cylinder if the temperature is raised to 38°C?

 A. 29.2 atm
 B. 42.5 atm
 C. 18.4 atm
 D. 26.8 atm

9. Ninety grams of water is brought from a temperature of 75°C to steam. How much energy is needed for this transformation? (ΔH_{vap} = 41 kJ/mol, C_{H2O} = 4.184 J/g•°C)

 A. 9.6 kJ
 B. 214 kJ
 C. 9619 kJ
 D. 9619 J

10. Water has a phase diagram in which the solid-liquid boundary line has a negative slope. How does the density change as pressure is increased?

 A. No change
 B. Decrease
 C. Increase
 D. This cannot be determined from the information given.

11. The fermentation of sucrose produces ethanol according to this equation:

$$C_{12}H_{22}O_{11}(aq) + H_2O(l) \rightarrow 4C_2H_5OH(aq) + 4CO_2(g)$$

Which expression shows the reaction rate for this process?

A. $\text{rate} = \dfrac{\Delta[\text{sucrose}]}{\Delta t}$

B. $\text{rate} = -\dfrac{\Delta[H_2O]}{\Delta t}$

C. $\text{rate} = \dfrac{\Delta[CO_2]}{\Delta t}$

D. $\text{rate} = -\dfrac{1}{4}\dfrac{\Delta[C_2H_5OH]}{\Delta t}$

12. A saturated lead chloride solution has a chloride concentration of 3.2×10^{-2} mol/L. What is the K_{sp} of lead chloride?

A. 1.6×10^{-5}
B. 3.3×10^{-5}
C. 5.1×10^{-6}
D. 5.1×10^{-4}

13. What is the pH of 50 mL of a 4.5×10^{-3} M aqueous solution of calcium hydroxide?

A. 2.05
B. 3.34
C. 10.65
D. 11.95

14. What is the pH of a solution containing 0.025 M HCO_2H and 0.032 M HCO_2Na? The pK_a of formic acid is 3.75.

A. 2.14
B. 2.64
C. 3.86
D. 6.75

15. Below are tabulated reduction potentials. Which substance reacts most readily with $Zn(s)$?

Half-Reaction	$E°$ (V)
$Zn^{2+}(aq) + 2e^- \rightarrow Zn(s)$	−0.76
$O_2(g) + H_2O(l) + 4e^- \rightarrow 4OH^-$	0.40
$Cl_2(g) + 2e^- \rightarrow 2Cl^-(aq)$	1.36
$Li^+(aq) + e^- \rightarrow Li(s)$	−3.04
$NO_3^-(aq) + 3H^+(aq) + 2e^- \rightarrow HNO_2(aq) + H_2O(l)$	0.93

A. O_2
B. Li^+
C. Cl_2
D. NO_3^-

16. Cold denaturation of a protein is exothermic and spontaneous. What is the driving force for this process?

A. A favorable increase in entropy
B. A favorable release of energy
C. A favorable change in temperature
D. Denaturation is a slow process

17. ^{201}Tl is a radioisotope used in medical imaging of the heart. It has a half-life of 3 days. How long will it take for ^{201}Tl to decay to 10% of its initial concentration?

A. 7 days
B. 9 days
C. 10 days
D. 15 days

Want More Practice?
Register your book online for more drill questions!

Answers and Explanations

1. **C** The ionization energies show a substantially large increase at I_4. This indicates an especially stable electron configuration after the loss of three electrons, I_{1-3}. Na has a noble gas configuration after the loss of one electron, and Mg after the loss of two, so eliminate choices (A) and (D). Si is expected to have stable oxidation states of +4 and −4, corresponding to noble gas configurations (Ne or Ar). We can therefore eliminate choice (B). Only Al has a noble gas configuration after the loss of three electrons, so choice (C) is correct.

2. **D** The question asks for the electron configuration of the silver ion. As a Group 11 element Ag has 11 valence electrons, so the ion has 10 (eliminate choices B and C). Moreover, as a Group 11 element Ag has an anomalous electron configuration. It is $[Kr]3d^{10}5s^1$ because of the additional stability associated with filled and half-filled subshells. Electrons are lost from the s subshell before the d, so Ag^+ has the electron configuration $[Kr]3d^{10}$ (eliminate A). Only choice (D) is correct.

3. **B** Ionic bonds are comprised of strong electrostatic forces between charged species, covalent bonds from electrons shared between two nuclei, and both dipole—dipole and H-bonding interactions from differences in electronegativity that give rise to bond polarization. H-bonding is a stronger subclass of dipole-dipole interactions. Of the IMFs listed, ionic bonds are strongest (eliminate choices C and D), and dipole-dipole the weakest (eliminate choice (A)). The correct answer is choice B.

4. **C** Sulfate is SO_4^{2-} with a formula mass of $32 + (4 \times 16) = 96$ g/mol. Nitrate is NO_3^-. Its formula mass is $14 + (3 \times 16) = 62$ g/mol. Phosphate is PO_4^{3-} with a formula mass of $31 + (4 \times 16) = 95$ g/mol, and dichromate is $Cr_2O_7^{2-}$ and has a formula mass of $(2 \times 52) + (7 \times 14) = 216$ g/mol. Choice (C) is correct.

5. **A** One mole of aspartame has a mass of $(14 \times 12) + 18 + (2 \times 14) + (5 \times 16) = 294$ g/mol. Of that total mass, $(14 \times 12)/294$ is carbon, which is 0.57, or 57%. One gram of aspartame × 0.57 = 0.57 g of carbon, choice (A).

6. **B** A balanced chemical equation must first be written for the reaction:

    $$2NH_3(g) + 2O_2(g) \rightarrow N_2O(g) + H_2O(g)$$

    Ammonia has a molecular mass of 17 g/mol, and oxygen of 32 g/mol. Given the nearly equivalent masses, this indicates that oxygen is the limiting reactant. Consequently, less than 46.5 g of product is expected (eliminate choice A). The number of moles of O_2 is 21.5 g/32 g/mol = 0.67 mol, or 2/3 mol. There is a 2:1 molar ratio between O_2 and N_2O, so $(2/3 \times \frac{1}{2}) = \frac{1}{3}$ mol N_2O (eliminate choice C). Only one answer can be correct, and that is choice B. To confirm, the molar mass of N_2O is 44 g/mol, so $\frac{1}{3}$ mol × 44 g/mol = 14.52 g (choice D is incorrect).

7. **D** Dichromate is $Cr_2O_7^{2-}$. Each oxygen has a charge of −2 for a total charge of −14. Because of the −2 charge on the ion, a +12 charge is needed (eliminate choice B). There are two Cr atoms, so each must have a charge of +6, choice (D).

8. **A** Using the ideal gas law, we can compare the initial conditions with the final conditions. The overall expression is $(P_1V_1)/(n_1T_1) = (P_2V_2)/(n_2T_2)$, where T is in Kelvin, not °C. The temperature has increased, so the pressure has increased (eliminate choices C and D). Neither n nor V changes, so the expression becomes $P_1/T_1 = P_2/T_2$. The initial temperature is 273 + 25°C = 298 K, and the final temperature is 273 + 38°C = 311 K. To solve for P_2, we now have 28 atm/298 K = P_2/311 K: P_2 = 29.2 atm, choice A.

9.   **C**   Two equations are needed to solve this problem. To raise the temperature of the liquid to the boiling point of water (100°C), the equation for q is needed: $q = mc\Delta T$. For the phase change from the liquid to the gas, $n\Delta H_{vap}$ is needed where n is the number of moles. The units are not the same, however; q is in joules and the phase change is in kJ, so a conversion is required. The value for ΔT is 25, so $q = (90\ g)(4.184\ J/g \bullet C)(25) = 9{,}414\ J$, or 9.14 kJ. The moles of water is 90 g/18 g/mol = 5 mol, so there are $(5\ mol)(41\ kJ/mol) = 205\ kJ$ of energy associated with the phase change. The total amount of energy needed for the transformation is 9.14 kJ + 205 kJ = 214 kJ, choice (C).

10.   **C**   The negative slope in the phase diagram of water indicates that as pressure increases the solid enters the liquid phase. The density of the liquid is not the same as the density of the solid, so eliminate choices (A) and (D). The density of ice decreases to maximize H-bonding distances, so the density of the liquid is greater (eliminate choice B). Only choice (C) is correct.

11.   **B**   Reaction rates are negative for reactants and positive for products, so choices (A) and (C) can be eliminated. The concentration is multiplied by 1/molar coefficient, so choice (D) is incorrect; the concentration should be multiplied by ¼. Only choice B gives the correct expression.

12.   **A**   The balanced equation for the reaction is

$$PbCl_2(s) \rightarrow Pb^{2+}(aq) + 2Cl^-(aq)$$

Therefore, eliminating the solid $K_{sp} = [Pb^{2+}][Cl^-]$. The lead concentration is one-half the chloride concentration, so $K_{sp} = (1.6 \times 10^{-2})(3.2 \times 10^{-2})^2 = 1.6 \times 10^{-5}$, choice (A).

13.   **D**   The solution will be basic, so choices (A) and (C) can be eliminated. There are two ^-OH ions for each mol of $Ca(OH)_2$, so $[^-OH] = 9.0 \times 10^{-3}$. The pOH = $-\log[^-OH] = 2.05$. The pH is $14.0 - 2.05 = 11.95$, choice (D).

14.   **B**   The Henderson-Hasselbalch equation is used to solve this problem, in which pH = pK_a + log [base]/[acid]. The pH will be higher than the pK_a because $[B^-]/[acid] > 1$ (eliminate choices A and D). Here pH = 3.75 + log (0.032/0.025) = 3.86, choice (B). This is a buffered solution, so the pH should be close to the pK_a, as it is.

15.   **C**   Recall that $\Delta G° = -nFE°$. A large E° indicates a very negative $\Delta G°$. The largest difference in E° values is obtained with Cl_2, so of the substances listed Cl_2 reacts most readily with $Zn(s)$, choice (C).

16.   **B**   Cold denaturation has a $-\Delta H$ (it is exothermic), $-\Delta G$ (it is spontaneous), $-T$ (it is cold), and $-\Delta S$ (entropy decreases with a decrease in T). Because $\Delta G = \Delta H - T\Delta S$, and $-\Delta G$ indicates a spontaneous reaction, choices (A) and (C) can be eliminated. This is a question about thermodynamics, not kinetics, so eliminate choice (D). Only choice (B) is correct.

17.   **D**   Ten percent of one gram of material is 0.1 g. The first decay produces 0.5 g, the second 0.25 g, the third 0.125 g, and the fourth 0.0625 g. Between three and four half-lives are needed to reach 0.1 g, which corresponds to between 9 and 12 days. Only choice (D) is correct.

Quick Review

- The nucleus contains protons and neutrons, collectively called nucleons. Their sum corresponds to the atomic mass (A).

- The number of protons corresponds to the atomic number (Z) and is unique to each element.

- Atoms of the same element that differ in their numbers of neutrons are called isotopes.

- Each electron in an atom has a distinct set of four quantum numbers that describe the electronic structure of the atom. These numbers describe an electrons distance from the nucleus (n), the shape of the occupied region in space (l), the region's orientation in a magnetic field (m_l), and an electron's spin (m_s).

- The periodic table is organized into blocks based on electron configurations. Therefore, an element's valence electron configuration can be determined from the element's location in the table.

- In their ground state, electrons occupy the lowest energy orbitals available, and occupy the subshells within those orbitals singly before pairing.

- For an atom in the d block of period n, the d subshell has a principle quantum number of n − 1. An f subshell has a principle quantum number of n − 2.

- Half-filled and filled subshells are exceptionally stable.

- Transition metals populate the ns orbital before the (n − 1)d orbital, but when forming ions, transition metals lose their valence ns electrons before their (n − 1)d electrons.

- Electrons occupy discrete energy levels within an atom. Absorption spectra result from the absorption of energy as electrons are excited to a higher energy state; emission spectra result from energy emitted as excited electrons return to a lower energy state.

- Atoms and ions are most stable when they have an octet of electrons in their outer shell.

- Atomic radius increases to the left and down the periodic table; for an element that forms charged species, the radius increases in this order: cations < neutral atom < anions. For isoelectronic ions, the species with more protons will have the smaller radius.

- Ionization energy, electron affinity, and electronegativity increase up and to the right on the periodic table, while acidity increases to the right and down the periodic table.

- The relative electronegativities of common atoms in decreasing order are F > O > N > Cl > Br > I ~ S ~ C > H.

- The best Lewis dot or resonance structures have 1) octets around all atoms, 2) minimized formal charges, and 3) place negative charges on more electronegative atoms.

- Ionic bonds form between atoms with large differences in electronegativity (metals + nonmetals). The strength of that bond depends on Coulomb's Law; larger charges and smaller ions make the strongest ionic bonds.

- Covalent bonds form between elements with similar electronegativities (two nonmetals).

- Coordinate covalent bonds form between a Lewis base (e^- pair donor) and a Lewis acid (e^- pair acceptor); the bonding electrons come from the electron pair donor and are shared.

- Nonpolar bonding means equal electron sharing; polar bonding means asymmetrical electron sharing. Electron density is higher around the more electronegative atom.

- If bond dipoles are symmetrically oriented in a molecule, the molecule as a whole is nonpolar; if the dipoles are asymmetrical, the molecule will be polar.

- VSEPR theory predicts the shape of molecules. Angles between electron groups around the central atom are maximized for greatest stability.

- VSEPR is used to predict electron group geometry. Groups are placed around a central atom in a way that minimizes repulsions.

- Molecular geometry is based on VSEPR, but only bonded pairs determine the molecular geometry.

- Molecular geometry gives the spatial configuration of only the bonded pairs.

- Nonpolar molecules have London dispersion forces and polar molecules have dipole forces.

- Hydrogen bonding results when hydrogen is bonded to very electronegative elements, such as O, N, and F.

- Intermolecular forces are cohesive, and determine the physical properties (melting and boiling points, solubility, vapor pressure, etc.) of a compound based on the relative strength of the interactions.

- Changes in pressure and/or temperature of a substance can induce phase changes.

- In order of low-to-high entropy (S, the number of available microstates) and low-to-high internal energy (H, enthalpy), the three important phases are solid, liquid, and gas.

- Energy is absorbed in an endothermic reaction ($+\Delta H$) and is released in an exothermic reaction ($-\Delta H$).

- Specific heat (c) is an intrinsic property that defines how resistant a substance is to a temperature change.

- The relationship between a change in temperature and the specific heat of a substance is given by $q = mc\Delta T$, where m is the amount (either mass or moles, depending on the units of c).

- Heat capacity (C) is given by $C = mc$, where m is the mass of the sample. Heat capacity is a proportionality constant that defines how much heat is required to change the temperature of a sample by $1\,°C$.

- A substance cannot simultaneously undergo a phase change and a temperature change.

- The heat associated with a phase change is given by $q = n\Delta H_{phase\ change}$, where n is the number of moles of substance (or mass if ΔH is given in energy/mass).

- Lines on a phase diagram correspond to equilibria between phases and phase transitions. The triple point, which is the intersection of all three lines on a phase diagram, represents an equilibrium state between all three phases.

- The phase diagram of water is unusual in that its solid/liquid equilibrium line has a negative slope. This results in ice melting under increased pressure, and the density of ice being less than that of liquid water.

- An ionic solid is held together by the electrostatic attraction between cations and anions in a lattice structure and is described by Coulomb's Law.

- In a network solid, atoms form an interconnected lattice of covalent bonds.

- A metallic solid is held together by a high density of shared, delocalized valence electrons that are no longer exclusively associated with a single atom.

- The ideal gas law states that $PV = nRT$.

- Standard temperature and pressure (STP) conditions are defined as 1 atm and 273 K.

- Molecules of an ideal gas take up no volume and experience no intermolecular forces.

- Real gases approach ideal behavior under most conditions, but deviate most from ideal behavior under conditions of high pressure and low temperature.

- Dalton's Law of Partial Pressures states that the total pressure inside a container is equal to the sum of the partial pressures of each constituent gas.

- The partial pressure of a gas divided by the total pressure of all gases is equal to its mole fraction within the gaseous mixture.

- Temperature is a measure of the average kinetic energy of molecules within a sample.

- Graham's Law of Effusion states that the rate of effusion of a gas is inversely proportional to the square root of its molar mass. That is, lighter gases effuse more quickly than heavier gases.

- Kinetics is the study of how quickly a reaction occurs and the reaction mechanism, but it does not determine *whether or not* a reaction will occur.

- All reaction rates are experimentally determined by measuring a change in the concentration of a reactant or product compared to a change in time (by convention given in *M/s*).

- Molecules must collide in order to react, and the frequency and energy of these collisions determine how fast the reaction occurs, but the reactants must also have the correct geometric orientation.

- Increasing the concentration of reactants *often* increases the reaction rate due to an increased number of collisions.

- Increasing the temperature of a reaction *always* increases the reaction rate since molecules move faster and collide more frequently. The energy of collisions also increases.

- Activation energy (E_a) is the minimum energy required to initiate a reaction and decreases in the presence of a catalyst, which increases both the forward and reverse reaction rates.

- Transition states are at energy maxima, while intermediates are at local energy minima along a reaction coordinate.

- A reaction mechanism must agree with experimental data, and suggests a possible pathway by which reactants and intermediates form products in a chemical reaction.

- The sum of all elementary steps of a mechanism will add to give the overall chemical reaction.

- The slow step of the mechanism is the rate limiting step, which determines the rate of the overall reaction.

- A rate law has the general form Rate $= k$ [reactants]^x, where x is the order of the reaction with respect to a given reactant, and k is the rate constant. A rate law for an elementary reaction can be written directly from the elementary step. Otherwise, a rate law can only be determined from experimental data.

- The overall order of a reaction is the sum of all exponents in the rate law.

- The value of the rate constant, k, depends on temperature and activation energy, and its units will vary depending on the reaction order in order to give a rate in M/s.

- Coefficients of the reactants in the rate limiting step of a mechanism can be used to determine the order of a reaction in the rate law; coefficients from the overall reaction alone CANNOT be used to find the order of a reaction.

- The equilibrium constant, K_{eq}, dictates the relative ratios of products to reactants when a system is at equilibrium.

- For $aA + bB \rightarrow cC + dD$: $K_{eq} = ([C]^c[D]^d)/([A]^a[B]^b)$.

- Pure solids and liquids are not included in the equilibrium constant.

- If $K > 10^3$, products are favored. If $K < 10^{-3}$, reactants are favored.

- The reaction quotient, Q, is a ratio of products and reactants with the same math as K, but used when the reaction is not known to be at equilibrium. If $Q < K$, the reaction will proceed in the forward reaction, but if $Q > K$, the reaction will proceed in the reverse direction until equilibrium is achieved. If $Q = K$, the reaction is at equilibrium.

- The only factor that changes the equilibrium constant is temperature.

- Changing the concentrations of the products or reactants of a system at equilibrium will force the system to shift according to Le Châtelier's principle.

- Increasing the temperature of a system at equilibrium favors the products in an endothermic reaction and the reactants in an exothermic reaction. Decreasing the temperature will have the opposite effect on both types of reactions.

- In a gaseous reaction, increasing the pressure by decreasing the volume favors the side of the reaction with fewer moles of gas. Decreasing the pressure has the opposite effect.

- Solution concentrations are generally given in either molarity (mol solute/L solution, M) or molality (mol solute/kg solvent, m). Molality is independent of temperature, whereas molarity is not.

- An electrolyte is a solute that produces solvated ions in solution. Strong electrolytes produce more solvated ions than weak electrolytes.

- The van't Hoff (or ionizability) factor, i, tell us how many ions one unit of a substance will produce in solution.

- All Group 1, ammonium, nitrate, perchlorate, and acetate salts are completely soluble. All silver, lead, and mercury salts are insoluble, except when they are paired with nitrate, perchlorate, or acetate.

- The solubility of solids in liquids increases with increasing temperature.

- The solubility of gases in liquids decreases with increasing temperature and increases with increasing pressure.

- The amount of a salt that can be dissolved in a solute is given by its solubility product constant (K_{sp}).

- Colligative properties depend on the number of particles in solution. These properties include vapor pressure depression, boiling point elevation, freezing point depression, and osmotic pressure.

- In the context of PCAT questions, the colligative strength of a substance can usually be determined based on its van't Hoff factor (i).

- Energy flow into a system has a positive sign. Energy flow out of a system has a negative sign.

- The first law of thermodynamics states that energy cannot be created or destroyed. Thus, $\Delta E = q + w$.

- The internal energy of an object is proportional to its temperature.

- Work can be calculated using $w = -P_{ext} \Delta V$ or $w = Fd$.

- The second law of thermodynamics states that all processes tend toward maxi•mum disorder, corresponding to the maximum number of microstates, represented by entropy (S).

- Enthalpy (H) is a measure of the heat energy.

- Breaking bonds requires energy [$+\Delta H$] and is an endothermic process, while forming bonds releases energy [$-\Delta H$] and the reaction is exothermic.

- $\Delta H_{reaction} = H_{products} - H_{reactants}$. This equation can also be applied to ΔG and ΔS.

- ΔG, the Gibbs free energy, is the amount of energy in a reaction available to do chemical work.

- Standard state conditions for G and H are 1 atm, 298 K, and 1 M concentrations, and are measured in kJ/mol. For entropy, standard state condition are 1 atm, 273 K, and 1 M concentrations, and are measure in J/mol. Standard state conditions are denoted by the superscript "o".

- For a reaction under any set of conditions, $\Delta G = \Delta H - T\Delta S$.

- If $\Delta G < 0$, the reaction is spontaneous in the forward direction. If $\Delta G > 0$, the reaction is nonspontaneous in the forward direction but is spontaneous in the reverse direction. If $\Delta G = 0$, the reaction is at equilibrium. Only ΔG can determine whether or not a reaction is spontaneous.

- For a reaction at equilibrium under standard state conditions, $\Delta G^\circ = -RT\ln K_{eq}$.

- For a reaction under nonequilibrium conditions, ΔG can be calculated using $\Delta G = \Delta G^\circ + RT\ln Q$.

- According to the Brønsted-Lowry definition, a cids are proton donors and electron acceptors; bases are proton acceptors and electron donors.

- Strong acids completely dissociate in water [$K_a > 1$]. [You should memorize the list of strong acids and bases.]

- For any conjugate acid and base pair, $K_a K_b = K_w$. Therefore, the stronger the acid, the weaker its conjugate base, and the stronger the base, the weaker its conjugate acid. Conjugates of strong acids and bases have no significant acid/base properties in water.

- Amphoteric substances may act as either acids or bases.

- Water is amphoteric, and autoionizes into OH^- and H_3O^+. The equilibrium constant for the autoionization of water is $K_w = [OH^-][H_3O^+]$. At 25°C, $K_w = 1 \times 10^{-14}$.

- pH = $-\log[H_3O^+]$. For a concentration of H_3O^+ given in 10^{-x} M notation, take the negative of the exponent to find the pH. The same is true for the relationship between $[OH^-]$ and pOH, K_a and pK_a, and K_b and pK_b.

- The higher the K_a [lower the pK_a], the stronger the acid. The higher the K_b [lower the pK_b], the stronger the base.

- At 25°C, $pK_a + pK_b = 14$.

- If a salt is dissolved in water and the cation is a stronger acid than water, the resulting solution will have a pH < 7. If the anion is a base stronger than water, the resulting solution will have a pH > 7.

- A buffer consists of equal molar amounts of a weak acid and its conjugate base, and has a pH equal to its pK_a.

- Buffers resist a change in pH upon the addition of a small amount of strong acid or base. A higher concentration of buffer resists a pH change better than a lower concentration of buffer (i.e., the solution has a higher buffering capacity).

- The Henderson-Hasselbalch equation can be used to determine the pH of a buffer solution.

- In a titration, the equivalence point is the point at which all of the original acid or base has been neutralized.

- Indicators are weak acids that change color when converted to their conjugate base. An indicator should be selected that changes color in the range +/− one pH unit from the equivalence point.

- When a strong acid is titrated against a weak base, the pH at the equivalence point is < 7. When a strong base is titrated against a weak acid, the pH at the equivalence point is > 7. When a strong base is titrated against a strong acid, the pH at the equivalence point is 7.

- At the half equivalence point of a titration of a weak plus a strong acid or base, the solution has equal concentrations of acid and conjugate base, and $pH = pK_a$. This is the buffer region of the titration curve.

- Oxidation is electron loss; reduction is electron gain (remember "OIL RIG").

- A species that is oxidized is a reducing agent (reductant), and a species that is reduced is an oxidizing agent (oxidant).

- In all electrochemical cells, oxidation occurs at the anode and reduction occurs at the cathode.

- Electrons always flow from the anode to the cathode.

- To preserve electrical neutrality, salt bridge anions always migrate toward the anode, and cations always migrate toward the cathode.

- The free energy of an electrochemical cell can be calculated from its potential using the relationship $\Delta G° = -nFE°$.

- A galvanic cell spontaneously generates electrical power ($-\Delta G$, $+E$).

- An electrolytic cell consists of nonspontaneous reactions and requires an external electrical power source ($+\Delta G$, $-E$).

- In a galvanic cell, electrons spontaneously flow from the negative ($-$) terminal to the positive ($+$) terminal. Therefore, in a galvanic cell, the anode is negatively charged ($-$) and the cathode is positively charged ($+$).

- In an electrolytic cell, electrons flow from the positive ($+$) terminal to the negative ($-$) terminal by applying an external voltage to drive a nonspontaneous reaction. Therefore, the anode is positively charged ($+$) and the cathode is negatively charged ($-$).

- Standard reduction potentials are intrinsic values and therefore should not be multiplied by molar coefficients in balanced half-reactions.

- For a given reduction potential, the reverse reaction, or oxidation potential, has the same magnitude of E but the opposite sign.

- Faraday's Law of Electrolysis states that the amount of chemical change is proportional to the amount of electricity that flows through the cell.

- Under nonstandard conditions, the potential of an electrochemical cell can be calculated using the Nernst equation: $E = E° - [\frac{RT}{nF}]\ln Q$, where n is the net transfer of electrons. Combining constants, this becomes $E = E° \frac{-0.059}{n} \log Q$. At equilibrium, $E°_{cell} = [\frac{RT}{nF}]\ln K$, or $0.059/n \log K$.

- Unstable nuclei can result from an overabundance of either protons or neutrons. The nuclei decay by emitting various particles.

- For nuclear decay reactions, the sum of all masses and atomic numbers in the products must equal the same sum of the corresponding numbers in the reactants.

- The rate of nuclear decay is governed by a species' half-life, $t_{1/2}$.

- Nuclear decay is a first order reaction. The shorter the half-life, the more rapidly the sample decays.

Chapter 10

Organic Chemistry

10.1   INTRODUCTION

Organic Chemistry Question Strategies

1. Remember that Process of Elimination is paramount! The erasable noteboard allows you to eliminate answer choices; this will improve your chances of guessing the correct answer if you are unable to narrow it down to one choice.
2. Answer the straightforward questions first. Leave questions that require analysis of experiments and graphs for later.
3. Make sure that the answer you choose actually answers the question, and isn't just a true statement.
4. Try to avoid answer choices with extreme words such as "always," "never," etc. In O-Chem, there is almost always an exception and answers are rarely black and white.
5. Math: Any questions that involve calculations should be left for last (there aren't many in O-Chem, but they happen). You should always round numbers and estimate while working out calculations on your whiteboard.
6. Again, don't leave any question blank.

Background and Introduction

This section covers the fundamentals of nomenclature in organic chemistry. Although this section will require memorization as your primary study technique, it is in your best interest to be comfortable reading, hearing, and using this terminology. Although most of the terminology that appears on the PCAT is IUPAC, some common nomenclature is also used.

n-Alkanes

An *n*-alkane is an open chain hydrocarbon that consists of hydrogen and singly bonded carbon atoms. It has the general formula C_nH_{2n+2}. Table 1 lists the names of the first ten n-alkanes.

Carbon Chain Prefixes and Alkane Names			
Number of carbon atoms in a row	Prefix	Alkane	Name
1	meth-	CH_4	methane
2	eth-	CH_3CH_3	ethane
3	prop-	$CH_3CH_2CH_3$	propane
4	but-	$CH_3CH_2CH_2CH_3$	butane
5	pent-	$CH_3(CH_2)_3CH_3$	pentane
6	hex-	$CH_3(CH_2)_4CH_3$	hexane
7	hept-	$CH_3(CH_2)_5CH_3$	heptane
8	oct-	$CH_3(CH_2)_6CH_3$	octane
9	non-	$CH_3(CH_2)_7CH_3$	nonane
10	dec-	$CH_3(CH_2)_8CH_3$	decane

Table 1

In the case of an all-carbon containing ring, these are preceded by the prefix **cyclo-**. Hence, a six-membered ring containing all $-CH_2-$ units is called *cyclohexane*. These have the general formula C_nH_{2n}.

Hydrocarbon Substituents

A substituent is an atom or group of atoms on a molecule that substitute for a hydrogen atom. Table 2 lists the nomenclature for hydrocarbon substituents commonly found on the PCAT.

Nomenclature for Substituents	
Substituent	**Name**
$-CH_3$	methyl
$-CH_2CH_3$	ethyl
$-CH_2CH_2CH_3$	propyl
$H_3C-\overset{\displaystyle H}{\underset{\displaystyle |}{C}}-CH_3$	isopropyl
$-CH_2CH_2CH_2CH_3$	butyl (or *n*-butyl)
$\underset{\displaystyle |}{CH_3}CHCH_2CH_3$	*sec*-butyl
$-\overset{\displaystyle CH_3}{\underset{\displaystyle CH_3}{\overset{\displaystyle |}{\underset{\displaystyle |}{C}}}}-CH_3$	*tert*-butyl (or *t*-butyl)

Table 2

10.2   STRUCTURES AND NOMENCLATURE

Common Functional Groups

Figure 1 shows the structures and names of functional groups commonly encountered on the PCAT. Be sure you are familiar with the contents shown.

R = alkyl group = hydrogen substituents group (or H), X = halogen (F, Cl, Br, I)

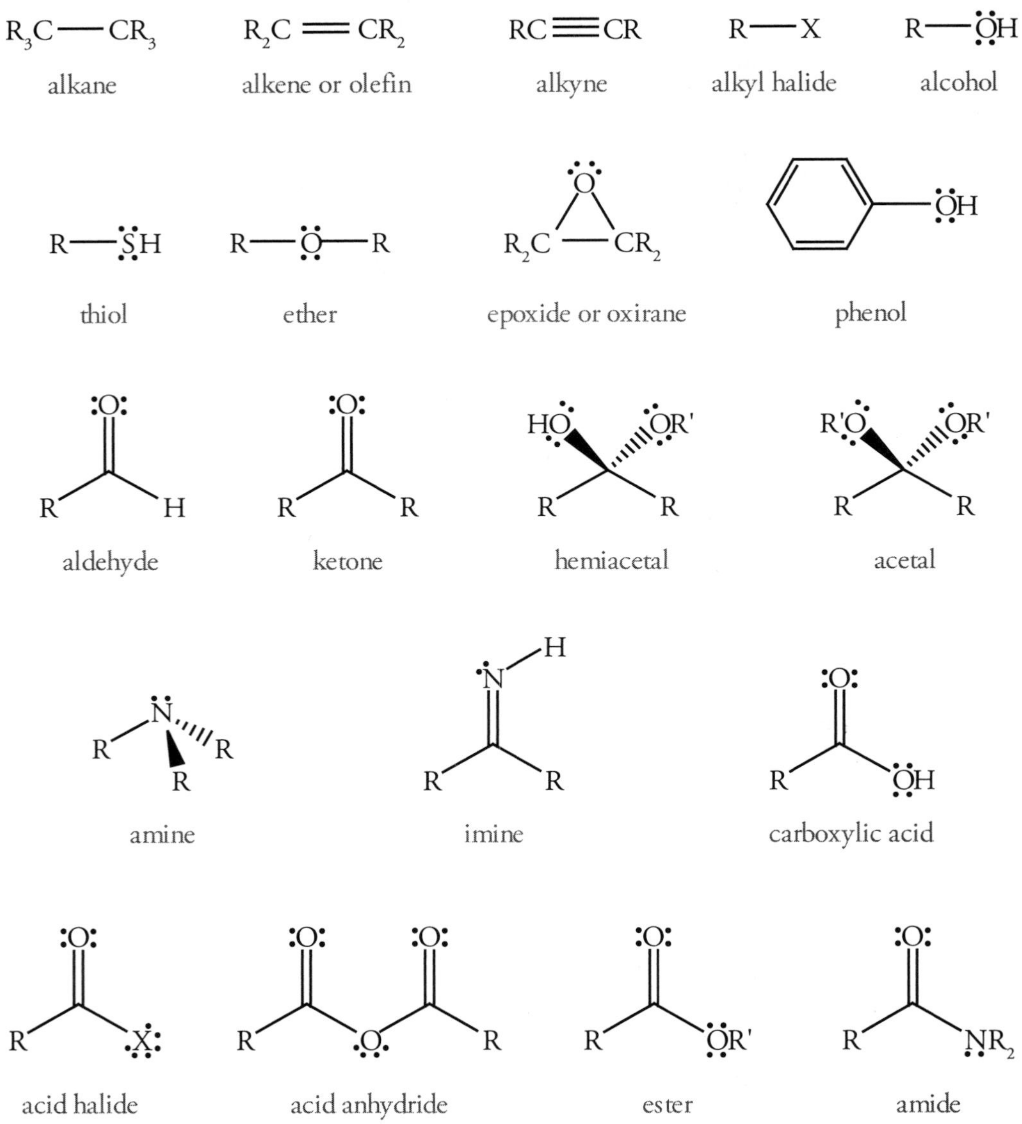

R_3C —— CR_3 R_2C === CR_2 RC ≡≡ CR R — X R — $\ddot{O}H$

alkane   alkene or olefin   alkyne   alkyl halide   alcohol

R — $\ddot{S}H$ R — $\ddot{O}$ — R R_2C ◁ CR_2 (O)   phenol ring — $\ddot{O}H$

thiol   ether   epoxide or oxirane   phenol

aldehyde   ketone   hemiacetal   acetal

amine   imine   carboxylic acid

acid halide   acid anhydride   ester   amide

Figure 1

Abbreviated Line Structures

The prevalence of carbon-hydrogen (C—H) bonds in organic chemistry has led chemists to use an abbreviated drawing system, merely for convenience. Called *abbreviated line structures*, they use only a few simple rules:

1. Carbons are represented as vertices.
2. C–H bonds are not drawn.
3. Hydrogens bonded to any atom *other* than carbon must be shown.

To illustrate rules 1 and 2, pentane can be represented using the full line structure,

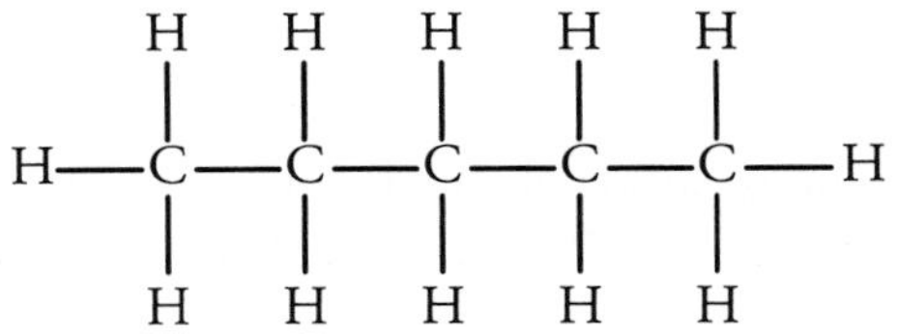

or using the abbreviated line structure.

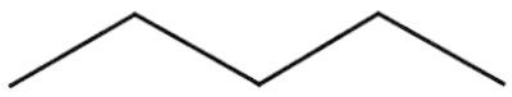

Although C—H bonds are not explicitly drawn, the number of hydrogens required to complete carbon's valency are bonded to carbon at each vertex but not shown. To clarify this, let's look more closely at the abbreviated line structure of pentane:

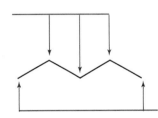

These three carbon atoms are each bonded to two other carbon atoms. In order to complete carbon's valency, we assume there are two hydrogens bonded to each of these carbons.

These two carbon atoms are each bonded to one other carbon atom. In order to complete carbon's valency, we assume there are three hydrogens bonded to each of these carbons.

To illustrate rule 3, consider dimethyl amine:

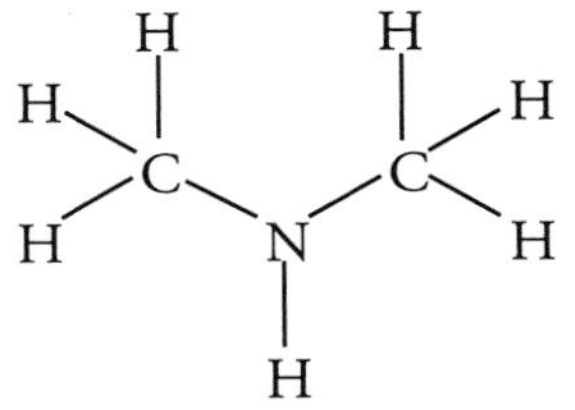

full Lewis structure

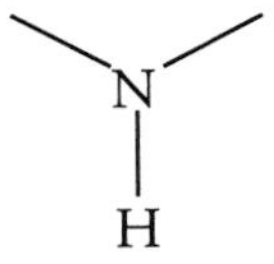

abbreviated line structure

Remember that hydrogens bonded to any other atom must be shown. Lone pairs of electrons are often omitted.

10.2

Nomenclature of Alkanes

Alkanes are named by a set of simple rules. One particular alkane (shown below) will be used to illustrate this process:

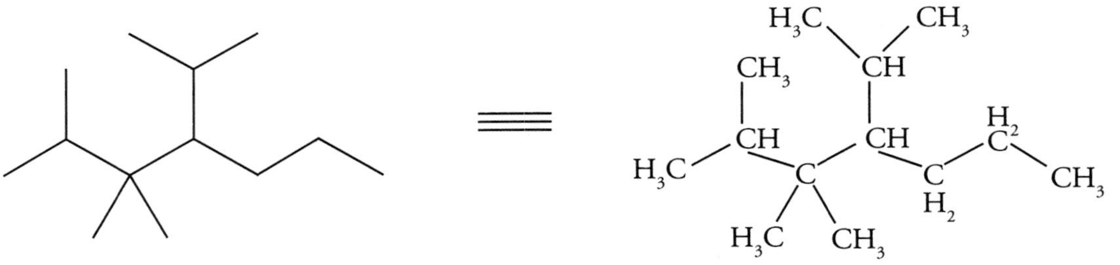

1. Identify the longest continuous carbon chain. The names of these chains are given in the first table in this chapter ("Carbon Chain Prefixes and Alkane Names").

    The longest chain in the compound above is a 7-carbon chain, which is called *heptane*. (This chain is shown below, outlined by dashed lines.)

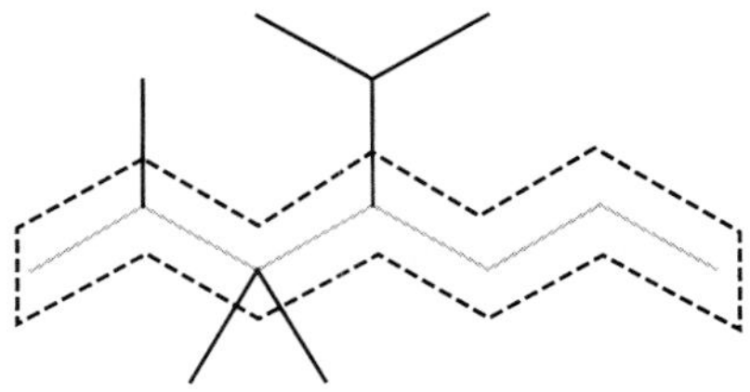

2. Identify any substituents on this chain. The names of some common hydrocarbon substituents are given in the second table in this chapter ("Nomenclature for Substituents").

    There are four substituents in this example: three methyl groups and one isopropyl group.

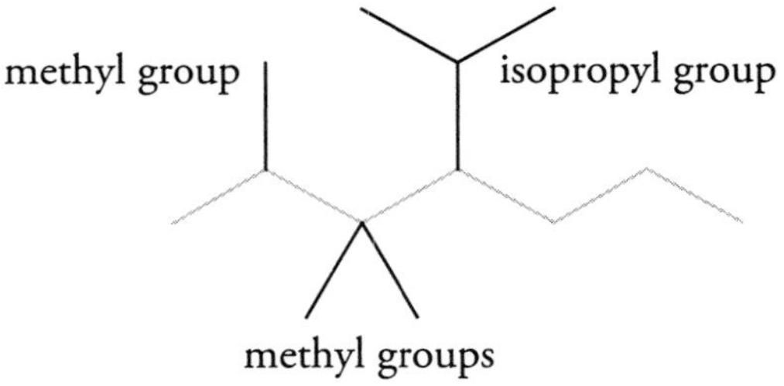

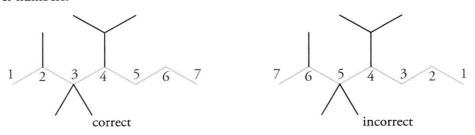

3. Number the carbons of the main chain such that the substituents are on the carbons with lower numbers.

Now each substituent can be associated with the carbon atom to which it's attached:

    2 – methyl
    3 – methyl
    3 – methyl
    4 – isopropyl

4.   Identical substituents are grouped together; the prefixes **di-**, **tri-**, **tetra-**, and **penta-** are used to denote how many there are, and their carbon numbers are separated by a comma.

In this case, we have

$$\left. \begin{array}{l} 2 - \text{methyl} \\ 3 - \text{methyl} \\ 3 - \text{methyl} \end{array} \right\} \longrightarrow 2,3,3\text{-trimethyl}$$

5.   Alphabetize the substituents, ignoring the prefixes di-, tri-, etc. and *n-*, *sec-*, *tert-*, and separate numbers from words by a hyphen and numbers from numbers by a comma.

The complete name for our molecule is therefore **2,3,3-trimethyl-4-isopropylheptane.**

Let's do another example and find the name of this molecule:

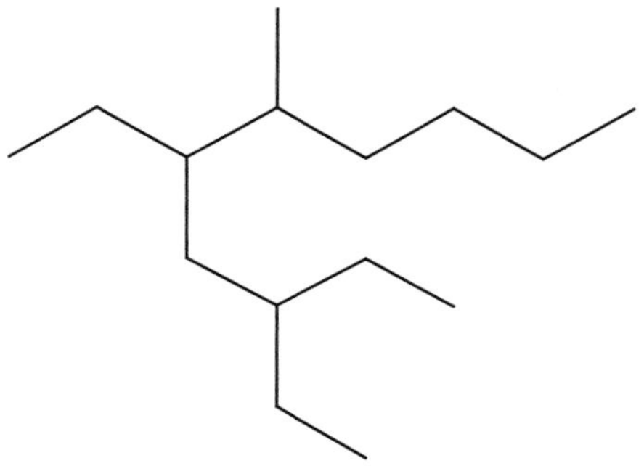

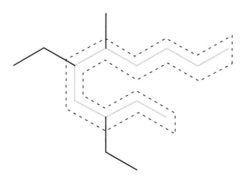

1.   The longest continuous carbon chain is a 10-carbon chain, called **decane**.

10.2

2. There are three substituents on this chain: two ethyl groups and a methyl group.

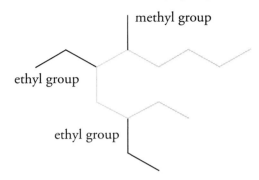

methyl group

ethyl group

ethyl group

3. The correct numbering of the carbons in the main chain is as follows:

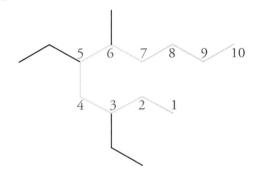

4. The substituents are now identified as
    3,5-diethyl
    6-methyl

5. The complete name of the molecule is therefore **3,5-diethyl-6-methyldecane**.

Nomenclature of Haloalkanes

Alkanes with halogen (F, Cl, Br, I) substituents follow the same set of rules as simple alkanes. Halogens are named using these prefixes:

Halogen	Prefix
fluorine	fluoro-
chlorine	chloro-
bromine	bromo-
iodine	iodo-

Table 3

By applying the same rules as for naming simple alkanes, verify the following names:

Structure   Name

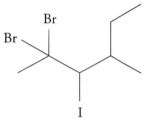

2-chlorobutane

2-chloro-1-fluoro-4-methylpentane

2,2-dibromo-3-iodo-4-methylhexane

Figure 2

Nomenclature of Alcohols

Alcohols also follow many of the same nomenclature rules as alkanes. Hydroxyl groups (–OH), however, are typically denoted by a suffix on the main alkyl chain. The table of straight-chain alcohols given below shows that to denote a hydroxyl group, the suffix **–ol** replaces the last **–e** in the name of the alkane.

Alkanes		Alcohols	
Structure	**Name**	**Structure**	**Name**
CH_4	methane	CH_3OH	methanol
CH_3CH_3	ethane	CH_3CH_2OH	ethanol
$CH_3CH_2CH_3$	propane	$CH_3CH_2CH_2OH$	propanol
$CH_3CH_2CH_2CH_3$	butane	$CH_3CH_2CH_2CH_2OH$	butanol

Table 4

When the position of the hydroxyl group needs to be specified, the number is placed after the name of the longest carbon chain and before the *–ol* suffix, separated by hyphens. For example,

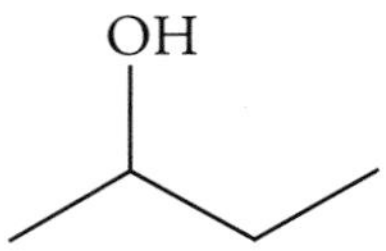

butan-2-ol
(or 2-butanol)
or *sec*-butanol

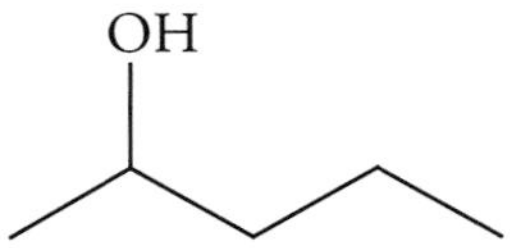

pentan-2-ol
(or 2-pentanol)

Priorities are assigned to give the lowest number to the hydroxyl group. For example,

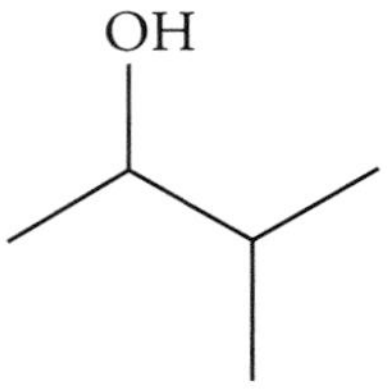

3-methylbutan-2-ol
(3-methyl-2-butanol)
not
2-methylbutan-3-ol

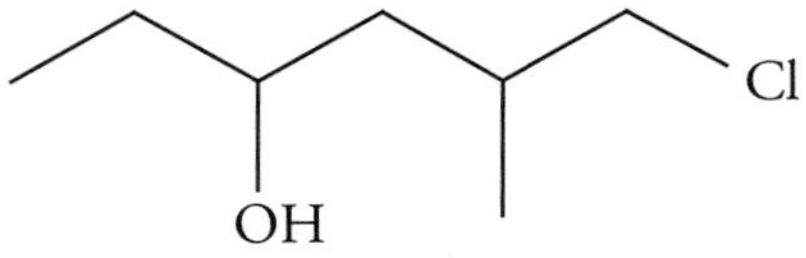

6-chloro-5-methylhexan-3-ol
(6-chloro-5-methyl-3-hexanol)

Nomenclature of Alkenes

"Alkene" means a hydrocarbon that contains a carbon-carbon double bond. A double bond is a site of unsaturation, so an alkene is an unsaturated hydrocarbon.

Naming the alkenes involves the same prefixes used for the alkanes, and the suffix "*-ene*" instead of "*-ane*." We number carbons by beginning at the molecular end closest to the double bond. Or, if the double bond is at the midpoint of the carbon chain, numbering begins at the end closest to the first branch point.

With the carbons thus numbered, the name shows, from left to right:

1. the site and nature of branches
2. the site of the double bond
3. a prefix corresponding to the length of the (longest possible) carbon chain
4. the alkene suffix ("*-ene*")

Sites of the branch points and double bond are located by counting carbons, beginning at the molecular end closest to the double bond. Or, if the double bond is at the midpoint of the carbon chain, counting begins at the end closest to the first branch point.

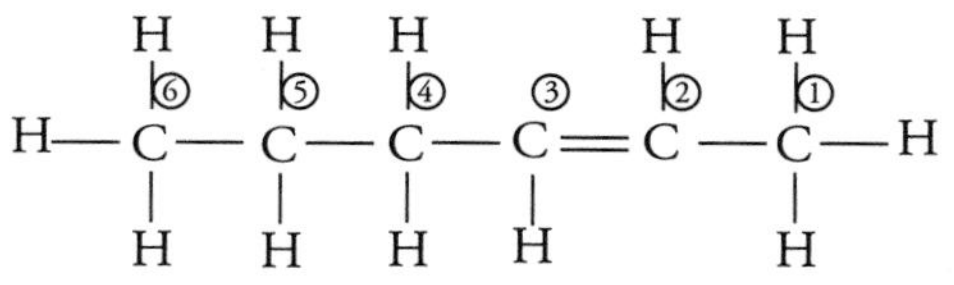

2-hexene

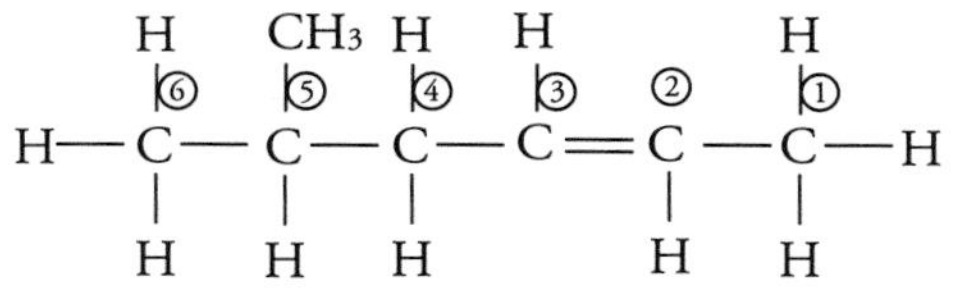

5-methyl-2-hexene

Figure 3

10.3 BONDING

Bonding in Organic Molecules

The chemistry of organic molecules is dominated by the reactivity of covalent bonds, in which electrons are shared between two atoms. An understanding of the fundamentals of covalent bonding can provide the intuitive grasp necessary to answer a wide range of questions in organic chemistry. These include hybridization, sigma (σ) bonding, pi (π) bonding, structural formulas, electron delocalization, resonance stabilization, bond length, bond energy, isomerism, chirality, and optical activity.

Hybridization

In order to rationalize observed chemical and structural trends, chemists developed the concept of orbital hybridization. In this model, imagine a mathematical combination of atomic orbitals centered on the same atom to produce a set of composite, **hybrid** orbitals. For example, consider an *s* and a *p* orbital on an atom.

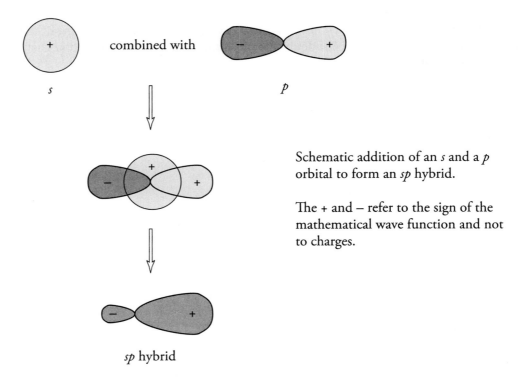

Schematic addition of an *s* and a *p* orbital to form an *sp* hybrid.

The + and − refer to the sign of the mathematical wave function and not to charges.

sp hybrid

Figure 4

Notice that the new orbital is highly directional; this allows for better overlap when bonding.

There will be two such *sp* hybrid orbitals formed because two orbitals (the *s* and the *p*) were originally combined; that is, the total number of orbitals is conserved in the formation of hybrid orbitals. For this reason, the number of hybrid orbitals is the sum of the superscripts (1 + 1 for *sp*, 1 + 2 for sp^2, and so on).

The percentages of the *s* character and *p* character in a given sp^x hybrid orbital are listed below:

sp^x hybrid orbital	s character	p character
sp	50%	50%
sp^2	33%	67%
sp^3	25%	75%

Table 5

To determine the hybridization for most atoms in simple organic molecules, add the number of atoms bonded to a central atom to the number of non-bonding electron pairs (non-delocalized) and use the following table (which also gives the ideal bond angles and molecular geometry). The number of bonded atoms to a central atom plus the number of lone pairs is equal to the number of orbitals that combined to make the new hybridized orbitals.

# of bonded atoms to a central atom + # of lone pairs	Hybridization	Bond Angles (ideal)	Molecular Geometry
2	sp	180°	linear
3	sp^2	120°	trigonal planar
4	sp^3	109.5°	tetrahedral

Table 6

Notice that the electron group geometry described by VSEPR (Chapter 9, Section 9.4) gives the hybridization, whereas the molecular geometry is described only by the bonded atoms. For example, NH_3, with four electron groups, is sp^3 hybridized. Its electron group geometry is tetrahedral, but with one lone pair its molecular geometry is trigonal pyramidal.

Sigma (σ) Bonds

A σ **bond** consists of two electrons that are localized between two nuclei. It is formed by the end-to-end overlap of one hybridized orbital (or an s orbital in the case of hydrogen) from each of the two atoms participating in the bond. Below, we show the σ bonds in ethane, C_2H_6:

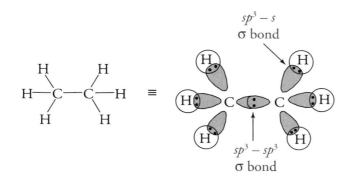

Figure 5

Remember that an sp^3 carbon atom has 4 sp^3 hybrid orbitals, which are derived from one s orbital and three p orbitals.

Pi (π) Bonds

A π **bond** is formed by a side-to-side overlap of two unhybridized p orbitals on adjacent atoms. (An sp^2 hybridized atom has three sp^2 orbitals—which come from one s and two p orbitals—plus one p orbital that remains unhybridized.) Below, we show the π bonds in ethene (ethylene), C_2H_4:

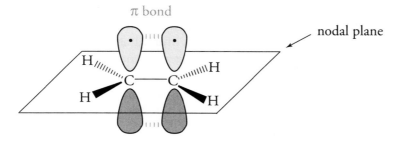

Figure 6

In any multiple bond, *there is only one σ bond; the remainder are π bonds.* Therefore,

a single bond: composed of 1 σ bond along the internuclear axis
a double bond: composed of 1 σ bond along the internuclear axis and 1 π bond
a triple bond: composed of 1 σ bond along the internuclear axis and 2 π bonds

Structural Formulas

By definition, an organic molecule is said to be **saturated** if it contains no π bonds and no rings; it is **unsaturated** if it has at least one π bond or a ring. A saturated compound with n carbon atoms has exactly $2n + 2$ hydrogen atoms, while an unsaturated compound with n carbon atoms has fewer hydrogens.

The formula below is used to determine the **degree of unsaturation** (d) of simple organic molecules and is used to predict molecular structure:

n = number of carbons
x = number of hydrogens*

$$\text{degree of unsaturation} = \frac{(2n + 2) - x}{2}$$

* x represents the number of hydrogens and any monovalent atoms (such as the halogens: F, Cl, Br, or I).
Since the number of oxygens has no effect, it is ignored.
For nitrogen-containing compounds, replace each N by 1 C and 1 H when using this formula.

One degree of unsaturation indicates the presence of one π bond or one ring; two degrees of unsaturation means there are two π bonds (two separate double bonds or one triple bond), or one π bond and one ring, or two rings, and so on. The presence of heteroatoms can also affect the degree of unsaturation in a molecule. This is best illustrated through a series of related molecules that all have one degree of unsaturation.

4-Chloro-1-butene (C_4H_7Cl) also has one degree of unsaturation, but the number of hydrogens is different. Each halogen atom (fluorine, chlorine, bromine, iodine) or other monovalent atom "replaces" one hydrogen atom, so $d = [(2 \bullet 4 + 2)-(7 + 1)]/2 = 1$:

Cl

Methoxyethene (C_3H_6O) also has one degree of unsaturation. Each oxygen (or other divalent atom) "replaces" one carbon and two hydrogen atoms (CH_2 groups are sometimes referred to as methylene groups), so $d = [(2(3 + 1) + 2)-(6 + 2)]/2 = 1$. Since a divalent atom can take the place of a methylene group, it doesn't affect the degree of unsaturation, and can be ignored.

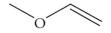

10.3

Bond Length and Bond Dissociation Energy

The term *bond length* describes the distance between two nuclei whose atoms have formed a bond. **Bond dissociation energy (BDE)** is the energy required to break a bond *homolytically*. In **homolytic bond cleavage**, one electron of the bond being broken goes to each fragment of the molecule. In this process two radicals form. This is *not* the same thing as **heterolytic bond cleavage** (also known as *dissociation*). In heterolytic bond cleavage, both electrons of the electron pair that make up the bond end up on the same atom; this forms both a cation and an anion.

$$(H_3C)_3C \longrightarrow H \longrightarrow C(CH_3)_3{}^{\bullet} + H^{\bullet}$$

homolytic bond cleavage

$$(H_3C)_3C \longrightarrow Cl \longrightarrow C(CH_3)_3{}^{\oplus} + Cl^{\ominus}$$

heterolytic bond cleavage

Figure 7

These two processes are very different and hence have very different energies associated with them. Here, we will consider only homolytic bond dissociation energies.

Bond order refers to the number of chemical bonds between two atoms and is a measure of the stability of a bond. In $H_2C = CH_2$, for example, the carbon-carbon bond order is two, whereas in H_3C-CH_3 it is one. When one examines the relationship between bond length and bond dissociation energy for a series of similar bonds, an important trend emerges: for similar bonds, *the higher the bond order, the shorter and stronger the bond*. The following table, which lists the bond dissociation energies (BDE, in kcal/mol) and the bond lengths (r, in angstroms, where $1 \text{ Å} = 10^{-10}$ m) for carbon-carbon and carbon-oxygen bonds, illustrates this trend:

	C—C	C=C	C≡C	C—O	C=O	C≡O
BDE	83	144	200	86	191	256
r (in Å)	1.54	1.34	1.20	1.43	1.20	1.13

Table 7

An important caveat arises because of the varying atomic radii: *bond length/BDE comparisons should be made only for <u>similar bonds</u>*. Thus, carbon-carbon bonds should be compared only to other carbon-carbon bonds; carbon-oxygen bonds should be compared only to other carbon-oxygen bonds, and so on.

Recall the shapes of unhybridized atomic orbitals about the atomic nucleus: *s* orbitals are spherical, while *p* orbitals are elongated "dumbbell"-shaped.

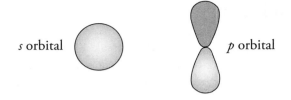

Figure 8

When comparing the same type of bonds, the greater the *s* character in the component orbitals, the shorter the bond (because *s*-orbitals are closer to the nucleus than *p*-orbitals). A greater percentage of *p* character also leads to a more directional hybrid orbital that is farther from the nucleus and thus a longer bond. In addition, when comparing the same types of bonds, *the longer the bond, the weaker it is; the shorter the bond, the stronger it is*. Moreover, the greater the overlap, the stronger the bond. In the following diagram, compare all the C–C bonds and all the C–H bonds:

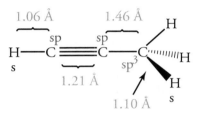

Figure 9

Bond	Bond length	Bond	Bond length
C—C ($sp - sp$)	1.21 Å	C–H ($sp - s$)	1.06 Å
C—C ($sp - sp^3$)	1.46 Å	C–H ($sp^3 - s$)	1.10 Å

Table 8

Isomerism

Constitutional Isomerism

Constitutional (or, less precisely, *structural*) **isomers** are compounds that have the same molecular formula but whose atoms are connected together differently. These compounds are also known as **tautomers.** Pentane (C_5H_{12}), for example, is a fully saturated hydrocarbon that has three constitutional isomers:

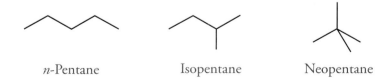

n-Pentane   Isopentane   Neopentane

Conformational Isomerism

Conformational isomers are compounds that have the same molecular formula and the same atomic connectivity, but which differ from one another by rotation about a (single) σ bond. In truth, they are the exact same molecule. For saturated hydrocarbons, there are two orientations of σ bonds attached to adjacent sp^3 hybridized carbons on which we will concentrate. These are the **staggered** conformation and the **eclipsed** conformation. In staggered conformations, a σ bond on one carbon bisects the angle formed by two σ bonds on the adjacent carbon. In an eclipsed conformation, a σ bond on one carbon directly lines up with a σ bond on an adjacent carbon. Both conformations can be visualized using either the flagged bond notation as shown in the representations on the left, or the Newman projection, which uses a vertex and a circle to represent two adjacent carbon atoms. The conformational isomers of ethane (C_2H_6) are shown here:

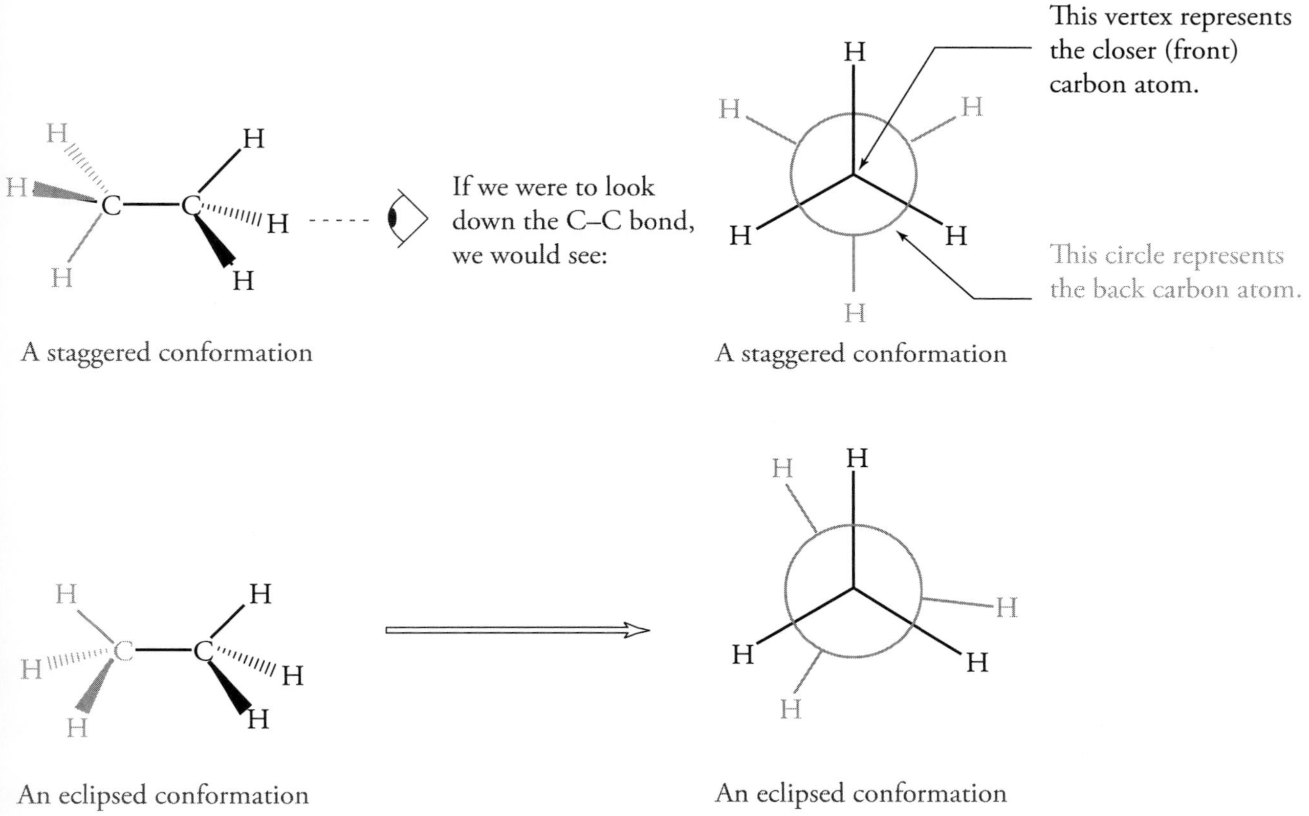

This vertex represents the closer (front) carbon atom.

If we were to look down the C–C bond, we would see:

This circle represents the back carbon atom.

A staggered conformation

A staggered conformation

An eclipsed conformation

An eclipsed conformation

Figure 10

Now we turn our attention to the conformational analysis of hydrocarbons such as *n*-butane.

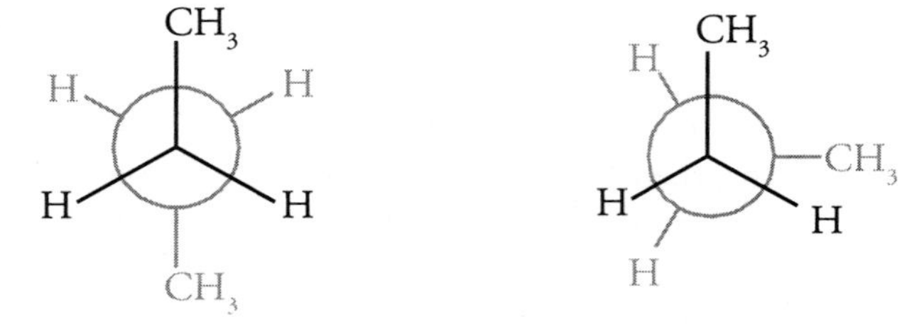

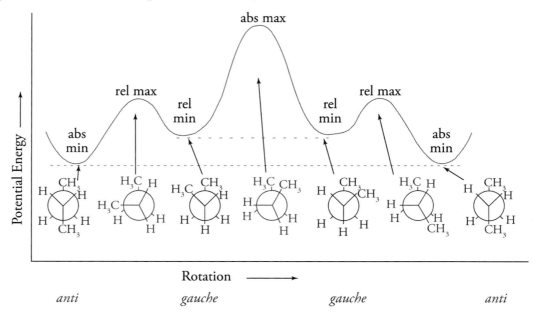

10.3

The σ bonds should actually directly line up with each other. For clarity here, they are not directly aligned.

staggered conformation

eclipsed conformation

less crowded
more stable

more crowded
electronic repulsion
less stable

Figure 11

It's important to note, however, that there are an infinite number of conformations for a molecule that has free rotation around a C–C bond, and that all of these other conformations are energetically related to the staggered and eclipsed conformations described here. For example, relative to the carbon atom in the rear of a Newman projection, the front carbon atom could be rotated *any number of degrees*. Any change in the rotation of one carbon, relative to its adjacent neighbor, is a change in molecular conformation.

The difference in stability among the various conformations can largely be attributed to electron repulsion and steric hinderance. Covalent bonds repel one another because they are composed of negatively charged electrons. The staggered conformation is more stable than the eclipsed, because in the staggered conformation the σ bonds are as far apart as possible, while in the eclipsed conformation they are directly aligned with one another. Moreover, it is more favorable to have bonded atoms assume the roomier staggered conformation where they are 60° apart, rather than the eclipsed conformation where they are directly aligned with one another. There are further aspects to consider in conformational analysis, however. Not all staggered conformations are of equal energy, and neither are all eclipsed conformations. There are particularly stable staggered conformations and particularly unstable eclipsed conformations. Using this information we can predict the stability of various conformations for *n*-butane.

Figure 12

Beginning with the most stable conformation of *n*-butane, the staggered conformation is referred to as the **anti conformation** and arises when the two largest groups attached to adjacent carbons are 180° apart. This produces the most sterically favorable, and hence the most energetically favorable (lowest energy) conformation. As the methyl groups and hydrogen atoms come into closer proximity to each other, potential energy increases because of electron repulsions and steric hinderance. The potential energy decreases in the **gauche conformation** because the hydrogen atoms are now in a staggered position, so their repulsions are minimized. As rotation continues, the maximum potential energy is reached when both the methyl groups and the hydrogen atoms are in close proximity to those on the adjacent carbon. Further rotation repeats this pattern.

It is generally the case that the *anti* conformation is the more stable. However, if the two groups are not too large and can form intramolecular hydrogen bonds with one another, then the *gauche* conformation can be more stable.

Thus far we've limited our discussion of conformational isomers to molecules with unrestricted rotation around σ bonds. Let's now consider the conformational analysis of two very common cycloalkanes, cyclopentane (C_5H_{10}) and cyclohexane (C_6H_{12}).

In cyclopentane, bond angles are 108° (close to normal tetrahedral angle of 109.5 °), so we might expect cyclopentane to be a planar structure. If all of the carbons of cyclopentane were in a plane, however, all of the carbon-hydrogen σ bonds on adjacent carbons would eclipse each other. In order to lower the energy of the system, cyclopentane has one carbon out of the plane of the other carbons and so adopts a puckered conformation. This puckering allows the carbon-hydrogen σ bonds on adjacent carbons to be somewhat staggered, and thus reduces the energy of the compound. This puckered form of cyclopentane is referred to as the "envelope" form.

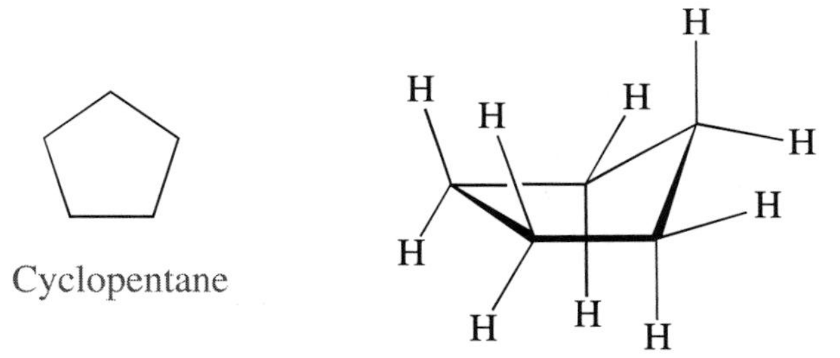

Cyclopentane

Figure 13

If cyclohexane were planar, it would have bond angles of 120°. This would produce considerable strain on sp^3 hybridized carbons as the ideal bond angle should be around 109°. Instead, the most stable conformation of cyclohexane is a very puckered molecule called the **chair form**. In the chair conformation, four of the carbons of the ring are in a plane with one carbon above the plane and one carbon below the plane. There are two chair conformations for cyclohexane, and they easily interconvert at room temperature:

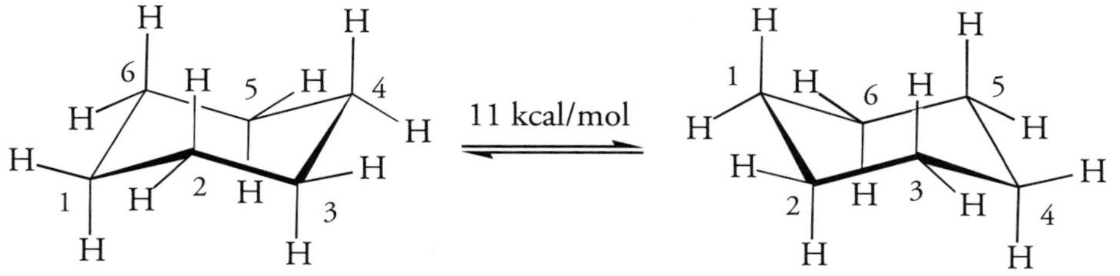

Figure 14   Chain Representations of Cyclohexane

As one chair conformation flips to the other, it must pass through several other less stable conformations including some (referred to as *half-chair* conformations) that reside at energy maxima and one (the *twist boat* conformation) at a local energy minimum (but still of much higher energy than the chair conformations). The boat conformation represents a transition state between twist boat conformations. It is important to remember, however, that all of these conformations are much more unstable than the chair conformations and thus do not play an important role in cyclohexane chemistry.

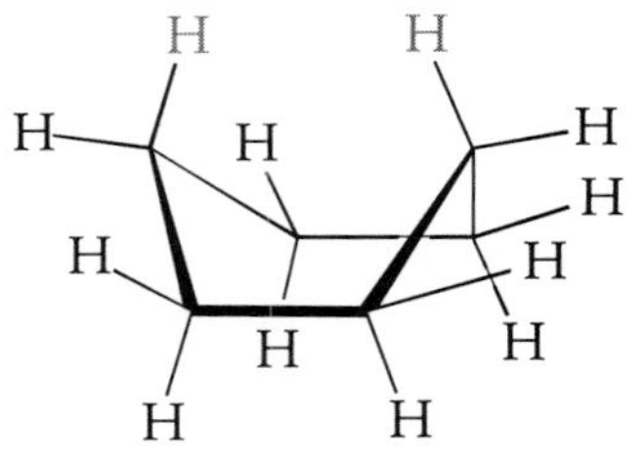

Figure 15   Boat Conformation

Notice that there are two distinct types of hydrogens in the chair forms of cyclohexane. Six of the hydrogens lie on the equator of the ring of carbons; they are in an **equatorial** position. The other six hydrogens lie above or below the ring of carbons, three above and three below; they are in an **axial** position.

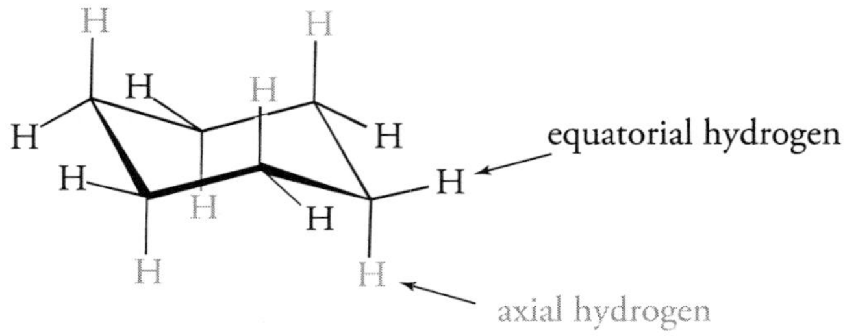

equatorial hydrogen

axial hydrogen

Figure 16

There is an energy barrier of about 11 kcal/mol between the two equivalent chair conformations of cyclohexane. At room temperature, there is sufficient thermal energy to interconvert the two chair conformations about 10,000 times per second. Note that when a hydrogen (or any substituent group) is axial in one chair conformation, it becomes equatorial when cyclohexane flips to the other chair conformation. The same is also true for an equatorial hydrogen, which flips to an axial position when the chair forms interconvert. This property is demonstrated for deuterocyclohexane:

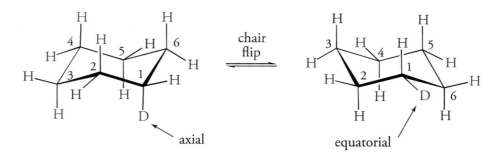

chair flip

axial

equatorial

Figure 17

These factors become important when examining substituted cyclohexanes. Let's first consider methyl-cyclohexane. The methyl group can occupy either an equatorial or axial position:

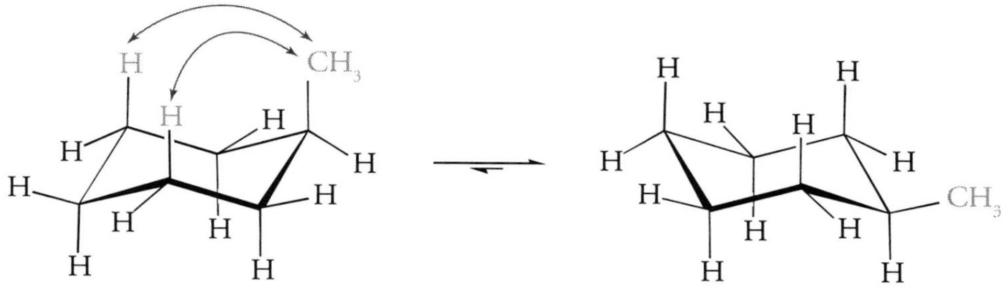

two 1,3-diaxial CH_3–H
interactions

no 1,3-diaxial CH_3–H
interactions

Figure 18

It is more favorable for large groups to occupy the equatorial position rather than a crowded axial position. For a methyl group, the equatorial position is more stable by about 1.7 kcal/mol over the axial position. This is because in the axial position, the methyl group is crowded by the other two hydrogens that are also occupying axial positions on the same side of the ring. It is more favorable for methyl to be in an equatorial position where it is pointing out, away from other atoms.

Stereoisomerism

Stereoisomerism is particularly important when looking at biological molecules, so several questions relating to stereochemistry routinely appear on the PCAT. **Stereoisomers** are molecules that have the same molecular formula and connectivity but that differ from one another only in the spatial arrangement of the atoms. They cannot be interconverted by rotation of σ bonds. For example, consider the following two molecules:

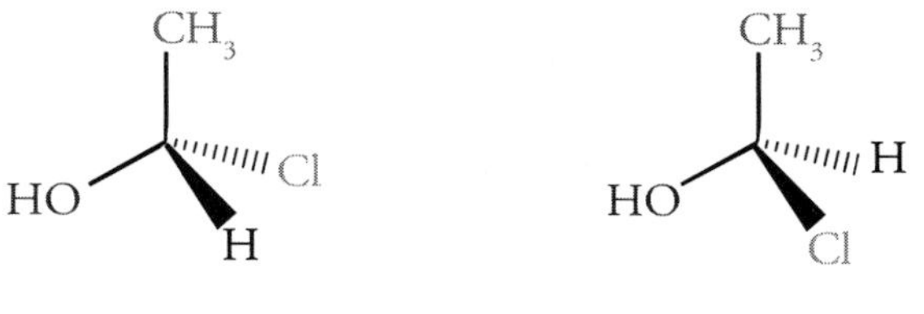

Molecule I   Molecule II

Both molecules have the same molecular formula, C_2H_5ClO, with the same atoms bonded to each other. However, if one superimposes II onto I without any rotation, the result is

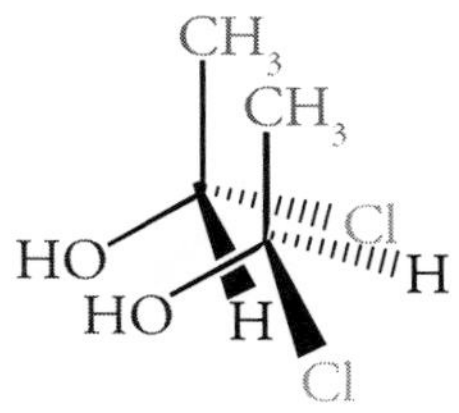

Note that while the –CH₃ and –OH groups superimpose, the –Cl and –H do not. Likewise, if we rotate Molecule II so that the –OH is pointing directly up (12 o'clock) and the –CH₃ is pointing at about 7 o'clock, and then attempt to superimpose II on I, the result is

While the –Cl and the –H groups are now superimposed, the –CH₃ and the –OH are not. No matter how Molecules I and II are rotated, two of the substituent groups will be superimposed, while the other two will not. Hence they are indeed different molecules: They are stereoisomers.

Chirality

Any molecule that cannot be superimposed on its mirror image is **chiral**, while a molecule that *can* be superimposed on its mirror image has a plane of symmetry and is said to be **achiral**. It's important that you be able to identify **chiral centers**. For carbon, a chiral center will have four different groups bonded to it and be *sp³* hybridized with (approximately) 109° bond angles and tetrahedral geometry. Such a carbon atom is also sometimes referred to as a **stereocenter**, a **stereogenic center**, or an **asymmetric center**.

Absolute Configuration

Chiral centers (carbon atoms that are *sp³* hybridized and bear four different substituents) can be assigned an **absolute configuration**. There is an arbitrary set of rules for assigning absolute configuration to a stereocenter (known as the **Cahn-Ingold-Prelog rules**), which can be illustrated using Molecule A:

Molecule A

1. Priority is assigned to the four different substituents on the chiral center according to increasing atomic number of the atoms directly attached to the chiral center. Going one atom out from the chiral center, bromine has the highest atomic number and is given highest priority, #1; oxygen is next and is therefore #2; carbon is #3, and the hydrogen is the lowest priority group, #4:

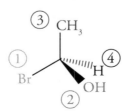

If isotopes are present, then priority among these is assigned on the basis of atomic weight with the higher priority being assigned to the heavier isotope (since they are all of the same atomic number). For example, the isotopes of hydrogen are ^{1}H, ^{2}H = D (deuterium), and ^{3}H = T (tritium), and for the following molecule, we'd assign priorities as shown:

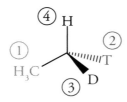

If two identical atoms are attached to a stereocenter, then the next atoms in both chains are examined until a difference is found. Once again, this is done by atomic number. Note the following example:

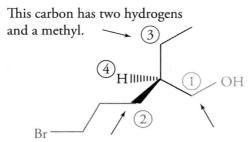

This carbon has two hydrogens and a methyl.

This carbon has two hydrogens followed by a –CH$_2$CH$_2$Br.

This carbon has two hydrogens and an –OH.

2. A multiple bond is counted as two single bonds for both of the atoms involved. For example,

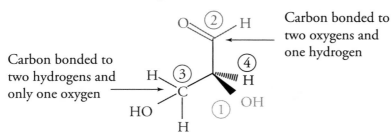

Carbon bonded to two oxygens and one hydrogen

Carbon bonded to two hydrogens and only one oxygen

3. Once priorities have been assigned, the molecule is rotated so that the lowest priority group points directly away from the viewer. A path is then traced from the highest priority group to the lowest remaining priority group. If the path traveled is *clockwise*, then the absolute configuration is **R** (from the Latin *rectus*, right). Conversely, if the path traveled is *counterclockwise*, then the absolute configuration is **S** (from the Latin *sinister*, left).

10.3

The Fischer projection is a simplification of the actual three-dimensional structure. It is a two-dimensional representation of a molecule. Vertical lines are assumed to go back into the page, and horizontal lines are assumed to come out of the page, as shown on the right in Figure 19.

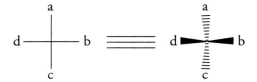

Figure 19

Enantiomers

It is important to be able to identify chiral centers because, as we have seen, when there are four different groups attached to a centralized carbon, there are two distinct arrangements or configurations possible for these groups in space. Consider the following two molecules:

Molecule A   mirror plane   Molecule B

Both have a chiral center. Molecules A and B are mirror images of each other, but they are not superimposable; therefore, they are chiral molecules.

or

These molecules are **enantiomers**: non-superimposable mirror images.

Note that two molecules that are enantiomers will always have opposite absolute configurations; for example,

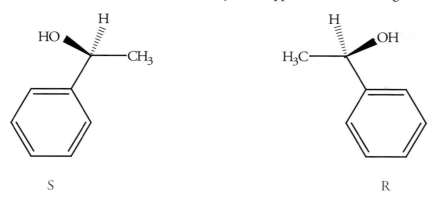

S   R

Figure 20

Physical properties such as melting point, boiling point, dipole moment, and dielectric constant are the same for both pure enantiomers of an enantiomeric pair.

Optical Activity

One important property that differs between enantiomers is the manner in which they interact with plane-polarized light. A compound that rotates the plane of polarized light is said to be **optically active**. A compound that rotates plane-polarized light clockwise is said to be **dextrorotatory** (*d*), also denoted by (+), while a compound that rotates plane-polarized light in the counterclockwise direction is said to be **levorotatory** (*l*), denoted by (−). The magnitude of rotation of plane-polarized light for any compound is called its **specific rotation**. This property is dependent on the structure of the molecule, the concentration of the sample, and the path length through which the light must travel.

A pair of enantiomers will rotate plane-polarized light with equal magnitude, but in opposite directions. For example, pure (+)-2-bromobutanoic acid has a specific rotation of +39.5°, while (−)-2-bromobutanoic acid has a specific rotation of −39.5°.

(+) and (−)-2-bromobutanoic acid

The specific rotation of a 50/50 mixture of enantiomers—a **racemic mixture**—is 0° because the rotations cancel one another. Therefore, a racemic mixture of enantiomers, also known as a *racemate*, is not optically active.

The magnitude of rotation cannot be predicted; it must be experimentally determined. In this case, the *R* enantiomer has the (+) rotation, while the *S* enantiomer has the (−) rotation. But be careful: *this is only coincidental. (+) and (−) say nothing about whether the absolute configuration is R or S.* There is no correlation between the sign of rotation and the absolute configuration.

Diastereomers

When there are multiple chiral centers, the number of possible stereoisomers is 2^n, where n is the number of chiral centers. If there is one chiral center, then there are two possible stereoisomers: the enantiomeric pair R and S. Two chiral centers means there are four possible stereoisomers. Consider the following molecule (3-bromobutan-2-ol, or 3-bromo-2-butanol), for example, where chiral centers are indicated with an asterisk:

$$Br-\overset{\overset{\displaystyle H}{|}}{\underset{\underset{\displaystyle CH_3}{|}}{C^*}}-\overset{\overset{\displaystyle H}{|}}{\underset{\underset{\displaystyle CH_3}{|}}{C^*}}-OH$$

Each of the two chiral centers can have either an R or S absolute configuration. This leads to four possible combinations of absolute configurations at the chiral centers, shown here:

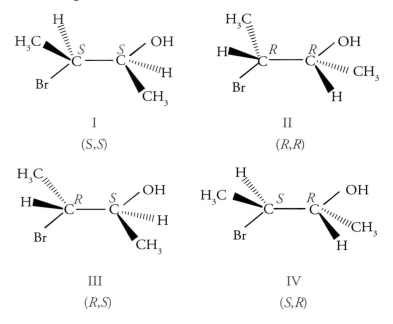

Figure 21

Each of the two chiral centers in Molecule I is of the opposite configuration of Molecule II: *S, S* vs. *R, R*. Note that they are non-superimposable mirror images:

I

II

Therefore, these molecules are enantiomers, as are Molecules III and IV. Is there a relationship between Molecules I and III?

I

III

These molecules are diastereomers. **Diastereomers** are stereoisomers that are non-superimposable, but not mirror images. The same is true for Molecules I and IV. One of the chiral centers has the same absolute configuration, while the other chiral center has the opposite configuration:

I

IV

The following figure summarizes all possible stereochemical relationships between isomers containing two stereocenters. Inverting at least one, but not all, of the chiral centers within a molecule will form a diastereomer. Enantiomers can be formed by inverting *every* stereocenter within the molecule.

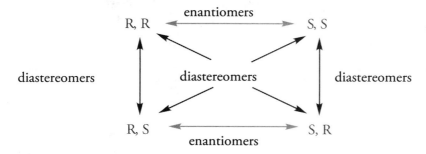

Figure 22

Racemic Mixtures

A **racemic mixture** is any 50/50 mixture of enantiomers. A polarimeter will show no rotation of polarized light because the enantiomers rotate light with equal magnitudes but in opposite directions.

Epimers

Epimers are a subclass of diastereomers that differ in their absolute configuration at a single chiral center (only *one* stereocenter is inverted). To illustrate, let's look at the Fischer projections of some sugars:

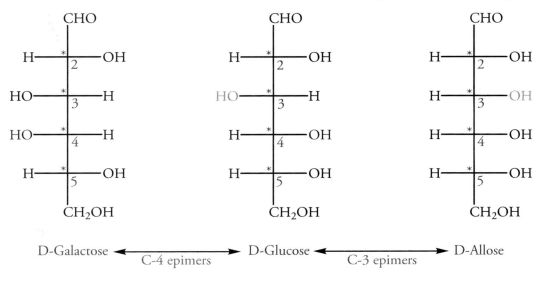

Figure 23

The prefix D on the name of these molecules refers to the orientation of the hydroxyl group (–OH) on the highest-numbered chiral center in a Fischer projection (C-5 in these cases). When the hydroxyl group is on the *right* of this carbon in the Fischer projection, the molecule is a D sugar. If the hydroxyl group is on the *left*, the molecule is an L sugar.

You must understand that D and L, like *R* and *S*, are entirely unrelated to optical activity, (+) or (–). Distinctions between D and L (or between *R* and *S*) can be made just by looking at a drawing of the molecule, but distinctions between (+) and (–) can be made only by running experiments in a polarimeter.

- *R* or *S* = absolute configuration (structure)
- D or L = relative configuration (structure)
- (+) or (–) = observed optical rotation (property)

In the structures above, D-glucose and D-galactose differ in stereochemistry at only one chiral center (C-4). Thus, they are said to be C-4 epimers, and C-4 is called the **epimeric carbon**. Likewise, D-glucose and D-allose differ in structure at a single chiral center (C-3). D-Glucose and D-allose are C-3 epimers, with C-3 being the epimeric carbon.

Notice that D-galactose and D-allose differ at two chiral centers (C-3 and C-4). At least one, but not all, of the stereocenters has been inverted. Therefore, they are diastereomers but *NOT* epimers. Note that all epimers are diastereomers, but not all diastereomers are epimers.

Anomers

Epimers that form as a result of ring closure are called **anomers**. For the PCAT, anomers will be encountered only with regard to sugar chemistry. To illustrate anomerism, consider D-glucose. Open-chain glucose exists in equilibrium with cyclic glucose, known as *glucopyranose*, where the term **pyranose** denotes a 6-membered ring. Cyclization occurs when the C-5 hydroxyl group attacks the carbonyl (C=O) carbon, C-1. This converts a carbon with three substituents to a carbon with four different substituents. Thus, a new stereocenter is formed (C-1). Because (C-1) forms a trigonal plane, it can be attacked from above or below. This gives rise to two possible forms: with the hydroxyl group *down*, it is α; with the hydroxyl group *up*, it is β. In the α position the hydroxyl group is opposite to the CH$_2$OH group on the ring structure, whereas in the β position the two groups are on the same side of the ring. It is the orientation at C-1 that distinguishes the two anomers. C-1 is known as the **anomeric center** (or **anomeric carbon**).

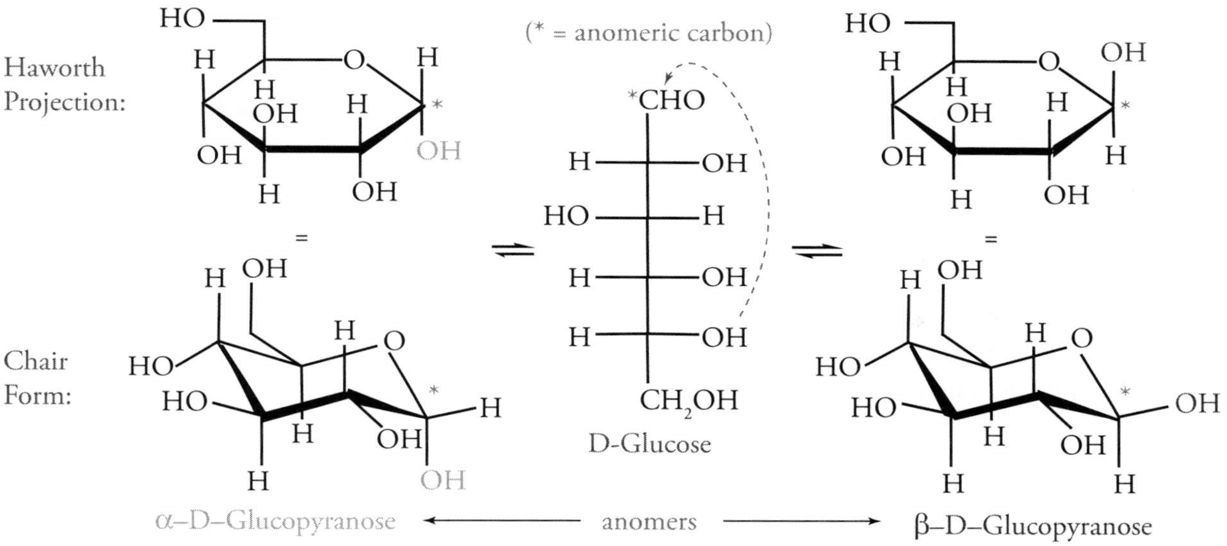

Figure 24

Meso Compounds

Let's look at another molecule with more than one stereocenter. Consider 2,3-butanediol:

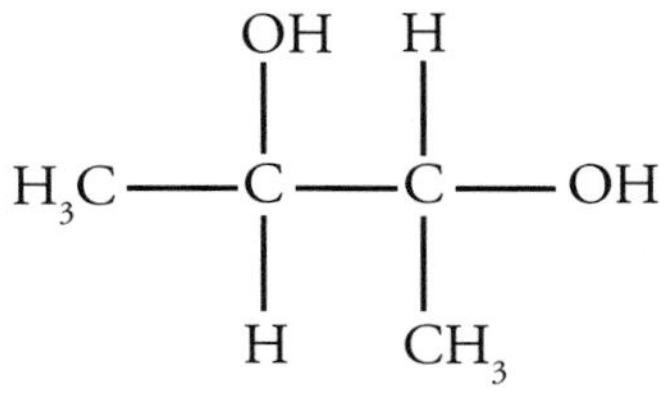

There are two chiral centers and therefore four possible stereoisomers. Notice that both chiral centers have the same groups attached to them: $-H$, $-CH_3$, $-OH$, and $-CH(OH)CH_3$. When the same four groups are attached to two chiral centers, the molecule can have an internal plane of symmetry. Consider, for example, the two stereoisomers of 2,3-butanediol:

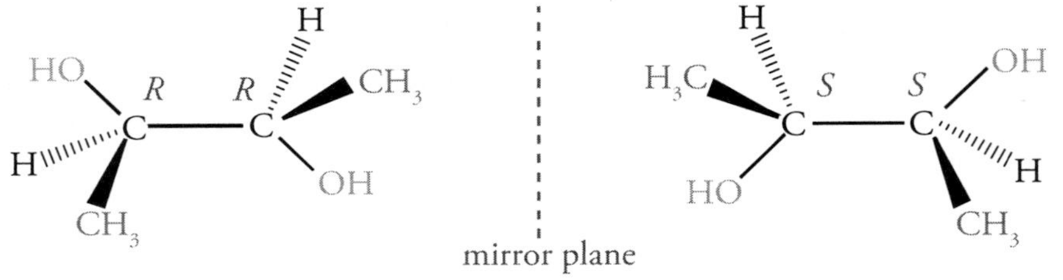

I   II

Molecules I and II are non-superimposable mirror images and therefore enantiomers. Also, neither has an internal plane of symmetry. This is demonstrated for Molecule II:

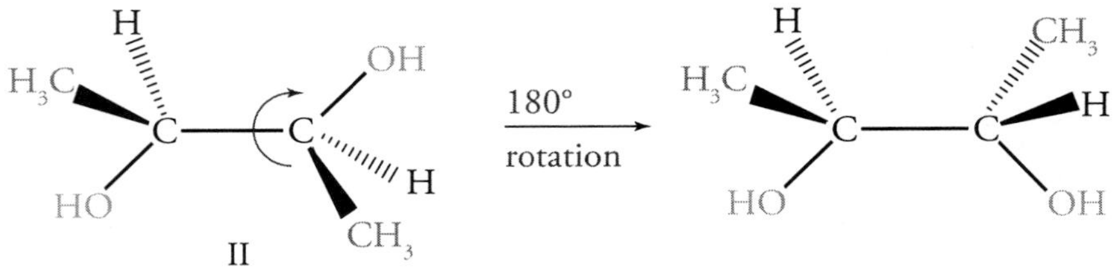

The $-OH$'s line up on the two chiral centers, but the $-CH_3$'s and $-H$'s do not. There is zero optical rotation because this is a racemic mixture.

Now look at the R, S stereoisomer and its mirror image:

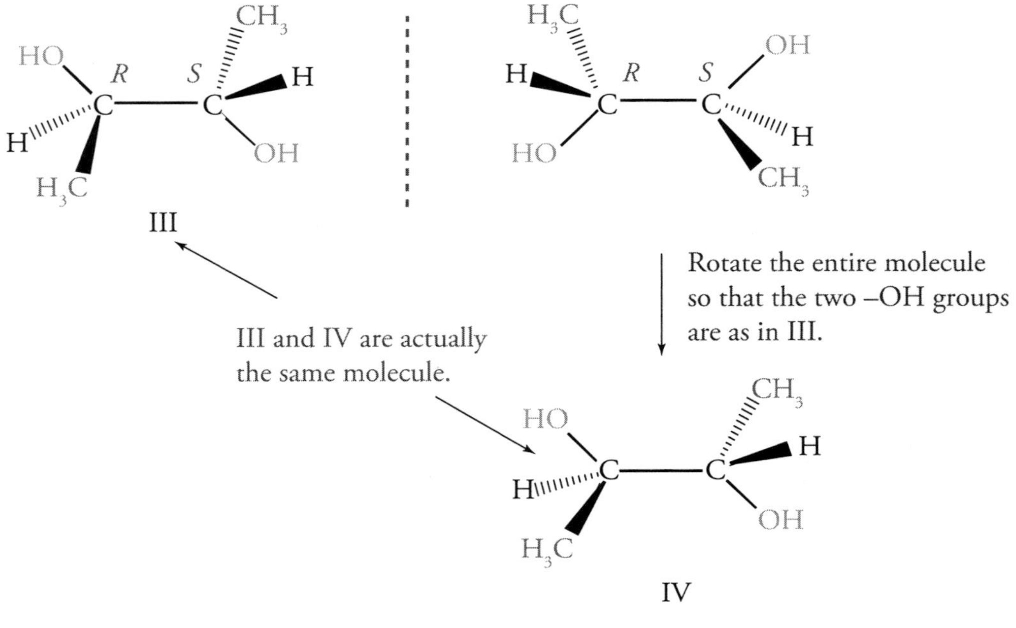

III

III and IV are actually the same molecule.

Rotate the entire molecule so that the two $-OH$ groups are as in III.

IV

Molecules III and IV are directly superimposable and therefore identical. This is because there is an internal plane of symmetry within the molecule.

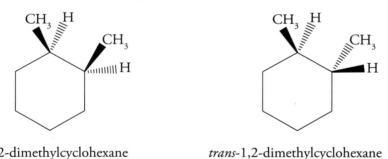

III

Rotate 180° about the C_2–C_3 σ bond →

One side of the molecule is the mirror image of the other side. This is a *meso* compound.

When there's an internal plane of symmetry in a molecule that contains chiral centers, the compound is called a **meso** compound. Actually then, 2,3-butanediol has only *three* stereoisomers, not four. Molecules I and II are enantiomers, while III and IV are the same molecule. Meso compounds are not optically active because one side of the molecule is a mirror image of the other. In a sense, the optical activity imparted by one side of the molecule is canceled by its other side.

Geometric Isomers

Geometric isomers are diastereomers that differ in the orientation of substituents around a ring or a double bond. Cyclic hydrocarbons and double bonds (alkenes) are constrained by their geometry. That is, they do not rotate freely about all bonds, so there's a difference between having substituents on the same side of the ring (or of the double bond) and having substituents on opposite sides. For example, the following are geometric isomers of 1,2-dimethylcyclohexane:

cis-1,2-dimethylcyclohexane   *trans*-1,2-dimethylcyclohexane

Figure 25

Priority of substituent groups is assigned the same way as for absolute configuration. On C-1, the methyl group is given higher priority than the H, and the same is true on C-2. The molecule in which the two higher-priority groups are on the same side is *cis*, and the molecule in which the two higher-priority groups are on opposite sides of the ring is *trans*.

For double bonds, the stereochemistry is designated by (*Z*) or (*E*). A high and low priority group are assigned at each carbon of the double bond based on atomic number, just as with absolute configuration. If the two high priority groups are on the *same* side, the configuration at the double bond is *Z* (from the German *zusammen*, meaning *together*). On the other hand, if the two high priority groups are on opposite sides of the double bond, the configuration is *E* (from the German *entgegen*, meaning *opposite*). Be aware, that the PCAT may also use the terms *cis* and *trans* when referring to double bonds. However, this is usually reserved for cases when there is one H attached to each carbon of the double bond, as shown below. The geometric isomers of 2-bromo-1-chloropropene and of 1,2-dibromoethene are shown below:

Highest priority groups (Br and Cl) on same side, so *Z*.

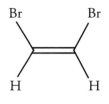

(*Z*)-2-bromo-1-chloropropene

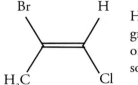

Highest priority groups (Br and Cl) on opposite side, so *E*.

(*E*)-2-bromo-1-chloropropene

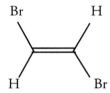

cis-1,2-dibromoethene

trans-1,2-dibromoethene

Figure 26

Summary of Isomers

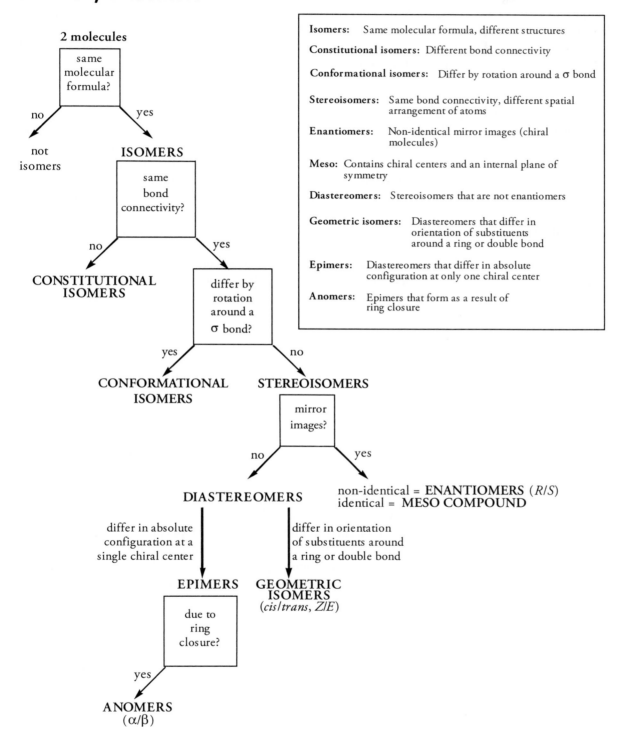

10.3

Isomers: Same molecular formula, different structures

Constitutional isomers: Different bond connectivity

Conformational isomers: Differ by rotation around a σ bond

Stereoisomers: Same bond connectivity, different spatial arrangement of atoms

Enantiomers: Non-identical mirror images (chiral molecules)

Meso: Contains chiral centers and an internal plane of symmetry

Diastereomers: Stereoisomers that are not enantiomers

Geometric isomers: Diastereomers that differ in orientation of substituents around a ring or double bond

Epimers: Diastereomers that differ in absolute configuration at only one chiral center

Anomers: Epimers that form as a result of ring closure

Figure 27

Physical Properties of Hydrocarbons

The physical properties of organic molecules that you need to know for the PCAT are **melting point**, **boiling point**, and **solubility**. For melting point and boiling point, consider the interactions between identical molecules. For solubility, we'll consider interactions between the solute (the dissolved substance) and the solvent (the dissolving liquid).

Melting and Boiling Points

Melting point (mp) and **boiling point (bp)** are indicators of how well identical molecules interact with (attract) each other. Nonpolar molecules, like hydrocarbons, interact principally because of an attractive London dispersion force, one of the intermolecular (van der Waals) forces. This force exists between temporary dipoles formed in nonpolar molecules that arise from a temporary asymmetric electron distribution. Such intermolecular forces must be overcome to melt a nonpolar compound (solid → liquid) or to boil a nonpolar compound (liquid → gas). The greater the attractive forces between molecules, the more energy will be required to overcome them. The weaker these forces, the lower the melting or boiling point.

Many factors determine the degree to which molecules of a given compound will interact. For hydrocarbons, the most significant of these factors is *branching*. Branching tends to inhibit London dispersion forces by reducing the surface area available for intermolecular interaction. Thus, it tends to reduce attractive forces between molecules, lowering both melting and boiling points. Consider the following two constitutional isomers:

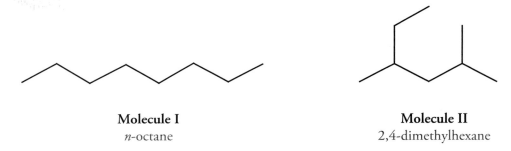

Molecule I
n-octane

Molecule II
2,4-dimethylhexane

Molecule I, *n*-octane, is unbranched. Molecule II, 2,4-dimethylhexane, is a branched isomer of *n*-octane. Although each compound has the same molecular formula, C_8H_{18}, these two constitutional isomers have dramatically different melting points and boiling points. *n*-Octane requires much more energy to melt or boil, because unbranched, it experiences greater London dispersion forces than does the branched isomer 2,4-dimethylhexane. Therefore, of the two, *n*-octane has both a higher melting point and a higher boiling point.

The second factor influencing the melting and boiling points of hydrocarbons is molecular weight. The greater the molecular weight of a compound, the more surface area there is to interact, the greater the number of van der Waals interactions, and the higher the melting point and boiling point. Therefore, hexane—a six-carbon alkane—has a higher mp and bp than propane, a three-carbon alkane.

The influence of molecular weight on melting point and boiling point is readily seen when considering the following trends for hydrocarbons:

- Small hydrocarbons (1 to 4 carbons) tend to be gases at room temperature.
- Intermediate hydrocarbons (5 to 16 carbons) tend to be liquids at room temperature.
- Large hydrocarbons (more than 16 carbons) tend to be (waxy) solids at room temperature.

Melting Point / Boiling Point Rules
1. Increasing branching decreases mp and bp.
2. Increasing molecular weight increases mp and bp.

Solubility

Solubility depends on the polarity of the solute and of the solvent. When it comes to solubility, *like dissolves like*. Polar molecules are soluble in polar solvents, and nonpolar molecules are soluble in nonpolar solvents. Long-chain hydrocarbons have either a zero or a very small dipole moment. Water, on the other hand, with its significant dipole moment, is a polar molecule. We can therefore predict that heptanoic acid, with its long saturated hydrocarbon chain, will not be very soluble in water.

10.4 MOLECULAR REACTIVITY

Several fundamental principles are needed to understand the reactivity of organic molecules. These principles are described here.

Reaction Intermediates

Most organic reactions proceed through one of the following three types of intermediate species:

1. carbocations (carbonium ions)
2. alkyl radicals
3. carbanions

Carbocations

Carbocations, or **carbonium ions**, are positively charged species with a full positive charge on carbon. The reactivity of these species is determined by the type of carbon that bears the positive charge. On the PCAT, carbocations will be sp^2 hybridized with an empty p orbital. Recall that according to VSEPR an empty orbital does not count as a group, so carbocations are planar species. Nucleophilic attack can occur from above or below the plane. This means that if the product has four different substituents on the carbon, there will be a racemic mixture.

Alkyl Radicals

Alkyl radicals are reaction intermediates that contain one unpaired electron. Even though these species are not positively charged, they are electron deficient, like carbocations. Consequently, the reactivity trends for alkyl radicals are the same as those for carbocations. Alkyl radicals on the PCAT will probably be sp^2 hybridized with the unpaired electron in an unhybridized p orbital. According to VSEPR, the molecular geometry of alkyl radicals will therefore be planar.

Carbanions

Carbanions are negatively charged species with a full negative charge localized on carbon. The reactivity of these species is determined by the type of carbon that bears the negative charge. On the PCAT, carbanions may be sp^2 hybridized with the lone pair in an unhybridized p orbital, or they may be sp^3 hybridized with the lone pair in an sp^3-hybridized orbital. Thus, carbanions can be either planar (sp^2 hybridized) or tetrahedral (sp^3 hybridized).

Stability				
Carbocations	3°	2°	1°	methyl
Alkyl Radicals	3°	2°	1°	methyl
Carbanions	methyl	1°	2°	3°
	more stable	→		less stable
	less reactive	→		more reactive
	lower energy	→		higher energy

Table 9

It's essential to understand the stabilities of reaction intermediates, because generally the major product of a reaction is derived from the most stable intermediate. Organic intermediates are stabilized in two major ways: **inductive effects** stabilize charge through σ bonds (the *sigma framework*), while **resonance effects** stabilize charge by delocalization through π bonds (the *pi framework*).

Inductive Effects

All substituent groups surrounding a reaction intermediate can generally be classified as electron-withdrawing groups or electron-donating groups. **Electron-withdrawing** groups pull electrons toward themselves through σ bonds. **Electron-donating** groups donate (push) electron density away from themselves through σ bonds. Groups *more* electronegative than carbon tend to withdraw, while groups *less* electronegative than carbon tend to donate. On the PCAT, alkyl substituents are generally considered to be electron-donating groups.

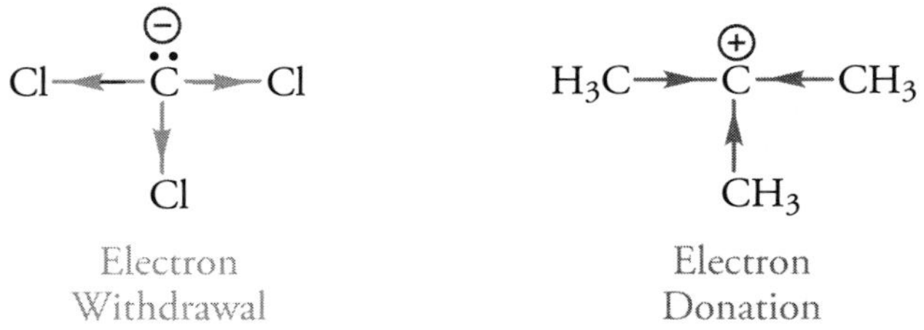

Figure 28

Electron-donating groups tend to stabilize electron-deficient intermediates (carbocations and radicals), while electron-withdrawing groups tend to stabilize electron-rich intermediates (carbanions). The stabilization of reaction intermediates by the sharing of electrons through σ bonds is called the **inductive effect**.

Resonance Stabilization

While induction works through σ bonds, resonance stabilization occurs in conjugated π systems. A **conjugated system** is one containing three or more atoms that each bear a p orbital. These orbitals are aligned so they are all parallel, creating the possibility of electron delocalization through the pi framework.

Consider the allyl cation:

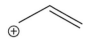

The electrons in the π bond can interact with the empty p orbital on the carbon bearing the positive charge. This is illustrated by the following resonance structures:

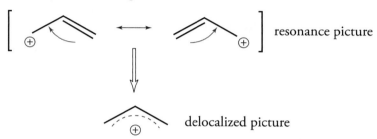

resonance picture

delocalized picture

The electron density is delocalized over the entire 3-carbon framework, which stabilizes the carbocation. In the localized structures, notice that there is a single bond (bond order = 1) and a double bond (bond order = 2). In the delocalized structure, each bond has an equivalent bond order of 1.5.

It is important to remember that resonance structures are just multiple representations of the actual structure. The molecule does not become one resonance structure or another; it exists as a combination of all resonance structures, although all may not contribute equally. All resonance structures must be drawn to give an accurate picture of the real nature of the molecule. In the case of the allyl cation, the two structures are identical and will have equivalent energy. They will also contribute equally to the delocalized picture of what the molecule really looks like. This average of all resonance contributors is called the **resonance hybrid**.

Benzene (C_6H_6) is another common molecule that exhibits resonance. Looking at a Lewis representation of benzene might lead you to believe that there are two distinct types of carbon-carbon bonds: single σ bonds (this structure of benzene has three such bonds) and double bonds (of which there are also three):

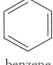

benzene

Thus, one might expect two distinct carbon-carbon bond lengths: one for the single bonds, and one for the double bonds. Yet experimental data clearly demonstrates that all the C–C bond lengths are identical in benzene. All the carbons of benzene are sp^2 hybridized, so they each have an unhybridized p orbital. Two

10.4

structures can be drawn for benzene, which differ only in the location of the π bonds. The true structure of benzene is best pictured as a resonance hybrid of these structures. Perhaps a better representation of benzene shows both resonance contributors, like this:

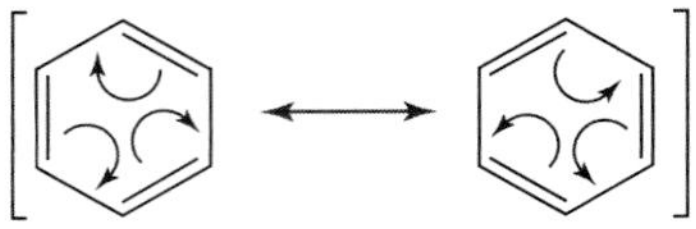

Notice that these resonance structures differ only in the arrangement of their π electrons, not in the locations of the atoms. All six unhybridized *p* orbitals are aligned parallel with one another. This alignment of adjacent unhybridized *p* orbitals allows for delocalization of π electrons over the entire ring. Whenever we have a delocalized π system, resonance structures can be drawn.

1. Resonance structures usually involve electrons that are adjacent to a π bond or an unhybridized *p* orbital. Here are some examples of molecules that are stabilized by resonance delocalization:

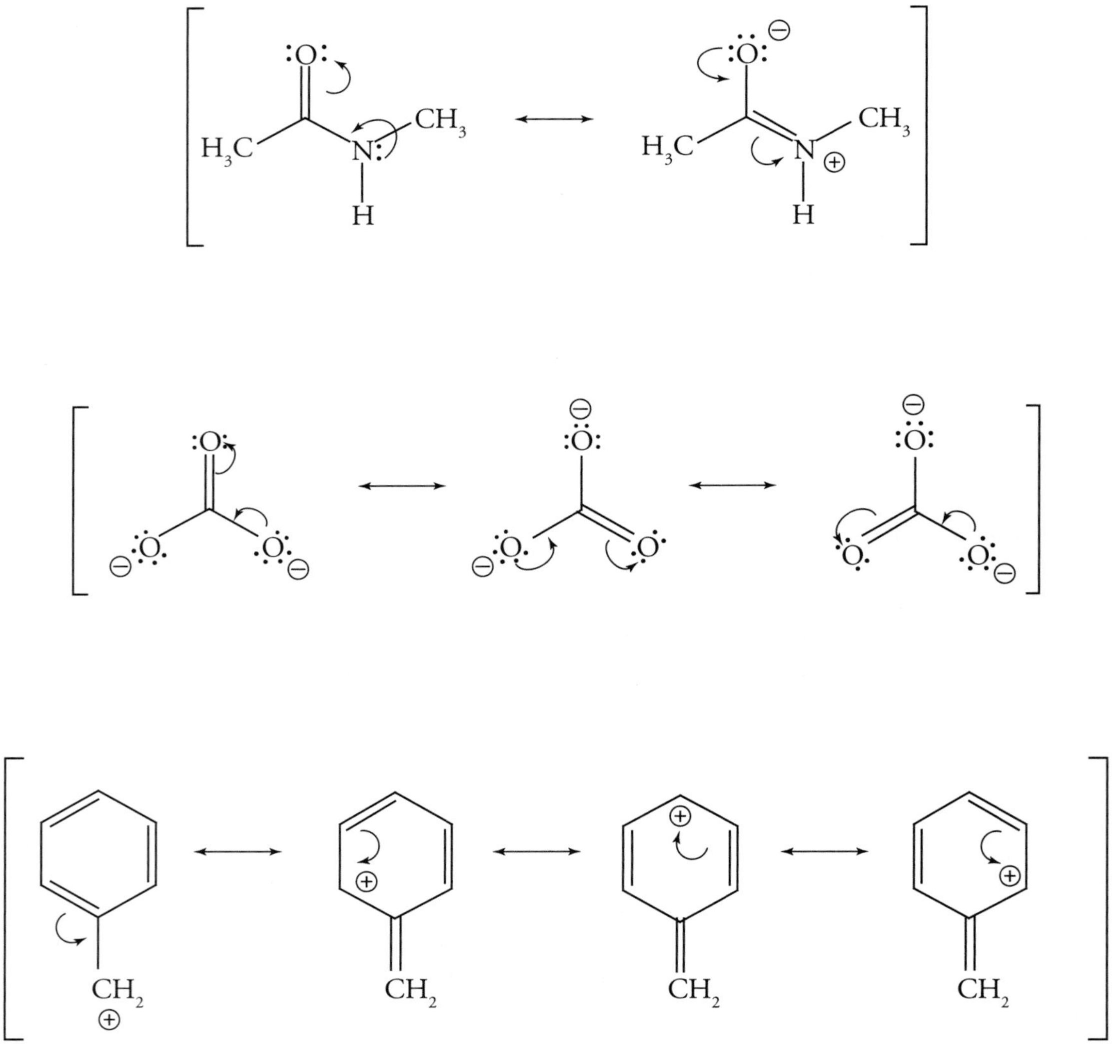

Figure 29

2. The evaluation of resonance structures involves primarily three criteria:
    (i) Resonance contributors in which the octet rule is satisfied, as it should be for all atoms, are more important than ones in which it is not.
    (ii) Resonance contributors that minimize separation of charge are better than those with a large separation of charge.
    (iii) In structures that have separation of charge, the more important resonance contributor has the negative charge on the more electronegative atom, and the positive charge on the less electronegative atom.
3. Resonance occurs through the pi framework of adjacent atoms, so resonance structures can never be drawn through atoms that are truly sp^3 hybridized.

| No resonance structures possible! | No resonance structures are possible with these electrons. | No resonance structures are possible with these electrons. |

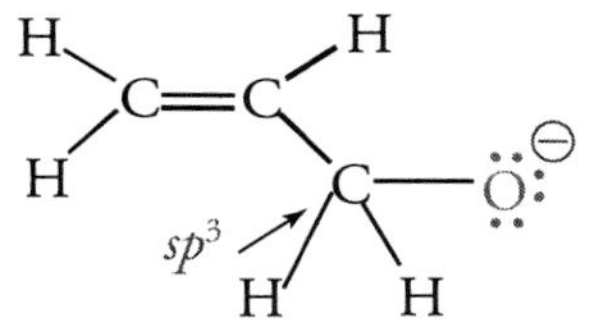

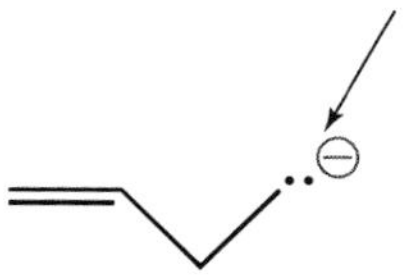

Resonance can affect the acidity of functional groups. Recall that a Brønsted-Lowry acid is a molecule that donates a proton (H^+). Since H^+ is donated, it is usually the case that the atom which donates the proton takes on a negative charge. The extent to which that negative charge is stabilized determines the relative acidity of the compound. Consider these examples:

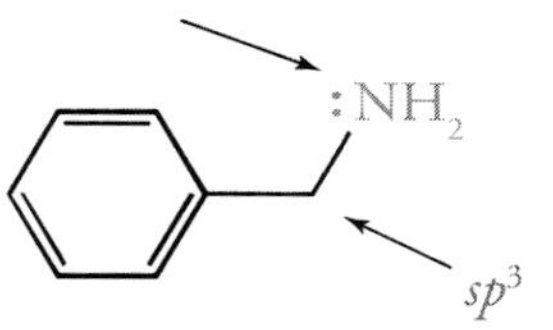

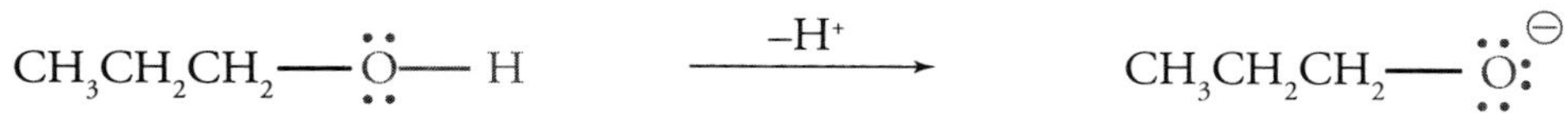

an alcohol $\xrightarrow{-H^+}$ *an alkoxide ion*

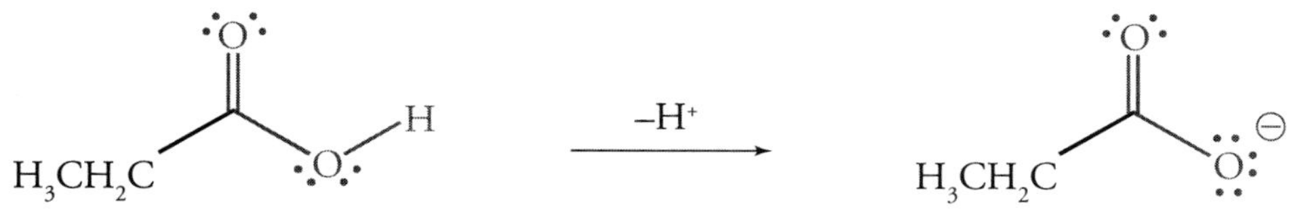

a carboxylic acid $\xrightarrow{-H^+}$ *a carboxylate ion*

an alkoxide ion

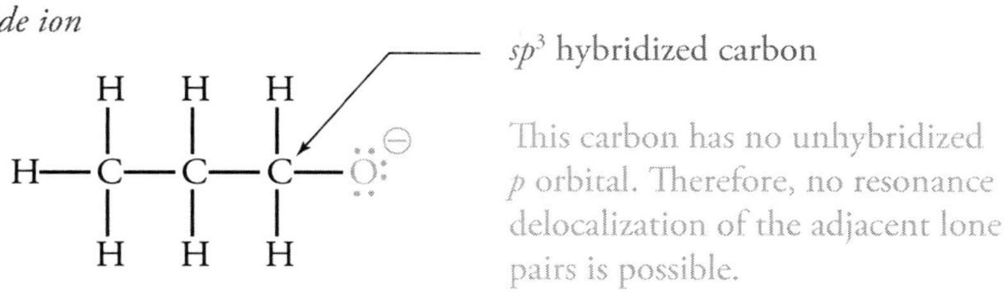

sp^3 hybridized carbon

This carbon has no unhybridized p orbital. Therefore, no resonance delocalization of the adjacent lone pairs is possible.

n-Propoxide

Figure 30

10.4

The electrons on the oxygen in the alkoxide ion above have no adjacent empty p orbital or π system. Therefore, the negative charge is localized and the molecule is highly reactive. This makes the alkoxide ion a very strong base (much like OH^-).

In the carboxylate ion, the electrons on the negatively charged oxygen are adjacent to a π bond and can therefore be delocalized. The carboxylate anion is resonance stabilized, which makes the carboxylic acid, the conjugate acid of the carboxylate anion, a stronger acid than it would be without resonance stabilization of the anion because of the higher tendency to lose its proton. (*Note:* These two resonance structures are identical and therefore of equal energy.)

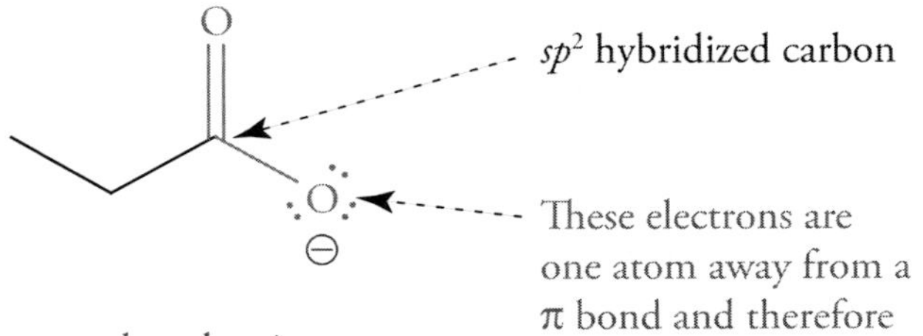

sp² hybridized carbon

These electrons are one atom away from a π bond and therefore can be delocalized.

a carboxylate ion

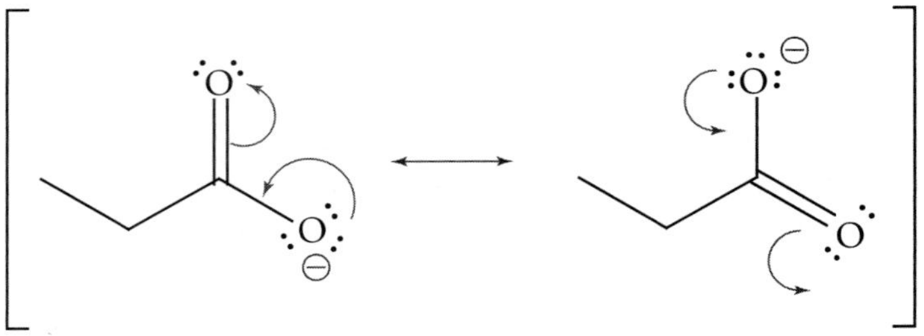

resonance structures for carboxylate ion

Let's examine the resonance structures for the phenoxide and the acetate ions:

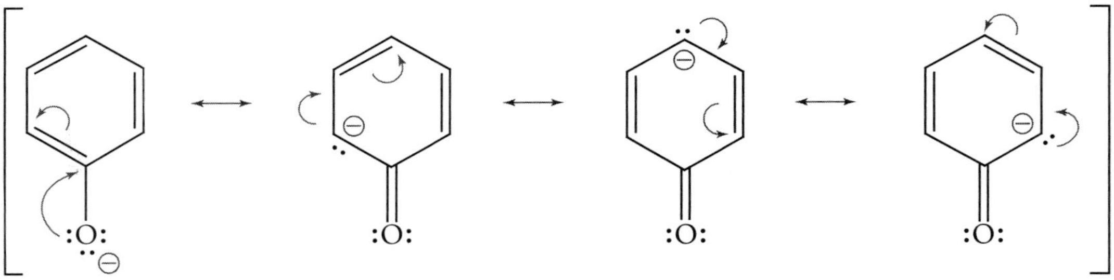

resonance structures for
the phenoxide ion

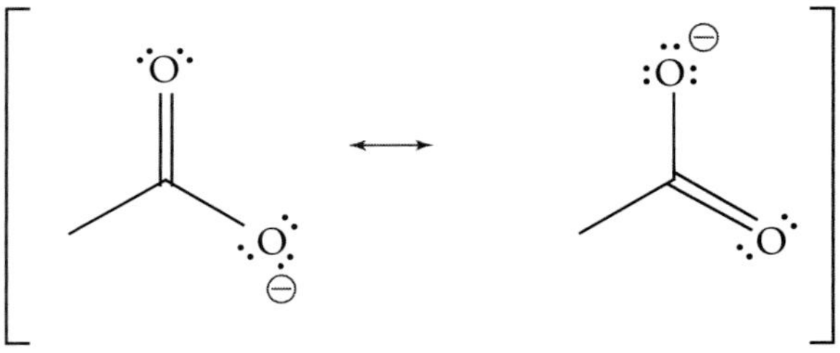

resonance structures for
the acetate ion

The resonance structures for the acetate ion are of equivalent energy with the negative charge on the electronegative oxygen. In examining the resonance structures for the phenoxide ion, notice that although there are four resonance structures, three of them have the negative charge on carbon rather than on the electronegative oxygen. Moreover, the three phenoxide resonance structures with a negative charge on carbon disrupt the aromaticity of the aromatic ring. Thus, the acetate ion is the more resonance stabilized, which makes acetic acid the stronger acid. The acidity of carboxylic acids is discussed further in section 10.9.

10.4

Ring Strain

The last item in our toolbox is **ring strain,** a feature of organic molecules that, unlike inductive and resonance effects, contributes to instability in a molecule. Ring strain arises when bond angles between ring atoms deviate from the ideal angle predicted by the hybridization of the atoms. Let's examine several cycloalkanes in turn.

Cyclopropane (C_3H_6) is very strained because the carbon-carbon bond angles are 60° rather than the idealized 109° for sp^3 hybridized carbons. Because of its instability, it reacts with H_2 to form propane. Similarly, cyclobutane undergoes hydrogenation to form butane.

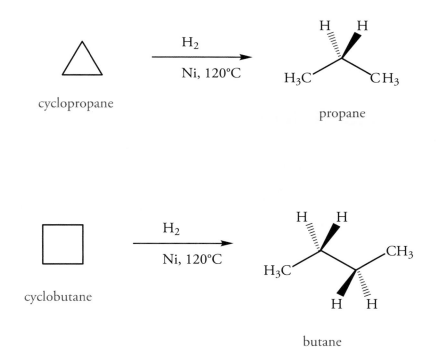

Figure 31

Unlike cyclopropane and cyclobutane, cyclopentane has a low degree of ring strain, and cyclohexane is strain free. Both molecules have near-tetrahedral bond angles due to the conformations they adopt. Consequently, these cycloalkanes do not undergo hydrogenation reactions under normal conditions, and react similarly to straight chain alkanes.

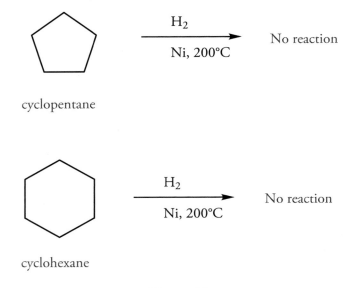

Figure 32

10.5 CLASSIFICATION OF COMMON REACTIONS

Free Radical Halogenation

The most important reaction of alkanes on the PCAT is **free-radical halogenation,** a reaction that proceeds by a multistep mechanism that includes **initiation**, **propagation**, and **termination** (and is often subject to **inhibition** by molecular oxygen).

Initiation

A free radical reaction can be initiated by light or heat. In a light-initiated reaction, a photon $(E = hf)$ typically interacts with a molecular halogen such as Cl_2 or Br_2, causing homolytic cleavage of a bond. This results in the formation of two halogen radicals.

Homolytic Cleavage: One electron goes with each atom of the bond being broken. This produces two radicals.

$$X-X \xrightarrow{hf} X\cdot \ + \ \cdot X$$

Propagation

For every halogen radical formed in the initiation step, about 10,000 alkyl halide molecules are formed in the propagation steps of this chain reaction. First, a halogen radical collides with an alkane molecule (R—H) causing homolytic cleavage of a C—H bond with formation of a molecule of hydrogen halide (H—X) and an alkyl radical (R·).

In the next step, the alkyl halide product is formed. This is accomplished by the collision of an alkyl radical (R·) with molecular halogen (X—X). This collision results in the homolytic cleavage of the molecular halogen so that a molecule of alkyl halide (R—X) product is formed and a halogen radical (X·) is regenerated.

$$R\text{—}H \ + \ ·X \longrightarrow R· \ + \ H\text{—}X$$

$$R· \ + \ X\text{—}X \longrightarrow R\text{—}X \ + \ ·X$$

The halogen radical then proceeds to collide with another alkane molecule, continuing the propagation of the chain reaction. Therefore, one halogen radical is able to lead to the production of many alkyl halide products since the halogen radical is always regenerated in the process.

Termination

Eventually, one of the radicals of the propagation steps reacts with another radical, terminating the chain reaction as shown here:

$$X· \ + \ ·X \rightarrow X\text{—}X$$

$$R· \ + \ ·R \rightarrow R\text{—}R$$

$$R· \ + \ ·X \rightarrow R\text{—}X$$

Inhibition

The free-radical halogenation reaction is inhibited by molecular oxygen. This occurs when an alkyl radical reacts with a molecule of molecular oxygen to form a less reactive alkyl peroxy radical (R—O—O·). The reaction slows down because the concentration of the more reactive alkyl radical intermediate is reduced.

$$R· \ + \ O\text{=}O \ \rightleftharpoons \ R\text{—}O\text{—}O·$$

Stereochemistry of Free-Radical Halogenation

As the hydrogen radical is abstracted during free-radical halogenation, the resulting carbon radical rehybridizes to place the single electron in an unhybridized p orbital. The geometry is planar with 120° bond angles. The lone electron resides above and below the plane of the molecule in the unhybridized orbital.

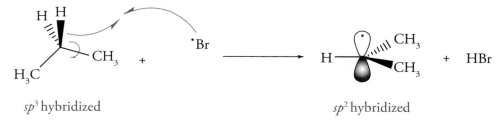

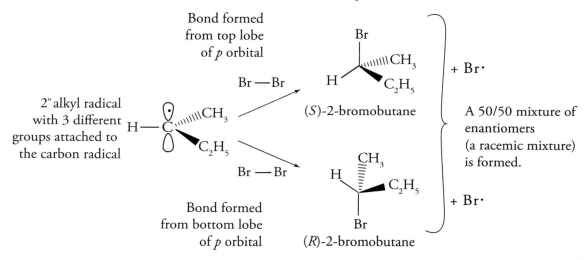

Figure 33

When the alkyl radical then reacts with a molecule of molecular halogen in the next step of the reaction, the carbon-halogen bond can form on either side of the plane defined by the sp^2 hybridized atom. Racemization can result since attack can occur on either side of the plane:

Figure 34

Stability of Alkyl Radicals

Next we examine the relative stability of carbon alkyl radicals. Free radicals are like carbocations in the sense that they have an unfilled p orbital (one electron for a radical versus zero electrons for a carbocation). Also, like carbocations, alkyl substituents on carbon increase the relative stability of the radical.

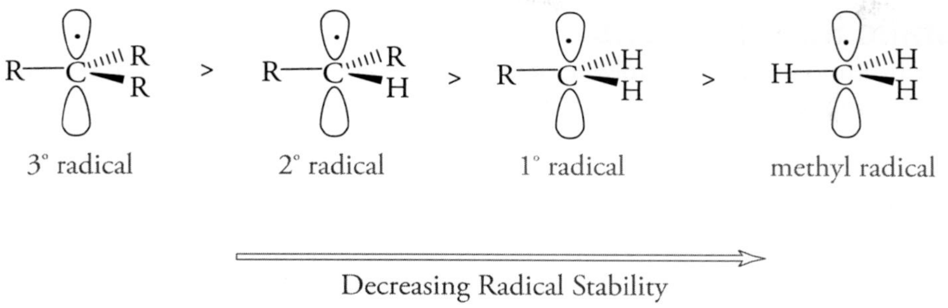

3° radical > 2° radical > 1° radical > methyl radical

Decreasing Radical Stability

Figure 35

Bromination of alkanes is much more selective than chlorination, as demonstrated in the following table.

Reaction Rate

	R_3CH (3°)		R_2CH_2 (2°)		RCH_3 (1°)
Bromination:	1,640.0	>	82.0	>	1
Chlorination:	5.3		3.9		1

The reason for the lower selectivity in the chlorination of an alkane is that the reaction is more exothermic than the corresponding bromination reaction. In the bromine case, only one of the two propagation steps is exothermic (the other is endothermic). For this reason, bromination is slower and more selective than chlorination.

Propagation Steps of Radical Bromination of Methane

Step	ΔH (kcal/mol)
$CH_4 + Br^{\cdot} \rightarrow CH_3^{\cdot} + HBr$	+18
$CH_3^{\cdot} + Br_2 \rightarrow CH_3Br + Br^{\cdot}$	-25

From the enthalpy values in the table above, fluorine should be a very unselective reagent. This is, in fact, experimentally observed.

Nucleophilic Substitutions

Nucleophilic substitution reactions involve a leaving group and a nucleophile. We begin this discussion by looking at the two types of molecules involved in all nucleophilic substitution reactions.

Nucleophiles and Electrophiles

Most organic reactions occur between nucleophiles and electrophiles. **Nucleophiles** are electron pair donors; they are also Lewis bases. Here are some common examples of nucleophiles:

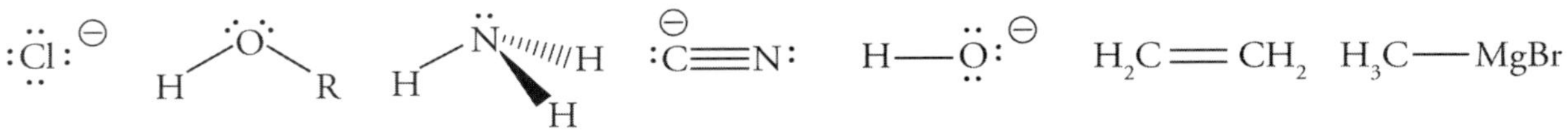

The relative strengths of nucleophiles follow these patterns:

1. **Nucleophilicity increases as negative charge increases.** For example, NH_2^-, a very strong base, is more nucleophilic than NH_3, a far weaker base.
2. **Nucleophilicity increases going down the periodic table within a particular group.** For example, $F^- < Cl^- < Br^- < I^-$.
3. **Nucleophilicity increases going left in the periodic table across a particular period.** For example, NH_2^- is more nucleophilic than OH^-.

Trend #2 is directly related to a periodic trend introduced in general chemistry: **polarizability**. As you go down any group in the periodic table, atoms become larger and generally more polarizable and more nucleophilic.

Trend #3 is related to the electronegativity of the nucleophilic atom. The less electronegative the atom in a given row, the higher its nucleophilicity.

Electrophiles are electron-deficient species or have strong positive dipoles, and therefore are Lewis acids. Here are some common examples of electrophiles:

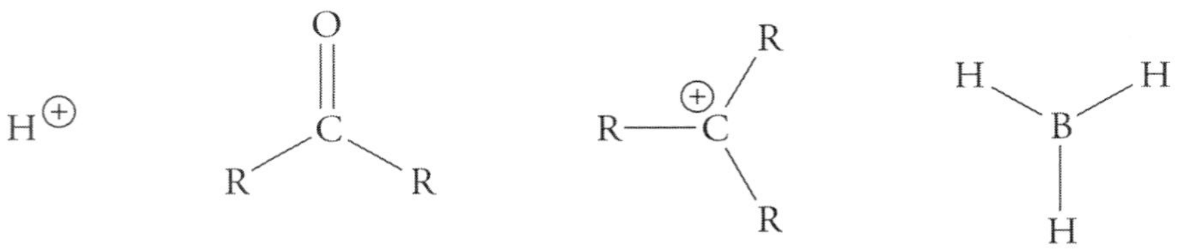

Reactions occur when a nucleophile reacts with an electrophile. A new covalent bond forms between the two species, as shown here. Notice that the arrow is drawn from the nucleophile to the electrophile.

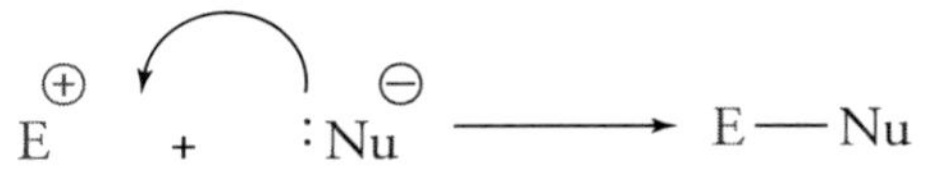

Substitution Reactions: S$_N$1 and S$_N$2

The S$_N$1 Mechanism

Over the course of S$_N$1 substitution reactions, a carbocation (carbonium ion) forms. Here the "1" indicates a unimolecular process. For alkyl cations, the relative stabilities are given below.

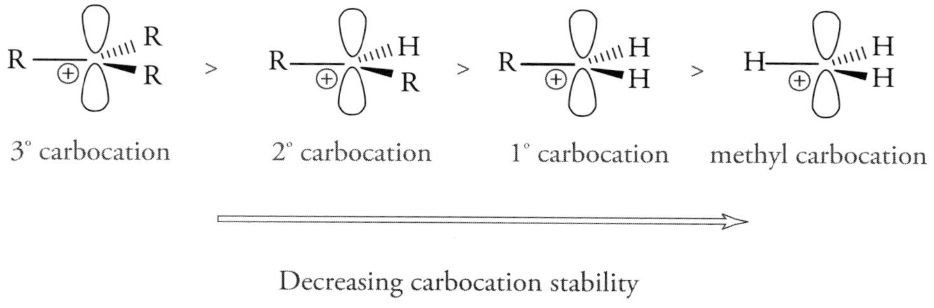

3° carbocation   2° carbocation   1° carbocation   methyl carbocation

Decreasing carbocation stability

Figure 36

The order of stabilities is associated with the electron-donating ability of alkyl groups, which stabilize the positive charge.

When (R)-3-bromo-3-methylhexane is treated with H$_2$O, a racemic mixture of 3-methylhexan-3-ol is formed:

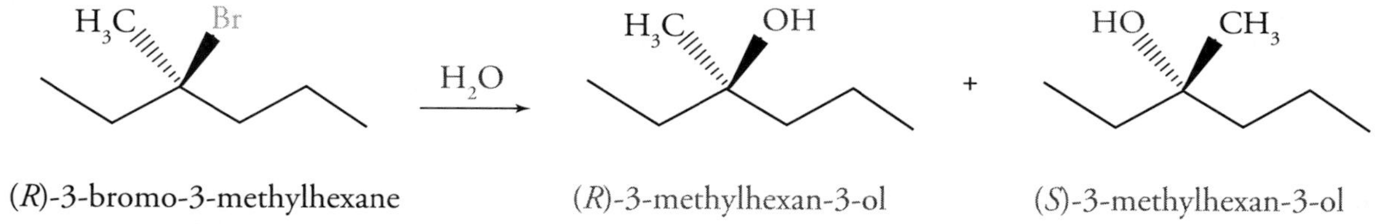

(R)-3-bromo-3-methylhexane   (R)-3-methylhexan-3-ol   (S)-3-methylhexan-3-ol

Figure 37

S$_N$1 substitution occurs in *two distinct steps*. In the first step of the S$_N$1 reaction, a *planar carbocation* with 120° bond angles forms. This is the slow step of the mechanism, or the rate limiting step. In the final step of this reaction, *racemization* occurs as the nucleophile attacks equally *on either side* of the carbocation. The result is a racemic mixture.

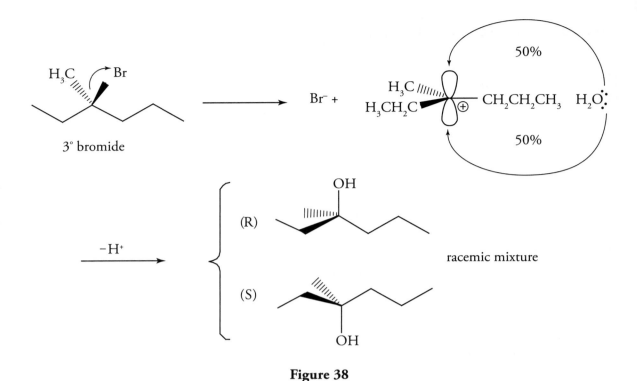

Figure 38

The rate of the S_N1 reaction depends only on the concentration of the electrophile (the species that dissociates). The rate of the reaction is equal to the product of the rate constant (k), and the electrophile concentration ([R-Br]):

$$\text{reaction rate} = k[\text{electrophile}]$$

Since the dissociation of the leaving group is the slow step of the mechanism, anything that makes that step more favorable will speed up the reaction. The more substituted the carbocation intermediate, the more stable it, so carbocation rearrangements can occur. Keep in mind that, more substituted substrates will dissociate to make more stable intermediates faster, speeding up the rate of the entire reaction.

To favor an S_N1 mechanism, strongly protic solvents such as water and alcohols should be used. The role of the solvent is twofold. The protic solvent helps to stabilize the carbocation and solvate the leaving group, thereby facilitating the first, or slow, step of the mechanism. Secondly, the solvent then behaves as the nucleophile in a **solvolysis** reaction, attacking the carbocation intermediate. This produces an alcohol if water is used as the solvent and an ether if the solvent is an alcohol. This reaction favors a weak nucleophile because the attack is occurring at a strongly reactive carbocation.

Key Features of an S$_N$1 Reaction

Reactivity of substrate:	3° > 2° >> 1° (Due to stabilization of the carbocation)
Stereochemistry:	Almost complete racemization due to nucleophilic attack on either side of a p orbital
Kinetics:	reaction rate = k[electrophile]
Solvent:	S$_N$1 reactions are favored by protic solvents.
Rearrangements:	Carbocation rearrangement is possible.
Favoring conditions:	Non-basic, weaker nucleophiles

The S$_N$2 Mechanism

Let us first consider an example of an S$_N$2 substitution reaction of an alkyl halide, where the "2" indicates a bimolecular process. When 1-iodobutane is treated with a Br$^-$ nucleophile, bromide replaces the I$^-$ group (the *leaving group*) to yield 1-bromobutane.

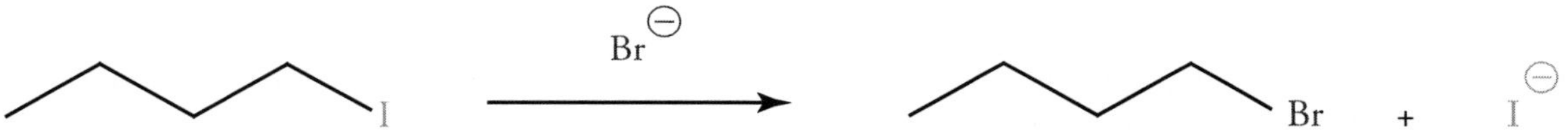

1-iodobutane

1-bromobutane

The nucleophilic bromide anion attacks the electrophilic carbon at the *same time* that the leaving group leaves in a concerted reaction. The attack must occur *from the backside* of the substrate.

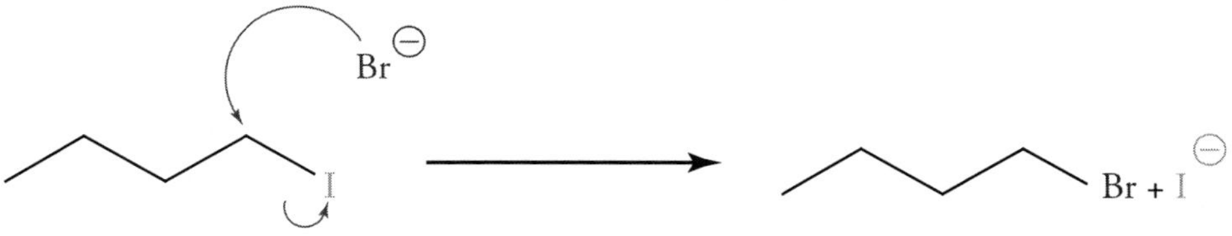

The reaction proceeds through a *pentavalent transition state.* As you can see in Figure 39, there is complete *inversion of configuration* at the carbon being attacked by the nucleophile. This is always the case in an S$_N$2 reaction, here shown on a chiral substrate. Notice that S$_N$2 substitution occurs in one step, unlike S$_N$1 reactions that occur in two steps.

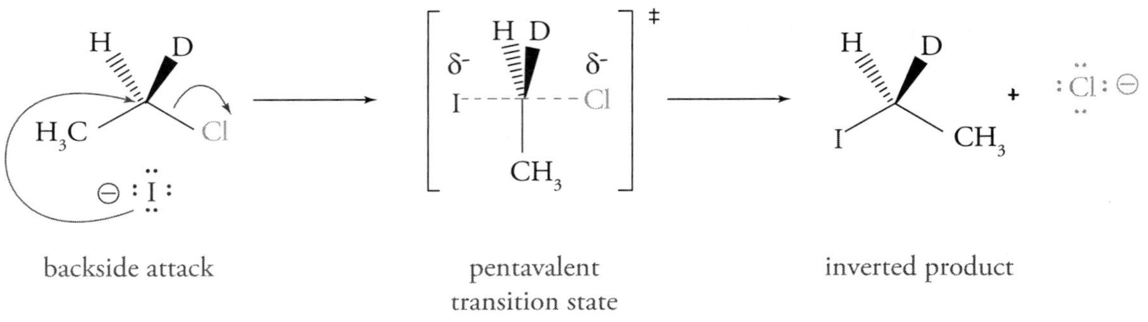

backside attack   pentavalent transition state   inverted product

Figure 39

The rate of the reaction depends on the concentrations of both the nucleophile and the electrophile, and is equal to the product of the rate constant (k), the concentration of the nucleophile ($[I^-]$), and the concentration of the electrophile ($[R\text{-}Cl]$).

$$\text{reaction rate} = k[\text{nucleophile}][\text{electrophile}]$$

Since the transition state is sterically crowded with five groups attached, the bulkier the group, the harder it is for the nucleophile to gain access to the reactive site. Therefore, less substituted substrates react faster than more substituted ones.

To favor an S_N2 mechanism, strongly polar solvents should be avoided. They solvate the nucleophile, hindering the backside attack needed for the concerted reaction to occur. To prevent this interference, polar, *aprotic* solvents such as acetone, DMF (dimethylformamide), or DMSO (dimethylsulfoxide) should be used. Their polar nature allows the charged nucleophiles and leaving groups to remain dissolved, but they are not as efficient at completely solvating the nucleophile.

Key Features of an S_N2 Reaction

Reactivity of substrate:	$CH_3 > 1° > 2° \gg 3°$ (Because of steric hindrance)
Stereochemistry:	Complete stereochemical inversion of the carbon that is attacked by the nucleophile
Kinetics:	reaction rate = $k[\text{nucleophile}][\text{electrophile}]$
Solvent:	S_N2 reactions are favored by polar, aprotic solvents.
Rearrangements:	Not possible due to the concerted mechanism
Favoring Conditions:	Strong, non-bulky nucleophiles

Alcohols undergo substitution reactions just as alkyl halides do. They can undergo either S_N1 or S_N2 reactions depending upon the degree of substitution of the alcohol. Alcohols are treated with strong acids to protonate the –OH and convert it into a good leaving group (H_2O). In S_N2 reactions, the base will attack while the leaving group dissociates. In S_N1 reactions, the water will first dissociate, followed by nucleophilic attack of the halide ion on the carbocation intermediate.

Substitution Reactions with Other Functional Groups

Ethers

Ethers are weak Lewis bases that are generally quite chemically unreactive in the absence of strong acids. In the presence of a strong acid, the acid protonates the oxygen of the ether, converting a poor leaving group into a good leaving group.

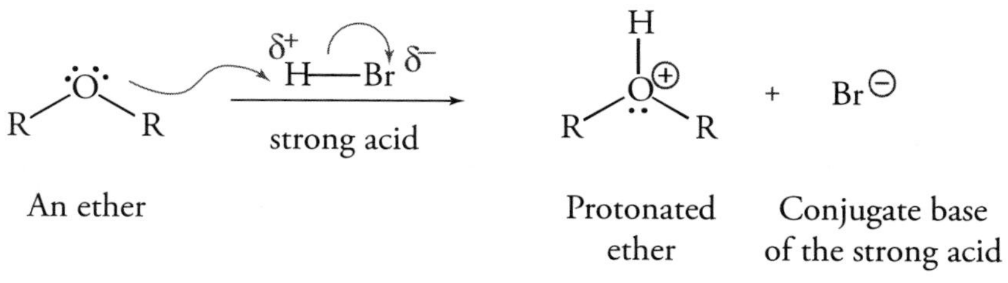

An ether   Protonated   Conjugate base
                   ether   of the strong acid

Figure 40

The reaction can proceed by either an S_N1 or S_N2 mechanism, where the halide (X^-) from the acid acts as the nucleophile. The ether cleavage reaction ultimately yields two molecules of haloalkane.

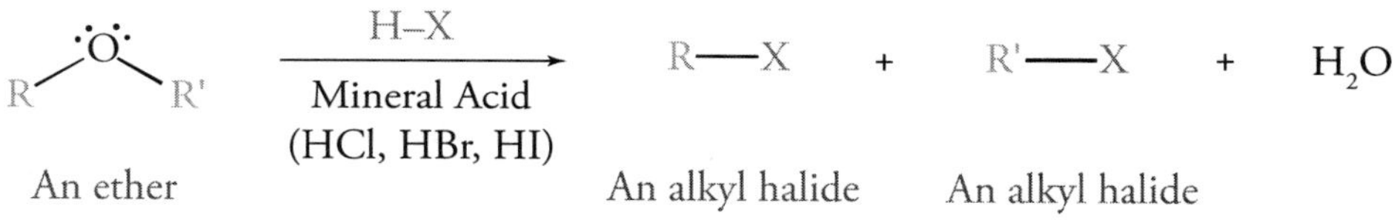

An ether   An alkyl halide   An alkyl halide

Figure 41

Alkylation

In this S_N2 substitution reaction, the lone pair of electrons on the nitrogen of an alkyl amine attacks the electrophilic, sterically-unhindered carbon atom of methyl iodide, as shown in Figure 42. The primary amine, methylamine with one alkyl group, first reacts with methyl iodide, to form a 2° amine, with two alkyl groups. The 2° amine then reacts with another molecule of methyl iodide to form a 3° amine, with three alkyl groups. Finally, the 3° amine reacts with yet another molecule of methyl iodide to yield a quaternary ammonium ion with four alkyl groups.

Notice that the quaternary ammonium ion no longer has a lone electron pair and can no longer act as a nucleophile.

10.5

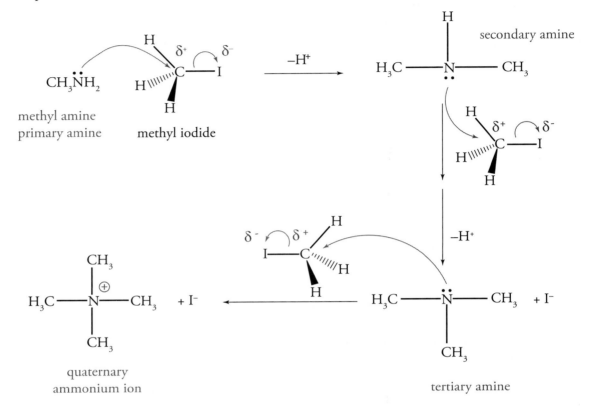

Figure 42

Elimination Reactions

Elimination reactions are defined by the bonding changes that occur over the course of a reaction. In an elimination reaction, two σ bonds in the starting material are converted into a π bond in the product. Notice that this is the reverse pathway of an addition reaction.

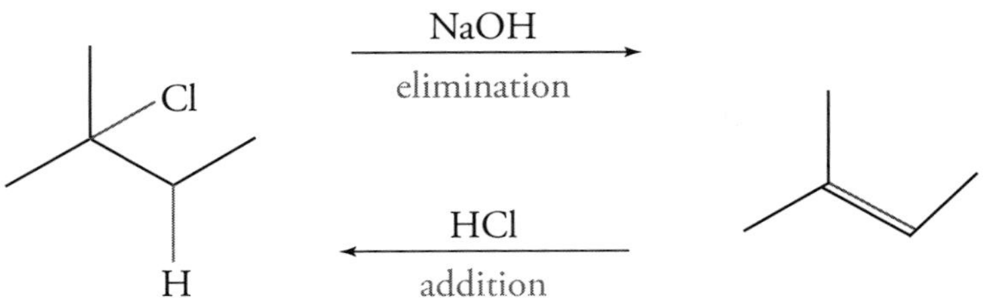

Figure 43

In the example above, the two σ bonds in the starting material that are broken are the C—Cl and the adjacent C—H bond. The π bond that forms in the product is the C=C double bond.

The E1 Mechanism

Like substitution, elimination can be either a unimolecular (E1) or a bimolecular (E2) process. E1 elimination, like S_N1 substitution, occurs via a 2-step mechanism.

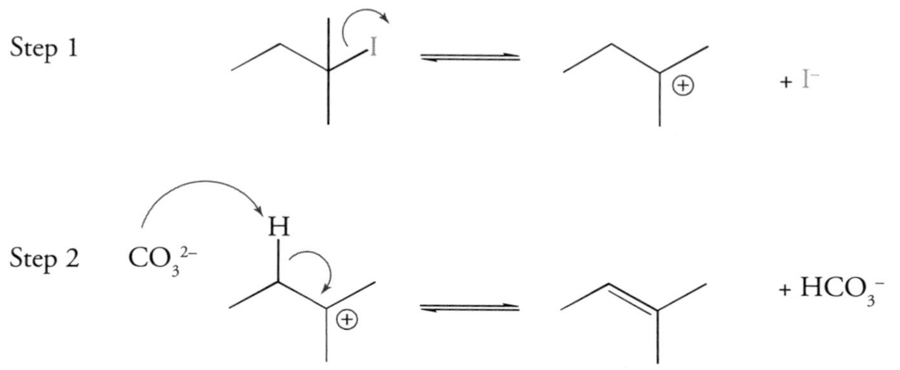

Step 1

Step 2 $CO_3{}^{2-}$

Figure 44

In step 1, iodide is a good leaving group (it is a very weak base), leaving behind a carbocation. A weak base then removes a proton on the adjacent carbon, and the electrons form a C=C double bond.

The positive charge is stabilized in the order 3° > 2° > 1°. Furthermore, in the E1 mechanism, the overall rate of the reaction is proportional only to the concentration of the substrate: rate = k[R-LG], where R represents the hydrocarbon substituent. It's important to note that the base must remove a proton that is adjacent to the leaving group for elimination to proceed.

Dehydration reactions of alcohols involve the loss of a molecule of water to form an alkene. This reaction requires a strong acid and is favored by high temperatures. Dehydration of alcohols is simply the reverse of acid-catalyzed hydration of alkenes, and is an example of an E1 mechanism. Let's investigate this reaction by looking at the dehydration of *tert*-butanol under anhydrous conditions.

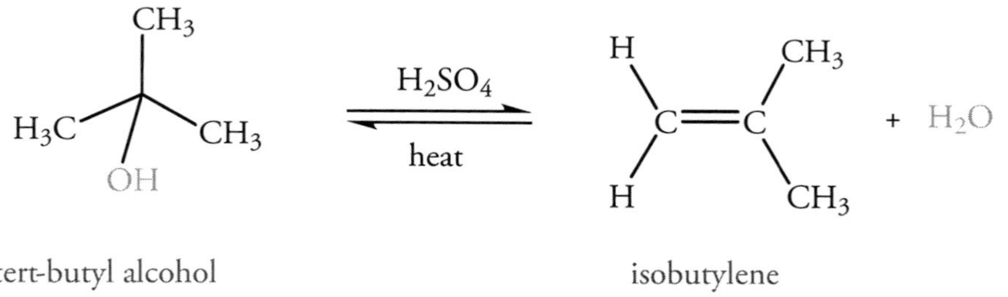

tert-butyl alcohol   isobutylene

In the first step of this reaction, protonation of the oxygen converts a poor leaving group (–OH) into a good leaving group (H_2O), and a carbocation is formed. The mechanism is completed when the conjugate base of the acid removes a proton from a carbon atom adjacent to the carbocation. The electrons from the C—H bond form a carbon-carbon π bond.

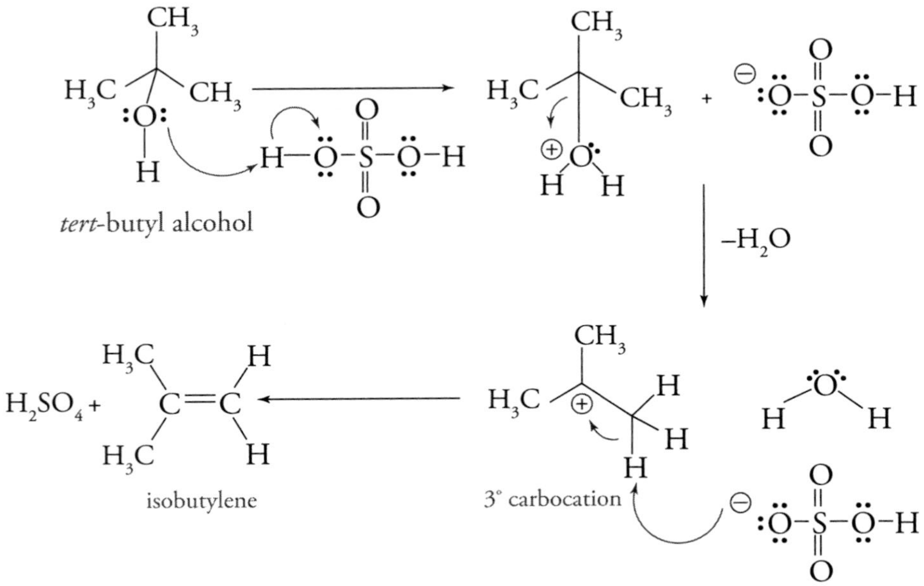

Figure 45

Rearrangements

A carbocation will rearrange to a more thermodynamically stable position, as shown here, where the 2° carbocation migrates to the more highly substituted 3° position:

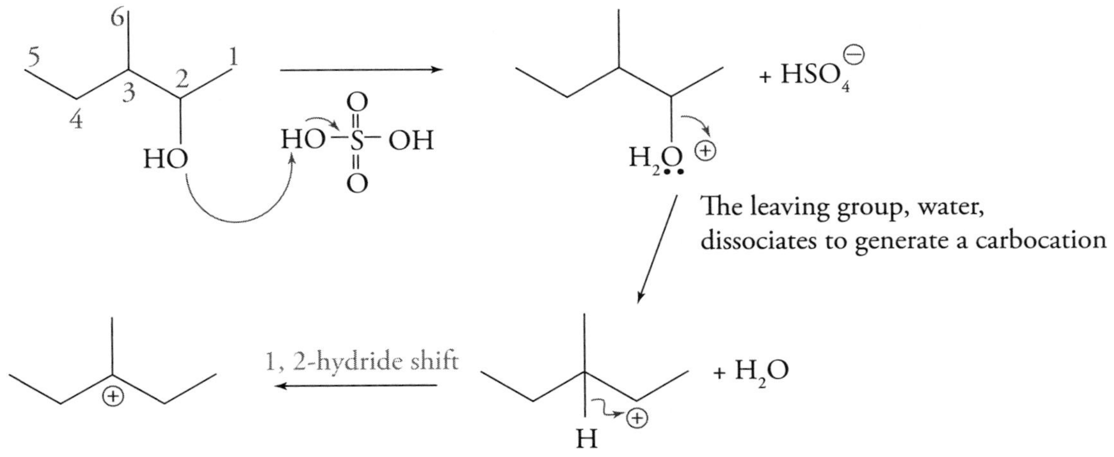

Figure 46

A carbocation will never rearrange to form a less stable carbocation.

The E1 mechanism is also favored by a protic solvent since it shares the same rate limiting step as the S_N1 reaction. After the carbocation has formed, the solvent may then act as a base if no other weak base is present in solution. Since this reaction generally occurs under conditions identical to the S_N1 reaction, these two mechanisms often compete with each other. It is rare to see 100% of either the S_N1 product or the E1 product for a given reaction. Instead, mixtures of products usually form.

Key Features of an E1 Reaction

Reactivity of substrate: 3° > 2° >> 1°

Stereochemistry:	Most substituted double bond forms—*trans* is favored over *cis*
Kinetics:	reaction rate = k[haloalkane]
Solvent:	E1 reactions are favored by protic solvents.
Rearrangements:	Carbocation rearrangement is possible.
Favoring Conditions:	Elimination reactions are favored over substitution reactions by using weak bases and high temperatures.

The E2 Mechanism

E2 elimination, just like S_N2 substitution, proceeds via a 1-step mechanism. A strong nucleophile removes a proton from the carbon adjacent to a leaving group. The carbon-carbon double bond forms at the same time. All three changes happen in a concerted fashion.

Due to steric considerations, small nucleophiles produce the most highly substituted alkenes, whereas bulky nucleophiles favor the least substituted one. The reaction rate is proportional to both the concentration of the alkyl halide and the concentration of the base, giving a bimolecular reaction: rate = $k[RX][HO^-]$.

The elimination pathway in many instances may compete with the substitution pathway. This is because a base can also act as a nucleophile. Generally speaking, strong bases such as OH^- or OR^- yield exclusively the elimination product(s) unless the substrate is primary.

Key Features of an E2 Reaction

Reactivity of substrate: $3° > 2° > 1°$	
Stereochemistry:	Small nucleophiles yield the most substituted alkene; bulky nucleophiles favor the least substituted one.
Kinetics:	reaction rate = $k[nuc][substrate]$
Solvent:	E2 reactions are favored by polar, aprotic solvents.
Rearrangements:	Not possible due to concerted mechanism
Favoring Conditions:	E2 reactions are favored over E1 reactions by the use of strong bases. High temperatures favor eliminations over substitutions, but primary substrates will substitute.

Summary of S_N1, S_N2, E1, and E2 Reactions

Figure 47 summarizes substitution and elimination reactions, where E^+ represents the electrophile.

Reaction dominance with increasing electrophilic substitution →

↑ Reaction dominance with increasing nucleophile strength

S_N2
- rate = $k[E^+][Nu^-]$
- one step
- backside attack
- requires strong Nu^-
- inversion of configuration
- methyl > 1° > 2° >> 3°

S_N1
- rate = $k[E^+]$
- two steps
- carbocation intermediate
- requires good Nu^-
- results in racemization
- 3° > 2° >> 1° > methyl

E2
- rate = $k[E^+][B^-]$
- one step
- antiperiplanar geometry
- requires strong base (B^-)
- small base gives most substituted alkene; bulky base gives least substituted
- 3° > 2° > 1°

E1
- rate = $k[E^+]$
- two steps
- carbocation intermediate
- requires weak base (B^-)
- major product is most substituted alkene; *trans* > *cis*
- 3° > 2° >> 1°

Figure 47

10.6 UNSATURATED HYDROCARBONS: ALKENES AND BENZENE

Reactions of the Alkenes

Alkenes undergo a wide variety of reactions. Most significant to the PCAT are the **electrophilic addition** reactions in which the carbon-carbon double bond, acting as a nucleophile (Lewis base), donates electrons to an atom or ion, the electrophile.

Markovnikov's Rule

A hydrogen halide adds to an alkene's double bond to form an alkyl halide. With "X" standing generically for a halide, the reaction is depicted like this:

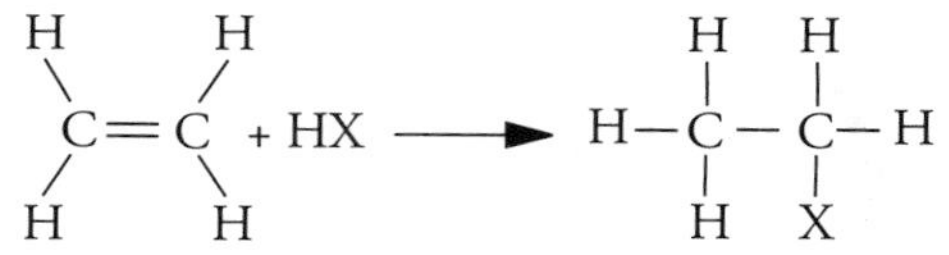

Electrophilic addition to an alkene involves two steps, the first of which is the rate-determining step. In that first step, π electrons from the carbon-carbon double bond attack the HX molecule's electropositive component to generate a **carbocation**.

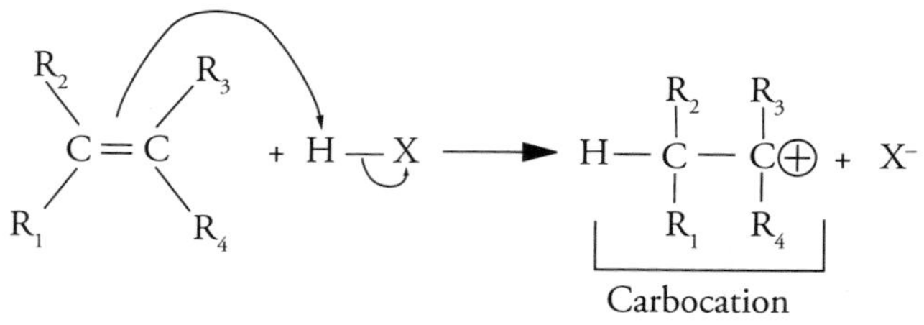

In the second step, the X^- ion rapidly reacts with the carbocation, and the product is formed.

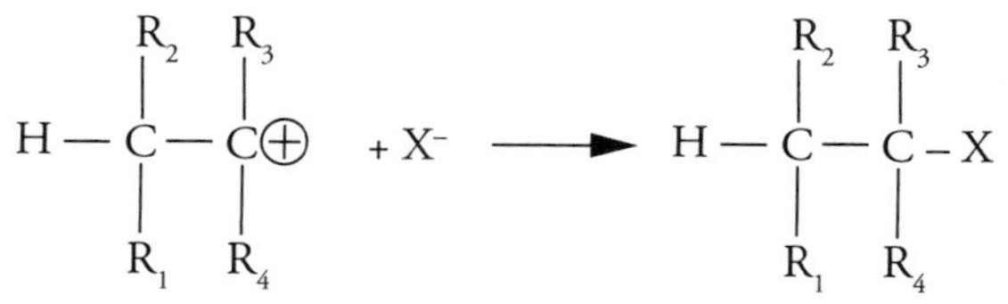

Electrophilic addition to an alkene normally follows the pattern of stability described previously, which is further described by **Markovnikov's rule:** *electrophilic addition to an alkene molecule yields, preferentially, a product in which the nucleophile is bound to the more highly substituted of the two doubly bonded carbons.* Markovnikov's addition is *normally* the favored route of electrophilic addition to alkenes, and it follows from the fact that the intermediate carbocation with the greatest stability is that in which the positive charge is located on the more highly substituted carbon. The positive charge can migrate to a position of greater stability, causing a rearrangement of the carbocation intermediate as shown here, where the positive charge in the second product migrated to the more highly substituted carbon:

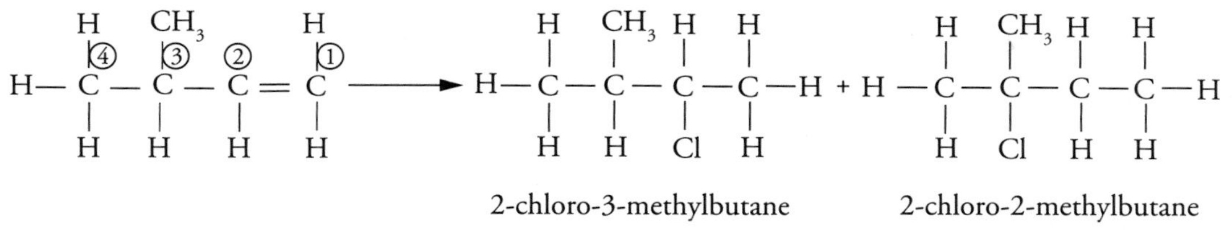

2-chloro-3-methylbutane   2-chloro-2-methylbutane

Electrophilic Addition Reactions

Anti-Markovnikov Addition in the Presence of Peroxides

When HBr adds to a double bond in the presence of *peroxides*, Markovnikov addition is not the norm. Electrophilic addition occurs by a different mechanism, involving not a carbocation but a carbon free radical. The new substituent appears at the *least* substituted carbon. That process is called an **anti-Markovnikov addition**:

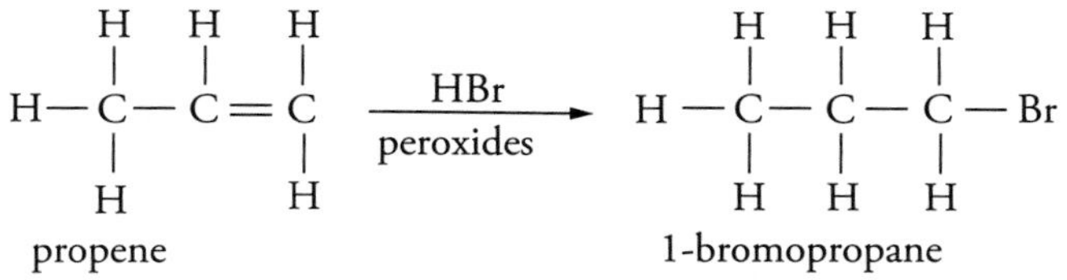

propene   1-bromopropane

Anti-Markovnikov addition
in the presence of peroxides:
addition occurs at the least
substituted carbon.

With respect to alkene electrophilic addition as it appears on the PCAT, you should know that:

- Normally, Markovnikov addition is the favored reaction, involving
  a. a carbocation in which a positive charge is carried on the more highly substituted carbon and, consequently,
  b. a final product in which the electronegative species binds to that same carbon.
- In the presence of peroxides, addition of HBr to an alkene occurs in anti-Markovnikov fashion via a carbon free radical intermediate. The most favored product will be that in which addition occurs at the alkene molecule's *least* substituted carbon.

Addition of Water: Hydration

With an acid catalyst, water will add to an alkene's double bond to form an alcohol:

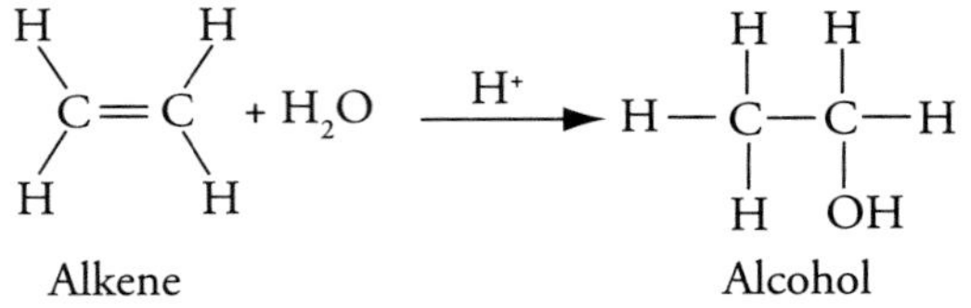

The reaction proceeds through a carbocation intermediate whose formation here, as with the addition of hydrogen halide, is the rate-determining step. The reaction is favored by a stable carbocation and *follows Markovnikov's rule.*

Hydration of an alkene competes with the reverse process—dehydration of an alcohol. Equilibrium will lie toward hydration if the acid is relatively dilute and the temperature is low. Equilibrium will lie toward *de*hydration if the acid is relatively concentrated and temperature is relatively high.

Hydroboration-Oxidation

Addition of borane (or its dimeric form, B_2H_6) to a double bond produces an organoborane, which, in turn, can undergo oxidation to form an alcohol. The transition state for the hydroboration reaction dictates a **syn addition** in which the hydrogen and boron add to the same side of the carbon-carbon double bond.

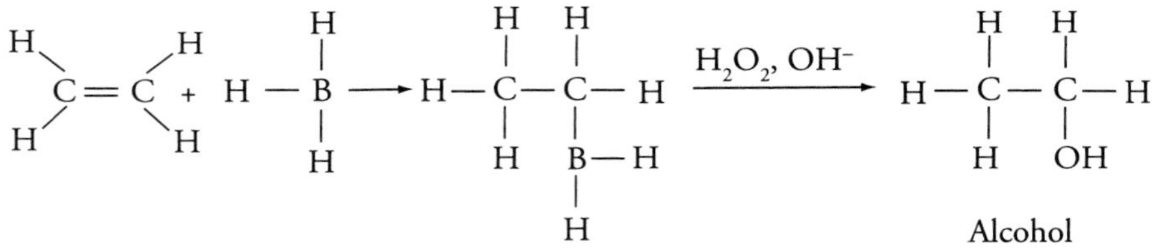

The ultimate product is an *anti-Markovnikov* addition of water.

Epoxide Formation and Hydrolysis

The next reaction we examine is **epoxide formation** and subsequent formation of *trans*-diols. In this type of reaction, a π bond in an alkene reacts with a peroxy acid [$RC(=O)O_2H$] to form an epoxide and a carboxylic acid. One such peroxycarboxylic acid used to form an epoxide is mCPBA. The π bond of the alkene, again, acts as the nucleophile, and the peroxy oxygen furthest from the carbonyl oxygen acts as the electrophile. We will not look at this reaction in any further mechanistic detail. The key point is that when an alkene reacts with a peroxy acid, an epoxide is formed.

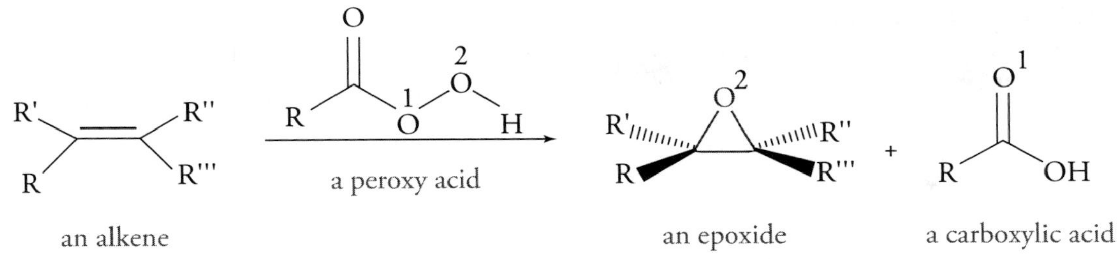

Figure 48

A specific example of an epoxidation followed by acidic or basic hydrolysis is shown here.

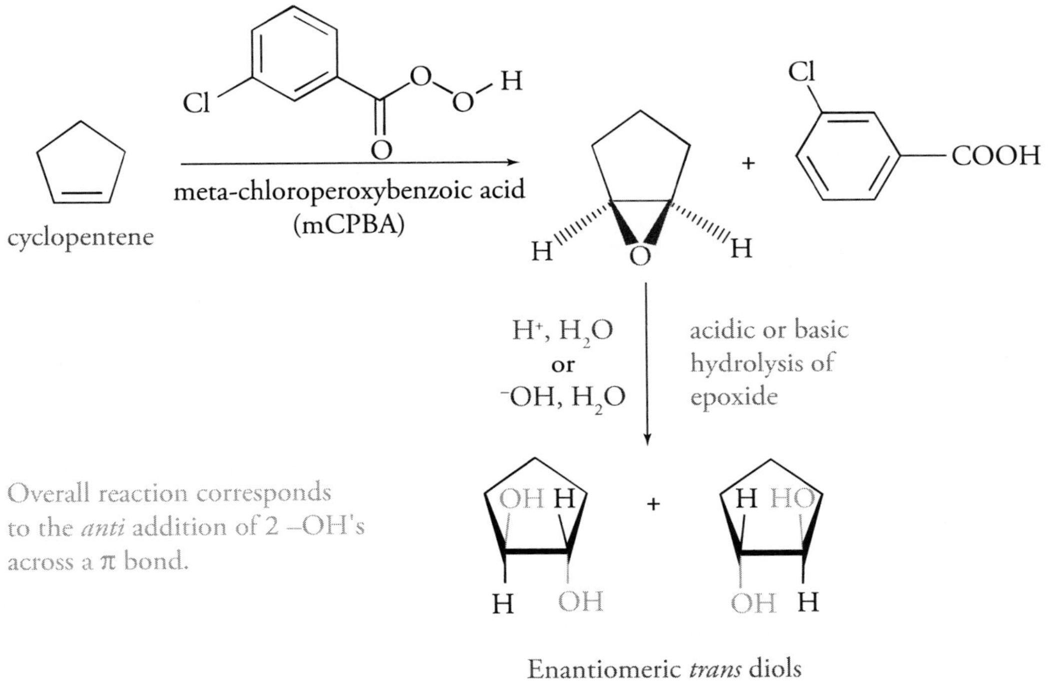

Overall reaction corresponds to the *anti* addition of 2 –OH's across a π bond.

Enantiomeric *trans* diols

Figure 49

Oxidation of π Bonds

When alkenes are treated with dilute $KMnO_4$ (potassium permanganate) or OsO_4 (osmium tetraoxide), *cis*-diols are formed. The stereochemistry of this reaction requires *syn* addition of two –OH's across the π bond.

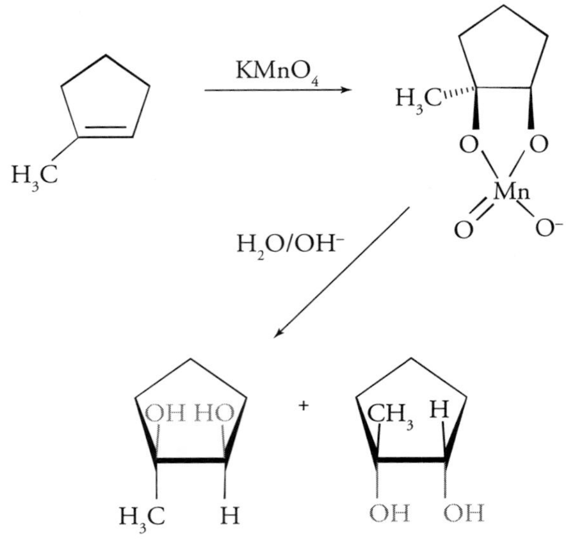

Figure 50

The geometry of the metal complex that is the product in the first step forces both oxygen atoms to bond to the same side of the alkene. When they are replaced by OH^-, these remain on the same side, *cis* to one another.

Hydrogenation

Another common reaction of π bonds is the hydrogenation reaction. Unsaturated hydrocarbons can be reduced by molecular hydrogen (H_2) in the presence of a metal catalyst. The stereochemistry of this reduction reaction is *syn* with the two hydrogens added to the same side of the π bond. A variety of metals (mostly from the right half of transition metal series) and metal-containing compounds can act as catalysts for this type of reaction. Don't allow a strange-looking metal catalyst to fool you on the PCAT; alkenes react with H_2 in the presence of any one of a variety of catalysts to make saturated alkanes as indicated here:

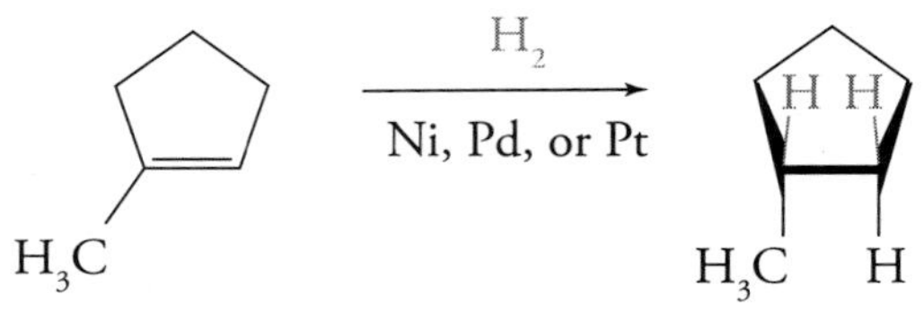

Next, we will explore hydrogenations of alkynes, compounds that have carbon-carbon triple bonds. If an alkyne is reduced by molecular hydrogen (H_2) in the presence of a metal catalyst, it will be reduced all the way to the alkane. This is demonstrated by the reduction of 2-pentyne all the way to the fully saturated pentane.

It is possible to stop the reduction of an alkyne at the alkene stage.

Cycloaddition Reactions

Concerted reactions are reactions that occur in one step without the formation of any intermediates. They usually occur with a high degree of stereoselectivity. Concerted reactions often occur via cyclic transition states by the reorganization of σ and π bonds. A typical concerted reaction is the **Diels-Alder reaction**.

In this reaction, a cyclohexene ring is formed from the cycloaddition of a diene with a dienophile:

a diene   a dienophile

The mechanism of the reaction is shown for both an alkene and an alkyne:

Due to its high degree of selectivity, the Diels-Alder reaction is a powerful tool in synthetic chemistry.

Polymerization of Alkenes

Alkenes can undergo polymerization reactions through addition (chain-growth) reactions, or through condensation (step-growth) reactions. In chain growth, the chain has only one growth point and individual units, called *monomers*, add one-by-one to the growing chain. The concentration of monomer decreases gradually. During a step-growth process, a chain has at least two growth points. The amount of monomer is quickly consumed, producing a possible mixture of compounds with intermediate molecular weights.

Chain polymerization requires chain initiation and propagation. The free radical polymerization of ethylene produces polyethylene, as shown in this overall reaction.

$$H_2C = CH_2 \xrightarrow[\text{initiator}]{\text{R–O–O–R}} (-CH_2 - CH_2 -)n$$

Ethylene   Peroxide   Polyethylene

In this reaction, homolytic cleavage of the peroxide bond produces two radicals that can add to a carbon-carbon double bond. The addition product results in a second radical that can then add to another carbon-carbon double bond, increasing the carbon chain.

$$R–O\bullet \quad H_2C{=}CH_2 \rightarrow R–O–CH_2–CH_2\bullet$$

The process continues until chain termination reactions occur.

Aromaticity and Substitution on the Benzene Ring

Hückel's Rule

Benzene, the aromatic prototype, is a planar, cyclic structure with six π electrons.

Benzene
6 π electrons

To be aromatic, all carbons in a ring must be sp^2 hybridized and follow Hückel's Rule, which states that a compound is particularly stable if all of its bonding orbitals are filled with paired electrons. To apply this rule, we first count the number of π electrons in the molecule and then set this number equal to $4n + 2$. If n is 0 or any positive integer, the compound is aromatic. All of the carbons in benzene, for example, are sp^2 hybridized, *and* benzene has 6π electrons, which gives $4n + 2 = 6$ and $n = 1$. Having fulfilled both criteria, benzene is classified as an aromatic compound. Aromatic compounds may also have N, O, or S in the ring in addition to C.

Because of their alternating double bonds, aromatic compounds form a planar ring and the delocalized π electrons form cyclic clouds above and below the plane. They are resonance stabilized due to the delocalization of the π electrons. As a result, aromatic compounds are generally very unreactive.

Benzene has two resonance forms, so it is a hybrid between the two, with π electrons fully delocalized:

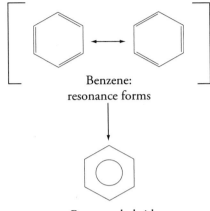

Benzene:
resonance forms

Benzene: hybrid

The benzene ring tends to undergo reactions in which the ring is preserved. Consequently—and this is important for the PCAT—*benzene tends to undergo substitution rather than addition.*

Nomenclature

For substituted benzene rings, the positions on the aromatic ring are identified relative to a substituent, and may be *ortho* (*o*), *meta* (*m*), or *para* (*p*). The positions are shown for toluene, which has a methyl substituent:

Toluene

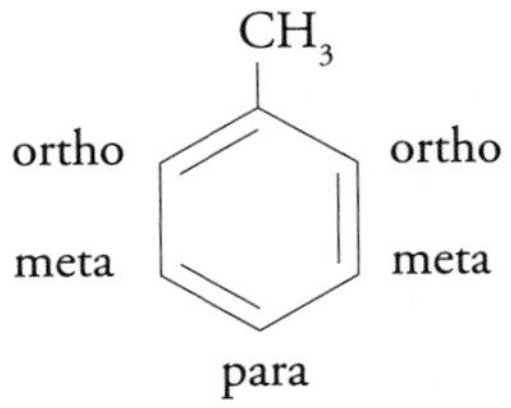

CH_3

ortho   ortho

meta   meta

para

The IUPAC naming system for substituted aromatic rings uses numbers for ring positions rather than the designations ortho, meta, and para. A single group attached to a ring is given the #1 carbon position; then other ring positions are numbered from 2 to 6. They can be numbered either clockwise or counterclockwise. As with chain compounds, the name chosen is the one with the smallest possible numbers. For example, 2-chloromethylbenzene has a methyl group in position 1 and a chloro group in position 2 (the ortho position). The compound 3-chloromethylbenzene has the chloro group in the meta position, and 4-chloromethylbenzene in the para position. Here are IUPAC names for other compounds:

2-hydroxybenzoic acid   benzene-1,4 dicarboxylic acid   2,4,6-trichlorophenol

Electrophilic Aromatic Substitution

A single substitution of a benzene ring raises or lowers the likelihood that the ring will undergo a *second substitution*.

In that regard, for the PCAT, it is important to know that:

- A group that donates (or "releases") electrons to the ring tends to increase the likelihood of additional substitution. It is said to activate the ring, and is termed a **ring activating group.** You can recognize most activating groups since they all have a lone pair of electrons on the atom directly attached to the ring.
- A group that withdraws electrons from the ring decreases the likelihood of additional substitution. Since this group is said to **deactivate** the ring, it is termed a **ring deactivating group**. You can recognize most deactivating groups since they have a + or δ+ charge on the atom directly attached to the ring.

A single benzene ring substituent affects not only the likelihood that a next substitution will occur, but also the *site* at which it will occur. Consider, for example, the associated resonance structures when the substituent is an electron donating group, symbolized as "D":

Now look at the resonance structures when the substituent is an electron withdrawing group, symbolized as "W":

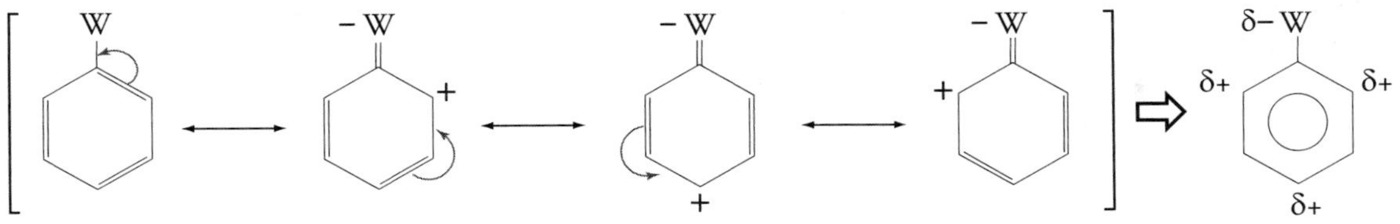

Notice that in the case of an electron donating group, a partial negative charge is localized on the ortho and para positions of the ring. Those positions are susceptible to electrophilic attack, and the substituent is an *ortho, para director*. In contrast, an electron withdrawing group *deactivates* the ring to electrophilic attack. Instead, attack occurs at the meta position because it is the least electropositive position on the ring. However, it does not carry a partial negative charge, so it is only weakly reactive. Here, the substituent is a *meta director*.

Halogens are an exception. They are highly electronegative and therefore electron withdrawing substituents. With their lone pairs of electrons, however, they are also electron donating. In actuality, they are deactivating but still *ortho, para* directors.

Friedel-Crafts Reactions with Benzene

Benzene reacts with alkyl halides in the presence of aluminum chloride to produce alkyl benzenes in a reaction known as a **Friedel-Crafts alkylation**. Aluminum chloride acts as a Lewis acid catalyst to enhance the electrophilicity of the alkylating agent by producing a carbocation and $AlCl_4^-$. The carbocation then reacts with the benzene ring.

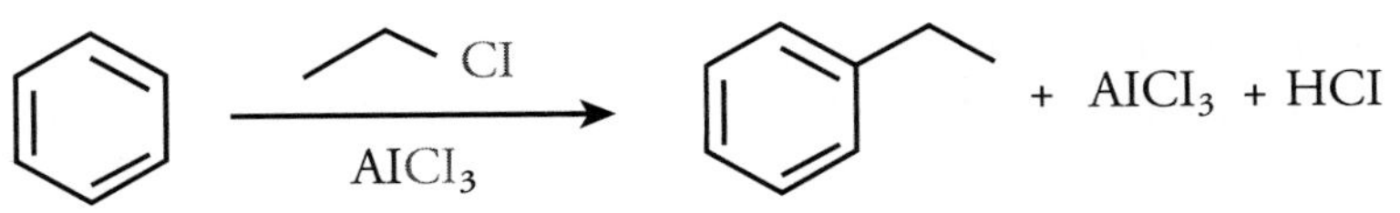

In a Friedel-Crafts acylation, $AlCl_3$ promotes the reaction of an acyl halide with benzene. This reaction yields an aromatic ketone, as shown here:

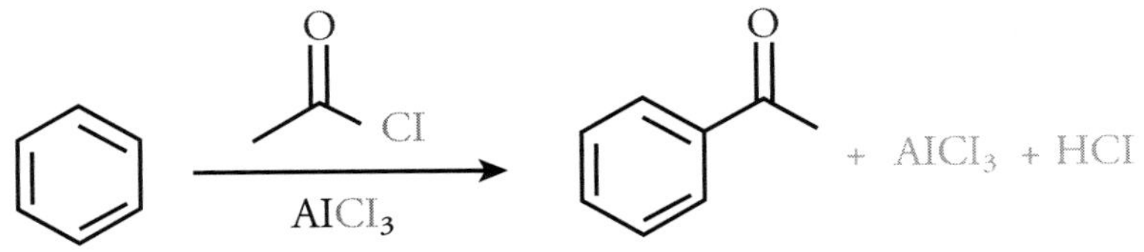

The product, an aryl ketone, can be reduced to an alkyl benzene. Because both the Friedel-Crafts alkylation and **Friedel-Crafts acylation** reactions proceed through formation of a carbocation, rearrangements can occur.

Reduction

Benzene and its aromatic derivatives can also undergo a reduction reaction. The **Birch Reduction** converts the arene to 1,4-cyclohexadiene using sodium (or lithium) as a reducing agent. Liquid ammonia is used as a solvent in the presence of an alcohol such as ethanol, methanol or *t*-butanol.

10.7 ALCOHOLS

We've seen that alcohols are a very useful class of chemicals because of their diverse reactivity. Let's review a few other properties of this important functional group, such as their intermolecular interactions and acidity.

Hydrogen Bonding

In order to examine the effect of hydrogen bonding in alcohols, let's examine two molecules that are isomers of one another, *n*-butanol and diethyl ether. Both have the same molecular formula ($C_4H_{10}O$), yet there is a dramatic difference in their boiling points (117°C for *n*-butanol vs. 34.6°C for diethyl ether). This difference arises from the ability of *n*-butanol to form intermolecular hydrogen bonds, while diethyl ether cannot. Alcohols form intermolecular hydrogen bonds because they have hydroxyl (–OH) groups. These create a strong dipole in which the hydroxyl group's proton acquires a substantial partial positive charge (δ^+) and the oxygen acquires a substantial partial negative charge (δ^-). The partial positive hydrogen can interact electrostatically with a non-bonding pair of electrons on a nearby oxygen, producing the hydrogen bond. On the other hand, in diethyl ether the hydrogens cannot participate in hydrogen bonding. It's important to remember that a hydrogen bond is *not* a covalent bond; it is an intermolecular hydrogen bonding interaction between a lone pair of electrons on an electron-rich donor atom, such as N, O, and F, and a H bonded to a more electronegative atom or group.

Intermolecular hydrogen bonding between molecules of *n*-butanol

molecular weight = 74
b.p. = 117°C

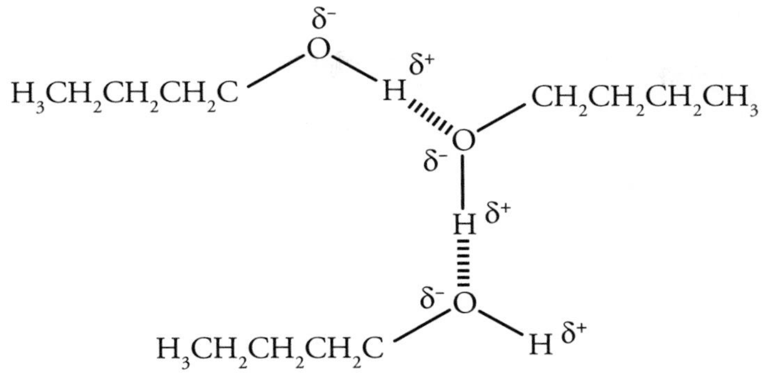

Intermolecular hydrogen bonding is not possible between molecules of diethyl ether.

molecular weight = 74
b.p. = 34.6°C

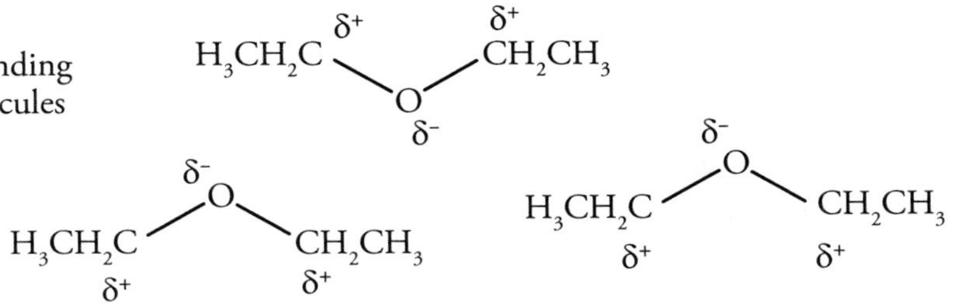

Figure 51

Now notice the hydrogen bonding pattern in *para*-nitrophenol (Figure 52), where the nitro group is opposite to the OH group. Hydrogen bonding can occur with both the nitro and the hydroxyl groups in this molecule, and the bonding is exclusively intermolecular. These hydrogen bonding interactions hold molecules of *para*-nitrophenol together and increase their boiling and melting points. In the hydrogen bonding pattern in *ortho*-nitrophenol, the nitro group and the hydroxyl group are in close proximity. Consequently, intramolecular hydrogen bonding can occur between the hydrogen of the hydroxyl group and a lone pair of electrons on the nitro group *on the same molecule*. These intramolecular hydrogen bonding interactions decrease the amount of intermolecular hydrogen bonding interactions that can occur between molecules, so the melting and boiling points of *ortho*-nitrophenol are lower than those of *para*-nitrophenol.

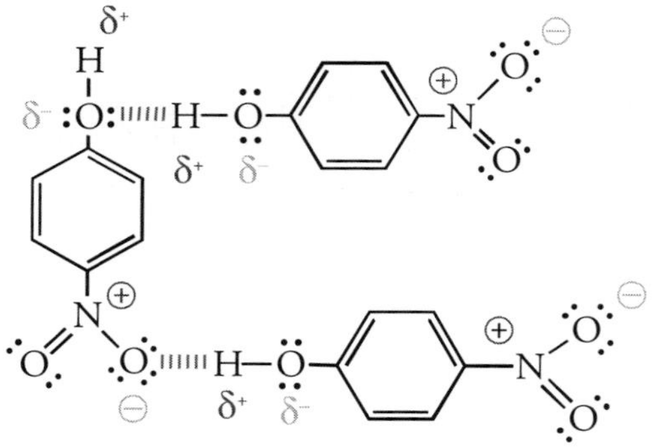

para-nitrophenol
Intermolecular hydrogen bonding

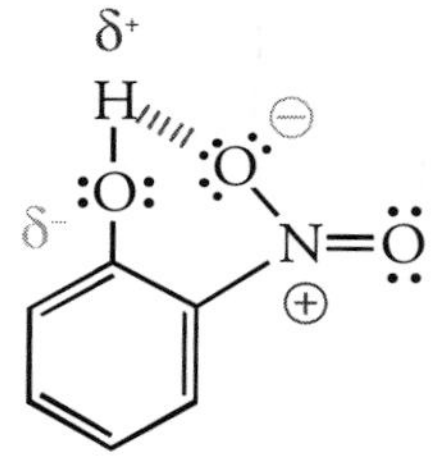

ortho-nitrophenol
Intramolecular hydrogen bonding

Figure 52

Nucleophilic Substitution

A variety of compounds undergo nucleophilic aliphatic substitution, but the alkyl halides serve as a good basis on which to study the process generically. "Nucleophilic substitution" means a reaction, conducted in a solvent, between an aliphatic compound (the substrate) and a **nucleophilic reagent**. The substrate:

a. gives up a **leaving group**, and
b. is attacked by a nucleophile, which substitutes for the leaving group.

$$\underset{\text{substrate}}{R-W} \ + \ \underset{\text{nucleophile}}{Z} \ \xrightarrow{\text{solvent}} \ R-Z \ + \ \underset{\text{leaving group}}{W}$$

The key to nucleophilicity is *the presence of an unshared electron pair.*

Here, for instance, is a reaction in which methyl bromide is the substrate, bromide ion the leaving group, and hydroxide ion the nucleophile.

$$CH_3Br \ + \ OH^- \ \longrightarrow \ CH_3OH \ + \ Br^-$$

The reaction of methylbromide with hydroxide ion occurs because bromide is a relatively good leaving group, and because the hydroxide ion is the stronger nucleophile (the stronger Lewis base).

10.7

Primary, Secondary, and Tertiary Alcohols

"Alcohol," generically written R-OH, means an alkyl or substituted alkyl group (including an aryl group) bound to an OH group. An alcohol is designated as primary, secondary, or tertiary depending on its alkyl group. An OH group bound to a carbon with one hydrocarbon substituent (R) gives a **primary alcohol**, an OH group bound to a carbon with two R groups gives a **secondary alcohol**, and an OH group bound to a carbon with three R groups gives a **tertiary alcohol**.

Primary

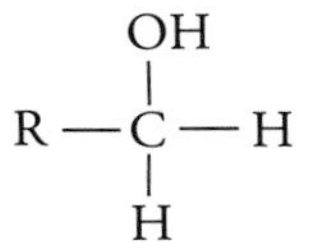

Secondary

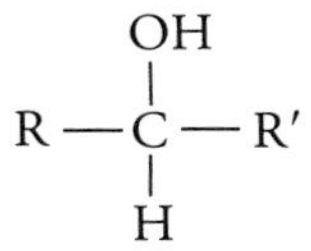

Tertiary

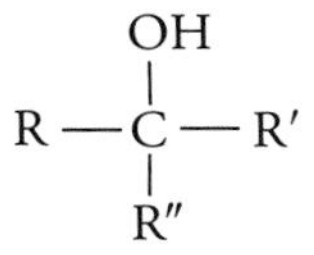

Here are the names and structures of some common alcohols:

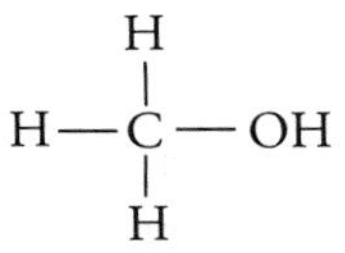

Methanol (1°)

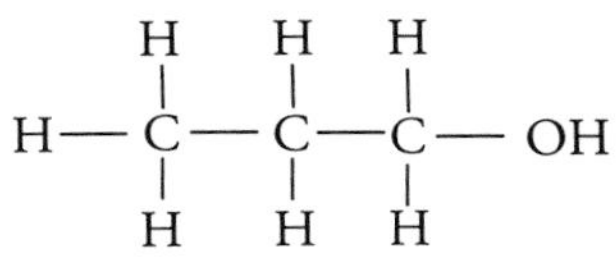

1-Propanol (1°)

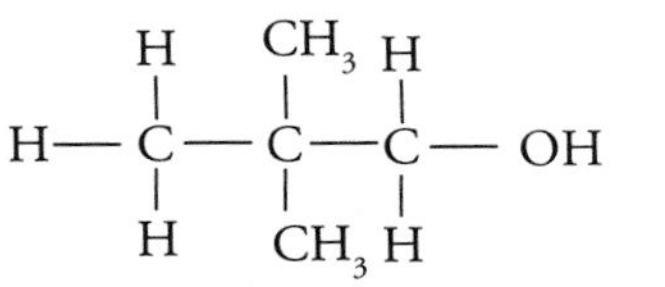

2,2-Dimethyl-1-propanol (1°)

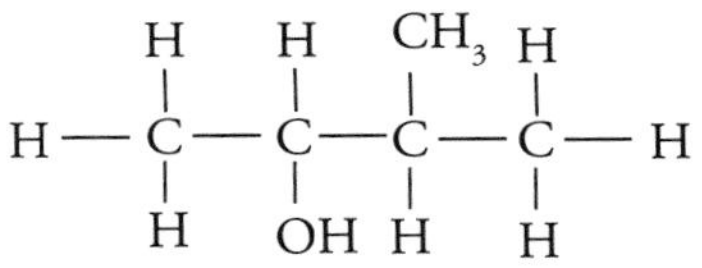

3-Methyl-2-butanol (2°)

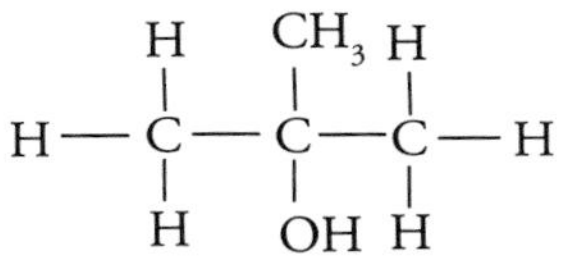

2-Methyl-2-propanol (3°)

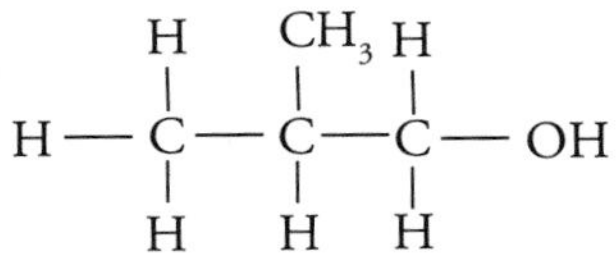

2-Methylpropanol (1°)

Figure 53

Physical Properties

Boiling Point, Solubility, and Hydrogen Bonding

The boiling points of alcohols generally follow trends associated with the other hydrocarbons. Increasing molecular weight tends to increase boiling point, and increased branching tends to reduce boiling point. When comparing an alcohol and a hydrocarbon of similar molecular weight, the *alcohol will have a much higher boiling point* because the hydroxyl group makes an alcohol susceptible to *hydrogen bonding*. Unshared electrons on the oxygen atom of the OH group on one alcohol molecule hydrogen bond to the hydrogen atom on the next.

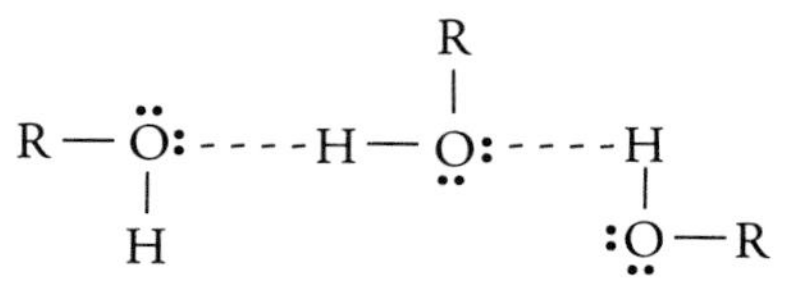

Alcohols with five carbons or fewer are soluble in water, but as the carbon chain grows, and the OH group represents a smaller portion of the molecule, water solubility decreases.

Acidity and Basicity

Just like water, an alcohol can behave both as an acid or a base. The OH group can lose a proton to form an **alkoxide ion**, hence acting as an acid, or acquire a proton to form an **oxonium ion**, thereby acting as a base.

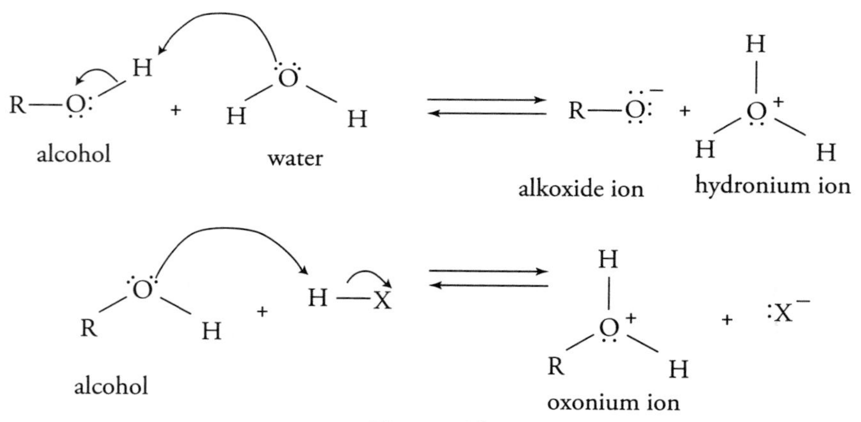

Figure 54

Strong acids form weak conjugate bases, and weak acids form strong conjugate bases. With a pK_a approximately equal to that of H_2O, alcohols are essentially non-acidic, so alkyl oxides are very strong bases (and hence very strong nucleophiles). The negative charge is localized on the electronegative oxygen atom:

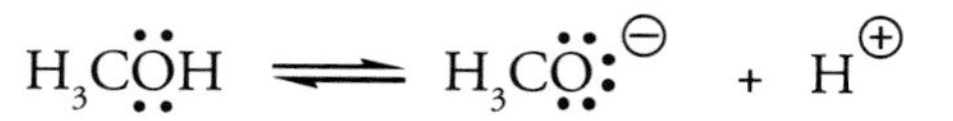

Phenols are considerably more acidic than alcohols due to resonance stabilization of the conjugate base, but are not as acidic as carboxylic acids. Resonance structures for the phenoxide ion are shown here:

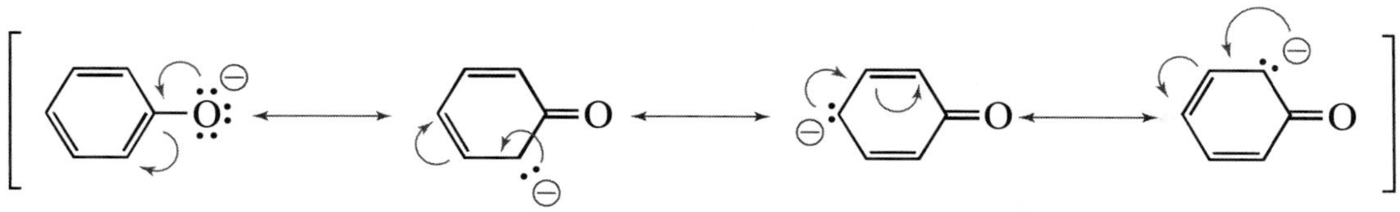

The general trend of acidities is the following:

General Rule of Thumb for Organic Compound Acidity.

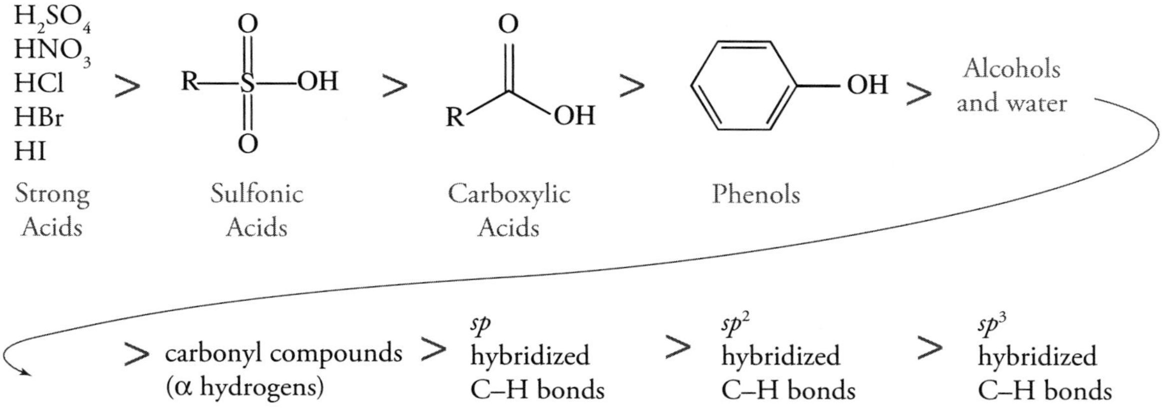

Preparation of Alcohols

Alcohols can be prepared by hydration of an alkene, but they can also be prepared by other methods including the following:

- Reduction of a Carbonyl. For this purpose, sodium borohydride ($NaBH_4$) and lithium aluminum hydride ($LiAlH_4$), both sources of H⁻, are the most frequently used reducing agents. Reduction of an aldehyde, ester, or carboxylic acid produces a primary alcohol, and reduction of a ketone produces a secondary alcohol.

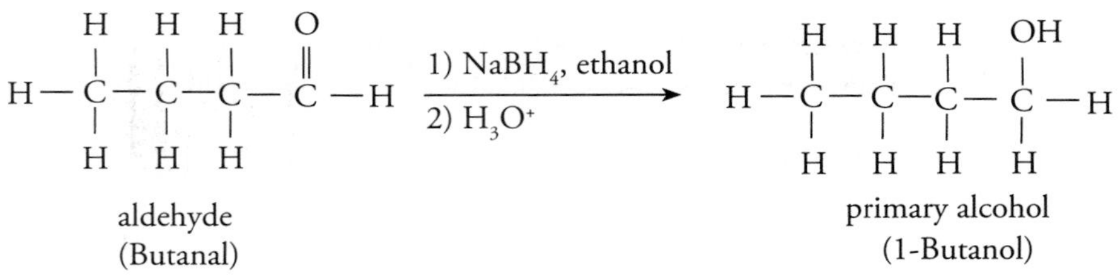
1) NaBH$_4$, ethanol
2) H$_3$O$^+$
aldehyde
(Butanal)
primary alcohol
(1-Butanol)

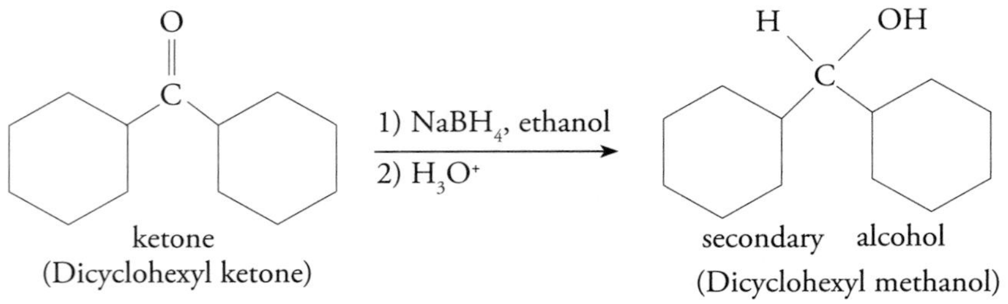
1) NaBH$_4$, ethanol
2) H$_3$O$^+$
ketone
(Dicyclohexyl ketone)
secondary alcohol
(Dicyclohexyl methanol)

- Reduction of a Carboxylic Acid

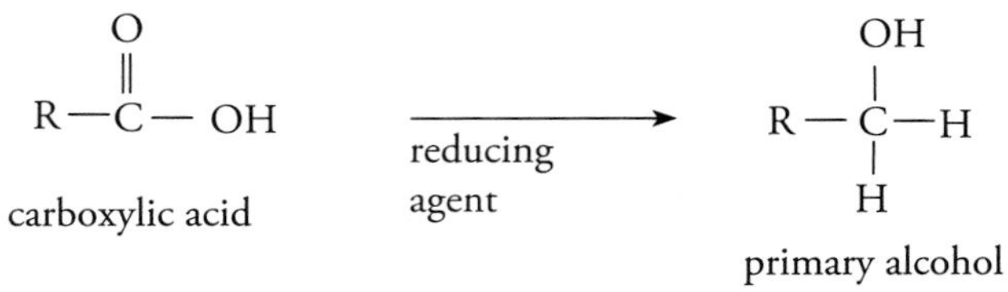
carboxylic acid
reducing
agent
primary alcohol

- Reduction of an Ester

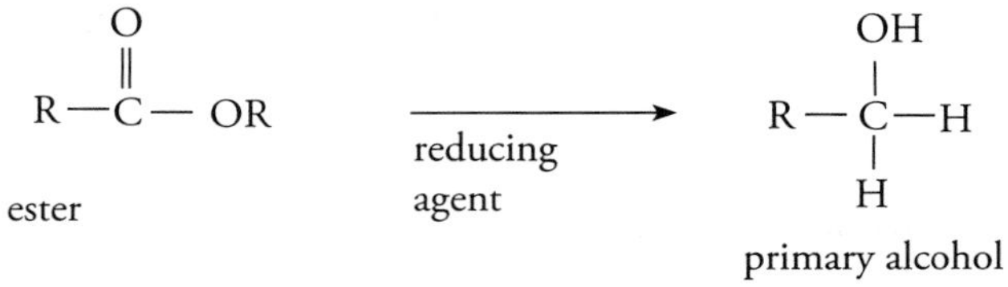
ester
reducing
agent
primary alcohol

Figure 55

Grignard Reagent

A **Grignard reagent**, also called alkylmagnesium halide, means a molecule with general structure RMgX, where X is chlorine, bromine, or iodine. The Grignard reagent is highly reactive and useful in a wide variety of organic reactions, including the synthesis of an alcohol by reaction with an aldehyde or ketone. Grignard reagents offer one of the few ways in which a carbon chain can be lengthened, which makes the Grignard reaction an extremely useful synthetic process in organic chemistry. The general mechanism is shown here, where bond polarization produces a nucleophilic R$^-$ group that attacks the positive dipole of the carbonyl carbon, followed by a second step involving protonation of the negatively charged oxygen, producing an alcohol:

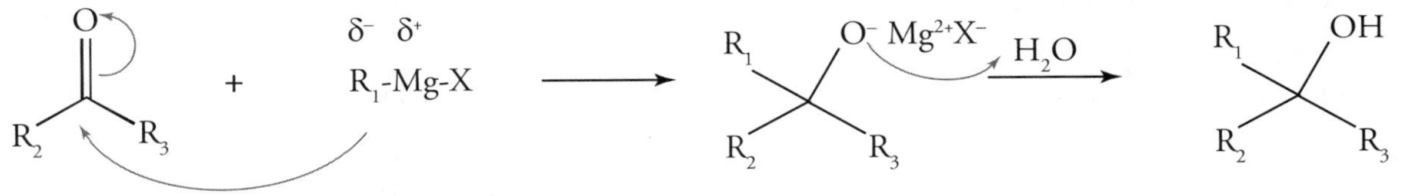

The Grignard reagent reacts with formaldehyde to give a primary alcohol, with aldehydes to give secondary alcohols, and with ketones to give tertiary alcohols.

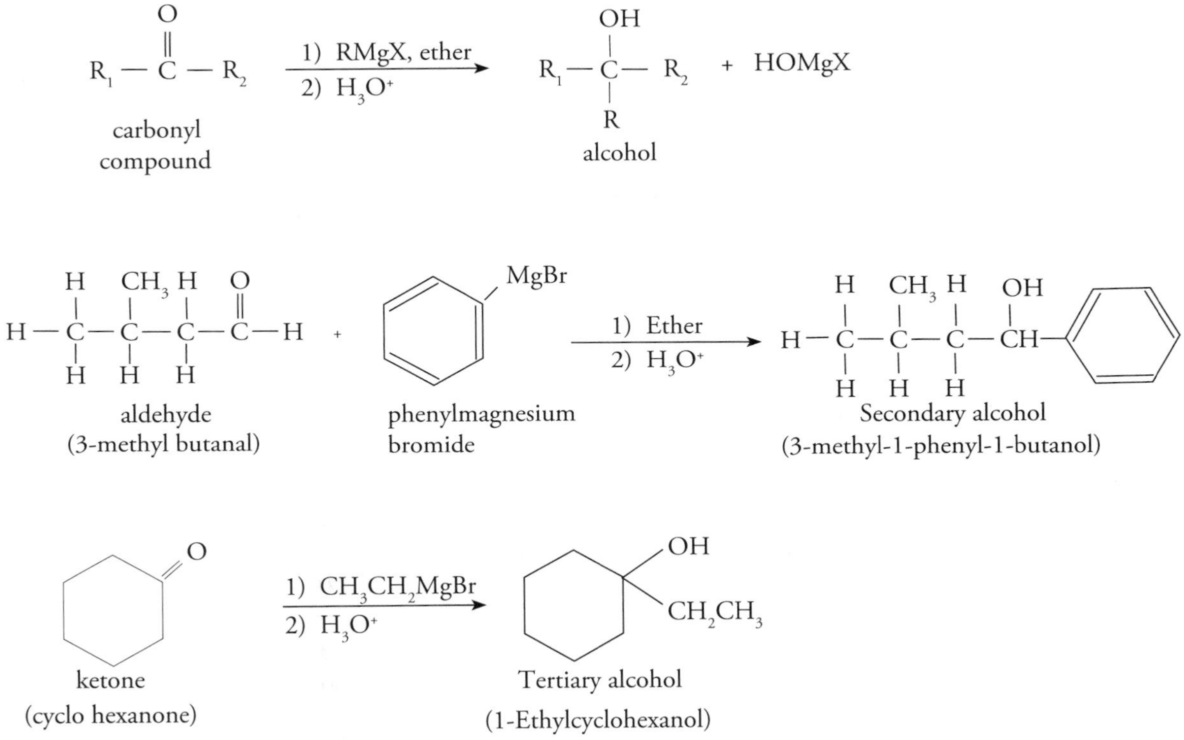

Figure 56

Reactions of Alcohols

Reaction with Halides to Form Alkyl Halides: Acid Catalyzed Substitution

Recall that substitution calls first for a leaving group, and that OH$^-$ (a strong base and a strong nucleophile) is a very *poor* leaving group. For that reason, substitution of OH by a halide requires that the OH group first be converted to a *good* leaving group. The role of the acid catalyst is to protonate the OH group so that it becomes OH$_2^+$, which means that the ultimate group to be lost is water (an excellent leaving group).

Oxidation of Primary and Secondary Alcohols to Form Aldehydes, Ketones, and Carboxylic Acids

In the presence of an oxidizing agent, such as PCC or a compound containing a metal in a high oxidation state—KMnO$_4$ or Cr(VI)—alcohols lose one or more of the hydrogens bound to the alcoholic carbon. These are designated as alpha (α) hydrogens because they are attached to the carbon that is bound to the functional group.

Consider a primary alcohol. Reacted with a relatively mild oxidizing agent (like pyridinium chlorochromate, PCC), it loses one of its alpha hydrogens (and the H from the OH group) to form an aldehyde.

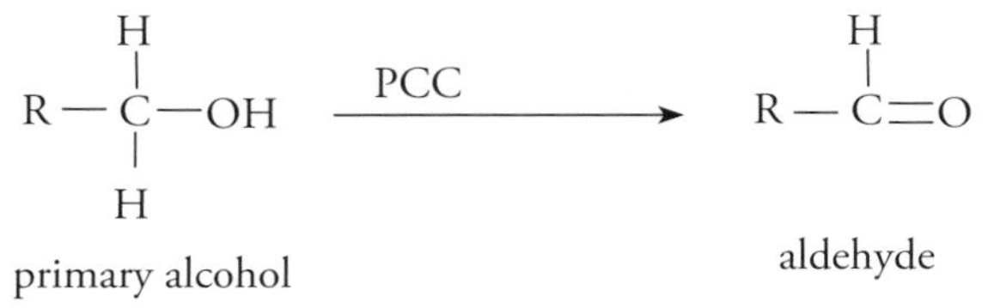

```
        H                              H
        |                              |
  R — C — OH    ──PCC──▶        R — C = O
        |
        H
  primary alcohol                  aldehyde
```

Reacted with a stronger oxidizing agent (like potassium permanganate or potassium dichromate), a primary alcohol loses both of its alpha hydrogens to form a carboxylic acid.

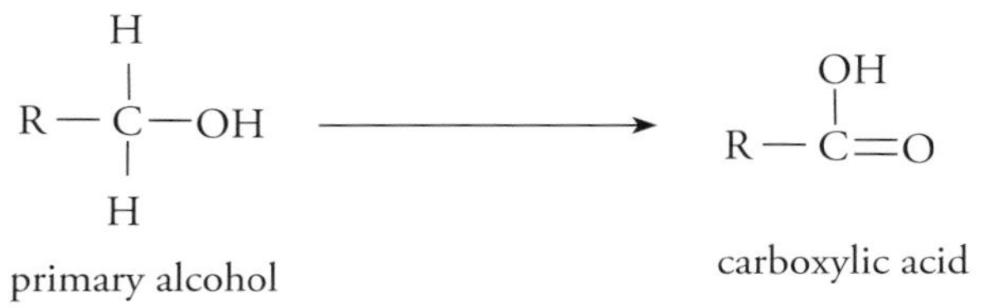

```
        H                              OH
        |                              |
  R — C — OH    ────────▶        R — C = O
        |
        H
  primary alcohol                  carboxylic acid
```

A secondary alcohol has only one alpha hydrogen. Oxidation produces a ketone.

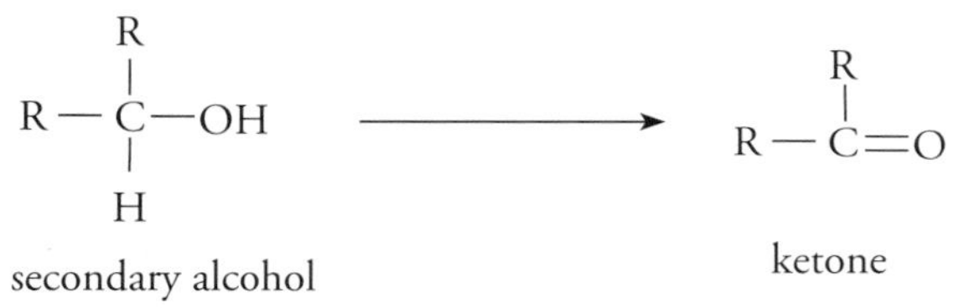

```
        R                              R
        |                              |
  R — C — OH    ────────▶        R — C = O
        |
        H
  secondary alcohol                ketone
```

A tertiary alcohol has no alpha hydrogens and thus does not undergo oxidation to form aldehydes, ketones, or carboxylic acids.

Protecting Groups

When synthesizing an organic compound, one of the reactants could contain a functional group that is not compatible with the reaction conditions. An unexpected product can be avoided by using a *protecting group* that can then be removed once the desired reaction has taken place. An example of a protecting group is trimethylsilyl chloride (TMSCl), which is commonly used to protect the –OH functional group of alcohols. Once the desired reaction is complete, the protecting group can be removed with an aqueous acid or fluoride, as shown here.

If a halide were present on the ring, for example, by using a protecting group on the –OH functional group, the halo alcohol could be converted to a Grignard reagent. Otherwise, an acid-base reaction would occur and the products would be ROMgCl and an alkane.

10.8   ALDEHYDES AND KETONES

Carbonyl group means a carbon atom doubly bound to an oxygen atom. Any compound with a carbonyl group is a **carbonyl compound**. Carbonyl compounds can be divided into (1) carboxylic acids and their derivatives and (2) the **aldehydes** and **ketones**.

In a ketone (R_2CHO), the carbonyl carbon is bound to two organic substituents. In an aldehyde, the carbonyl carbon is bound to one organic substituent and a hydrogen atom (RCHO). In one particular aldehyde, formaldehyde (IUPAC name: methanal), the carbonyl carbon is bound only to the oxygen atom and to two other hydrogen atoms; it is not bound to an organic substituent.

Ketone   Aldehyde   Formaldehyde

Properties of Aldehydes and Ketones

The carbonyl bond is polar: the more electronegative oxygen atom carries a partial negative charge, and the carbonyl carbon a partial positive one. Hence, the boiling points of aldehydes and ketones exceed those of nonpolar compounds of similar weight. However, because there is no intermolecular hydrogen bonding, their boiling points are not as high as those of alcohols of similar molecular weight.

As polar compounds, aldehydes and ketones of five or fewer carbons are water soluble.

Reactivity

Nucleophilic Addition Reactions to Aldehydes and Ketones

Because of the polarized nature of the C=O double bond in carbonyl compounds, the carbon in aldehydes and ketones is susceptible to nucleophilic attack and can readily be reduced. This nucleophilic addition reaction is shown below with a generic nucleophile (Nu:).

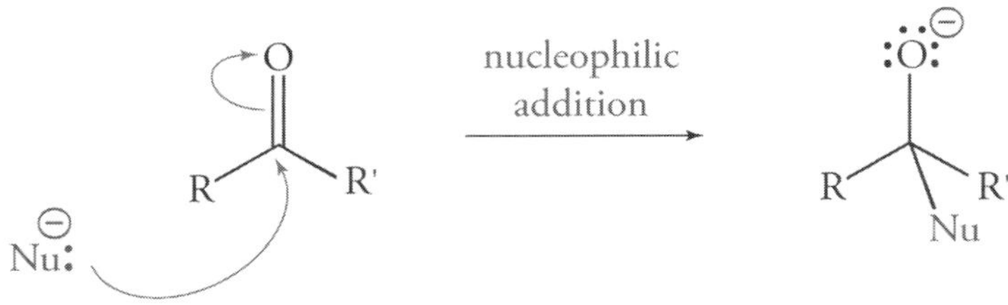

Nucleophilic addition reactions are defined by the bonding changes that occur over the course of the reaction, just as in electrophilic additions. In these reactions, a π bond in the starting material is broken, and two σ bonds in the product result. This very general reaction allows for the conversion of aldehydes or ketones into a variety of other functional groups such as alcohols via hydride reduction:

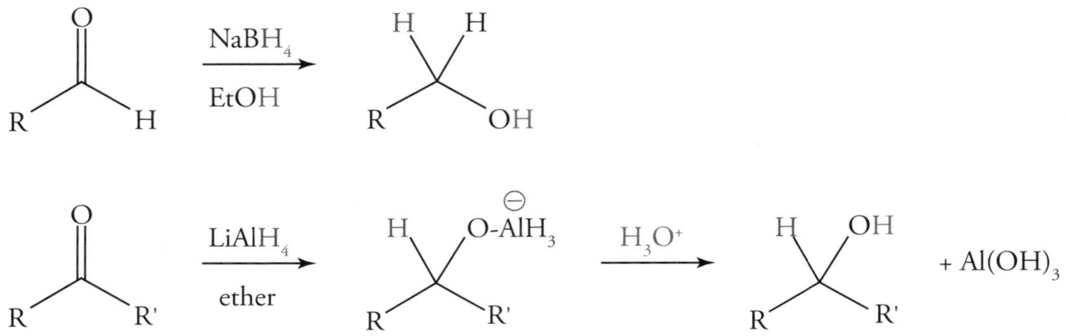

Note: Sodium borohydride ($NaBH_4$) and lithium aluminum hydride ($LiAlH_4$) are common reducing agents seen on the PCAT. In general, strong reducing agents easily lose electrons by adding hydride (H^-) to the carbonyl.

Acidity and Enolization

Carbon atoms are designated as α, β, or γ, depending on their positions relative to a carbonyl carbon.

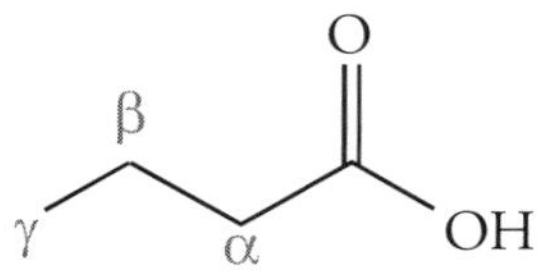

The alpha carbon is acidic because the conjugate base is resonance stabilized. A resonance-stabilized carbanion of this type is referred to as an **enolate ion**. *An enolate ion is negatively charged and nucleophilic.* The nucleophilic character of an enolate ion lies predominately at the carbon at which the proton was abstracted, *not* the oxygen atom of the carbonyl. This is why the α-carbon atom of enolates is the nucleophile in most common enolate reactions.

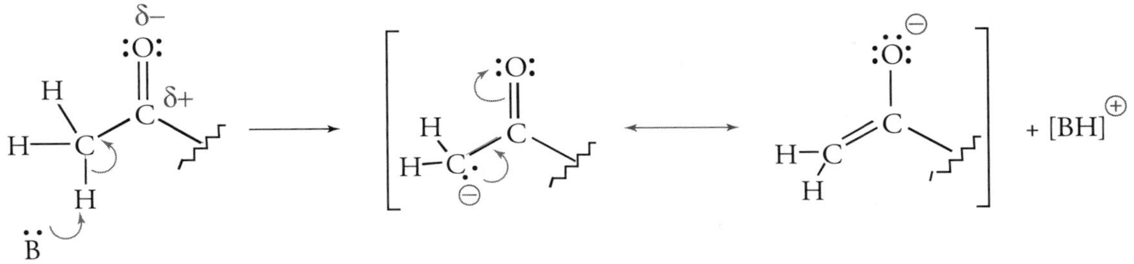

resonance forms of enolate anion

If the α-proton is between two carbonyl groups, its acidity is greatly enhanced.

Keto-Enol Tautomerism

A ketone is converted into an enol by deprotonation of an α-carbon and subsequent protonation of the carbonyl oxygen. These two forms are very similar to one another and differ only by the position of a proton and a double bond. This is referred to as **keto-enol tautomerism**. Two molecules are **tautomers** if they are readily interconvertible constitutional isomers in equilibrium with one another.

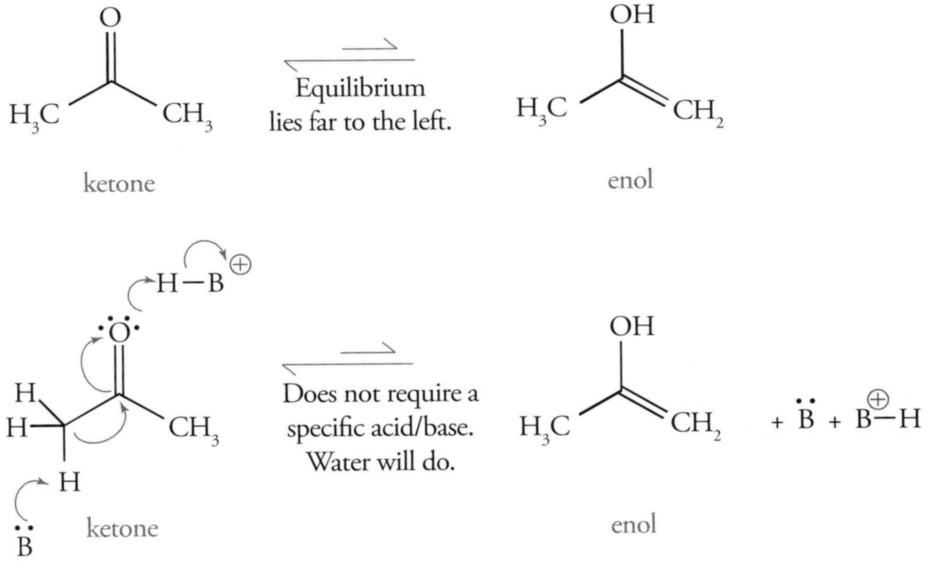

Figure 57

Organometallic Reagents

Organometallic reagents are commonly used to perform nucleophilic addition to a carbonyl carbon. The basic structure of an organometallic reagent is R⁻ M⁺. They act as a source of electron rich, or anionic carbon atoms and therefore function as either strong bases or nucleophiles. Grignard and lithium reagents are the most common organometallic reagents.

Grignard reagents, discussed previously, are generally made via the action of an alkyl or acyl halide on magnesium metal, as depicted below. To avoid unwanted protonation of the very basic Grignard reagent, the reaction is carried out in an aprotic solvent such as diethyl ether.

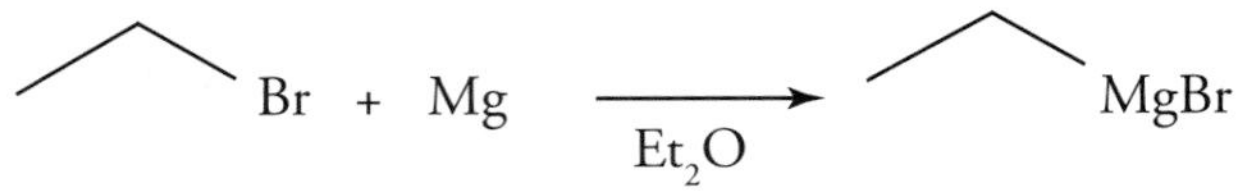

The carbonyl containing compounds are then added to the Grignard reagents in order to yield alcohol products. In the reaction below, the methyl magnesium bromide acts as a nucleophile and adds to the electrophilic carbonyl carbon. An intermediate alkoxide ion is formed that is rapidly protonated to produce the alcohol when aqueous acid is added in a second step.

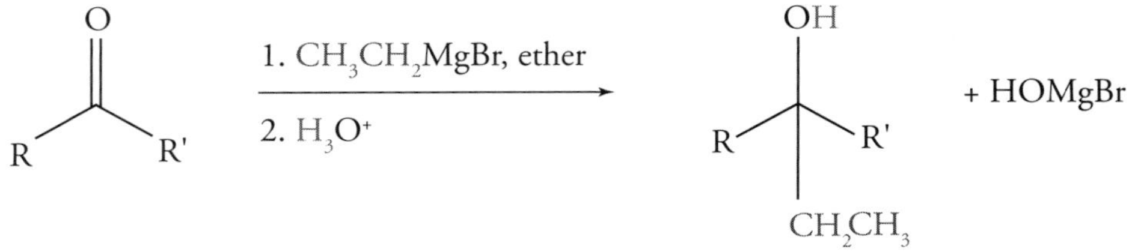

Organolithium reagents are generally made by the reduction of alkyl halides with Li metal as shown below. The reagents are prepared by reacting alkyl halide and lithium in a 1:2 molar ratio. Organolithium reagents react as bases or nucleophiles in the same manner as Grignard reagents.

$$CH_3I + 2Li \xrightarrow{\text{Et}_2O} CH_3Li + LiI$$

Wittig Reaction

While the *mechanism* of the Wittig reaction is not important for the PCAT and is fairly different from the standard nucleophilic addition reaction mentioned above, it is important to be able to *recognize* this reaction. **Wittig reagents** react with aldehydes and ketones to form alkenes, as seen in the reaction below. Since the reaction involves both an addition and an elimination step in its mechanism, there is still a π bond in the product.

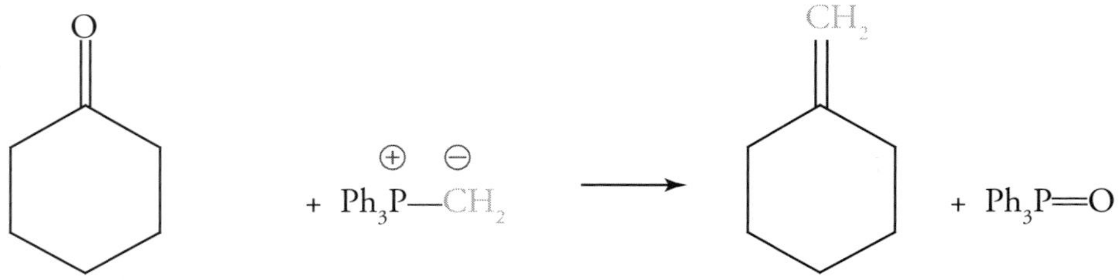

Acetals and Hemiacetals

Acetals and hemiacetals are of fundamental importance in biochemical reactions that occur in living organisms. They can be synthesized from nucleophilic addition reactions to aldehydes or ketones. There are many examples of these molecules in common biochemical pathways. Here are two:

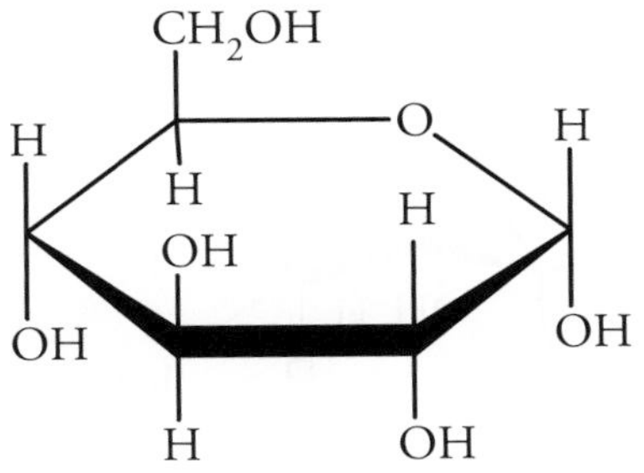

α-D-glucose

a hemiacetal

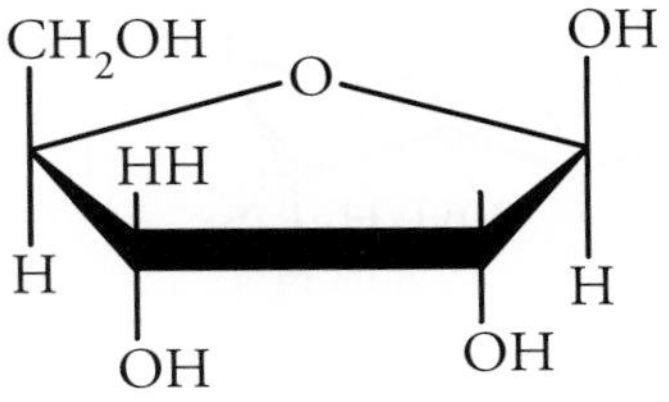

β-D-ribose

a hemiacetal

Acetals and hemiacetals have these general formulas:

acetals

hemiacetals

Figure 58

Acetals are formed when aldehydes or ketones react with alcohols in the presence of acid. This occurs by a nucleophilic addition mechanism. Notice that one (hemiacetal) or two (acetal) –OR groups from the alcohol form bonds to the carbonyl carbon, with subsequent protonation of the carbonyl oxygen. The aldehyde or ketone, the hemiacetal, and the acetal are all in equilibrium with one another. In order for the hemiacetal to form the acetal, a molecule of water must be lost.

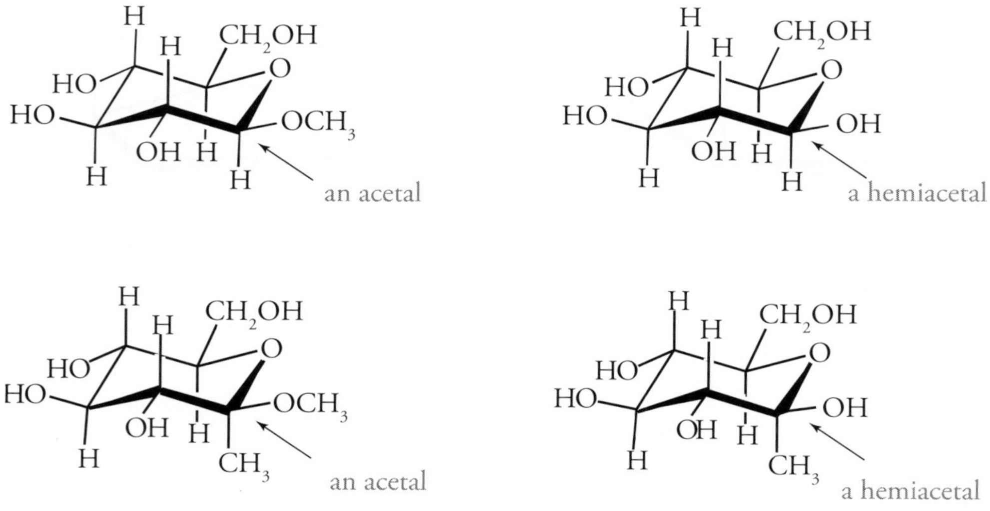

Figure 59

Acetal Formation

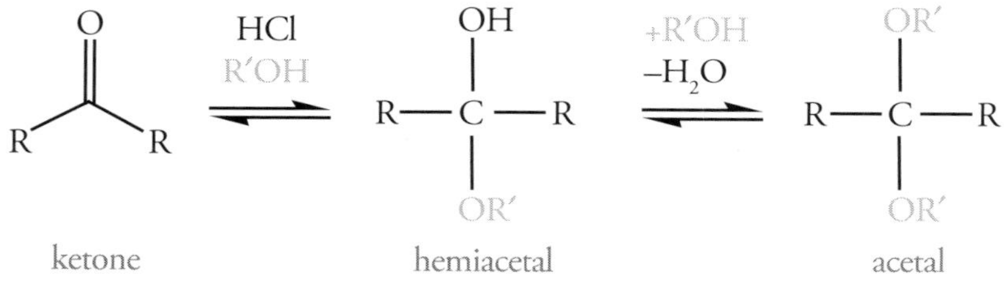

Figure 60

The mechanism of the reaction is shown here, which is initiated by protonation of the oxygen of the carbonyl. The alcohol is the nucleophile.

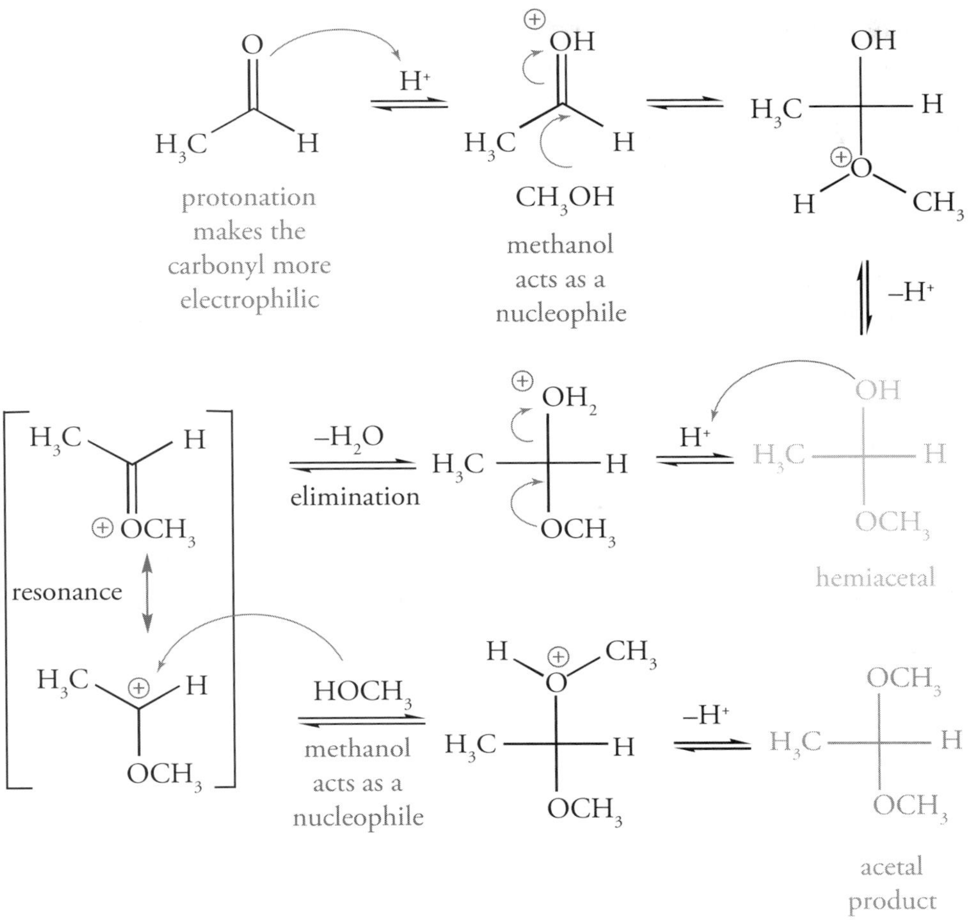

Figure 61

Imine Formation

A reaction that closely resembles acetal formation is the reaction of aldehydes or ketones with primary amines (R–NH$_2$). In this reaction, an aldehyde or ketone reacts with a primary amine (R–NH$_2$) to form an imine:

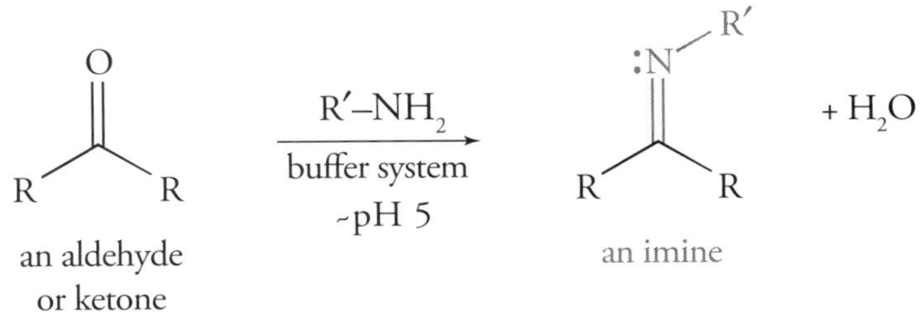

Again, the reaction begins with protonation of the oxygen of the carbonyl, but this time followed by nucleophilic attack by an amine rather than an alcohol.

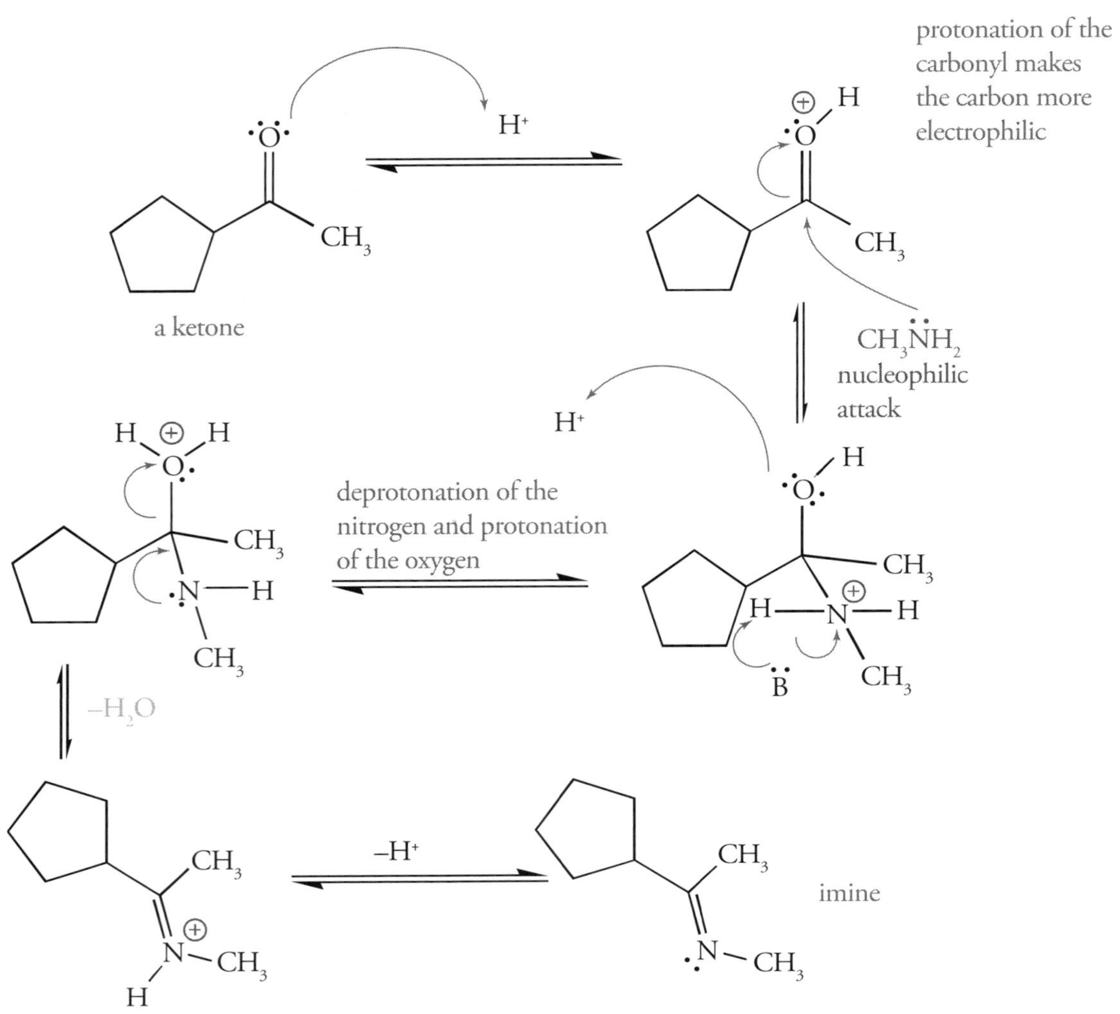

protonation of the
carbonyl makes
the carbon more
electrophilic

a ketone

CH_3NH_2
nucleophilic
attack

deprotonation of the
nitrogen and protonation
of the oxygen

$-H_2O$

imine

Figure 62

Aldol Condensation

A classic reaction in which the enolate anion of one carbonyl compound reacts with the carbonyl group of another carbonyl compound is called the *aldol condensation*. This reaction combines the two types of aldehyde/ketone reactivities: the acidity of the α-proton, and the electrophilicity of the carbonyl carbon.

In the first step of this reaction, a strong base removes an α-proton from the aldehyde, resulting in the formation of a resonance-stabilized enolate anion. Next, the α-carbon of the enolate anion attacks the carbonyl carbon of another aldehyde molecule, thereby generating an alkoxide ion that is subsequently protonated by a molecule of water. This results in the formation of a general class of molecules referred to as β-hydroxy carbonyl compounds. When two different α-hydrogens are present, the result is a **crossed aldol condensation**. On the PCAT, there is typically only one reactant that contains an α-hydrogen.

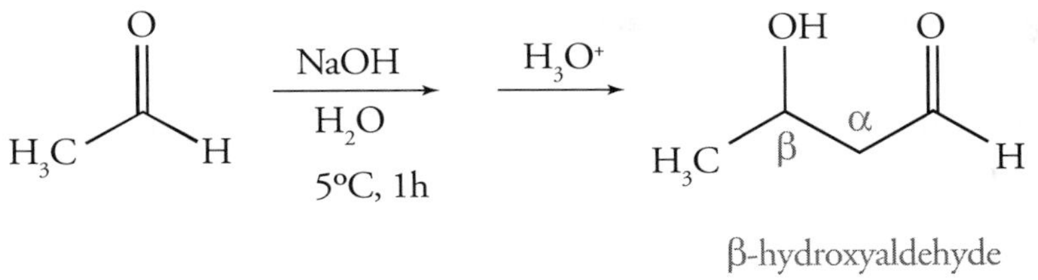

β-hydroxyaldehyde

The Mechanism

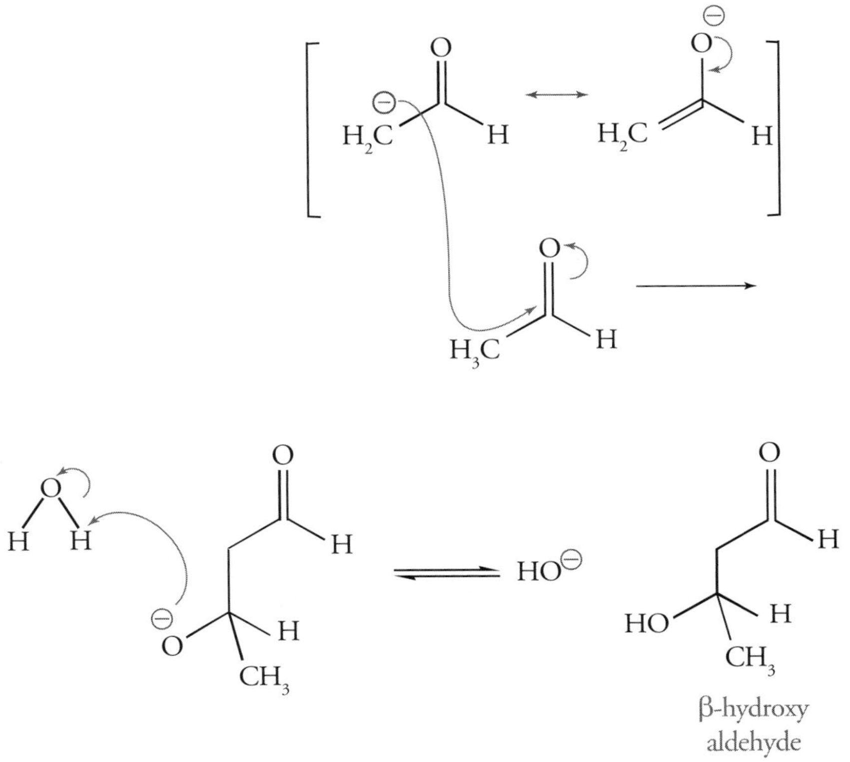

β-hydroxy
aldehyde

Figure 63

If the β-hydroxyaldehyde or ketone products are heated, they will undergo an elimination reaction (dehydration) to form an α,β-**unsaturated carbonyl compound**. Notice that with the newly formed carbon-carbon π bond, the molecule is resonance stabilized:

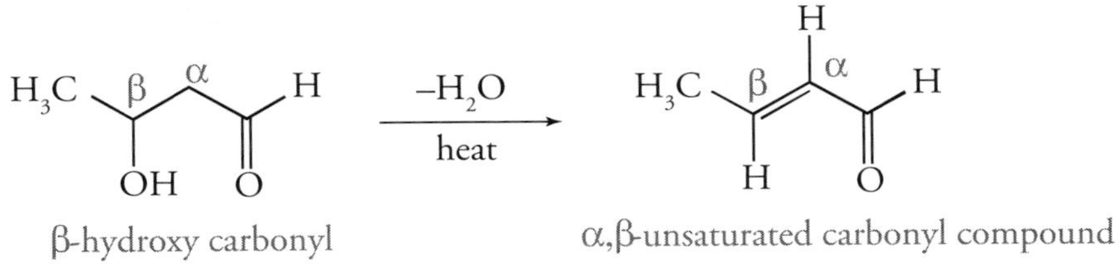

β-hydroxy carbonyl

α,β-unsaturated carbonyl compound

Wolff-Kishner Reduction

The carbonyl groups of an aldehyde or ketone can be converted to a $-CH_2$ group via a Wolff-Kishner reduction. The aldehyde or ketone is heated with hydrazine (H_2NNH_2) and NaOH or KOH in a high-boiling alcohol, such as a glycol. A typical reaction is outlined below.

A Wolff-Kishner reduction will not reduce a carbonyl group of a carboxylic acid.

10.9 CARBOXYLIC ACIDS

Carboxylic acid means an organic molecule with a terminal **carboxyl group**:

The compounds are generically designated RCOOH for aliphatic acids or ArCOOH for aromatic (benzoic) acids.

Carboxylic acid molecules can be large and complex. A single molecule might carry two or three carboxyl groups, such as **dicarboxylic acids** $R(COOH)_2$ and **tricarboxylic acids** $R(COOH)_2$:

Malonic Acid (Propanedioic Acid)

Citric Acid (Tricarboxylic Acid)

Naming Carboxylic Acids

Naming the *open chain* carboxylic acids involves the same prefixes used for the alkanes and the suffix "oic acid" instead of "ane." We number carbons by beginning at the carbon of the carbonyl.

With the carbons thus numbered, the name shows, from left to right:

1. The sites and nature of branches
2. A prefix corresponding to the length of the (longest possible) carbon chain
3. The suffix "oic acid"

$$H-\overset{\overset{H}{|}}{\underset{\underset{H}{|}}{C}}-\overset{\overset{H}{|}}{\underset{\underset{H}{|}}{C}}-\overset{\overset{O}{||}}{C}-OH \qquad : \qquad \text{Propanoic acid}$$

$$H-\overset{\overset{H}{|}}{\underset{\underset{H}{|}}{C}}-\overset{\overset{CH_3}{|}}{\underset{\underset{H}{|}}{C}}-\overset{\overset{H}{|}}{\underset{\underset{H}{|}}{C}}-\overset{\overset{H}{|}}{\underset{\underset{H}{|}}{C}}-\overset{\overset{O}{||}}{C}-OH \qquad : \qquad \text{4-Methylpentanoic acid}$$

$$HO-\overset{\overset{O}{||}}{C}-\overset{\overset{H}{|}}{\underset{\underset{H}{|}}{C}}-\overset{\overset{H}{|}}{\underset{\underset{CH_2CH_3}{|}}{C}}-\overset{\overset{H}{|}}{\underset{\underset{H}{|}}{C}}-\overset{\overset{H}{|}}{\underset{\underset{H}{|}}{C}}-\overset{\overset{CH_3}{|}}{\underset{\underset{H}{|}}{C}}-\overset{\overset{H}{|}}{\underset{\underset{H}{|}}{C}}-\overset{\overset{O}{||}}{C}-OH \quad : \quad \text{3-Ethyl-6-methyloctanedioic acid (a \underline{di}carboxylic acid)}$$

Naming the ring-based carboxylic acids involves the whole phrase "carboxylic acid" (not the little "oic acid" shorthand). We number carbons on the ring beginning with the one to which the COOH group is attached. With the carbons thus numbered, the name shows, from left to right:

1. The sites and nature of branches
2. The name of the ring structure
3. The words "carboxylic acid"

Acyl Groups and Common Names

3-Bromocyclohexane carboxylic acid

"Acyl group" (image of acyl group R) means a carbonyl group bound to some organic structure. An acyl group, therefore, is part and parcel of carboxylic acids, just as it is part of any carbonyl compound—aldehyde/ketone, carboxylic acid, and carboxylic acid derivative. Acyl groups vary, depending on the nature of "R" (which could be a hydrogen atom). Many acyl groups have "common names" not drawn from the IUPAC system. The acyl group that has one carbon in its structure where R is hydrogen, is indicated as "form," so methanoic acid HCOOH is often called "formic acid." Two carbons are indicated as "acet," so acetic acid is formally known as ethanoic acid. Table 10 lists a few carboxylic acids with their IUPAC names.

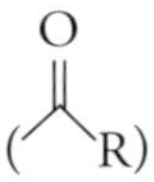

Carboxylic Acid	IUPAC Name
HCOOH	methanoic
CH_3COOH	ethanoic
CH_3CH_2COOH	propanoic
$CH_3(CH_2)_2COOH$	butanoic
$CH_3(CH_2)_3COOH$	pentanoic
$CH_3(CH_2)_4COOH$	hexanoic

Table 10

Physical Properties of Carboxylic Acids

The acyl carbon shares properties with the carbonyl carbon of aldehydes and ketones. That is, it is sp^2 hybridized and has planar geometry. Unlike aldehydes and ketones, but *like* alcohols, carboxylic acid molecules form hydrogen bonds with one another. Boiling points for carboxylic acids, therefore, are much higher than they are for alkanes of similar molecular weight, and they are higher, even, than alcohols of similar molecular weight. This is because carboxylic acid molecules can form *two* hydrogen bonds. These intermolecular interactions form a **cyclic dimer,** as shown here:

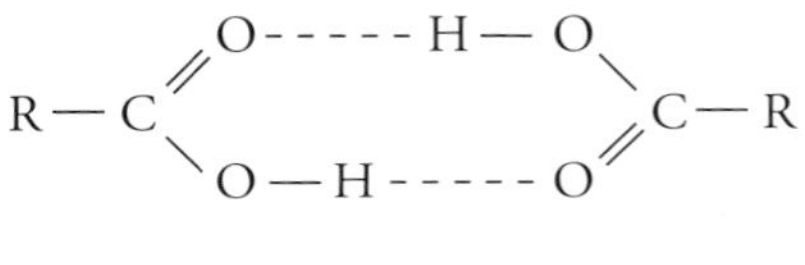

Acidity

A carboxylic acid loses a proton because of the stability of the carboxylate anion RCOO⁻, which is *stabilized by resonance.* The negative charge is delocalized, giving a partial negative charge and partial double bond character to both oxygen atoms bound to the acyl carbon.

For the PCAT, it is important to know that the *stability of the carboxylate ion makes carboxylic acids more acidic than alcohols.*

Inductive Effects

Consider a molecule of 2-chloro-3-phenylpropanoic acid:

2-chloro-3-phenylpropanoic acid

If a halogen atom is bound to the alpha carbon, the corresponding carboxylate ion is stabilized. This is because the halogen atom is electronegative and as such is an electron withdrawing group. It stabilizes the anion, thereby increasing the acidity of the corresponding acid. An electron-releasing group bound to the alpha carbon has the opposite effect. It destabilizes the anion and reduces acidity.

Whether the acid does or does not contain a benzene ring, the inductive effects of alpha carbon substitution are the same.

For the PCAT, remember that:

- Alpha carbon substitution by an electron-withdrawing group tends to increase acidity.
- Alpha carbon substitution by an electron-releasing group tends to decrease acidity.

Preparing Carboxylic Acids

Oxidation of Alcohols, Aldehydes, and Alkylbenzenes

Oxidation of primary alcohols with a strong oxidizing agent ($KMnO_4$ or CrO_3) will cause the alcohol to lose both its alpha hydrogens and produce a carboxylic acid. (A weaker oxidizing agent will produce an aldehyde, and secondary alcohols can be oxidized to ketones.) Oxidation of aldehydes will produce carboxylic acids as well. **Tollens reagent** $Ag(NH_3)_2^+$ is preferred as an oxidizing agent because it minimizes side reactions.

$$RCH_2OH \xrightarrow[\text{heat}]{\substack{(1)\ KMnO_4, OH^- \\ (2)\ H_3O^+}} RCO_2H$$

$$R\text{--}CHO \xrightarrow{CrO_3} RCO_2H$$

Hydrolysis of Nitriles

Primary and secondary alkyl halides can be converted to carboxylic acids through a two-step process involving cyanide. In the first step, a nitrile (alkyl cyanide) is prepared by an S_N2 reaction. This step is then followed by hydrolysis in aqueous acid, which produces the carboxylic acid.

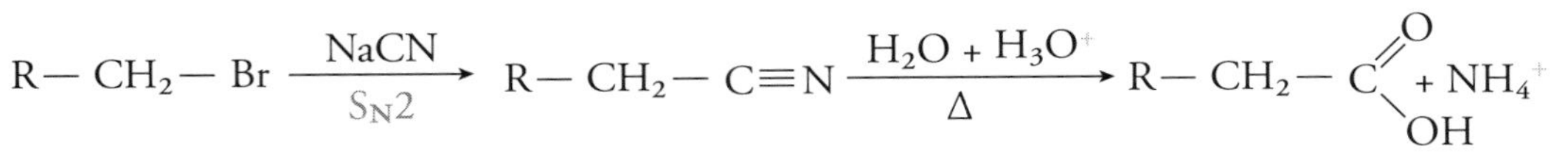

$$R-CH_2-Br \xrightarrow[S_N2]{NaCN} R-CH_2-C\equiv N \xrightarrow[\Delta]{H_2O + H_3O^+} R-CH_2-C\overset{O}{\underset{OH}{<}} + NH_4^+$$

Reactions of Carboxylic Acids

Reduction to Yield Primary Alcohols

With a powerful reducing agent like $LiAlH_4$ followed by treatment with acid, carboxylic acids can be reduced to primary alcohols. Two examples are shown here:

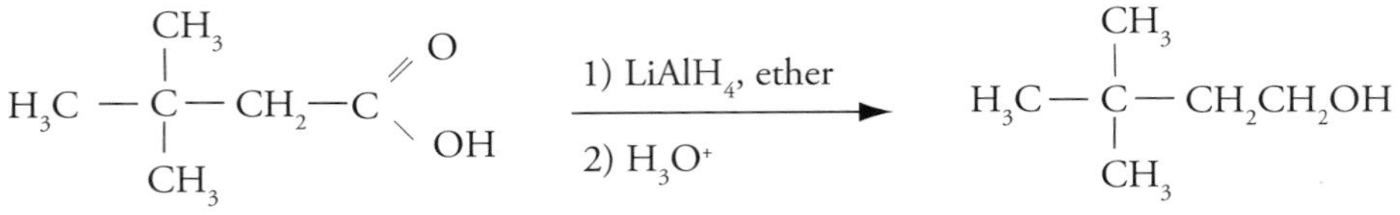

3,3-dimethylbutanoic acid → 3,3-dimethyl-1-butanol

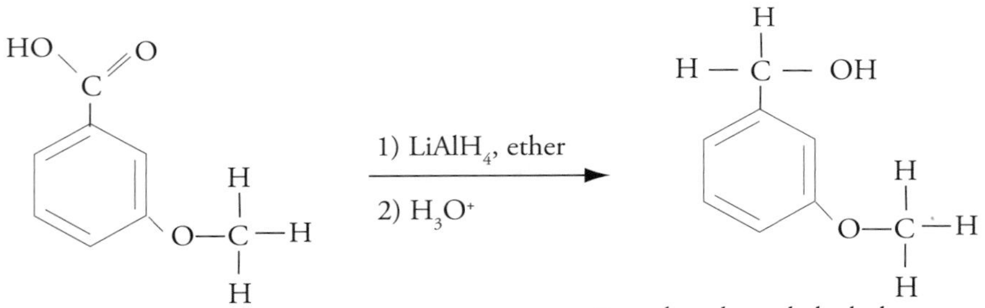

3-methoxybenzoic acid → 3-methoxybenzyl alcohol

Figure 64

Reduction to Yield Aldehydes or Ketones

Carboxylic acids are less reactive to nucleophiles than aldehydes or ketones. A carboxylic acid can be reduced to an aldehyde or ketone using a potent reducing agent, such as LiH, alkyl lithium, or $LiAlH_4$. The aldehyde or ketone can then be respectively reduced to a primary or secondary alcohol. In contrast, when a carboxylic acid reacts with $NaBH_4$, an aldehyde is produced that cannot be isolated because it is more reactive than the carboxylic acid.

10.9

Decarboxylation

Decarboxylation is the loss of a CO_2 molecule. The reaction is slow, however, unless the β carbon forms a carbonyl. The acid is then called a β-keto acid. The reaction proceeds through formation of an enolate ion that is a *resonance stabilized intermediate.* Protonation of the enolate ion then yields the ultimate decarboxylated product.

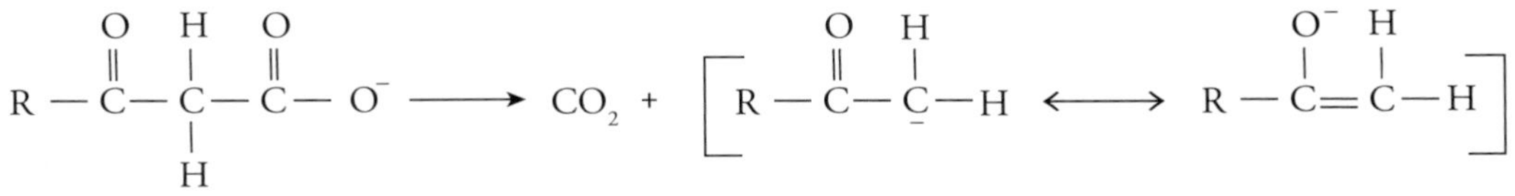

β-keto acid

enolate ion

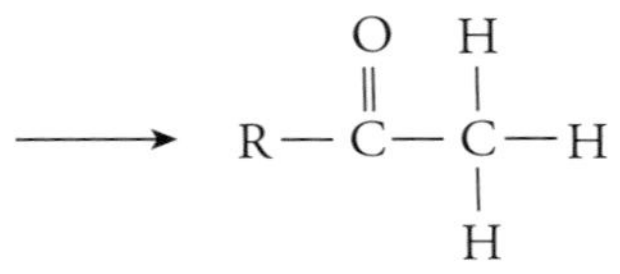

ketone

Formation of Carboxylic Acid Derivatives

Carboxylic acid derivatives are categories of compounds generated from carboxylic acids. The derivatives that are important for the PCAT are these:

- acid chlorides
- acid anhydrides
- esters
- amides

Carboxylic Acids to Acid Chlorides

Acid chlorides are prepared by the reaction between a carboxylic acid and either $SOCl_2$, PCl_3, or PCl_5.

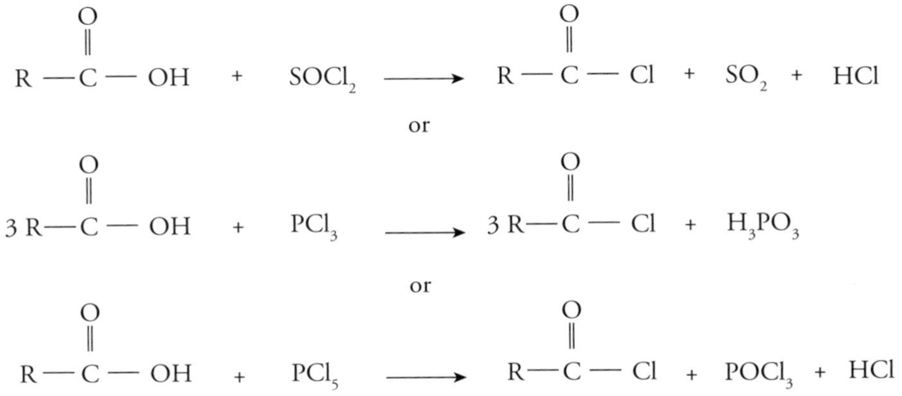

Figure 65

Carboxylic Acids to Acid Anhydrides

We might conceive of an acid anhydride as two carbonyl groups linked together by oxygen:

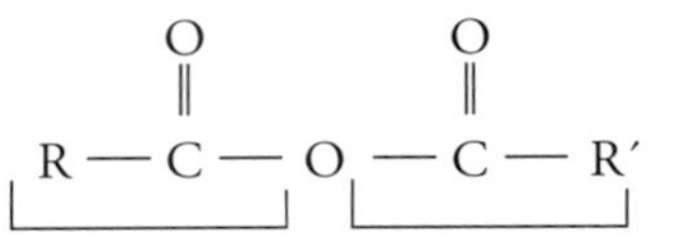

acid anhydride

In the presence of pyridine, an acid anhydride forms from the reaction of a carboxylic acid and an acid chloride, and yields an acetic anhydride when R and R′ are CH_3:

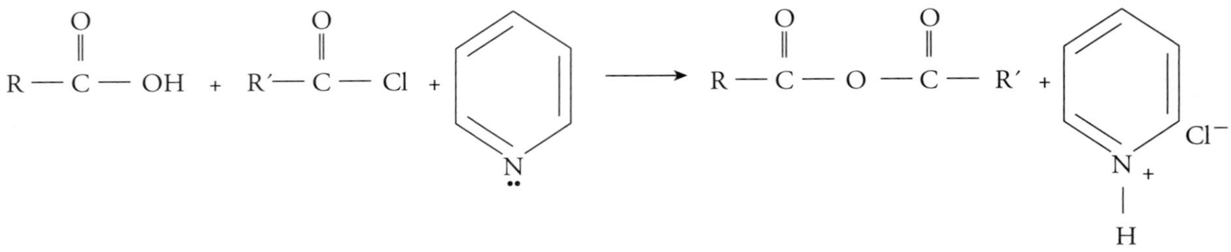

Carboxylic Acids to Esters

Ester means a molecule in which the carboxylic acid's OH group is replaced by an OR group. Esters are formed in an acid-catalyzed reaction between a carboxylic acid and an alcohol.

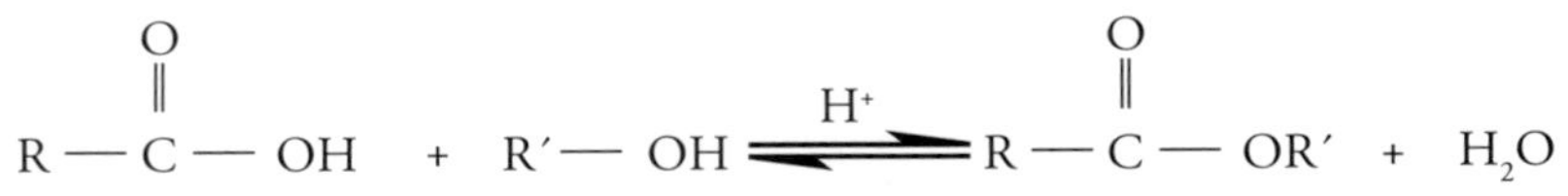

Acid Chlorides to Amides

The reaction between a carboxylic acid and an amine produces a salt (it is an acid-base reaction), but the reaction of an amine or NH_3 with an acid chloride produces an amide:

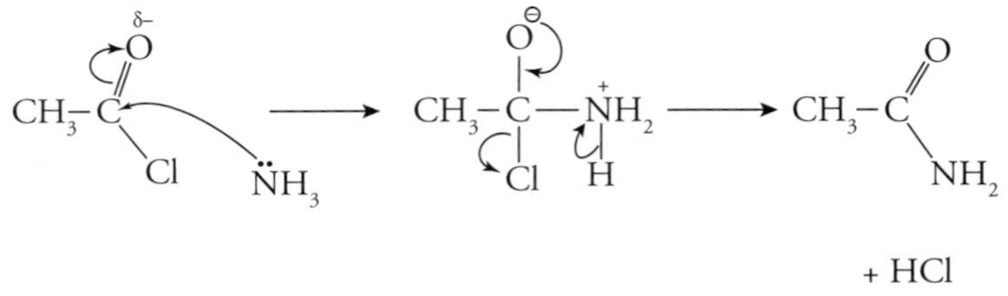

+ HCl

Esters to Amides

As shown above, carboxylic acids undergo nucleophilic attack to produce esters. If an ester is reacted with a primary amine, secondary amine, or ammonia, the product is an amide.

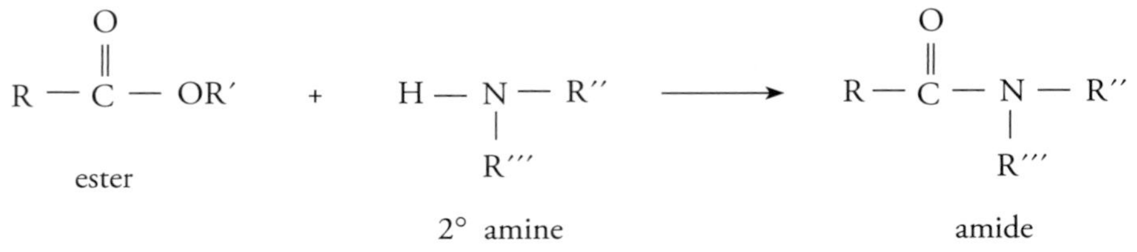

Many of the reactions of the carboxylic acid derivatives involve conversion from one derivative to another. It should be noted that the better the leaving group attached to the derivative, the more reactive the species. The relative reactivity of the four important derivatives for the PCAT is therefore

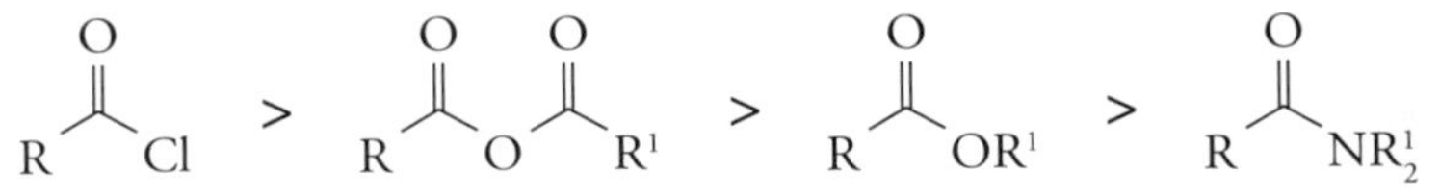

$$
\underset{R \quad Cl}{\overset{O}{\parallel}} > \underset{R \quad O \quad R^1}{\overset{O \quad\quad O}{\parallel \quad\quad \parallel}} > \underset{R \quad OR^1}{\overset{O}{\parallel}} > \underset{R \quad NR_2^1}{\overset{O}{\parallel}}
$$

10.10   ESTERS

Acid Catalyzed Hydrolysis

The acid catalyzed reaction of a carboxylic acid and an alcohol produces an ester. The reaction is, however, reversible, so choosing one reaction over the other is really a matter of manipulating equilibrium.

Base Promoted Hydrolysis of Esters: Soap

The reaction of an ester with sodium hydroxide involves nucleophilic attack on the electropositive acyl carbon, followed by proton transfer which forms a good leaving group:

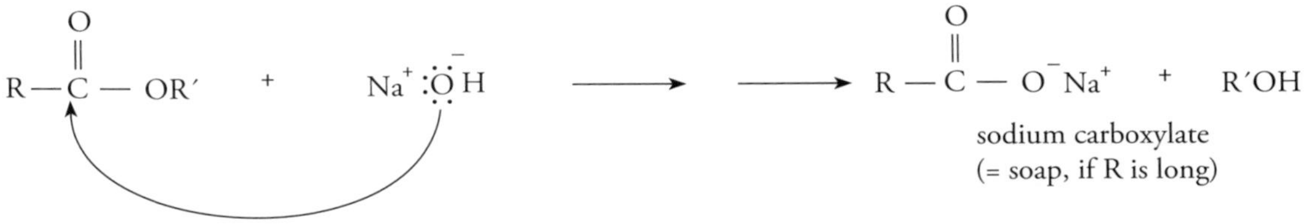

If the carboxylate portion of the salt is long (12 to 18 carbon atoms) the salt is a *soap*. When added to water, individual soap molecules are not dissolved as are true water-soluble substances. Rather, the molecules (hundreds of them, perhaps) coalesce to form a spherical *micelle* in which the outward directed polar heads are solvated by water. Nonpolar substances, such as oils, dissolve in the nonpolar center. Thus, the soap removes oils, which are then washed away in the polar solvent, water. We will return to a discussion of soaps when we discuss lipids in Chapter 11.

Transesterification and Reduction

In a **transesterification** reaction, one OR group of an ester is replaced by another:

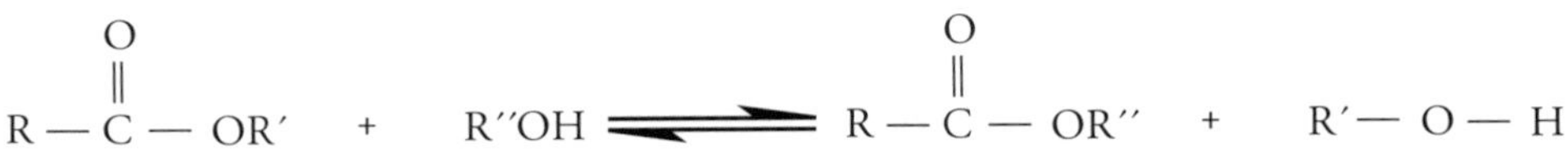

In the presence of a reductant, an ester is reduced to a primary alcohol, as shown here:

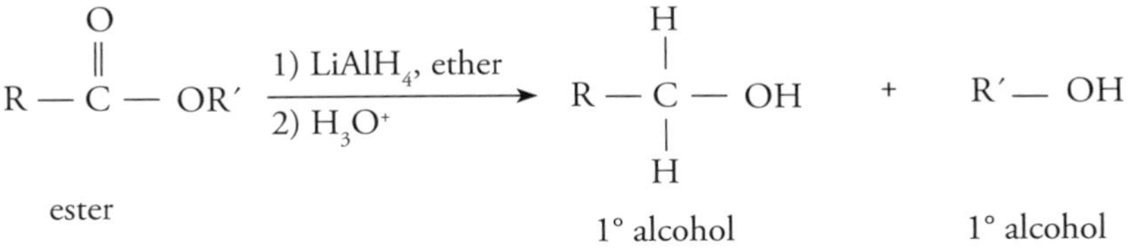

10.11 AMINES

Amines are organic derivatives of ammonia and, like, ammonia, are weak bases. In their reactions they behave as nucleophiles due to their lone pair of electrons. An *alkylamine* has a nitrogen attached to an sp^3 hybridized carbon, whereas in an *arylamine* the nitrogen is attached to an sp^2 hybridized carbon of an aromatic ring.

Naming Amines

Amines are classified according to the degree of substitution at the nitrogen atom. A **primary amine** has nitrogen attached to a single carbon, a **secondary amine** to two carbon atoms, and a **tertiary amine** to three.

Primary amine   Secondary amine   Tertiary amine

A nitrogen with four substituents is positively charged and is the *ammonium* ion. One example is ethylammonium chloride, $CH_3CH_2NH_3^+Cl^-$.

Primary amines are named as alkylamines and use the same numbering convention as alcohols. Arylamines are named as **arene amines** . Aniline is a name used for amino-substituted derivatives of benzene, where the carbon bearing the amino group is designated as C-1. Compounds with two amino groups have the suffix *diamine*.

1-methylbutylamine   p-fluoroaniline   1,4-benzenediamine

Amines are named as a substituent when a hydroxyl or carbonyl group is present. Secondary and tertiary amines become *N*-substituted derivatives of primary amines.

3-aminopropanol   N-ethylbutylamine

Physical Properties of Amines

With their lone pair of electrons, amines are more polar than alkanes but less polar than alcohols. They engage in dipole-dipole interactions and primary and secondary amines in H-bonding. Consequently, amines have elevated boiling points. All amines can act as Lewis bases and are frequently found in coordinate covalent compounds, such as hemoglobin, where the two electrons on each nitrogen atom form a covalent bond to a metal center.

Although amines are weak bases, they are the strongest bases of all neutral molecules. Alkylamines are stronger bases than ammonia and are consistent in their pK_a's, which range from approximately 10–11. Arylamines are weaker bases than alkylamines or arylamines, with pK_a's ranging from 4–5. Because amines are electron donors, this weak basicity is a result of conjugation of the unshared pair of electrons with the aromatic ring. Conjugation of an arylamine with more than one aromatic ring reduces the basicity even further.

Preparing Amines

Alkylation of Ammonia

In principle, alkylamines can be prepared by nucleophilic substitution reactions of alkyl halides with ammonia. While this method can be used to prepare α-amino acids, it generally leads to a complex mixture of products because the product, a primary amine, competes with ammonia for the alkyl halide. Competitive alkylation with secondary and tertiary amines can occur in a similar manner. Aryl halides normally do not react with ammonia.

$$RX + 2NH_3 \rightarrow RNH_2 + NH_4X$$
Primary amine

$$RX + RNH_2 + NH_3 \rightarrow RNHR + NH_4X$$
Secondary amine

$$RX + R_2NH + NH_3 \rightarrow R_3NH + NH_4X$$
Tertiary amine

Gabriel Synthesis

The formation of biproducts can be avoided through the use of the **Gabriel synthesis**. The reagent for this reaction is the potassium salt of phthalimide, which has a negatively charged nitrogen atom that acts as a nucleophile in an S_N2 process:

Phthalimide

The Gabriel synthesis can only be used to prepare amines of the type RCH_2NH_2. Formation of secondary and tertiary amines does not occur because phthalimide can only undergo a single alkylation.

Reduction

Organic compounds containing nitrogen can generally be reduced to an amine. Suitable precursors are **alkyl azides**, **nitriles**, or nitro groups followed by reduction through catalytic hydrogenation or the use of $LiAlH_4$. Examples of these types of reactions are shown here:

Alkyl azides:

$$R-N=N^+=N^- \quad \xrightarrow[\text{2) } H_2O]{\text{1) } LiAlH_4} \quad RNH_2$$

Nitriles:

$$R-C\equiv N \quad \xrightarrow[\text{2) } H_2O]{\text{1) } LiAlH_4} \quad RNH_2$$

Nitro groups:

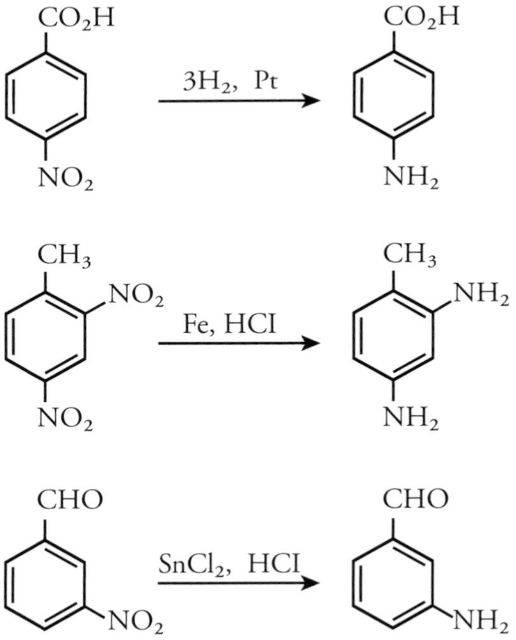

The reaction of an aldehyde or ketone with ammonia produces an imine that can be reduced to primary amines through catalytic hydrogenation:

| Aldehyde or ketone | Ammonia | Imine | Primary amine |

Reactions of Amines

Hofmann Elimination

The **Hofmann elimination**—a synthetic method used to prepare alkenes—can be used for structure determination. The overall reaction involves the use of a quaternary ammonium iodide in an aqueous slurry of silver oxide. The quaternary ammonium hydroxide is formed in solution and silver iodide precipitates:

$$2(R_4N^+I^-)(aq) \; + \; Ag_2O(s) \; + \; H_2O(l) \; \rightarrow \; 2(R_4N^+\,{}^-OH)(aq) \; + \; 2AgI(s)$$

Quaternary ammonium iodide   Silver halide   Quaternary ammonium hydroxide   Silver iodide

10.11

When heated, the soluble product undergoes β elimination in a concerted E2 mechanism to form an alkene and an amine. The less sterically hindered β hydrogen is removed by the base.

The unique aspect of the Hofmann elimination is that elimination gives the *less* substituted alkene. It is used to prepare alkenes that are not synthetically accessible by dehydrohalogenation of alkyl halides.

10.12 STRUCTURAL ANALYSIS

Infrared Spectroscopy: Identifying Functional Groups

Infrared spectroscopy (IR) is a physical method used to characterize functional groups in a compound or mixture of organic compounds. It uses electromagnetic radiation that lies between microwaves and visible light to excite molecular vibrations. The energy absorbed produces a unique molecular fingerprint, called a *spectrum*, that is measured in **wavenumbers** (cm^{-1}), the number of waves in 1 cm. High frequencies, large wavenumbers, and short wavelengths are all associated with high energy. A compound must have a dipole to be IR active.

A typical IR spectrum shows the **mid-IR** region, which is between 4,000 and 400 cm^{-1}. The functional group region is from 4,000 to 1,400 cm^{-1}, and the fingerprint region, which is characteristic of the compound as a whole, is from 1,400 to 600 cm^{-1}.

More energy is needed to stretch a bond than bend it, so stretching is typically in the functional group region, whereas bending is in the fingerprint region. The greater the change in dipole moment, or polarity, the more intense the absorption. The energy required to stretch a bond depends on two factors:

1. Bond strength: Stronger bonds require more energy to stretch, so bond strength is proportional to bond order. For example, $C=N$ absorbs at approximately 1,600 cm^{-1}, whereas $C-N$ absorbs at around 1,100 cm^{-1}.
2. Masses: Heavier atoms vibrate at lower frequencies. Thus, $C-H$ absorbs at about 3000 cm^{-1}, but $C-O$ absorbs at approximately 1,100 cm^{-1}.

Resonance lowers the bond order, so corresponding frequencies are lowered. Also, hydrogen bonding lowers the frequency. Here is the spectrum of propan-1-ol (*n*-propanol), showing a significant OH bond at 3,350 cm^{-1}. The absorption peak is broad because of intermolecular hydrogen bonding.

Infrared spectrum of propan-1-ol, $CH_3CH_2CH_2OH$

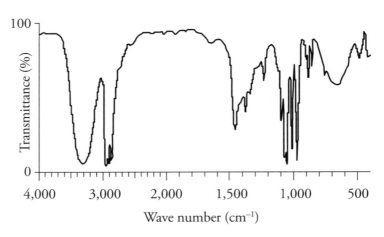

The PCAT expects you to know key IR frequencies, tabulated here:

Type of bond	Wavenumber (cm^{-1})
$C\equiv N$	2,260–2,220
$C\equiv C$	2,260–2,100
$C=C$	1,680–1,600
$C=N$	1,650–1,550
	~1,600 and ~1,500–1,430
$C=O$	1,780–1,650
$C-O$	1,250–1,050
$C-N$	1,230–1,020
O–H (alcohol)	3,650–3,200
O–H (carboxylic acid)	3,300–2,500
N–H	3,500–3,300
C–H	3,300–2,700

It's not necessary to memorize specific frequencies, but you should be able to identify the approximate frequencies of functional groups.

Nuclear Magnetic Resonance: Identifying Molecular Structure

10.12

Nuclear magnetic resonance spectroscopy focuses on the absorption of energy when an atom's nucleus is excited from a low energy spin state to the next higher one. Proton nuclear magnetic resonance (^{1}**NMR**) provides information about the environments of the various hydrogens in a molecule.

As with an electron, a proton has two spin states: $+\frac{1}{2}$ and $-\frac{1}{2}$. Electromagnetic energy can be absorbed only when the two spin states have different energies, which can occur when a proton is placed in an external magnetic field, B_0. The spin state that aligns with B_0 has a lower energy than the one aligned against B_0. The difference in energy is proportional to the strength of the applied field.

A single proton will feel the full strength of the external magnetic field, but a proton in an organic molecule responds to the external field and any local fields in its environment. Local fields reduce the effect of the applied field, causing the proton to be **shielded**. If shielding is reduced, the proton is said to be **deshielded**.

Different protons produce signals at different applied field strengths. The molecular environment determines whether a proton absorbs energy at a higher field strength (*upfield*), or at a lower field strength (*downfield*). This dependence is called a **chemical shift** (δ). A chemical shift is measured against tetramethylsilane [$(CH_3)_4Si$], abbreviated TMS, because its protons are more shielded than those in most organic compounds. Here are some examples of chemical shifts relative to TMS:

downfield shift

←─────────────────────────────

	$CHCl_3$	CH_2Cl_2	CH_3Cl
δ	7.3	5.3	3.1

Hydrogens that are bonded to double bonds or aromatic rings are significantly deshielded, as are those bonded to electronegative atoms, so they have a downfield chemical shift. Chemically equivalent protons have identical electronic environments. Their signal strength is proportionally enhanced.

Spin-spin splitting occurs when nonequivalent protons interact, and is most significant when hydrogens are bonded to adjacent carbon atoms. The number of adjacent protons determines the number of peaks in the splitting pattern. The number of peaks associated with chemically equivalent protons in the NMR spectrum is $n + 1$ where n is the number of nonequivalent, neighboring protons, called **nearest neighbors**. Here, for example, is the NMR spectrum of ethanol.

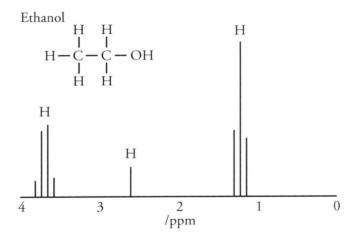

Notice that the proton directly bonded to oxygen has no nearest neighbors and forms a *singlet*, whereas the two protons on C1 have three nearest neighbors that produce a splitting pattern with four peaks (a *quartet*), and the protons on C2 have two nearest neighbors, producing three peaks (a *triplet*). The single –OH proton is shifted downfield due to deshielding effects from the electronegative oxygen.

10.12

The PCAT expects you to know these commonly encountered chemical shifts:

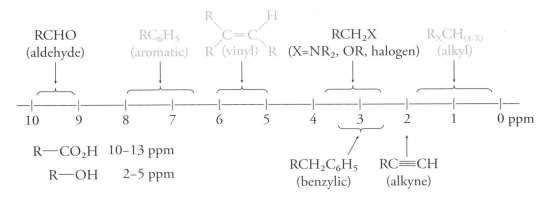

R—CO₂H   10–13 ppm

R—OH   2–5 ppm

Mass Spectrometry: Identifying Mass and Structures

Mass spectrometry does not involve the absorption of electromagnetic radiation, but instead bombards a molecule with high energy electrons that are able to break chemical bonds. The electron impact produces positively charged molecular ions with essentially the same mass as the fragments from which they were formed. The fragments are propelled through a magnet causing them to deflect and separate according to their mass-to-charge ratio (*m/z*). The lightest particles will be deflected the most, whereas the heaviest will be deflected the least. A detector produces a mass spectrum that shows a plot of the relative intensity of the fragments versus their ***m/z* ratio**.

The mass spectrum of pentane is shown below. Notice that the heaviest ion, known as the *molecular ion*, has a mass of 72, which corresponds to the mass of pentane. Clusters around a major peak occur from the gain or loss of protons, stability of the ion, and naturally occurring elemental isotopes.

$$CH_3\text{-}CH_2\text{-}CH_2\text{-}CH_2\text{-}CH_3$$

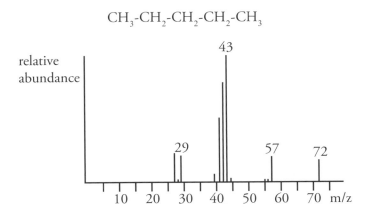

The structure of the molecule is deduced from its fragmentation pattern, and the molecular formula of the compound can be obtained.

Mass spectrometry also gives information about the number of unsaturated bonds in a fragment. This is accomplished by comparing the mass of a fragment to the formula for an alkane, C_nH_{2n+2}, or to an alkene or ring structure, C_nH_{2n}.

Ultraviolet-Visible (UV-VIS) Spectroscopy: Identifying π Systems

UV-VIS spectroscopy provides information on transitions between electronic energy levels and is primarily used to identify conjugated π systems. Transitions are measured in the 200–400 nm UV region of the electromagnetic spectrum and the 400–800 nm visible region, for a total range of 200–800 nm.

The presence of a solvent causes absorptions to be broad in a UV-VIS spectrum. There is a maximum absorption at λ_{max} that is characteristic of the electronic transitions occurring within the molecule. The absorption, or *band*, is called the **absorbance** (*A*). A **molar absorptivity**, ε, can be calculated by dividing *A* by the concentration *c* in moles per liter and the path length *l* in centimeters:

$$\varepsilon = \frac{A}{c \cdot l}$$

Adding substituents to a double bond or having a system with extended conjugation causes λ_{max} to shift to longer wavelengths.

The structure and UV spectrum of ATP is shown here:

ATP

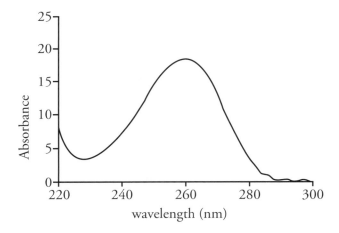

The absorption at 760 nm corresponds to electronic transitions that occur in the heterocycle.

CHAPTER 10 KEY TERMS

α,β-unsaturated carbonyl compound
π bond
σ bond
absolute configuration
absorbance
achiral
acyl group
aldehydes
alkoxide ion
alkyl azides
alkyl radicals
anomeric carbon
anomeric center
anomers
anti conformation
anti-Markovnikov addition
arene amine
asymmetric center
axial
Birch Reduction
bond dissociation energy (BDE)
bond order
Cahn-Ingold-Prelog rules
carbanions
carbocation
carbonium ions
carbonyl compound
carbonyl group
carboxyl group
carboxylic acid
chair form
chemical shift
chiral
chiral centers
conformational isomers
conjugated system
constitutional isomers
crossed aldol condensation
cyclic dimer
deactivate
decarboxylation
degree of unsaturation
deshielded
dextrorotatory
diastereomers
dicarboxylic acids
Diels-Alder reaction

eclipsed
electron-donating
electron-withdrawing
electrophiles
electrophilic addition
enantiomers
enolate ion
epimeric carbon
epimers
epoxide formation
equatorial
ester
free-radical halogenation
Friedel-Crafts acylation
Friedel-Crafts alkylation
Gabriel synthesis
gauche conformation
geometric isomers
Grignard reagent
heterolytic bond cleavage
Hofmann elimination
homolytic bond cleavage
hybrid
hydroboration
inductive effect
infrared spectroscopy (IR)
initiation
keto-enol tautomerism
ketones
leaving group
levorotatory
m/z ratio
Markovnikov's rule
mass spectrometry
meso
mid-IR
molar absorptivity
nearest neighbor
nitrile
NMR
nucleophiles
optically active
oxonium ion
polarizability
primary alcohol
primary amine
propagation

pyranose
racemic mixture
resonance effects
resonance hybrid
ring activating group
ring deactivating group
ring strain
secondary alcohol
secondary amine
shielded
solubility
solvolysis
specific rotation
spin-spin splitting
staggered

stereocenter
stereogenic center
stereoisomers
syn addition
tautomers
termination
tertiary alcohol
tertiary amine
the electrophile
Tollens reagent
transesterification
tricarboxylic acids
UV-VIS spectroscopy
wavenumber
Wittig Reagents

ORGANIC CHEMISTRY DRILL

1. How many σ and π bonds are present in 2-pentyne?

   A. 5 σ bonds and 2 π bonds
   B. 12 σ bonds and 1 π bond
   C. 14 σ bonds and 1 π bond
   D. 12 σ bonds and 2 π bonds

2. 1,3-dichloropentane reacts with a stoichiometric amount of NaI via nucleophilic substitution. What is the product?

   A. 1-chloro-3-iodopentane
   B. 1,3-iodopentane
   C. 3-chloro-1-iodopentane
   D. 3,3-chloroiodopentane

3. The reaction of 1,2-dimethylcyclohexene with diborane produces *cis*-1,2-dimethylcyclohexanol. What type of reaction is this?

   A. Markovnikov addition
   B. Birch reduction
   C. Anti-Markovnikov addition
   D. Grignard

4. Of these three species, which is aromatic?

   I. $C_8H_8^-$
   II. $C_8H_8^{2+}$
   III. $C_8H_8^{2-}$

   A. I only
   B. II only
   C. I and III only
   D. II and III only

5. When fluorobenzene reacts with benzyl chloride, the primary product is 4-fluorodiphenylmethane. This is an example of a(n):

   A. Wolff-Kishner reduction
   B. Friedel-Crafts alkylation
   C. Aldol condensation
   D. Gabriel synthesis

6. In the presence of KOH and H_2O, butanal reacts to form 2-ethyl-3-hydroxyhexanal. This is an example of what type of reaction?

   A. Aldol condensation
   B. Wittig reaction
   C. Markovnikov addition
   D. Hoffman elimination

7. Which of these compounds is more stable in the enol rather than the keto form?

   I. 2,4-cyclohexadienone
   II. 2,4-pentanedione
   III. 2-butanone

   A. I only
   B. III only
   C. I and III
   D. I and II

8. Order these carboxylic acids by increasing pK_a:

   fluoroacetic acid   propanoic acid   dichloroacetic acid

   A. propanoic acid, dichloroacetic acid, fluoroacetic acid
   B. dichloroacetic acid, fluoroacetic acid, propanoic acid
   C. fluoroacetic acid, dichloroacetic acid, propanoic acid
   D. propanoic acid, fluoroacetic acid, dichloroacetic acid

9. 4-chloro-1-butanol is oxidized to 4-chlorobutanoic acid. What reagent is most suitable for this conversion?

   A. $LiAlH_4$
   B. $K_2Cr_2O_7$
   C. HCl
   D. $NaBH_4$

10. The compound 2-phenylethylamine can be prepared from 2-phenylethylbromide using which synthetic method?

   A. Wolff-Kishner reduction
   B. Hoffman elimination
   C. Gabriel synthesis
   D. Nucleophilic addition

11. How many ^{1}NMR signals are there for the compound 1,3-dichloro-2-butene, and what is the splitting pattern?

   A. 3 signals; two doublets and a triplet
   B. 2 signals; a triplet and a doublet
   C. 2 signals; a singlet and a doublet
   D. 3 signals; a singlet, a triplet, and a doublet

Want More Practice?
Register your book online for more drill questions!

Answers and Explanations

1. **D** A ball-and-stick model of 2-pentyne is shown here:

    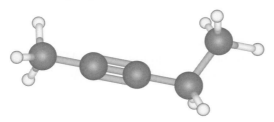

    The triple bond contains 1 σ bond and 2 π bonds (eliminate choices B and C). All bonds to H are σ bonds, and there are an additional three C-C σ bonds. The total number of σ bonds is 1 + 8 + 3 = 12, so choice (D) is correct.

2. **C** Nucleophilic attack favors the less hindered primary position, so substitution occurs at C-1. Choices (A) and (D), therefore, can be eliminated. The reaction is stoichiometric, so only one substitution reaction will occur (eliminate choice B). The correct answer is choice (C).

3. **C** This is a hydroboration-oxidation reaction that results in *syn* hydration of the double bond, so eliminate choices (B) and (C). In the presence of diborane and peroxide, the double bond is substituted symmetrically in a manner not consistent with a Markovnikov addition. Thus, choice (A) can be eliminated, and choice (C) is correct:

1,2-dimethylcyclohexene	*cis*-1,2-dimethylcyclohexanol

4. **D** Using Hückel's Rule for predicting aromaticity, in structure I, there are 9 π electrons: $4n + 2 = 9$. The value of n cannot be an integer, so I is not aromatic (eliminate choices A and C). Determining the aromaticity of structure III will allow us to decide between choices (B) and (D). The structure given in III has 10 π electrons: $4n + 2 = 10$, and $n = 2$, a whole number. Structure III is therefore aromatic, and choice (D) is correct. Note that II has 6 π electrons: $4n + 2 = 6$ where $n = 1$, so it, too, meets the Hückel Rule.

5. **B** Here is the reaction given:

    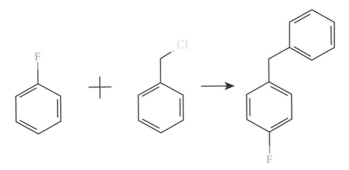

This is not a reduction reaction, and the Gabriel synthesis is used to prepare amines, so eliminate choices (A) and (D). In an aldol condensation, an enol or enolate reacts with a carbonyl compound (eliminate choice C). Choice (B) is correct.

6. **A** In the presence of a strong base, the α-carbon in butanal is abstracted forming an enolate. The enolate undergoes nucleophilic addition followed by protonation in H_2O. This sequence is typical of an aldol condensation, choice A. The reactant and product are shown below:

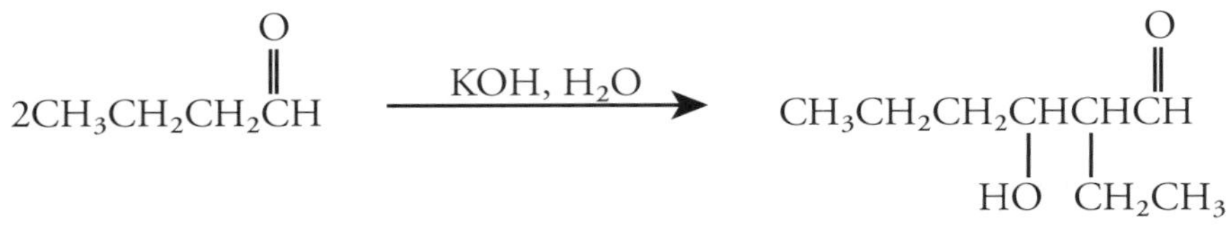

$$2CH_3CH_2CH_2\overset{\overset{\displaystyle O}{\|}}{C}H \xrightarrow{\text{KOH, } H_2O} CH_3CH_2CH_2\underset{\underset{\displaystyle HO}{|}}{C}H\underset{\underset{\displaystyle CH_2CH_3}{|}}{C}H\overset{\overset{\displaystyle O}{\|}}{C}H$$

butanal   2-ethyl-3-hyrdoxyhexanal

7. **D** The keto form of a compound is generally more stable than the enol. An enol becomes more stable if it can engage in resonance or intramolecular hydrogen bonding. The compound 2,4-hexadienone forms an enol that is phenol, which is stabilized by resonance, so choice (B) can be eliminated. The enol of compound II is stabilized by intramolecular H-bonding, so it is more stable. Thus, choice (D) is correct. The enol form of compound III is not stabilized, so the keto form is more stable than the enol (eliminate choice C).

8. **B** Propanoic acid will have the lowest K_a and therefore the highest pK_a: it does not have an electronegative group that withdraws electrons and increases its acidity. Both choices (A) and (D) (eliminate C) can be eliminated. Fluoroacetic acid has one electronegative substance that increases its acidity, but dichloroacetic acid has two. Dichloroacetic acid is therefore more acidic (eliminate choice A). The correct answer is choice (B). In order of increasing acidity the pK_a's are 4.9, 2.6, and 1.3.

9. **B** Both choices (A) and (D) are reductants, so both of those choices can be eliminated. A strong oxidant is needed to oxidize an alcohol to a carboxylic acid, so choice (C) can be eliminated. The correct answer is choice (B). Notice that chromium has a +6 oxidation state in $K_2Cr_2O_7$, which makes it a very strong oxidant.

10. **C** The Gabriel synthesis is used to convert an alkyl halide to an amine, choice (C). The potassium salt of phthalimide, whose structure is shown below, is used in the synthesis.

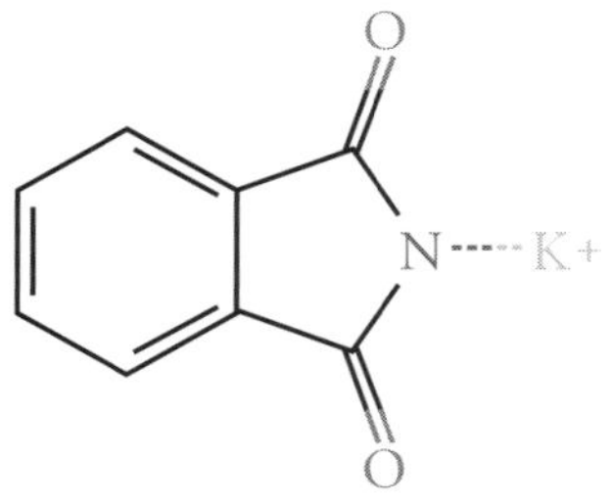

Potassium phthalimide

11.   **D**   The structure of 1,3-dichloro-2-butene is shown here:

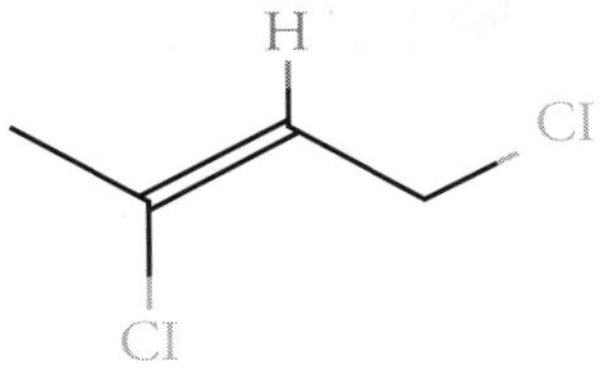

There are three sets of protons that are chemically inequivalent. These produce three signals, so choices (B) and (C) can both be eliminated. The signals correspond to the methyl group, the single proton on the double bond (the allylic proton), and the two adjacent protons (the methylene protons). The methyl protons produce a singlet because there are no adjacent protons. There is a proton adjacent to the methylene group, so the methylene group appears as a doublet. The allylic proton has two adjacent protons, so it appears as a triplet. The correct answer is choice (D).

Quick Review

- Sigma (σ) bonds generally form through the internuclear overlap of hybrid orbitals; pi (π) bonds form through the side-to-side overlap of unhybridized p orbitals.

- Saturated compounds have the general formula C_nH_{2n+2}; unsaturated molecules contain rings or π bonds.

- Compounds with the same molecular formula are known as isomers; structural, or constitutional, isomers differ by the connectivity of atoms in the molecule.

- Conformational isomers differ by rotation around a σ bond.

- Stereoisomers have the same connectivity, but differ in the spatial orientation of atoms.

- Chiral molecules have chiral centers that consist of an sp^3 hybridized carbon with four different substituents, are not superimposable on their mirror image, and rotate plane-polarized light.

- Enantiomers are non-superimposable mirror images that have an opposite absolute configuration at all chiral centers.

- Enantiomers rotate plane-polarized light with equal magnitude but in opposite directions. Therefore, a 50:50 mixture of enantiomers, or a racemic mixture, is not optically active.

- Diastereomers are stereoisomers that are not mirror images. They differ in absolute configuration for at least one, but not all chiral carbons.

- Epimers are diastereomers that differ in absolute configuration at only one stereocenter.

- Geometric isomers are diastereomers that are cis/trans (or Z/E) pairs on a ring or double bond. When highest priority groups are on the same side of a ring or bond, the molecule is *cis* (or Z); when they're on opposite sides, the compound is trans (or E).

- Meso compounds are achiral molecules with chiral centers and an internal plane of symmetry.

- As the substitution of carbocations and radicals increases, so does their stability due to an inductive effect. Carbanions are more stable when they are less substituted.

- Resonance stabilization results from the delocalization of electrons through a system of conjugated π bonds or unhybridized p orbitals. Multiple, equally valid structures can exist that together lower the energy of the system.

- Radical brominations are regioselective for tertiary bromides, while chlorinations yield mixtures of substitution products.

- All free radical halogenations are non-stereoselective, giving racemic mixtures of products when one new stereocenter is formed.

- Nucleophiles are Lewis bases and are electron rich, while electrophiles are Lewis acids and are electron deficient. A reaction occurs when a nucleophile reacts with an electrophile.

- Nucleophiles are stronger when negatively charged, less electronegative, or more polarizable.

- Good leaving groups are weak conjugate bases. Their stability in solution increases, such that uncharged and/or larger groups are usually better LGs.

- More substituted substrates and protic solvents favor an S_N1 reaction over S_N2.

- Carbocation intermediates formed in either S_N1 or E1 reactions will rearrange if possible to form a more stable carbocation.

- Second order reactions (S_N2 or E2) require specific spatial orientations of the reacting species (S_N2 = backside attack of Nuc; E2 = antiperiplanar conformation of H and LG).

- First order reactions (S_N1 or E1) do not depend on the concentration of the Nuc or base.

- Elimination reactions break two σ bonds and form one π bond.

- Non-nucleophilic bases and heat favor elimination reactions over substitutions. Strong bases favor E2 over E1.

- Elimination reactions favor the formation of the more substituted bond (E2 reactions must use small bases). Trans double bonds are favored over *cis*.

- The electrons in C=C π bonds can act as nucleophiles in addition reactions, which replace one π bond with two σ bonds.

- When π electrons attack electrophiles, the resulting carbocation will be on the more substituted carbon and yield the Markovnikov (more substituted) product.

- Addition reactions that place a non-hydrogen group on the less substituted carbon are termed anti-Markovnikov additions.

- Anti addition places two new substituents on opposite sides of the planar double bond, while *syn*-addition places them on the same side of the planar double bond.

- Addition reactions are usually not stereospecific since the alkene is planar. Electrophiles will add with equal frequency to both faces of the bond, giving a racemic mixture.

- Alkenes and alkynes can be hydrogenated with H_2 and metal catalysts.

- Alkenes can undergo cycloaddition reactions and polymerization through a free radical reaction.

- Aromatic compounds are cyclic, planar, conjugated (all sp^2 hybridized atoms), have $4n+2$ π electrons, and are exceptionally stable due to resonance. They adhere to Hückel's Rule.

- To preserve aromaticity, aromatic rings undergo substitution rather than addition reactions.

- A benzene ring with an electron donating substituent favors substitution at ortho and para positions.

- An electron withdrawing substituent on a benzene ring deactivates the ring to substitution. All but the halogens, which are both electron withdrawing and electron donating, favor substitution at meta positions.

- Alcohols engage in H-bonding interactions, and can be classified as primary, secondary, or tertiary.

- Alcohols can be prepared through the reduction of a carbonyl, of a carboxylic acid, of an ester, or through formation of a Grignard reagent.

- Alcohols undergo acid catalyzed substitution reactions; they can be oxidized to aldehydes, ketones, or carboxylic acids, and are protected from undesired reactions using protecting groups.

- The C=O bond is very polarized due to the high electronegativity of oxygen, resulting in the carbon of the carbonyl group being electrophilic.

- Protons α to a carbonyl are acidic and can be removed by a strong base to yield a nucleophilic carbanion, or enolate.

- Keto-enol tautomerism is the rapid equilibration of the more stable keto form of a carbonyl and the less stable enol form where the α-proton shifts to the carbonyl oxygen.

- Nucleophilic additions involve the attack of a nucleophile on the carbon of an aldehyde or ketone. These reactions break one π bond to form two σ bonds.

- Hydride reduction, a type of nucleophilic addition, can convert ketones or aldehydes into alcohols. Alcohols can be converted back to carbonyl compounds using oxidizing agents.

- Reactions of aldehydes and ketones include the Wittig reaction, formation of acetals and hemiacetals, imine formation, and Wolff-Kishner reduction.

- An aldol condensation forms a C—C bond where the carbonyl carbon of one molecule is the electrophile, and the α-carbon of another carbonyl is the nucleophile.

- α,β-Unsaturated carbonyl compounds are electrophilic at the β-carbon and undergo addition reactions.

- Carboxylic acids are acidic due to resonance stabilization of their conjugate base, the carboxylate anion.

- Electron withdrawing groups increase the acidity of carboxylic acids by stabilizing the negative charge of the carboxylate anion through an inductive effect.

- Carboxylic acids are prepared through oxidation of alcohols, aldehydes, and alkylbenzenes, and hydrolysis of nitriles.

- Reactions of carboxylic acids include reduction to primary alcohols, aldehydes, or ketones and decarboxylation.

- The reactivity of carboxylic acid derivatives decreases as follows: acid halide > acid anhydride > ester > amide.

- Nucleophilic addition to the carbonyl carbon in a carboxylic acid derivative is usually followed by elimination of a good leaving group.

- Organic compounds differ in their solubility in polar (aqueous) or nonpolar (organic) solvents. The more alkane-like the molecule, the lower the solubility in polar solvents.

- Soaps are formed from the base promoted hydrolysis of esters.

- A transesterification reaction replaces one OR group of an ester with another.

- Amines are weak bases that behave as nucleophiles. They are classified as alkyl-amines or arylamines.

- Amines are synthesized through alkylation of ammonia, the Gabriel synthesis, or by reduction of alkyl azides, nitriles, or nitro groups.

- Amines undergo Hofmann elimination reactions.

- IR spectroscopy identifies the functional groups present in molecules.

- The most common IR resonances tested on the PCAT are the C=O bond (~1,700 cm^{-1}), the C=C bond (~1,650 cm^{-1}), and the O—H bond (~3,600 cm^{-1}).

- NMR excites an atom's nucleus from a low energy spin state to the next higher one. ^{1}NMR provides information about a proton's environment.

- In mass spectrometry bonds are broken and molecular fragments identified by their mass-to-charge (m/z) ratios.

- UV-VIS spectroscopy is used to identify conjugated systems.

Chapter 11

Biochemistry

Biological chemistry, or Biochemistry, describes chemical processes within and relating to living organisms. As a bridge between biology and chemistry, it focuses on biologically relevant processes at a molecular level. Processes involving enzymes, DNA, and RNA were introduced to you in Chapter 6. In this chapter, we will describe amino acids, proteins, lipids, and steroids.

11.1   AMINO ACIDS

Structure

All amino acids contain an amino group ($pK_a \approx 9.5$) that is a base and a carboxyl group ($pK_a \approx 2.5$) that is an acid. When the charges balance, the amino acid forms a **zwitterion**, which has a net charge of zero, as shown here:

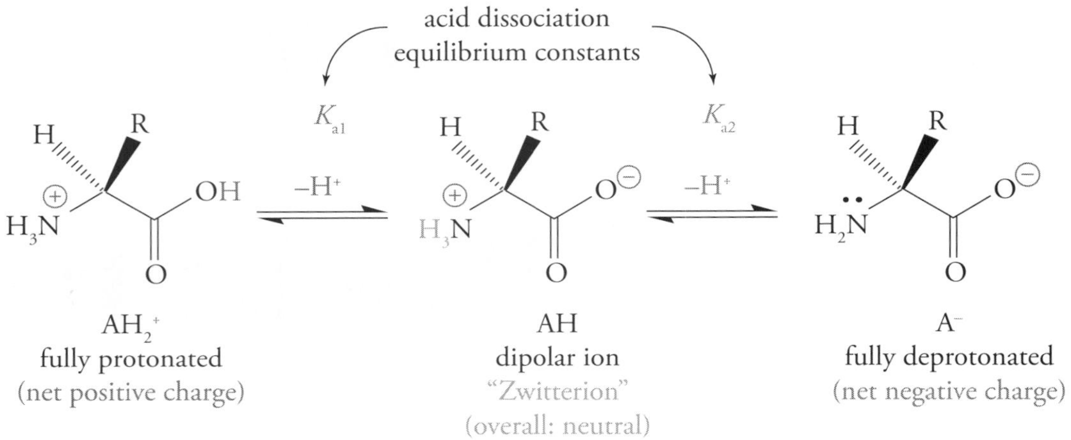

Figure 1

Notice that amino acids have an alpha hydrogen. The R group represents the **side chain** which is unique for each amino acid, and may be acidic, basic, or neutral, depending on its structure.

Chirality of Amino Acids

With the exception of glycine, the alpha carbon of an amino acid is chiral. The alpha carbon of glycine has two hydrogen atoms, making it achiral.

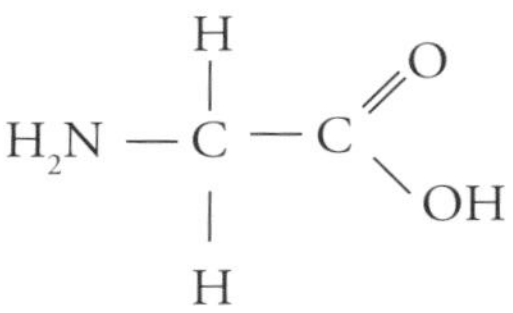

Glycine

Configuration of Amino Acids as "L" and "D"

By convention, a Fischer projection of an amino acid is drawn with the carboxylic acid group on top. This means that the amine group can be placed either on the left or the right of the projection. If it is on the left, the structure is an **L-amino acid**. Drawing the amine group on the right gives a **D-amino acid**. All animal amino acids are of the "L" type.

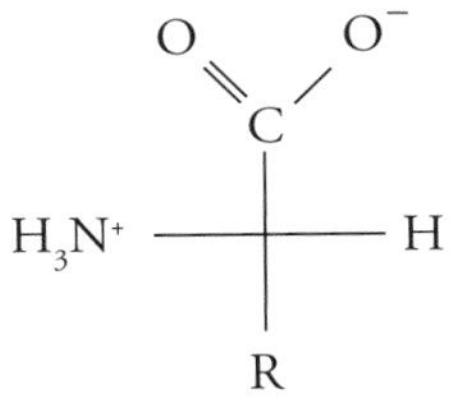

L-amino acid 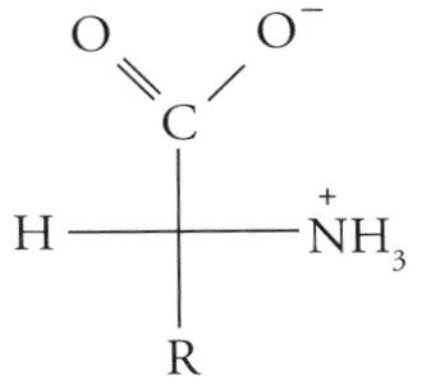   D-amino acid

Classification of Amino Acids as Neutral, Basic, and Acidic

We classify amino acids in terms of common characteristics associated with side chains. For example, look at L-aspartic acid:

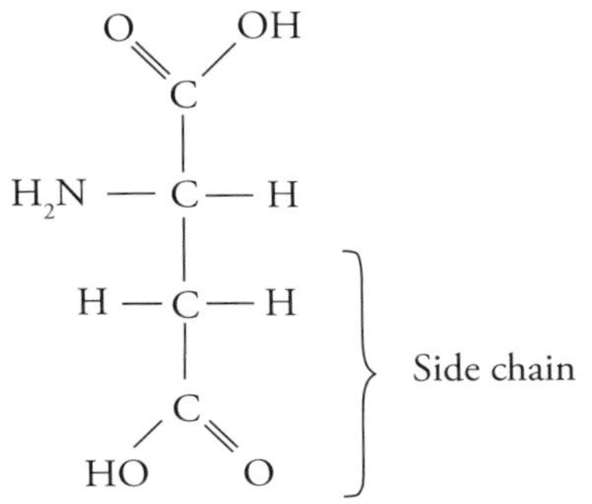

L-Aspartic acid

Because of the carboxylic acid functional group on the side chain, aspartic acid is an **acidic amino acid.** Look now at lysine:

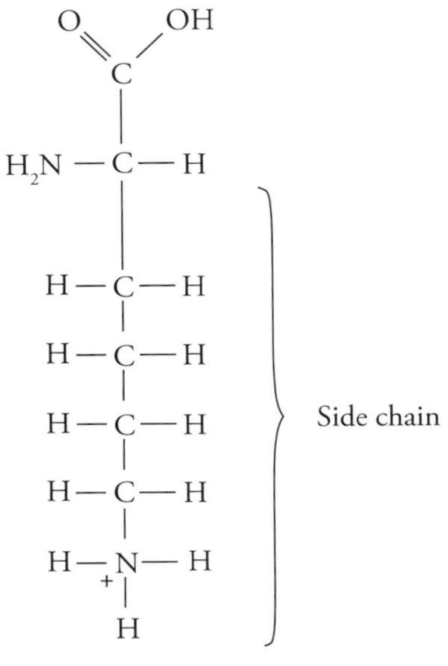

Lysine

Lysine has a basic group on the side chain, so it is a **basic amino acid.**

In cases in which the amine group and carbonyl group in the side chain can form resonance structures (such as when a carbonyl is adjacent to the lone pair of electrons on nitrogen), the amino acid is neutral:

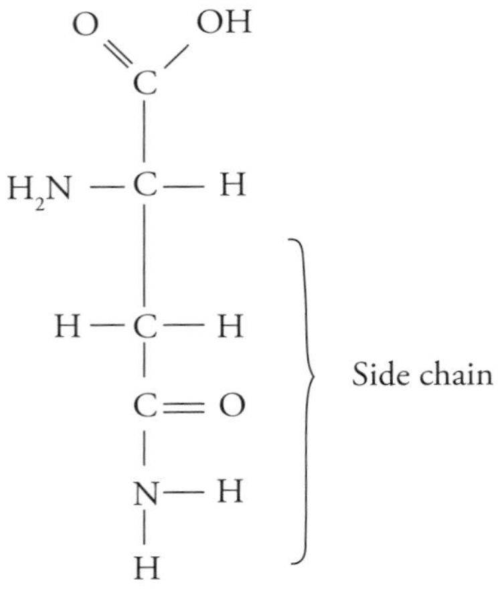

Asparagine

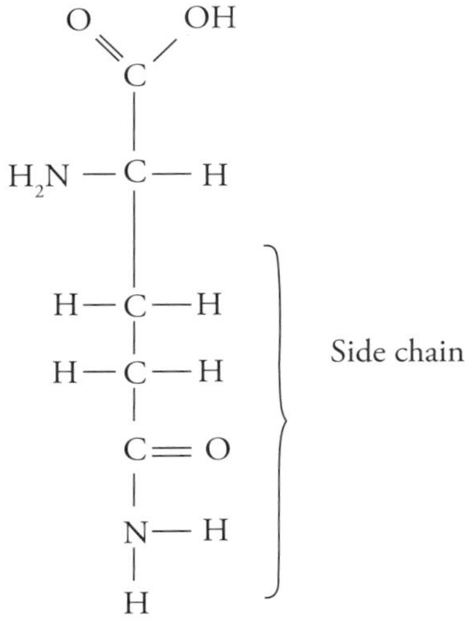

Glutamine

The Sulfur Side Chains
Three amino acids normally encountered in biological systems contain sulfur in their side chains. They are methionine, cysteine, and cystine. Cystine is formed when two molecules of cysteine are linked by a **disulfide bridge.** All three of these sulfur-containing amino acids are neutral.

Zwitterions
At low pH and in its fully protonated form, a neutral amino acid has a net charge of +1, as shown below. In its fully deprotonated form at high pH, it has a net charge of –1. Midway between the two is the **isoelectric point** (the **pI**), where the amino acid has a net charge of zero. This point corresponds to the formation of a zwitterion. Notice that the fully protonated form and the zwitterion form an acid/conjugate base pair (COOH/COO⁻), as do the zwitterion and deprotonated form (NH_3^+/NH_2). As with any conjugate acid-base pair, when the acid and conjugate base are in equilibrium, they form a buffered solution.

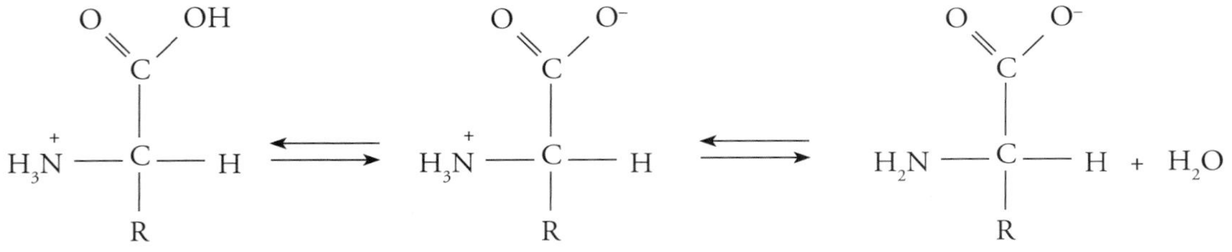

low pH:
net positive charge

Isoelectric point
pI

high pH:
net negative charge

Amino Acid Titration

We can titrate an amino acid solution and generate a titration curve that allows us to identify the corresponding pK_{a_1}, pI, and pK_{a_2}. Midpoints indicate buffer solutions, and the pI indicates the point where complete neutralization has occurred—that is, the isoelectric point and formation of a zwitterion. This can be illustrated by the titration curve of glycine, a neutral amino acid:

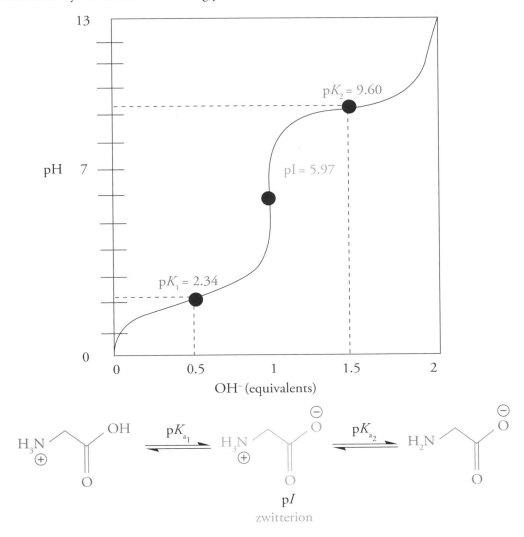

Figure 2

Classifying Amino Acids

Each amino acid has both a three-letter abbreviation and a one-letter abbreviation, which you do *not* need to memorize. Though they are all unique, many of them are similar in their chemical properties. For the PCAT, it is *not* necessary to memorize all 20 side chains, but it is important to understand the chemical properties that characterize them. The important properties of the side chains include their varying *shape, charge, ability to hydrogen bond, and ability to act as acids or bases*. These side group properties are important in the structure of proteins.

Here is a reference table of the 20 amino acids:

Nonpolar, Hydrophobic

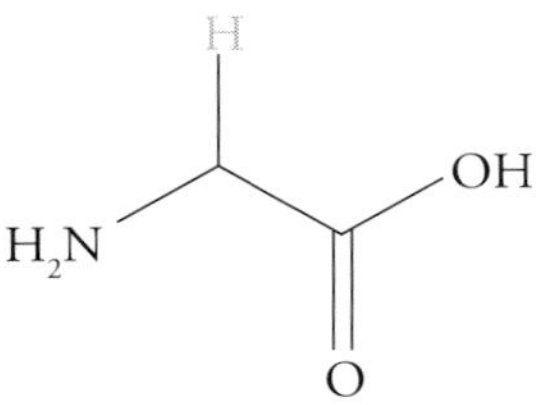

glycine

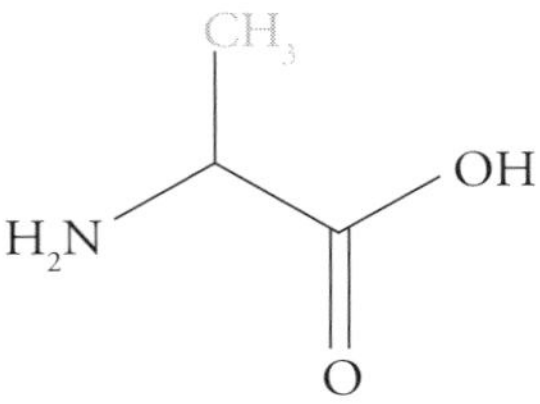

alanine

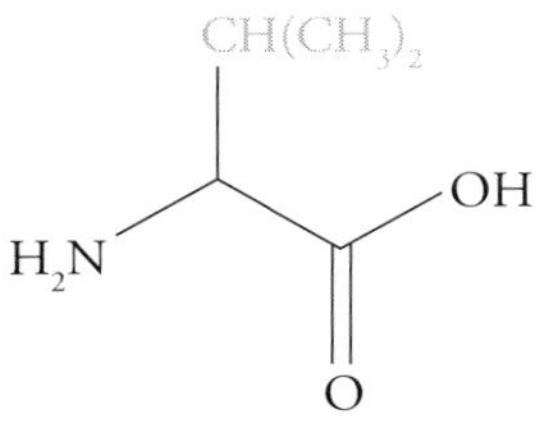

valine

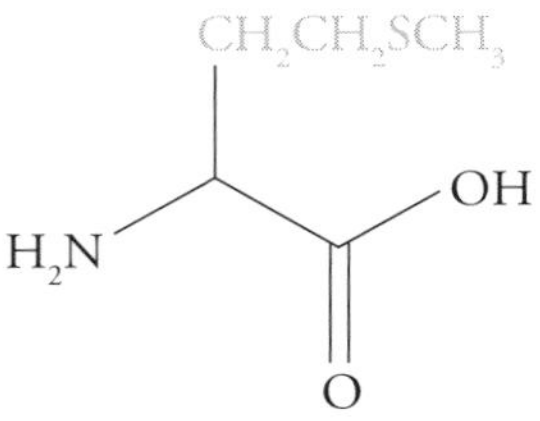

methionine

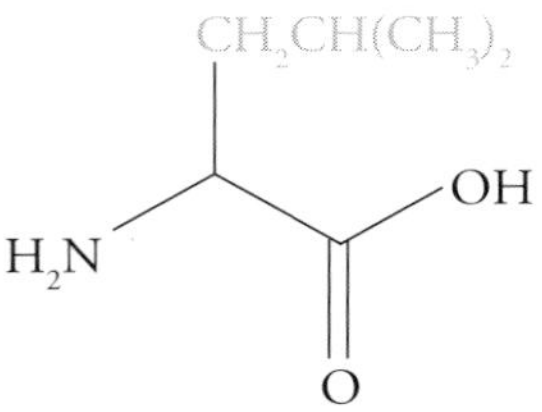

leucine

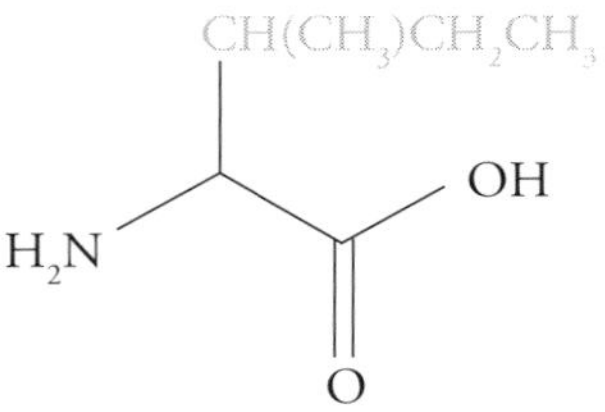

isoleucine

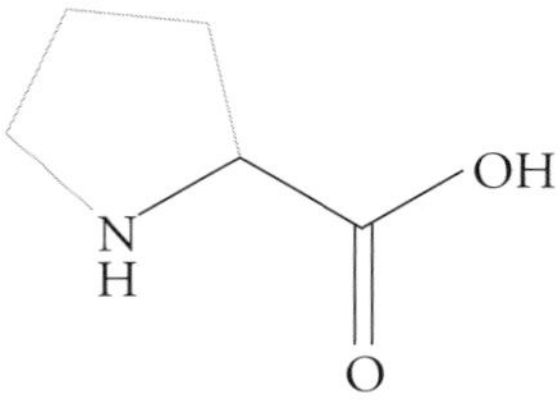

proline

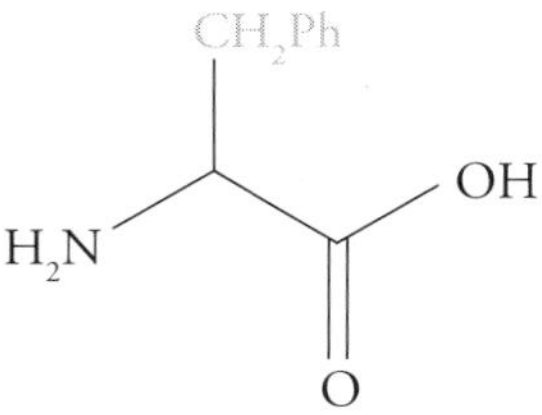

phenylalanine

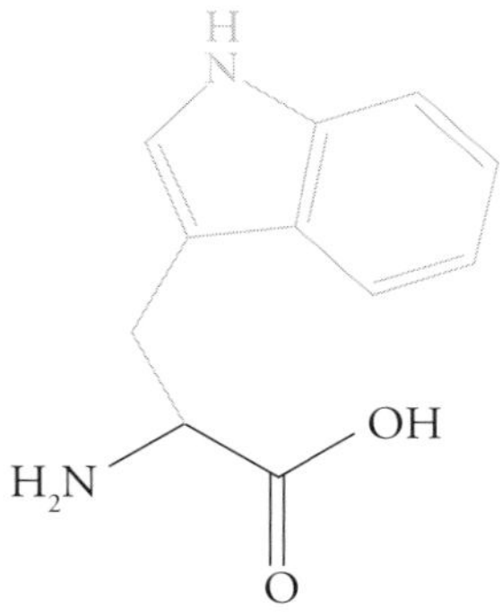

tryptophan

Polar, Neutral

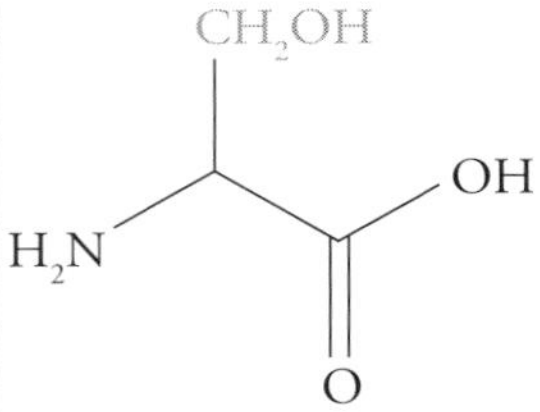

serine

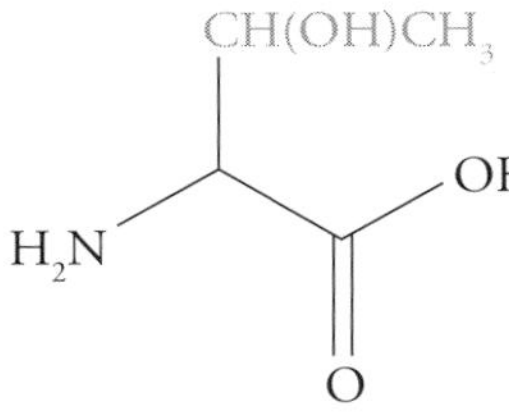

threonine

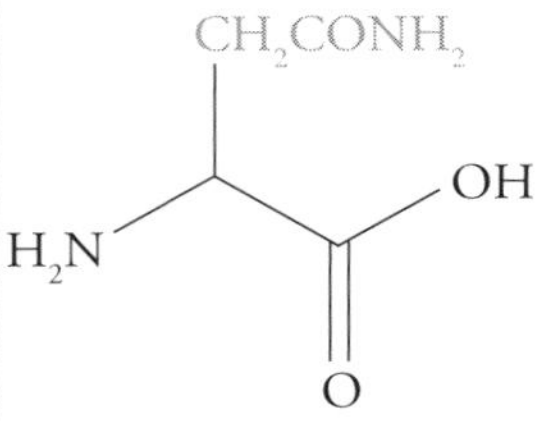

asparagine

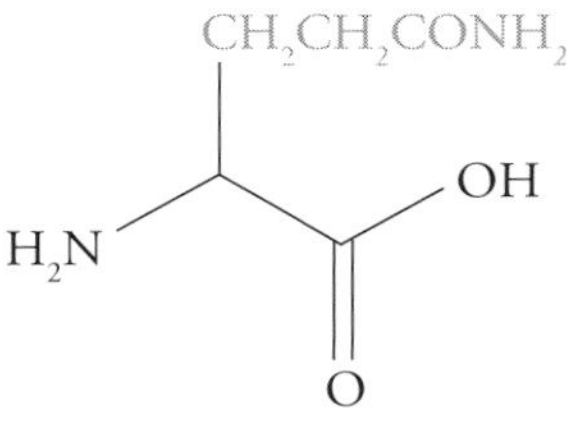

glutamine

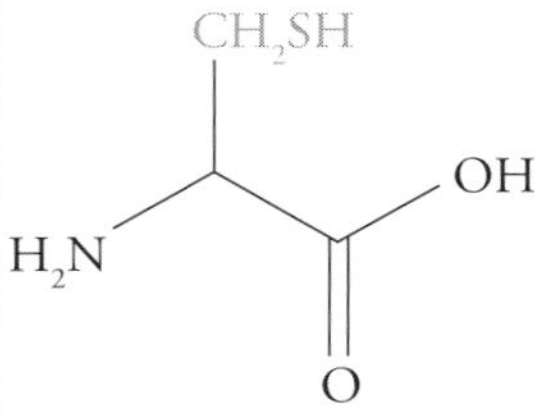

cysteine

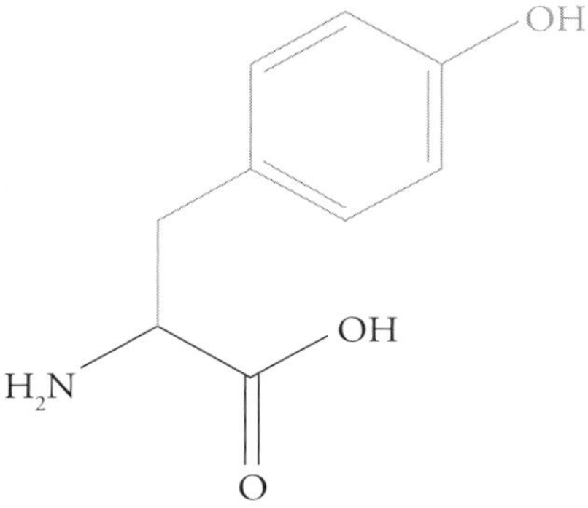

tyrosine

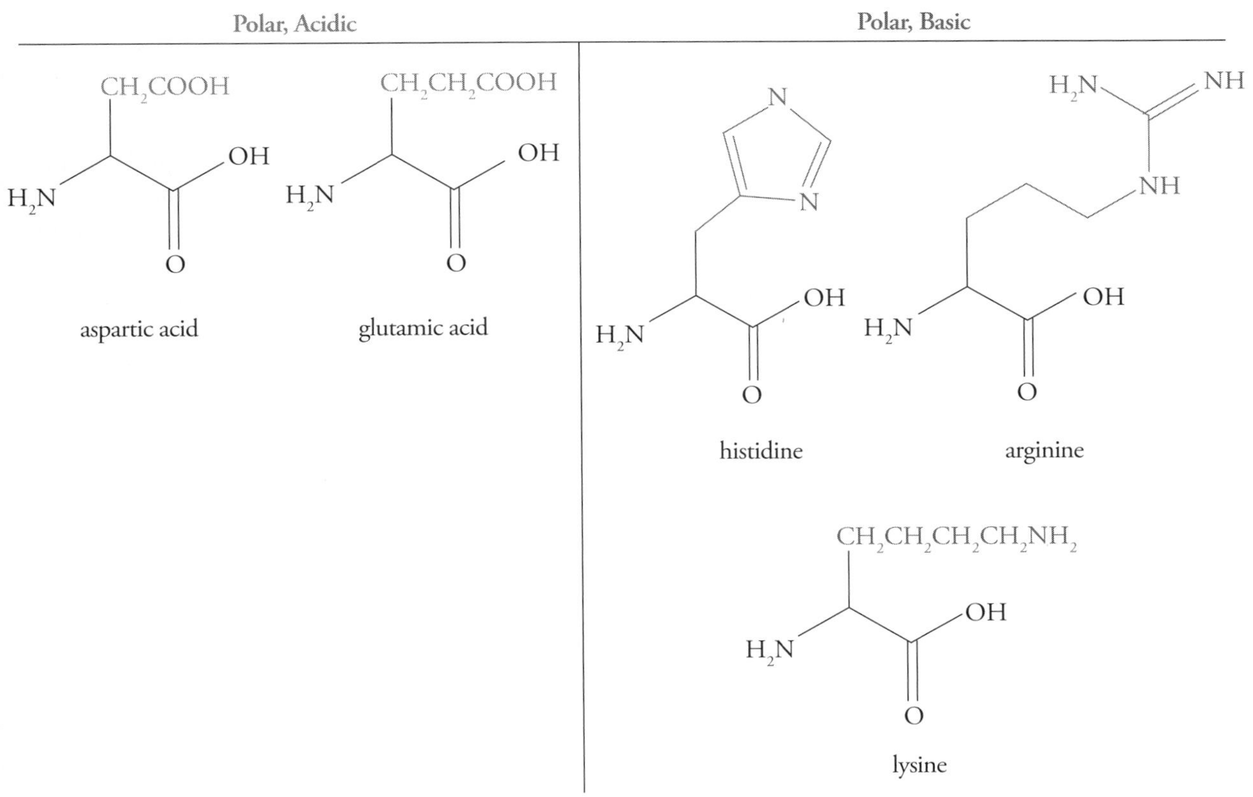
Polar, Acidic
Polar, Basic
CH2COOH
CH2CH2COOH
aspartic acid
glutamic acid
histidine
arginine
CH2CH2CH2CH2NH2
lysine

Figure 3

Amino Acid Separation—Gel Electrophoresis

Gel electrophoresis is a technique that separates amino acids based on their charge. In general, when employing this technique, amino acids are loaded onto a gel that is held at a constant pH and then exposed to an electric field. If the pH is different from their p*I*, each amino acid will bear an overall charge because the p*I* is specific to the unique structure of the side chain of each amino acid. The amino acids will therefore migrate through the gel based on their charge and the external electric field. The PCAT tends to ask about how specific amino acids will migrate relative to each other in these separation conditions. In order to answer these questions, we need to understand the relationship between pH, pK_a, and p*I* (as discussed previously). See the table below, which summarizes how pH will determine the direction of amino acid migration during an electrophoresis separation:

pH	Charge on Amino Acid	Direction of Migration
greater than p*I*	negative	toward positive electrode
lower than p*I*	positive	toward negative electrode
equal to p*I*	neutral (zwitterion)	no migration

Table 1

11.2 PROTEINS

Formation of Proteins from Amino Acids

There are two common types of covalent bonds between amino acids in proteins: the peptide bonds that link amino acids together into polypeptide chains, and disulfide bridges between cysteine R-groups. A **peptide bond** is formed between the carboxyl group of one amino acid and the α-amino group of another amino acid with the loss of water. This occurs by the same nucleophilic addition-elimination mechanism for formation of any one of the carboxylic acid derivatives from any other carboxylic acid derivative. Remember that a peptide bond is just an amide bond between two amino acids. By convention, the amine group is written on the left (the **N-terminus**) and the carboxylic acid group on the right (the **C-terminus**).

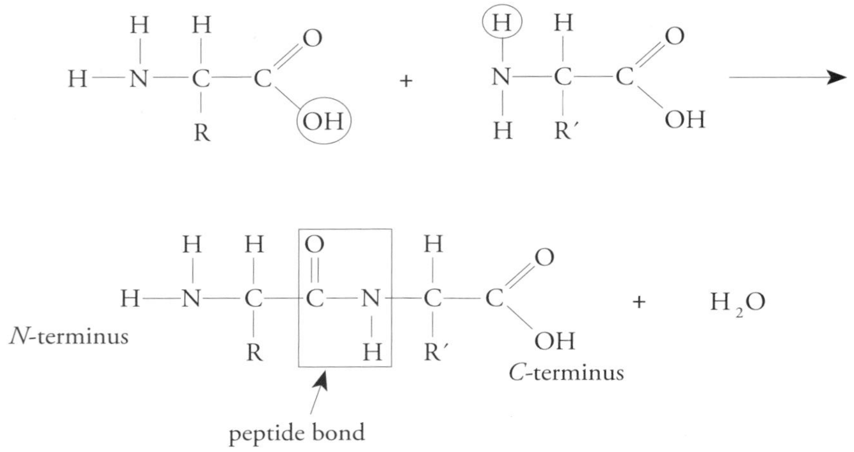

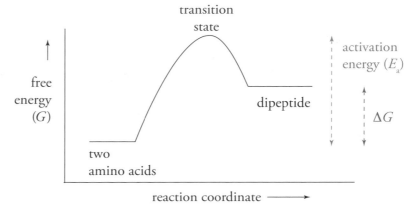

Figure 4   Formation of a Peptide Bond

A **peptide** consists of 2–50 amino acid residues. A **polypeptide** is a polymer of greater than 50 amino acid residues linked by peptide bonds that comprise part, or all, of a protein molecule. In a **protein**, a long polypeptide or combination of polypeptides are bound together by cross-links. "Protein" and "polypeptide," therefore, are not quite synonymous because some proteins contain more than one polypeptide.

As you can see in Figure 4, the formation of a peptide bond with two amino acids is not thermodynamically favorable and requires energy. This naturally occurring reaction, which takes place during translation in cells, involves enzyme catalysis, is RNA directed, and co-factor mediated (see Chapter 6).

Figure 5   Energetics of Peptide Bond Formation

Protein Structures

Proteins may be classified in terms of their primary, secondary, tertiary, and quaternary structure. Be sure you are familiar with the types of bonding characteristic of each structure.

Primary Structures

The **primary structure** is the sequence of amino acids that make up the protein, and there consists of covalent bonds. By convention, the amino acids that form the protein's primary structure are listed in order from the N-terminus (the end of the protein with a free $-NH_2$ group) to the C-terminus (the end of a free $-COOH$ group).

Secondary Structures

A **secondary structure** describes the three-dimensional folding of a polypeptide chain in the protein. These are local, folded structures that are caused by hydrogen bonding interactions between the polypeptide's amide "backbone" of $-NH$ and $>C=O$ groups and does *not* include the side chains. A secondary structure most often involves two particularly stable conformations: the alpha helix, or a β-pleated sheet.

- The **α-helix** is a clockwise (right-handed), spiral structure with the side chains on the outside of the central axis. Each turn of the helix is comprised of 3.6 amino acids. On each amino acid within the α-helix, the oxygen of the amide $>C=O$ group forms a hydrogen bond to the proton bonded to an amide nitrogen atom four residues away. Notice that the side chains, represented as $-R$ groups, are located on the outside of the helical structure.

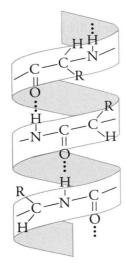

Figure 6 A Clockwise (right-handed) α-helix

- The **β-pleated sheet** is another form of secondary structure. In this structure, polypeptide chains align themselves in parallel. Hydrogen bonds form between $-NH$ and $>C=O$ groups on amino acid residues that are relatively far apart from one another, and/or between separate polypeptide chains. The side chains extend above or below the plane of the sheet.

  In a **parallel β-pleated sheet**, adjacent polypeptide chains run in the same direction (N to C and N to C), and in an **anti-parallel β-pleated**, adjacent polypeptide chains run in opposite directions (N to C vs. C to N).

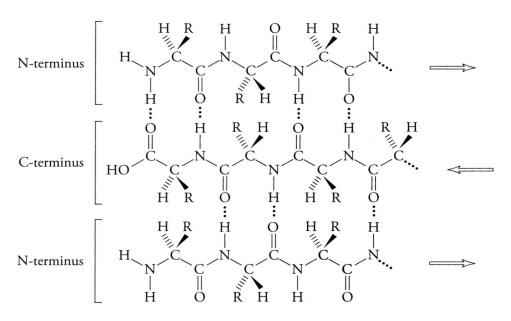

Figure 7 A β-pleated Sheet

Tertiary Structures

A tertiary structure describes the way in which interactions with solvent and between side chains distant from one another cause the protein molecule to fold. The folding characteristic of tertiary structure will cause nonpolar ("hydrophobic") side chains to closely pack in the interior of the structure, away from the aqueous solvent, with the polar ("hydrophilic") side chains exposing themselves at the surface. The polar side-chains are in contact with the aqueous solvent and curl in *three dimensions*. Frequently, the result is a *globular protein*:

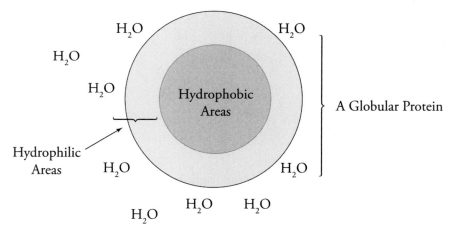

Figure 8 The Tertiary Structure of a Globular Protein

A common occurrence in tertiary structure is the formation of disulfide bonds between two cysteine residues that are in close spatial proximity. These bonds are not required, but often help to stabilize the three-dimensional structure.

Quaternary Structures

A quaternary structure refers only to proteins composed of more than one polypeptide chain. To refer to such a protein's quaternary structure is to refer to the way its several polypeptide chains form bonds and cross-links between and among its separate polypeptides. An example is hemoglobin, that consists of four subunits.

Figure 9   The Quaternary Structure of Hemoglobin

Hemoglobin is an example of a *conjugated protein*. The protein functions in concert with other chemical groups, called *prosthetic groups*, that form part of the structure but that are not polypeptides. In hemoglobin, the prosthetic group is the heme unit containing Fe(II), which is involved in oxygen transport. Prosthetic groups are important structural units of metalloproteins and vitamins, among other classes of quaternary compounds.

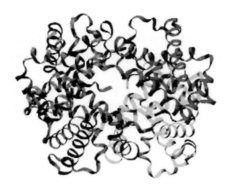

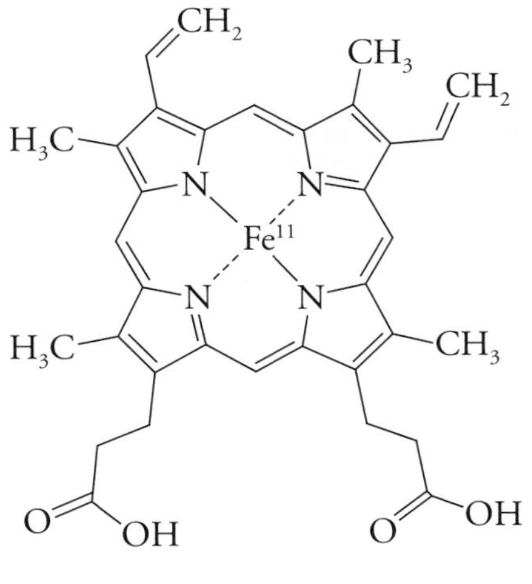

Figure 10   The Heme Prosthetic Group of Hemoglobin

Hydrolysis of the Peptide Bond

Denaturation involves breaking bonds within a protein, causing it to lose its quaternary, tertiary, and secondary structure that is responsible for the three-dimensional conformation of the protein in its native state. Changes in temperature or pH, for example, can disrupt the hydrogen-bonding interactions. **Hydrolysis** refers to any reaction in which water is a nucleophile, and converts proteins into their constituent amino acids and peptides.

Hydrolysis of the peptide bond to form a free amine and a carboxylic acid is thermodynamically favored but kinetically slow. There are two common means of accelerating the rate of peptide bond hydrolysis: strong acids and proteolytic enzymes.

Acid hydrolysis is the cleaving of a protein into its constituent amino acids with strong acid and heat. This is a non-specific means of cleaving peptide bonds. The amount of each amino acid present after hydrolysis can then be quantified to determine the overall amino acid content of the protein.

Hydrolysis of a protein by another protein is called **proteolysis** or **proteolytic cleavage**, and the protein that does the cutting is known as a **proteolytic enzyme** or **protease**. Proteolytic cleavage is a specific means of cleaving peptide bonds. Many enzymes only cleave the peptide bond adjacent to a specific amino acid. For example, the protease trypsin cleaves on the carboxyl side of the positively charged (basic) residues arginine and lysine, while chymotrypsin cleaves adjacent to hydrophobic residues such as phenylalanine. (You do *not* need to memorize these examples for the PCAT.)

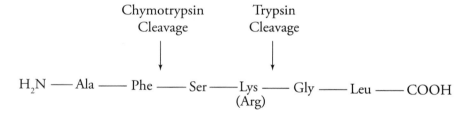

Figure 11   Specificity of Protease Cleavage

11.3   LIPIDS AND STEROIDS

Lipids

Lipids are oily or fatty substances that play three physiological roles, summarized here and discussed below.

- In cellular membranes, phospholipids constitute a barrier between intracellular and extracellular environments.
- In adipose cells, triglycerides (fats) store energy.
- Finally, cholesterol is a lipid that serves as the building block for the hydrophobic steroid hormones.

A lipid is characterized by its hydrophobicity because of the predominance of carbon-carbon bonds. A synonym for hydrophobic is **lipophilic** (which means lipid-loving); a synonym for hydrophilic is **lipophobic**.

Fatty Acid Structure

Fatty acids are composed of long unsubstituted alkanes that end in a carboxylic acid. The chain is typically 14 to 18 carbons long. Because they are synthesized two carbons at a time from acetate, only *even-numbered* fatty acids are made in human cells. A fatty acid with no carbon-carbon double bonds is **saturated** because every carbon atom in the chain is covalently bound to the maximum number of hydrogens. **Unsaturated** fatty acids have one or more double bonds in the chain, giving it a kinked structure. These double bonds are almost always Z or *cis*. The position of a double bond in the alkyl chain of a fatty acid is denoted by the symbol Δ, with carbons numbered starting with the carboxylic acid carbon. For example, a (Z) double bond between carbons 3 and 4 in a fatty acid would be referred to as (Z)-Δ^3 (or *cis*-Δ^3).

The drawing below illustrates how free fatty acids interact in an aqueous solution; they form a structure called a **micelle**. Water forms a shell around the spherical micelle, interacting with polar carboxylic acid head groups, while hydrophobic lipid tails form hydrophobic interactions inside the sphere.

Soaps, whose action was described when we discussed the hydrolysis of esters in Chapter 10, are the sodium salts of fatty acids (RCOO⁻Na⁺). They are **amphipathic**, which means they are both hydrophilic and hydrophobic.

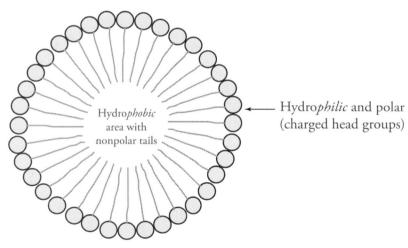

Hydro*phobic* area with nonpolar tails

Hydro*philic* and polar (charged head groups)

Figure 12   A Fatty Acid Micelle

Triacylglycerols

The technical name for fat is **triacylglycerol** or **triglyceride** (shown below). The triglyceride is composed of three fatty acids esterified to a glycerol molecule. Glycerol is a three-carbon triol with the formula $HOCH_2$–CHOH–CH_2OH. It has three hydroxyl groups that can be esterified to fatty acids.

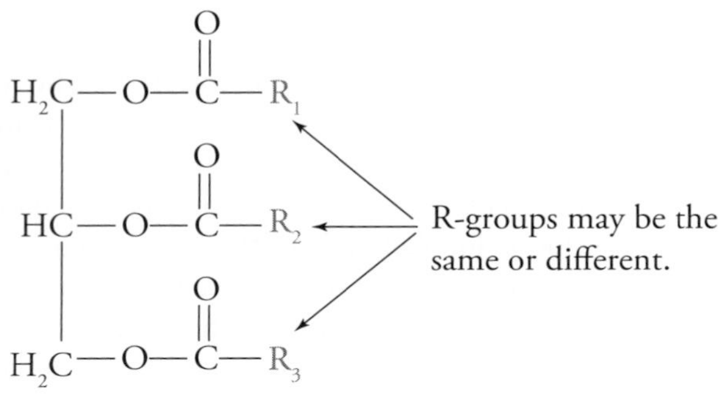

Figure 13   A Triglyceride (Fat)

The triacylglycerol undergoes reactions typical of esters, such as base-catalyzed hydrolysis. Soap is economically produced by base-catalyzed hydrolysis of triglycerides from animal fat into fatty acid salts (soaps). This reaction, called **saponification,** is illustrated below.

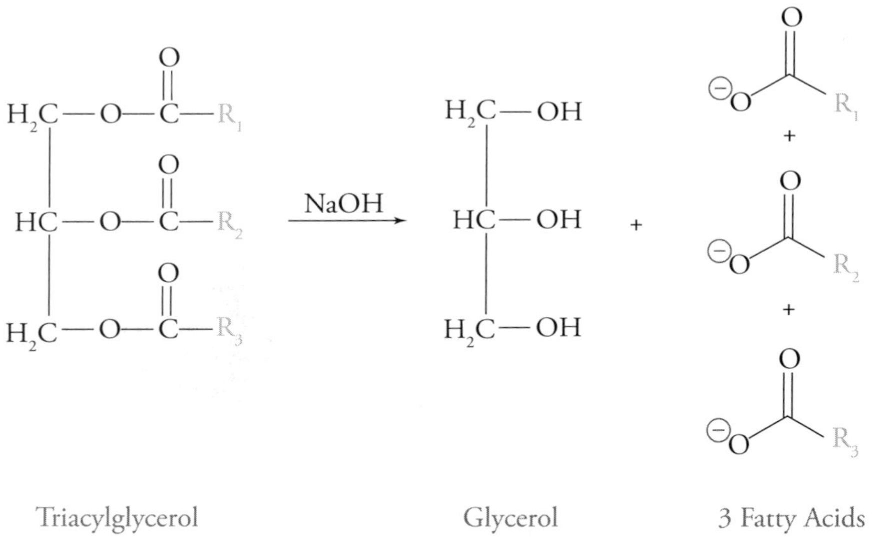

Triacylglycerol   Glycerol   3 Fatty Acids

Figure 14   Saponification

Fat molecules store much more energy than carbohydrates, because fats are much more *reduced*. Fats therefore undergo more oxidative reactions that release energy during metabolism.

Introduction to Lipid Bilayer Membranes

Membrane lipids are **phospholipids** derived from diacylglycerol phosphate or DG-P. Phospholipids are **detergents**, substances that efficiently solubilize oils while remaining highly water-soluble. Detergents are like soaps, but stronger.

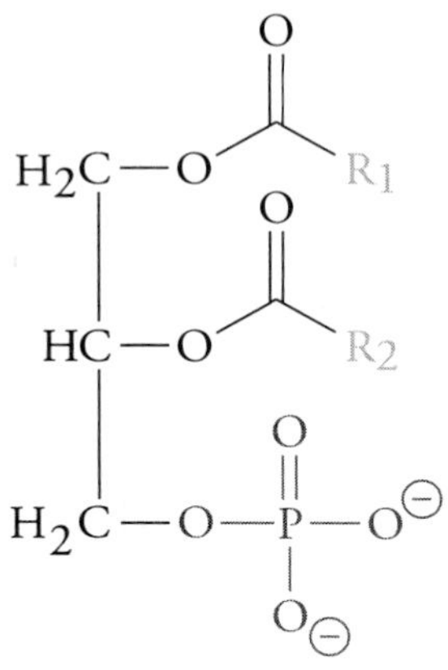

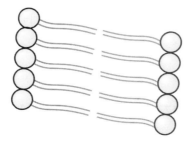

Figure 15   A Phosphoglyceride (Diacylglycerol Phosphate, or DGP)

We saw previously how fatty acids spontaneously form micelles. Phospholipids also minimize their interactions with water by forming an orderly structure—in this case, it is a **lipid bilayer** (below). Hydrophobic interactions drive the formation of the bilayer, and once formed, it is stabilized by van der Waals forces between the long tails.

Figure 16   A Small Section of a Lipid Bilayer Membrane

Since the membrane surrounding cells is impermeable to charged molecules such as Na^+, protein gateways such as ion channels are required for these species to enter or exit cells.

Steroids

All steroids have the basic tetracyclic ring system shown in Figure 17, which is based on the structure of **cholesterol**, a polycyclic amphipath.

The steroid cholesterol is an important component of the lipid bilayer. It is carried in the blood and combines with and transports fats and proteins in a unit called a **lipoprotein**. One type of lipoprotein has been implicated as the cause of atherosclerotic vascular disease, which refers to the buildup of cholesterol "plaques" on the inside of blood vessels.

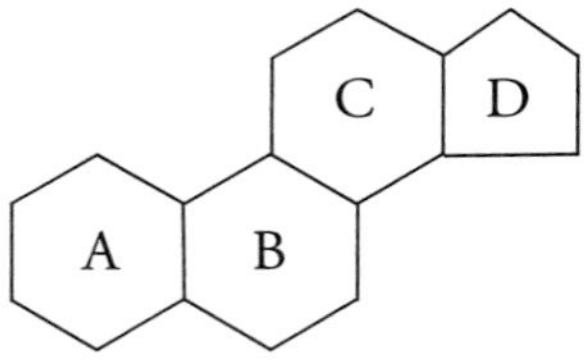

tetracyclic ring system

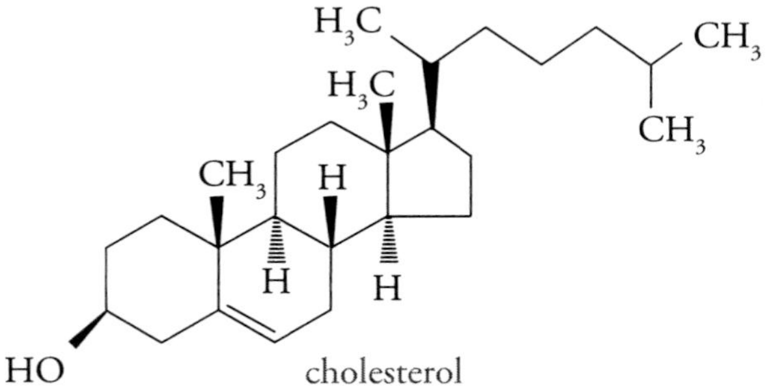

cholesterol

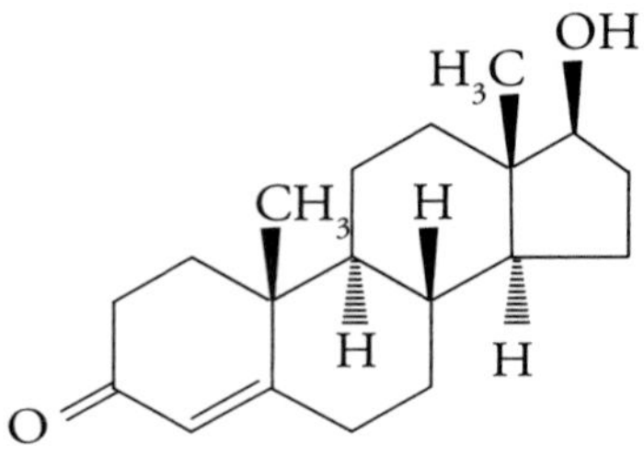

testosterone

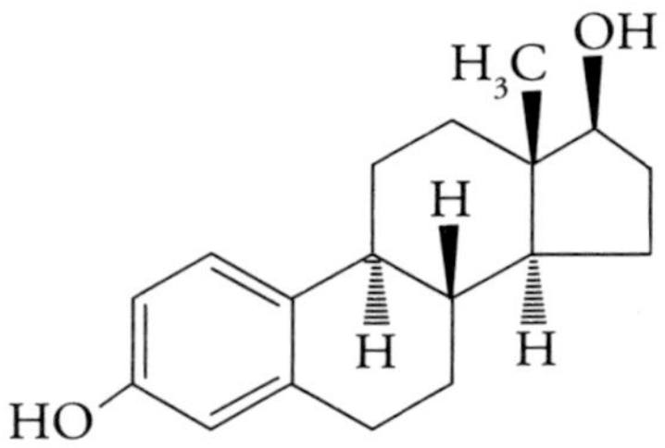

estrogen

Figure 17 Cholesterol-Derived Hormones

Steroid hormones are made from cholesterol. Be aware of the contrast between *peptide* hormones, such as insulin, which exert their effects by binding to receptors at the cell-surface, and *steroid* hormones, such as estrogen, which diffuse into cells to find their receptors.

CHAPTER 11 KEY TERMS

α-helix

β-pleated sheet

acidic amino acid

amphipathic

anti-parallel β-pleated

basic amino acid

cholesterol

D-amino acid

denaturation

detergents

disulfide bridge

gel electrophoresis

hydrolysis

isoelectric point

L-amino acid

lipid bilayer

lipophilic

lipophobic

lipoprotein

micelle

parallel β-pleated sheet

peptide

peptide bond

phospholipids

polypeptide

primary structure

protein

proteolysis or proteolytic cleavage

proteolytic enzyme or protease

saponification

saturated

secondary structure

side chain

soaps

triacylglycerol or triglyceride

unsaturated

zwitterion

BIOCHEMISTRY DRILL

1. Disulfide bonds are characteristic of which protein structure(s)?

    I.   Primary
    II. Secondary
    III. Tertiary
    IV. Quarternary

  A.   I, II, and III
  B.   II, III, and IV
  C.   III and IV
  D.   IV only

2. A peptide chain contains this sequence of amino acids: Leu–Val–Cys–Asp. Which –R groups would cross-link?

  A.   Leu and Val
  B.   Cys
  C.   Cys and Asp
  D.   Val and Asp

3. Here are tabulated pI values for several amino acids:

Amino Acid	pI
Glycine	5.97
Lysine	9.74
Glutamic acid	3.22
Proline	6.30
Cysteine	5.07

Electrophoresis of three amino acids in solution is carried out in a solution buffered at a pH of 4.5. The results are shown here:

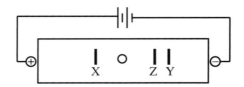

What are the identities of X, Y, and Z?

  A.   Pro, Gly, Lys
  B.   Glu, Gly, Lys
  C.   Pro, Lys, Gly
  D.   Cys, Gly, Glu

4. Subunits are encountered in which structure?

    I.   Secondary
    II. Tertiary
    III. Quaternary

  A.   II and III
  B.   I, II, and III
  C.   III only
  D.   II only

5. An unsaturated fatty acid can be converted to short-chain aldehydes, and then to short-chain carboxylic acids. What type of reactions are these?

  A.   Condensation
  B.   Reduction
  C.   Displacement
  D.   Oxidation

6. How is cholesterol best described?

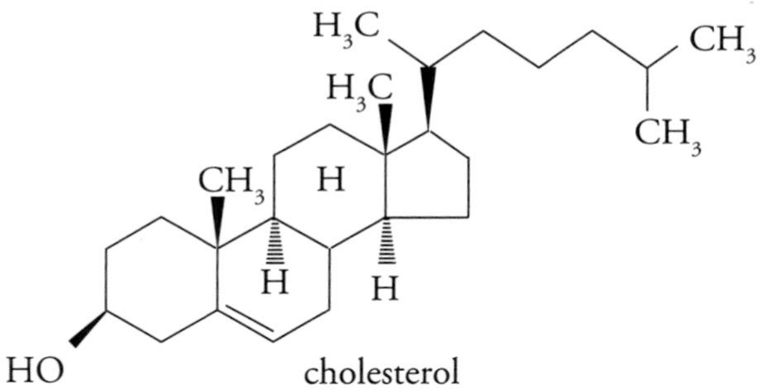

cholesterol

  A.   An alcohol
  B.   A steroid
  C.   A lipid
  D.   A polycyclic compound

Want More Practice?
Register your book online for more drill questions!

Answers and Explanations

1. **C**   Disulfide bonds form between –SH groups of cysteines in the polypeptide chain, producing cross-linking. This causes the chain to develop a three-dimensional shape, so you can eliminate I and choice (A). The cysteines are side chain groups, so II can be eliminated, which eliminates choice (B). The three-dimensional shape is characteristic of a tertiary structure, so choice (D) can be eliminated. Choice (C) is correct.

2. **B**   Cross-linking occurs between cysteine –R groups, which contain an –SH functional group. This functional group does not exist in Leu, Val, and Asp. Thus, the correct answer is choice B.

3. **B**   Below its pI an amino acid is positively charged, and above its pI it is negatively charged. The pH of the buffer is 4.5, so if the pI is above 4.5 the amino acid is positively charged. Otherwise, the amino acid is negatively charged. X has migrated towards the positive electrode, so it is negatively charged. Both Y and Z have migrated towards the negative electrode; they are positively charged. The only amino acid listed that has a pI below the pH is glutamic acid, so that is X. Only choice (B) is correct.

4. **C**   Secondary structures are characterized by hydrogen bonding interactions, so eliminate I and choice (B). Tertiary structure do not contain discrete subunits, so eliminate II and choices (B) and (D). Polypeptide subunits can form interactions that produce a quaternary structure Thus, only choice (C) is correct.

5. **D**   The fatty acid contains an –R component and a carboxylic acid functional group. Because the sequence is conversion to an aldehyde and then to a carboxylic acid, the reactions involve the –R component, not the $-CO_2H$. Short-chain aldehydes can be produced from a fatty acid by oxidation. The aldehydes can then be oxidized further to short-chain carboxylic acids, eliminating choices (A), (B), and (C). Thus, choice (D) is correct.

6. **B**   Cholesterol is not a lipid, so choice (C) can be eliminated. While cholesterol does have an –OH group, it also has a polycyclic structure. The polycyclic structure is characteristic of steroids, so of choices (A), (B), and (D), choice (B) is the correct choice.

Quick Review

- All amino acids contain an amino group that is a base with a pK_a of approximately 9.5, and a carboxyl group that is an acid with a pK_a of approximately 2.5. When the overall amino acid is neutral it forms a zwitterion.

- With the exception of glycine, all amino acids are chiral and can be designated as L- or D-. Animal amino acids are of the L- type.

- The isoelectric point (p*I*) corresponds to the formation of a zwitterion.

- Amino acids can be classified as acidic, basic, or neutral, depending on the chemical properties of the side chain.

- Gel electrophoresis is a physical method used to separate amino acids in an applied electric field based on their charge in a buffered medium.

- A peptide bond is an amide bond linking amino acids together into polypeptide chains. Disulfide bridges form cross-links between cysteine side chains.

- A peptide consists of 2–50 amino acid residues. A polypeptide is a polymer of greater than 50 amino acid residues, and a protein is a long polypeptide or combination of polypeptides bound together by cross-links.

- Formation of a peptide bond is not thermodynamically favored.

- Proteins may be classified in terms of their primary, secondary, tertiary, or quaternary structures.

- The primary structure is the sequence of amino acids that make up the protein.

- The secondary structure describes the three-dimensional folding of a polypeptide chain. This can form an α-helix that forms a clockwise spiral structure containing hydrogen bonds, or β-pleated sheets in which polypeptide chains align themselves in parallel with hydrogen bonds between them.

- A tertiary structure forms from interactions with solvent and between side chains distant from one another that cause the protein to fold. Disulfide bonds are common in tertiary structures.

- Quaternary structures are proteins composed of more than one polypeptide chain forming bonds and cross-links between them.

- Prosthetic groups are not polypeptides that can form part of the protein structure.

- Denaturation involves breaking bonds within a protein causing it to lose its three-dimensional conformation.

- In hydrolysis, water is a nucleophile that converts proteins into their constituent amino acids and peptides.

- Hydrolysis of a protein by another protein is called proteolysis (proteolytic cleavage). The protein that does the cutting is the proteolytic enzyme (protease).

- Lipids are oily or fatty substances that are characterized by their hydrophobicity.

- A fatty acid is composed of long, unsubstituted alkanes that end in a carboxylic acid. They are classified as saturated or unsaturated. Unsaturated fatty acids contain one or more double bonds between carbon atoms.

- Free fatty acids can form a micelle, which is a spherical structure with hydrophilic groups on the outside of the shell and hydrophobic groups inside of the structure.

- Soaps are amphipathic: they are both hydrophilic and hydrophobic.

- Triacylglycerols are composed of three fatty acids esterified to a glycerol molecule.

- Base catalyzed hydrolysis of triglycerides is called saponification.

- Membrane lipids are phospholipids derived from diacylglycerol phosphate. They form an orderly structure called a lipid bilayer.

- Steroids have a characteristic ring system based on the structure of cholesterol, a polycyclic amphipath.

- Cholesterol transports fats and proteins through the blood in a unit called a lipoprotein.

- Steroid hormones are made from cholesterol. They can be classified as peptide hormones that bind to receptors on a cell surface, or as steroid hormones that diffuse into cells.

Chapter 12

Critical Reading

12.1 CRITICAL READING OVERVIEW

The PCAT Critical Reading section is placed between the science and math sections and is 50 minutes long. It has six discrete passages with 7–9 multiple-choice questions each, which together total 48 questions. On average, you will have eight minutes per passage and approximately 30 seconds per question, so plan to set aside about 4 minutes to read the passage and another 4 to answer the questions.

For a successful outcome in this limited time, it is essential that you become familiar with the structure of the Critical Reading section and the kinds of questions asked prior to taking the PCAT. Remember that time management is key, so pace yourself accordingly and periodically check the clock. There is no guessing penalty on the PCAT, so be sure to fill in an answer for every question.

Passages range in length from approximately 400–700 words, which is about the length of two book pages. Topics are drawn from the natural sciences, social sciences, and humanities. The topics may be historical or current, and are considered to be of social, cultural, political, or ethical interest, or of technical interest to the natural sciences. They might include, for example, animal versus human behavior, music as therapy, the consequences of secondhand smoke or eating disorders, or historical government acts. The passages themselves can generally be categorized as informative, persuasive, or speculative, and they may be either practical or theoretical.

All question stems relate directly to the associated passage and test understanding of either parts of the passage or the passage in its entirety. There may be references to specific words, phrases, sentences, or paragraphs, or to the passage as a whole.

Content Objectives

There are specific content objectives to the Critical Reading section of the PCAT. You will be tested on your comprehension of a passage, your ability to analyze the passage content, and on how effectively you can evaluate the author's objective in writing the passage. Each of these three areas carries equal weight in the overall evaluation, which means that each contributes one-third to the overall score. The three areas are more fully described below.

Comprehension

Comprehension includes your ability to recognize and understand words in context, to identify or infer main ideas, to identify details in the passage that lend support to the author's stated position, and to draw logical conclusions. You may, for example, be asked to define a term, or to select the main idea of a passage or a group of related paragraphs. You may also be asked to select facts or ideas that are explicitly stated, or to draw a conclusion by inference.

Analysis

This metric tests your ability to infer and interpret. You are expected to be able to demonstrate how ideas presented in the passage are related and identify the author's intent in writing the passage. You should be able to recognize the author's tone or attitude through word usage or inference. You must be able to separate factual statements from opinions, and identify techniques the author uses to shape the reader's opinions through persuasion. Does the author present evidence, or simply make claims that are unsupported?

Evaluation

This third objective targets your ability to reasonably judge bias, to judge the effectiveness of supporting arguments, and to evaluate the author's conclusion or thesis. You will be asked to infer the author's underlying assumptions based on their viewpoint or preferences, and to determine if the supporting arguments are effective and used appropriately. This is where you distinguish between supporting statements that are used effectively and those that are not.

Identifying Passage Categories

Passages can generally be categorized as Informative, Persuasive, or Speculative. As you read through a passage, identify its category and read through it in the context in which it was written.

Informative Passages

These passages are meant to inform the reader about a particular event, topic, person, or phenomenon. The topic is explained in detail and is meant to educate. For example, an informative passage might explain the process for donating blood, or describe the social impacts of homelessness. There will be a list of important facts that allow the content to speak for itself. The passage will not express an opinion or try to convince the reader to follow a course of action. Rather, it will likely encourage the reader to learn more about the topic.

Persuasive Passages

In a persuasive passage, the author uses logic and reason to argue that a particular point of view is more legitimate than another, and to convince the reader to take a particular action. Arguments should be clear and supported by logical reasons and facts that are convincing. The author takes a stand on a particular issue and builds a strong argument to win over a reader.

A persuasive passage is designed to demonstrate not only why the writer's opinion is correct, but also why any other opinion is without merit. Criticisms, proposals, and editorials are all ways to use persuasion to influence a reader. Topics might include an opinion on universal health care, why it is important to socially distance in a pandemic, or why you should not be concerned about foreign influence shaping national foreign policy.

Speculative Passages

These are nonfiction passages, designed to hypothesize about future outcomes associated with a particular circumstance. Any speculations are supported by scientific fact. Rational events, observations, or personal experiences are also used to support speculations. An author will frequently use anecdotes and hypothetical stories in this type of passage, and a writing style that might include hyperbole. A topic for this type of passage might be how Jules Verne foresaw the use of computers for statistical acquisition, or how we might imagine a world without viruses. The passage should be logically structured and based on factual information.

How to Read a Passage

A Critical Reading passage should be approached very differently from the way you generally read a text. Do not try to thoroughly understand or memorize the content as you would a textbook, but rather look for the main points and how they are linked together to communicate a main idea.

The passages may be dense, convoluted, or even feel highly edited. You do not need to develop a deep understanding of the content, but rather be able to locate the information you need to answer the questions. Each paragraph will have a main point that you may want to rephrase into your own words. Link the main points together to find a common theme or idea, and decide if there is a particular tone.

Note the author's overall tone. Is the writer supportive, angry, or noncommittal, for example, or hesitant, perhaps? Does the author speculate or criticize? A PCAT question might ask, for example, how the conclusions that are drawn are affected by the author's attitude.

How to Tackle a Passage

There are six fundamental steps to approaching Critical Reasoning passages. These steps allow you to assess whether or not you want to immediately tackle a passage or skip it and return to it later. The steps will guide you through a systematic process for attacking a passage.

Step 1

The first step when taking the PCAT is to rank and order all of the passages, and decide whether you will read it *Now*, *Later*, or *Never*. This is an individual decision that will be based on the level of difficulty of the topic and language used in the text. Some readers, for example, may already be deeply familiar with the topic, whereas other may not. Some may find the language level too unapproachable, whereas others may be comfortable with the vocabulary and sentence structures used. Determine your level of comfort or familiarity and categorize each passage appropriately.

Step 2

Before reading a *Now* passage, read through all associated question stems, but ignore the answer choices. After all, wouldn't everyone want to know what questions will be asked before a test? On your erasable noteboard, indicate any words or phrases in the question stems that are particularly relevant to the passage content, such as references to definitions, trends, people, conclusions, or categories. Also indicate words such as *not* or *except*.

Step 3

Staying on the last question set saves valuable time, so don't go back to the first question set as you begin to work through the passage. As you read the passage, indicate important references, any words used to indicate support for an argument, transitional and exception words, and conclusions. Remember, you are deconstructing an essay, so jot down topic sentences and main points. This will allow you to relate pieces to each other and identify the overall structure.

Step 4
Sum up the main points and tone of the passage.

Step 5
Remember to answer the question sets in reverse order. For each one identify the question type, and if necessary translate the question into your own words. Find the relevant information in the passage, and select the "least wrong" answer.

Step 6
Give yourself five minutes before the end of the allotted time for the Critical Reasoning section to make sure you have left nothing blank. Remember, there is no guessing penalty on the PCAT! Also, *do not* review completed questions unless you have marked them for review.

Reading for Structure and Content
You can analyze the structure of a passage on three levels, described below. The individual sentences, paragraphs, and overall passage offer information that guides you in responding to questions.

Level 1

Individual Sentences
Look for words such as *however, for example, therefore,* and *although* that indicate a shift in perspective. These sentences are important in identifying an author's argument and the evidence supporting a claim.

Level 2

Paragraphs and Chunks of Information
Together, the sentences lead to the intent of the paragraph or chunk of information. They may introduce a different point of view, for example, or provide evidence, a new stage of development, or a new phase. If you are pressed for time, read the topic sentence and the last sentence of the paragraph, as these bring together the main point.

Level 3

The Passage as a Whole

The paragraphs create a logical structure of the author's intent in writing the passage. The reader should come away with a clear idea of the type of passage, the author's tone and purpose, and the methods used to support an argument. That is, the main point, the attitude, the purpose, and the evidence should be clear.

The Main Point

While the main point can often be found in the first or last paragraphs of a passage, this is not always the case. There are times when a main point is spread throughout the content, requiring the reader to piece together the main ideas of paragraphs or chunks of information.

Students will often infer too much from a passage and go beyond the scope of its main point, or they will restrict the content too narrowly by focusing on only a few points. These are traps to avoid!

The Attitude

This is the tone the author conveys. Is the author a neutral observer describing different points of view, using such words as *shamefully, distressingly, thankfully, with relief,* or *sadly,* or is the author presenting his or her own voice by criticizing, advocating, or praising? A PCAT question might ask how the author would respond to new information.

The Purpose

The purpose of the passage as a whole is the larger claim being supported. It defines the author's overall intent in writing the passage.

The Evidence

Evidence supporting or rejecting a thesis may be scattered throughout the content, so be sure to indicate words such as these: *as shown by, as evidenced by, as seen, given,* and so on. The PCAT may ask you to determine whether the evidence is presented convincingly and supports the author's purpose in writing the passage.

12.2 TYPES OF QUESTIONS ASKED

The PCAT asks questions about passages that fall into general categories. These are: 1) Purpose, or why the author wrote the passage; 2) Viewpoint, the author's position or perspective; 3) Tone, the author's attitude toward the subject or audience; 4) Implications, which are conclusions drawn from something not explicitly stated; 5) Arguments/Evidence that explicitly state reasons that support a thesis; 6) Relationships, or how elements relate to each other; 7) Language, how words are used to provide meaning; and 8) Organization, how the passage uses organizational patterns. Examples of each are listed below. The last category, Organization, includes the following subcategories: Chronological, Compare and Contrast, Order of Importance, Sequence, Spatial, Cause and Effect, and Problem and Solution.

Become familiar with these general categories and the types of questions that are typically associated with them. You do not need to memorize them, but you should practice asking these same questions in your own reading. The more you practice, the more adept you will become at extracting the correct responses on the actual test.

Remember that when answering PCAT questions, you can typically narrow the choices down to two answers rather quickly. Of the two remaining, the correct response in the Critical Reading section will be the one that is "least wrong."

As you drill down into the passage content, here are questions that the PCAT typically asks in each category. You can be sure that the PCAT will ask questions from each to test your comprehension, ability to analyze the passage, and your ability to evaluate its content.

I. Comprehension

Purpose
Why the author wrote this passage

What is the author's thesis or primary purpose in writing this passage?
Which statement best expresses the author's main point?
What is the main point of a given paragraph?
What is the focus of given paragraphs?
What is the author's intent in discussing a particular example?
What is the author's intent in including the information in a given paragraph?
What can the reader conclude from this passage?

Implications
Conclusions drawn from something not explicitly stated

How does information presented in a given passage imply an outcome or conclusion?
What information suggests a particular result.
What is the implication of a given statement?
How does a particular reference suggest the author's view?
How are similarities identified?

Language
How words are used to provide meaning

How is a given word used to suggest an attitude?
In the context used, what is the meaning of a given word?

II.   Analysis

Viewpoint
The author's position or perspective

What is the author's overall perspective?
What is the author's attitude towards a topic?
Which expression used in the passage best indicates the author's attitude toward the topic?
What are the author's claims?
How does the author use given information in a paragraph to illicit a reader's response?

Tone
The writer's attitude toward the subject or the audience

What is the author's tone throughout the passage?
What is the overall tone of a given paragraph?
What does the tone suggest about the author's attitude?
How does a particular statement reveal the author's tone?

Relationships
How elements relate to each other

How are the ideas presented in two paragraphs related?
How does the author relate two responses?
How does the author relate two models or situations?
What statement best expresses a particular characteristic?
How does a given quotation support a claim?
How does information given in a particular sentence or paragraph support a claim in another?
Why is a given topic mentioned?
How does a particular case study relate to the research?
How do paraphrases relate to stated facts?
How do multiple reasons or information connect to a conclusion?

Organization
How the passage uses organizational patterns
*Chronological, Compare and Contrast, Order of Importance, Sequence,
Spatial, Cause and Effect, and Problem and Solution*

What organizational strategy does the author use to relate ideas coherently?
What organizational strategy is used to support a main idea?
What method is used to discuss viewpoints?
What is the function of a given paragraph's topic sentence?
How does the author develop the information presented in two paragraphs?
What organizational pattern does the author use to support information in a given paragraph?
What does the author accomplish by concluding the passage as shown?
What strategies does the author use to support an overall thesis?
Does the author use questions, and if so, why?

III. Evaluation

Arguments/Evidence
Explicitly stated reasons that support a thesis

What statement expresses a fact to support the author's opinion?
What is the strongest evidence presented for supporting a position?
Which information adds the most credibility to the author's argument?
What is the connection between the passage topic and an argument?
How does the author support a point made in a given paragraph?
What insights provide the strongest support for the author's thesis?
Which reference is *not* intended for its rhetorical effect?
What statements represent or support assumptions?
What statements represent or support positions?
What conclusions are supported?
What evidence provides the strongest challenge to the author's thesis?
Which sentence in a given paragraph expresses the author's value judgment or opinion?
Which statement best summarizes the author's view?
How is an author's bias revealed?

Suggested Reading List and Online Sources

Practice your reading skills by choosing periodicals, books, and online sources that are at a fairly elevated level of difficulty. Use them to identify passage types and transitions and to practice reading for structure and content. As you read, ask yourself the types of questions the PCAT asks.

Here is a list of suggested material:

The New Yorker

Atlantic Monthly

Harper's Bazaar

Foreign Affairs

The Economist

Adam Smith, *An Inquiry into the Nature and Causes of the Wealth of Nations*

Henry David Thoreau, *Walden*

Plato, *The Republic*

Gutenberg.org

Authorama.com

CRITICAL READING DRILL

PASSAGE 1

A Killer Connection?

1.   The Transantarctic Mountains split our planet's southernmost continent into east and west, at times rising more than 14,000 feet high. Today, it's a barren landscape of inhospitable rock and ice. But for the scientists who hike and camp its rocky spine, it's also a portal to another Earth.

2.   Park University paleobotanist Patty Ryberg and her colleagues are uncovering the fossilized remains of a lush forest that thrived in the Antarctic Circle some 260 million years ago during the Permian period. One type of tree, called glossopterids, dominated much of a supercontinent. Then they vanished in a geological instant. The glossopterids didn't die alone. About 90 percent of life on Earth was snuffed out in our planet's biggest known extinction, called the Great Dying. What killed everything? Now, a global campaign to map Earth's ancient mega-eruptions, paired with advances in rock dating, is pushing us closer than ever to explaining why some volcanoes and asteroids kill and others don't. Those results show that the size of an eruption or asteroid isn't as important as the type of rocks incinerated.

3.   One suspect behind several mass extinctions is a kind of enormous volcanic zone called a large igneous province, or LIP. Picture a flattish, layer cake-like volcano big enough to cover a county—or a continent. Amid the seemingly endless oozing lava, its internal plumbing system rips open miles-deep cracks like something from a bombastic action flick. Every major extinction coincides with one of these eruptions. An LIP called the Siberian Traps formed just as the ancient forests disappeared in Antarctica. Some 50 million years later, an LIP called the Central Atlantic Magmatic Province coincided with another mass extinction—one that eventually led to the rise of the dinosaurs. But while those eruptions lasted for perhaps a million years, the extinctions happened in much shorter time periods. Why?

4.   Carleton University geoscientist Richard Ernst, who has studied LIPs for two decades, launched a large-scale effort in 2010 to find answers. Although ancient LIPs are now eroded and often hard to spot, Ernst found he could map the behemoths by examining their ancient magma plumbing systems. His results were surprising: 20 previously undiscovered LIPs, all over the world. Incredibly, many formed billions of years ago and left no signs of a mass extinction. By using high-tech dating techniques to examine crystals in the rock, Ernst's team has also narrowed down the timelines of these eruptions. These new discoveries also help explain what was happening at LIPs during mass extinctions. For example, as the Siberian Traps formed, huge ponds of lava pooled deep underground. This magma cooked surrounding sedimentary rocks as well as enormous seams of coal. As they burned, those organic matter-rich rocks released gases like sulfur and carbon dioxide. Once the pressure below was too much, miles-deep cracks ripped open on Earth's surface, freeing the greenhouse gases. Our planetary thermostat likely rose dozens of degrees Fahrenheit. Those same organics were burned and released in eruptions that wiped out Triassic life and gave rise to the dinosaurs, according to a *Nature* study last May.

5.   The type of rocks burned isn't just important for mega-eruptions. A recent drilling expedition to Mexico's dino-killing Chicxulub crater—the only mass extinction conclusively linked to an impact—found the asteroid hit sedimentary rock rich in sulfurs. And a November *Nature* study showed such rocks cover just 13% of Earth's surface. The dinosaurs might've survived if the space rock hit elsewhere. So really, mass extinctions often just boil down to bad luck. "My lesson from this is that Earth can go through dramatic changes," Ernst says. "The planet doesn't particularly care about the biology on it, including humans."

From "A Killer Connection?" *Discover*, Volume 39, #2, March, 2018 by Eric Betz

1. What is the focus of paragraph 2?

   A. To describe the Great Dying
   B. To discover the underlying cause of mass
      extinctions
   C. To explain how glossopterids vanished
   D. To describe the importance of rock dating

2. What does the author claim?

   A. More research into mass extinctions is needed.
   B. Extinctions are bad luck.
   C. Research into extinctions point to the release of
      toxic gases as a cause.
   D. LIPs lead to mass extinctions.

3. How does paragraph 5 reveal the author's tone?

   A. "The planet doesn't particularly care about the
      biology on it, including humans."
   B. "…mass extinctions often just boil down to bad
      luck."
   C. "…the asteroid hit sedimentary rock rich in
      sulfurs."
   D. "…the only mass extinction conclusively linked
      to an impact."

4. What is the strongest evidence presented for supporting
   the argument that toxic gases caused the Great Dying?

   A. Fissures developed on Earth's surface.
   B. Huge ponds of lava formed underground.
   C. Sedimentary rock rich in sulfurs only cover 13%
      of Earth's surface.
   D. Magma from the Siberian Traps burned organic
      matter-rich rocks.

5. How does examination of the Siberian Traps relate to the
   research?

   A. The Siberian Traps were implicated in the Great
      Dying.
   B. Seams of coal burned and released greenhouse
      gases, which coincided with a mass extinction.
   C. Every major extinction coincides with an
      eruption.
   D. Earth's thermostat rose dozens of degrees
      Fahrenheit.

6. What organizational strategy does the author use to relate
   paragraphs 4 and 5?

   A. Cause and effect
   B. Order of importance
   C. Problem and solution
   D. Sequence

7. What is the author's primary purpose in writing this
   passage?

   A. To describe the devastating effects of mass
      extinctions
   B. To show how nature is in control
   C. To present evidence that that the composition of
      rocks is implicated in mass extinctions
   D. To show how the formation of lava fields can
      have devastating consequences

8. In paragraph 3 *bombastic* means

   A. like a bomb.
   B. devastating.
   C. explosive.
   D. exaggerated.

PASSAGE 2
The Biology of Sugars Points to a Sweet Strategy for Treating Cancer

1. Over the last few decades, researchers tinkering with molecules that turn an immune cell on and off have created a revolutionary approach to fighting cancer. Instead of taking aim at the tumor directly, this new class of medicines harnesses the patient's own immune cells to tackle the disease. Immune-based cancer therapies are saving thousands of lives, and the science behind them earned the 2018 Nobel Prize in Physiology or Medicine.

2. These drugs, called checkpoint blockers, appeared after scientists discovered molecules that help cancer cells block immune processes that would otherwise attack a tumor. The secret lies with several "brake" proteins on white blood cells, T cells, that prevent the immune system from overreacting to microbial threats. Tumor cells have learned to survive by engaging the brake molecules, sending T cells into a stupor that allows cancer to gain a foothold. By thwarting this hijacking maneuver, checkpoint blockers release the brakes and awaken T cells to attack the tumor. A clever trick—except that so far, these immune-based drugs only work in about a fifth of cancer patients and for certain tumors, barely at all.

3. To push past those limits, a few companies are venturing into a new frontier—glycobiology, the science of the sugars that stud the surface of cells. Sugars act like switches and knobs that control where and when a cell's biological machines, proteins and lipids, do their jobs. Yet for all their fine-tuning finesse and power, sugars are highly complex molecules that have often eluded a deeper understanding of their workings because they are so hard to study in the lab.

4. Recently, though, the science has caught up and biotech companies have begun to build on these findings to develop anti-cancer drugs. In November at an American Association for Cancer Research meeting in Miami, Palleon Pharmaceuticals, a Massachusetts startup, unveiled new data from experiments in rodents on a profoundly different set of checkpoint blockers that target sugars.

5. These experimental drugs work by interfering with complex sugars called glycans that coat the surface of tumor cells and let them pass unnoticed by the otherwise vigilant immune system. It's an "under appreciated mechanism of immune evasion," says Michael O'Dwyer, a clinician-researcher at National University of Ireland, Galway, who has no ties to Palleon. Many researchers are going after the T cells' braking systems, he says, but "probably with diminishing returns." He adds: "There's only so much you can get out of the T cells."

6. Palleon launched in 2015 on the strength of research by a handful of labs suggesting that structured patterns of cell-surface glycans—a molecular fingerprint on virtually all cells—might hold the key to rousing a host of additional cancer-fighting immune cells. These macrophages, natural killer cells and other cells make up a different arm of the immune system. Known as innate immune cells, these cells form the body's first line of defense, which sets the stage for a subsequent T-cell attack.

7. One particular glycan, sialic acid, is sensed by a family of surface proteins found mostly on innate immune cells but also on activated T cells at tumor sites. These proteins, called Siglecs, act as molecular brakes. When Siglecs bind to sialic acids, coating the surface of a tumor, the immune cell goes to sleep. Several companies—including Innate Pharma in Marseille, France, and South San Francisco–based Alector—are hoping to wake those drowsy cells with therapies that block Siglecs.

8. A team of researchers led by Palleon co-founder Carolyn Bertozzi, a Stanford chemist, went after these same molecular pathways with a radically different approach. Rather researchers designed a therapeutic that stymies all Siglecs by trimming sialic acids off the tumor cell. In a 2016 proof-of-concept study, the team showed that treating a dish of breast cancer cells with the experimental drug exposed them to killing by natural killer cells.

9. At another immunotherapy meeting in Washington, D.C. in November, Palleon vice president Li Peng presented data showing this strategy can work in mice with implanted tumors—even in ones that draw weak responses with FDA-approved checkpoint-blocking drugs. In separate experiments, the team confirmed that T cells, macrophages and natural killer cells all contribute to the drug's benefit. Cancer cells "are like wolves in sheep's clothing—bad guys disguising themselves with the glycan code," Peng says. By removing sialic acids from glycans on the surface of tumor cells, the drug "reveals their real identity so immune cells can see the bad guys."

From "The Biology of Sugars Points to a Sweet Strategy for Treating Cancer" *Scientific American*, November 28, 2018, by Esther Landhuis

1. What organizational pattern does the author use in this passage?

    A. Compare and contrast
    B. Problem and solution
    C. Chronological
    D. Spatial

2. In paragraph 9, what information supports a claim that cancer cells, "…are like wolves in sheep's clothing…"?

    A. Glycans are coated with sialic acids.
    B. Siglecs bind to sialic acids.
    C. Sialic acids are coated with glycans.
    D. Sialic acids bind to Siglecs.

3. What is the author's thesis?

    A. FDA checkpoint-blocking drugs include those with weak responses.
    B. Blocking Siglecs is a promising approach to treating cancer.
    C. Removing sialic acids is key to developing anti-cancer treatments.
    D. Immune based cancer therapies are proving effective at treating cancer.

4. What does 'checkpoint-blocking' mean in paragraph 9?

    A. The coating on the surface of a tumor
    B. Siglec-binding
    C. Awakening T cells to attack tumors
    D. Proteins that act as molecular brakes

5. Why is glycobiology described as a new frontier?

    A. Sugars are complex and have eluded deep understanding.
    B. Sugars have little impact on proteins and lipids.
    C. Sugars are implicated in the functioning of proteins and lipids.
    D. Cellular surfaces are an important target of tumor therapies.

6. What is the main point of paragraph 5?

    A. To describe the immune system
    B. To express the opinion of someone with no ties to Palleon
    C. To describe the action of an alternative drug therapy
    D. To describe T cells' braking systems

7. What does the overall tone of paragraph 3 suggest about the author's attitude?

    A. Excitement
    B. Judgmental
    C. Skeptical
    D. Ambivalent

8. What impact did glycobiology have on Palleon's research?

    A. It provided a focus on T cells.
    B. It led to research into the role of sialic acids in tumor growth.
    C. It confirmed their findings on breast cancer cells.
    D. It led to the development of immune-based drugs.

Want More Practice?
Register your book online for more drill questions!

Passage 1 Answers

1. **B** The Great Dying and the disappearance of glossopterids are events that occurred, but are not the focus of the paragraph, so choices (A) and (C) can be eliminated. Rock dating is described as important, but it also is not the focus. Thus, choice (D) can be eliminated. The correct answer choice is (B)—this paragraph is about discovering the underlying causes of mass extinctions.

2. **C** The author never explicitly states that more research into mass extinctions is needed, nor do all LIPs lead to mass extinctions, so eliminate choices (A) and (D). While the author states both choices (B) and (C), choice (B) is an opinion, whereas choice (C) is a fact that arises from research. A claim is something that is proposed to be true based on an argument or line of evidence. An opinion is not open to proof or disproof. The question asks for a claim, so choice (C) is correct.

3. **A** A tone elicits an emotional response. Both choices (C) and (D) are stated facts, so they can be eliminated. Choice (A) expresses an attitude about how the considerable forces of nature regard living species, and to a lesser degree so does choice (B). Of choices (A) and (B), however, choice (A) is the better one.

4. **D** A response must be found that relates specifically to toxic gases. While choices (A), (B), and (C) are true, only choice (D) connects toxic gases to the Great Dying.

5. **B** The research is to find the cause of mass extinctions. Choices (A), (C), and (D) are true, but are not the underlying cause, which is the release of gases toxic to life. The correct answer is choice (B).

6. **A** The events are not described in order of importance, nor does the passage state a problem and propose a solution or list events sequentially. The passage describes how toxic gases were released and their effect on life, so choice (A) is correct.

7. **C** In paragraph 2 the author states, "Those results show that the size of an eruption or asteroid isn't as important as the type of rocks incinerated." Only choice (C) supports this claim. The author incorporates choices (A) and (D) in the discussion, and presents his opinion (choice B), but only choice (C) is correct.

8. **D** The word *bombastic* means overblown or inflated. Thus, choice (D) is correct.

Passage 2 Answers

1. **B** While the passage does compare and contrast techniques in different locations, the focus of the passage is on the development of a method for killing cancer cells. We can therefore eliminate choices (A) and (D). The timeline is not chronological, so choice (C) is wrong. We are presented with a problem and a possible solution, choice (B).

2. **A** When siglecs bind to sialic acids, the immune cells "go to sleep" (paragraph 7). Thus, choices (B) and (D) are wrong. Glycans coat sialic acids, so choice (C) is wrong. Only choice (A) is correct.

3. **D** While choice (A) is true, as is choice (B), neither is the author's thesis. Not all treatments may include removing sialic acids (choice C), and it also is not the author's thesis. Only choice (D) expresses the author's main idea in describing the research.

4. **C** "Checkpoint-blocking" does not refer to the coating on the surface of a tumor, so choice (A) is incorrect. Siglecs cause an immune cell to go to sleep, so choice (B) is wrong. Siglecs are referred to as molecular brakes, so eliminate choice (D). Only choice (C) is correct: T cells are "brake" proteins.

5. **C** The focus of choice (A) is on sugars, not why glycobiology is a new frontier (eliminate choice A). Choice (B) is wrong: sugars do have an impact on proteins and lipids. The connection between glycobiology and cellular surfaces is not made in choice (D). Only choice (C) connects proteins and lipids to glycobiology.

6. **C** The immune system is not described, so eliminate choice (A). While choice (B) is true, it is not the main point of the paragraph. T cells' braking systems are mentioned but not described, so choice (D) can be eliminated. Only (C) is correct.

7. **D** There are contradictory feelings, or ambivalence, in paragraph 3, centered around a new approach and its difficulties. The author is not excited, judgmental, or skeptical that the new approach will prove effective, but rather ambivalent, choice (D).

8. **B** Palleon's research focused on stymying "all Siglecs by trimming sialic acids off the tumor cell." They moved away from the previous approach of developing immune-based drugs, choices (A) and (D). Glycobiology did not confirm their findings on breast cancer cells, so choice (C) is wrong. Only choice (B) is correct.

Quick Review

- Passages are generally categorized as informative, persuasive, or speculative, and may either be practical or theoretical.

- Comprehension includes your ability to recognize and understand words in context, to identify or infer main ideas, to identify details in the passage that support a stated position, and your ability to draw logical conclusions.

- Effective analysis includes your ability to infer and interpret by relating ideas and the author's intent, separating facts from opinions, and identifying persuasive language.

- Effective evaluation involves judging bias, inferring underlying assumptions, and evaluating arguments based on their effectiveness.

- Informative passages encourage you to learn more about a topic and is meant to educate.

- Persuasive passages demonstrate why the writer's opinion is correct and why any other opinion is without merit.

- Speculative passages hypothesize about future outcomes associated with a circumstance and are supported by scientific fact.

- Rank the passage based on its level of difficulty, read associated question stems, highlight references in the passage, sum up the main points and tone of the passage, translate questions into your own words if necessary, and be sure to leave nothing blank.

- Analyze the structure of a passage based on individual sentences, paragraphs and chunks of information, and look for the author's overall intent.

  - The main point is generally found in the first or last paragraph of the passage.
  - The attitude is the tone the author conveys.
  - The purpose is the larger claim being supported.
  - Evidence may support or reject a thesis.

- Questions that are asked on the PCAT fall into these general categories:

  - Purpose: why the author wrote the passage
  - Viewpoint: the author's position or perspective
  - Tone: the writer's attitude toward the subject or the audience
  - Implications: conclusions drawn from something not explicitly stated
  - Arguments and Evidence: explicit reasons that support a thesis
  - Relationships: how elements relate to each other
  - Language: how words are used to provide meaning
  - Organization: how organizational patterns are used

- Attack answer choices that are disputable. Specific, strong statements are often wrong, and vague, wimpy statements are often correct.

- Practice your reading skills by reading sources that are at a fairly elevated level of difficulty.

Chapter 13

Quantitative Reasoning

13.1   MATH BASICS

Integers	Positive and negative whole numbers, and zero; NOT fractions or decimals.
Prime Number	An integer that has exactly two distinct factors: itself and 1. All prime numbers are positive; the smallest prime number is 2. Two is also the only even prime number. One is not prime.
Rational Numbers	All positive and negative integers, fractions, and decimal numbers; technically, any number that can be expressed as a fraction of two integers—which means everything except numbers containing weird symbols (such as $\sqrt{2}$), π, or e.
Irrational Numbers	Any number that does not end or repeat (in other words, any number that isn't rational). This includes all numbers with radicals that can't be simplified, such as $\sqrt{2}$ (perfect squares with radicals, such as $\sqrt{16}$, don't count because they can be simplified to integers, such as 4). Also, all numbers containing π or e. Note that repeating decimals like $0.33333\overline{3}$ are rational (they're equivalent to fractions, such as $\frac{1}{3}$).
Real Numbers	Any number on the number line; everything except imaginary numbers (see below).
Imaginary Numbers	The square roots of negative numbers, that is, any numbers containing i, which represents $\sqrt{-1}$.
Consecutive Numbers	The members of a set listed in order, without skipping any; consecutive integers: –3, –2, –1, 0, 1, 2; consecutive positive multiples of 3: 3, 6, 9, 12.
Distinct Numbers	Numbers that are different from each other.
Sum	The result of adding numbers.
Difference	The result of subtracting numbers.
Product	The result of multiplying numbers.
Quotient	The result of dividing numbers.
Remainder	The integer left over after dividing two numbers. For example, when 17 is divided by 2, the remainder is 1. Remember, on the PCAT, a remainder is ALWAYS an integer.
Reciprocal	The result when 1 is divided by a number. For example, the reciprocal of 2 is $\frac{1}{2}$, the reciprocal of $\frac{3}{4}$ is $\frac{4}{3}$, and the reciprocal of $\frac{1}{16}$ is 16.
Positive Difference	Just what it sounds like—the number you get by subtracting the smaller of two numbers from the bigger one. You can also think of it as the distance between two numbers on the number line.
Absolute Value	The positive version of a number. You just strike the negative sign if there is one. You can also think of it as the distance on the number line between a number and zero.
Arithmetic Mean	The average of a list of values; also simply referred to as the "mean."
Median	The middle value in a list when arranged in increasing order; in a list with an even number of members, the average of the *two* middle values.
Mode	The value that occurs most often in a list. If no value appears more often than all the others in a list, then that list has no mode.

Order of Operations

For problems that involve several different operations, you must perform the operations in a particular order. Here's an easy way to remember the order of operations.

Please **E**xcuse **M**y **D**ear **A**unt **S**ally

First, you perform operations enclosed in **P**arentheses; then you take care of **E**xponents; then you **M**ultiply, **D**ivide, and finally **A**dd, and **S**ubtract, working from left to right.

The Associative Law: When adding a string of numbers, you can add them in any order you like. The same thing is true when multiplying a string of numbers.

$$5 + 6 + 7 \text{ is the same as } 7 + 6 + 5$$

$$2 \times 3 \times 4 \text{ is the same as } 3 \times 4 \times 2$$

The Distributive Law: Some combinations of addition and multiplication can be written in two different formats, which often proves extremely useful in finding PCAT answers. The Distributive Law states that

$$a(b + c) = ab + ac$$

and that

$$a(b - c) = ab - ac$$

If a problem gives you information in factored format, which is $a(b + c)$, you should distribute it immediately. If the information is given in distributed form, which is $ab + ac$, you should factor it.

A PCAT problem might look like this.

What Comes First?
Perform all operations within parentheses first. The Distributive Law is something of an exception; it gives you two ways to get the same result.

For all x, $\dfrac{2x + 4}{x + 2} = ?$

A. $x + 2$
B. x
C. 2
D. $x + 4$

Here's How to Crack It

Let's use the distributive property on the numerator of this fraction and rewrite it in factored form.

$$\frac{2(x + 2)}{(x + 2)}$$

$\dfrac{(x + 2)}{(x + 2)}$ equals just 1. Therefore, we can cancel out both terms and the answer must be (C).

Factors and Multiples

The **factors** of a number are all of the numbers by which it can be divided evenly. The test sometimes refers to factors as **divisors**. Some questions on the PCAT will specifically require you to identify the factors of a given number. You may find factorizations useful for solving other questions, even if they don't specifically talk about factorizations. There are two forms of factorization: plain old factorization and prime factorization.

Factors

The **factorization** of a number is a complete list of its factors. The best way to compile a list of all of a number's factors is to write them in pairs, beginning with 1 and the number itself. Then count upward through the integers from 1, checking at each integer to see whether the number you're factoring is divisible by that integer. If it is, add that integer to the list of factors, and complete the pair.

Here is the factorization of 60:

> Remember that the largest factor of a number is that number!

1	60
2	30
3	20
4	15
5	12
6	10

Start with 1 and the original number as your first pair and move up (2, 3, 4, and so on) to ensure that you won't miss any. You'll know your list is complete when the two columns of factors meet or pass each other. Here, the next integer after 6 that goes into 60 is 10, so you can be sure that the factorization is complete. This is the most efficient way to get a complete list of a number's factors.

Prime Factors

The other kind of factorization is **prime factorization**. The prime factorization of a number is the unique group of prime numbers that can be multiplied together to produce that number. For example, the prime factorization of 8 is $2 \times 2 \times 2$. The prime factorization of 30 is $2 \times 3 \times 5$.

Prime factorizations are found by pulling a prime number out of a number again and again until you can't anymore. The prime factorization of 75, for example, would be found as follows:

$$75 =$$

$$3 \times 25 =$$

$$3 \times 5 \times 5$$

Multiples

The PCAT also expects you to know the definition of a **multiple**. The multiples of a number are simply all the numbers that are evenly divisible by your original number. An easy way to think of multiples is to recite the times tables for a number. For example, the positive integer multiples of 6 are simply 6 × 1, 6 × 2, 6 × 3, and so forth, that is, 6, 12, 18.... If the test asks you for the "fifth positive integer multiple of 6," that just means 6 × 5, or 30. It's easy to confuse factors and multiples, so here's a way to keep the two straight. If you look back at the factorization of 60, you'll see that there are only 12 factors of 60, which is few. But 60 has as many multiples as you like. So think "factors are few, multiples are many."

> Remember that the smallest multiple of a number is that number!

Also notice that factors are smaller than or equal to your original number, whereas multiples are larger than or equal to your original number.

> What is the largest factor of 180 that is NOT a multiple of 15 ?

To answer the question, just make the biggest number you can, using the prime factors of 180. The prime factorization of 180 is 2 × 2 × 3 × 3 × 5. Since 15 is the same as 3 × 5, just make sure your number doesn't have 3 *and* 5 as factors. The factor 2 × 2 × 5 may look tempting, but the largest number that fits the bill is 2 × 2 × 3 × 3, or 36.

Fractions

Fractions can be thought of in two ways. A fraction is just another way of expressing division. The expression $\frac{1}{2}$ means 1 divided by 2. The fraction $\frac{x}{y}$ is nothing more than x divided by y. A fraction is made up of a **numerator** and a **denominator**. The numerator is on top; the denominator is on the bottom. Just think, *denominator* starts with "d," just like *downstairs*.

$$\frac{1}{2} \quad \frac{\text{numerator}}{\text{denominator}}$$

The other way to think of a fraction is as a part over a whole.

$$\frac{1}{2} \quad \frac{\text{part}}{\text{whole}}$$

In the fraction $\frac{1}{2}$, we have one part out of a total of two parts. In the fraction $\frac{3}{7}$, we have three parts out of a total of seven parts.

Fraction Reduction

In any fraction involving large numbers, try to reduce the fractions before you do anything else.

Reducing Fractions

To reduce a fraction, see if the numerator and the denominator have a common factor. It may save time to find the largest factor they share, but getting this information isn't crucial. Whatever factor they share can now be canceled. Let's take the fraction $\frac{6}{8}$. Is there a common factor? Yes: 2.

$$\frac{6}{8} = \frac{\cancel{2} \times 3}{\cancel{2} \times 4} = \frac{3}{4}$$

Get used to reducing all fractions (if they can be reduced) before you do any work with them. It saves a lot of time and prevents errors that crop up when you try to work with large numbers.

Comparing Fractions

Sometimes a problem will involve deciding which of two fractions is larger. For example, which is larger, $\frac{2}{5}$ or $\frac{4}{5}$? Think of these as parts of a whole. Which is bigger, two parts out of five or four parts out of five? $\frac{4}{5}$ is clearly larger. In this case, it was easy to tell because they both had the same whole, or the same denominator.

If you're dealing with fractions that do not have the same denominator, just put the fractions next to each other and multiply diagonally. Whichever number is larger, is the larger fraction. Take a look.

$$\frac{2}{3} \qquad\qquad \frac{4}{7}$$

$$2 \times 7 = 14 \qquad 4 \times 3 = 12$$

Because 14 is larger than 12, $\frac{2}{3}$ is the larger fraction.

Adding and Subtracting Fractions

Now that we've reviewed finding a **common** denominator, adding and subtracting fractions is simple. Let's use the Bowtie to add $\frac{2}{5}$ and $\frac{1}{4}$.

$$\frac{2}{5} \bowtie \frac{1}{4} = \frac{8+5}{20} = \frac{13}{20}$$

Let's use the Bowtie to subtract $\frac{2}{3}$ from $\frac{5}{6}$.

$$\overset{\enclose{circle}{15}\quad\enclose{circle}{12}}{\frac{5}{6}\diagdown\!\!\!\!\diagup\frac{2}{3}} \rightarrow \frac{15-12}{18} = \frac{3}{18} \quad \text{or} \quad \frac{1}{6}$$

Multiplying Fractions

To multiply fractions, line them up and multiply straight across.

$$\frac{5}{6} \times \frac{4}{5} = \frac{20}{30} = \frac{2}{3}$$

Was there anything we could have canceled or reduced *before* we multiplied? Yes. We could cancel the 5 on

top and the 5 on the bottom. What's left is $\frac{4}{6}$, which reduces to $\frac{2}{3}$.

Sometimes students whose math skills are a bit rusty think they can cancel or reduce in the same fashion *across an equals sign.*

$$\frac{\cancel{5}x}{6} = \frac{4}{\cancel{5}} \qquad \text{NO!}$$

You *cannot* cancel the 5s or reduce the $\frac{4}{6}$ in this case. When there is an equals sign, you have to cross-multiply,

which yields $25x = 24$, so x in this case would equal $\frac{24}{25}$.

Dividing Fractions

To divide one fraction by another, just invert the second fraction and multiply.

$$\frac{2}{3} \div \frac{3}{4} \text{ is the same thing as } \frac{2}{3} \times \frac{4}{3} = \frac{8}{9}$$

Again, just invert and multiply. Try the next example.

$$\frac{6}{1} \div \frac{2}{3}$$

Just flip the second fraction and multiply.

$$\frac{6}{1} \times \frac{3}{2} = \frac{18}{2} = 9$$

Fractions, Decimals, and Percentages

On arithmetic questions, you will often be called upon to change fractions to decimal numbers, or decimal numbers to percentages, and so on. Be careful whenever you change the form of a number.

You turn fractions into decimals by doing the division represented by the fraction bar.

$$\frac{1}{8} = 1 \div 8 = 0.125$$

To turn a decimal number into a fraction, count the number of decimal places (digits to the right of the decimal point) in the number. Then place the number over a 1 with the same number of zeros, get rid of the decimal point, and reduce.

$$0.125 = \frac{125}{1,000} = \frac{25}{200} = \frac{1}{8}$$

Decimals

A fraction can be written as a decimal and vice versa. Take the fraction $\frac{3}{5}$. Remember what we said before: a fraction is just another form of division.

$$\frac{3}{5} = 3 \div 5 = .6 \qquad\qquad 5\overline{)3.0}^{.6}$$

You can also express any decimal as a fraction.

$$.4 = \frac{4}{10} = \frac{2}{5} \qquad\qquad .03 = \frac{3}{100}$$

The test-writers frequently ask questions using decimals but want answers as fractions, or vice versa, so the ability to go back and forth between the two is essential to succeeding on the test.

Adding and Subtracting Decimals

To add or subtract decimals, just line up the decimal points and proceed as if it were regular addition or subtraction. To add 9.25, 3.2, and 8.567

$$
\begin{array}{r}
9.250 \\
3.200 \\
+\ 8.567 \\
\hline
21.017
\end{array}
$$

It helps to add zeros to fill out the decimal places of the numbers with fewer digits. The decimal 3.2 is the same as 3.200.

Stay in Line
When adding or subtracting decimals, keep all decimal points lined up.

Multiplying Decimals

To multiply decimals, simply ignore the decimal points and multiply your numbers. When you've finished, count all the digits to the right of the decimal points in the original numbers you multiplied. Then, place the decimal point in your answer so that there are the same number of digits to the right of it.

Here's an example.

$$
\begin{array}{r}
2.32 \\
\times\ .03 \\
\hline
.0696
\end{array}
$$

$3 \times 232 = 696$. There are a total of four digits to the right of the decimal point in the original numbers. Therefore, we now place the decimal so that there are four digits to the right in the answer.

Dividing Decimals

The best way to divide one decimal by another is to convert the number you are dividing *by* (in mathematical terminology, the **divisor**) into a whole number. You do this simply by moving the decimal point as many places as necessary.

This works as long as you also remember to move the decimal point in the number that you are dividing (in mathematical terminology, the **dividend**) the same number of spaces.

To divide 12 by 0.6, set it up the way you would an ordinary division problem.

$$.6\overline{)\ 12}$$

To convert 0.6 into a whole number, move the decimal point over one place to the right. Now you must move the decimal point in 12 one place as well. The operation looks like this:

$$6\overline{)120} \qquad 6\overline{)120}^{\,20}$$

Converting Decimals to Percentages

Decimal numbers and percentages are essentially the same. The difference is the percent sign (%), which means "÷ 100." To turn a decimal number into a percentage, just move the decimal point two places to the right, and add the percent sign.

$$0.125 = 12.5\%$$

To turn percentages into decimal numbers, do the reverse; get rid of the percent sign and move the decimal point two places to the left.

$$0.3\% = 0.003$$

It's important to understand these conversions, and to be able to do them in your head as much as possible.

Watch out for conversions between percentages and decimal numbers—especially ones involving percentages with decimal points already in them (like 0.15%). Converting these numbers is simple, but this step is still the source of many careless errors. The value 0.15% is equal to the decimal 0.0015.

Percents

A **percentage** is a fraction in which the denominator equals 100. In literal terms, the word *percent* means "divided by 100." If a question asks for 40 percent of something, for instance, you can express the percentage as a fraction: $\dfrac{40}{100}$. To properly translate all percent questions, it is helpful to have a decoding table for the various terms you'll come across.

The Big Four: Fraction/Percent Equivalents You Should Know

$$\frac{1}{5} = 0.2 = 20\%$$

$$\frac{1}{4} = 0.25 = 25\%$$

$$\frac{1}{3} = 0.\overline{33} = 33\frac{1}{3}\%$$

$$\frac{1}{2} = 0.5 = 50\%$$

Word for Word
Use the English to math conversion chart to translate each word into math.

English	Math Equivalent
percent	/100
of	multiplication (×)
what	variable (y, z)
is, are, were	=
what percent	$\dfrac{y}{100}$

Using the above table, let's say you had a word problem in which you had to translate the following sentence into math terms: "What percent of 7 is 14?" Word for word, substitute the math terms above in the appropriate places. You should end up with

$$\frac{y}{100} \times 7 = 14$$

Now, solve for y to arrive at 200. Tack on your percent sign and call it a day.

Percent Change

Percent change is a way of talking about increasing or decreasing a number. The percent change is just the amount of the increase or decrease, expressed as a percentage of the starting amount.

For example, if you took a $100.00 item and increased its price by $2.00, that would be a 2% change, because the amount of the increase, $2.00, is 2% of the original amount, $100.00. On the other hand, if you increased the price of a $5.00 item by the same $2.00, that would be a 40% increase—because $2.00 is 40% of $5.00. If you ever lose track of your numbers when computing a percent change, just use this formula:

$$\% \text{ Change} = \frac{\text{Amount Change}}{\text{Original}} \times 100$$

Averages

The PCAT uses averages in a variety of question types. Remember, the **average** is the sum of all the values divided by the number of values you're adding. Looking at this definition, you can see that every average involves three quantities: the total, the number of things being added, and the average itself.

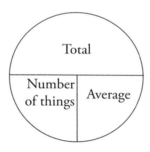

The chart above is called an Average Pie. It's The Princeton Review way of organizing the information found in an average problem. Cover up the "average" section with your thumb. In order to find the average, you divide the total by the "number of things." Now cover up the "number of things" section. You can find it by dividing the total by the average. Finally, you can find the total by multiplying the number of things by the average.

When you run into an average in a PCAT question, you'll be given two of the three numbers involved. Usually, solving the problem will depend on your supplying the missing number in the Average Pie.

The Average Pie becomes most useful when you're tackling a multiple-average question—one that requires you to manipulate several averages in order to find an answer.

Ways to Remember
To find the average, divide the total by the number of things. Think of the horizontal line in the average pie as one big division bar!

Here's an example:

A pharmacy disburses an average of 48 Zolpidem prescriptions during the first six months of the year. If the pharmacy averaged 54 prescriptions during the first eight months of the year, what was the average number of prescriptions of Zolpidem disbursed during the seventh and eighth months?

A. 60
B. 66
C. 72
D. 144

Here's How to Crack It

In this question, there are three separate averages to deal with: the pharmacy's average during the first six months of the year, the pharmacy's average during the entire eight months, and the average during the final two months. In order to avoid confusion, take these one at a time. Draw the first average pie.

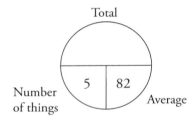

You have the number of things and the average, so you can find the total. You know that Sydney's total for the first 6 months is 288. Fill in that information and draw another pie. For your second pie, the question tells you that the pharmacy's average across all 8 months was 54, so you can multiply those numbers to find the total over 8 months, or 432. Fill in your second average pie below.

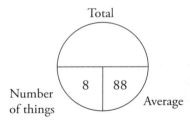

Since you know the total across all 8 months and the total of the first 6 months, you can figure out the total of the last two months:

$$432 - 288 = 144$$

Draw one last pie, using the information that you have:

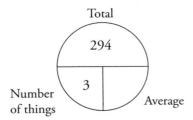

Accordingly, the pharmacy averaged a total of 72 prescriptions during the last two months; so the answer is (C).

———————————◯———————————

Multiple-average questions are never terribly difficult. Just draw an average pie every time you see the word *average* in the question. Organization is everything on these questions. It's easy to make careless errors if you get your numbers scrambled, so make sure you label the parts of the average pie. Notice that you can always add or subtract totals and numbers of things, but you can never add or subtract averages.

The Weighted Average

PCAT writers have a particular fondness for weighted average problems. First, let's look at a regular unweighted average question.

> If Sally received a grade of 90 on a test last week and a grade of 100 on a test this week, what is her average for the two tests?

Piece of cake, right? The answer is 95. You added the scores and divided by 2. Now let's turn the same question into a weighted average question.

> If Sally's average for the entire year last year was 90, and her average for the entire year this year was 100, is her average for the two years combined equal to 95?

The answer is "not necessarily." If Sally took the same number of courses in both years, then yes, her average is 95. But what if last year she took 6 courses while this year she took only 2 courses? Can you compare the two years equally? PCAT likes to test your answer to this question.

Here's an example.

The average number of courses that 12 first-year pharmacy students take is 8, while the average number of courses that 9 second-year pharmacy students take is 6. What is the average number of courses taken by both the first-year and second-year pharmacy students?

A. 7
B. 7.14
C. 7.98
D. 8.16

Here's How to Crack It

The PCAT test-writers want to see whether you spot this as a weighted average problem. If you thought the first-string team was exactly equivalent to the second-string team, then you merely had to take the average of the two averages, 8 and 6, to get 7. In weighted average problems, the PCAT test-writers always include the average of the two averages among the answer choices, and it is always wrong.

The two years are not equivalent because the students took a different number of courses each year. To get the true average, we'll have to find the total number of courses and divide by the total number of students. How do we do this? By going to the trusty average formula as usual. The first line of the problem says that the 12 first-year students take an average of 8 courses.

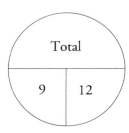

So the total is 12 × 8, or 96.

The second sentence says that the 9 second-year students that average 6 courses each.

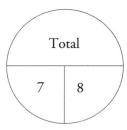

So the total is 9 × 6, or 54.

Now we can find the true average. Add all the courses taken by both first- and second-year pharmacy students to find that: 96 + 54 = 150. This is the true total. Next, divide it by the total number of students (12 + 9 = 21). Therefore, the answer is $\dfrac{150}{21}$ = 7.14, or (B).

Standard Symbols

Symbol	Meaning
=	is equal to
≠	is not equal to
<	is less than
>	is greater than
≤	is less than or equal to
≥	is greater than or equal to

Exponents

An **exponent**, or **power**, is a short way of writing the value of a number multiplied several times by itself. $4 \times 4 \times 4 \times 4 \times 4$ can also be written as 4^5. This is expressed aloud as "4 to the fifth power." The lower and larger number (4) is called the **base**, and the upper number (5) is called the **exponent**. There are several rules to remember about exponents.

Negative Powers

A negative power is simply the reciprocal of a positive power. (The reciprocal of 3 is $\dfrac{1}{3}$.)

$$3^{-1} = \frac{1}{3} \qquad 3^{-2} = \frac{1}{3^2} = \frac{1}{9} \qquad 3^{-3} = \frac{1}{3^3} = \frac{1}{27}$$

The Zero Power

Anything to the zero power is 1.

$$4^0 = 1 \qquad x^0 = 1$$

The First Power

Anything to the power of 1 is itself.

$$5^1 = 5 \qquad y^1 = y$$

Distributing Exponents

When several numbers are inside parentheses, the exponent outside the parentheses must be distributed to all of the numbers within.

$$(4y)^2 = 4^2 y^2 = 16y^2$$

Multiplying Exponents When Bases Are the Same

Exponential terms can be multiplied when their bases are the same. Just leave the bases unchanged and add the exponents.

$$n^3 \times n^5 = n^{3+5} = n^8 \qquad\qquad 3 \times 3^4 = 3^{1+4} = 3^5$$

Coefficients, if they are present, are multiplied normally.

$$2b \times 3b^5 = 6b^6 \qquad\qquad \frac{1}{2}c^3 \times 6c^5 = 3c^8$$

Dividing Exponents When Bases Are the Same

Exponential terms can also be divided when their bases are the same. Once again, the bases remain the same, and the exponents are subtracted.

$$x^8 \div x^6 = x^{8-6} = x^2 \qquad\qquad 7^5 \div 7 = 7^{5-1} = 7^4$$

Coefficients, if they are present, are divided normally.

$$6b^5 \div 3b = 2b^4 \qquad\qquad 5a^8 \div 3a^2 = \frac{5}{3}a^6$$

Multiplying and Dividing Exponents When *Exponents* Are the Same

There's one special case in which you can multiply and divide terms with different bases—when the exponents are the same. In this case you can multiply or divide the different bases. Then the bases change and the exponents remain the same.

For multiplication:

$$3^3 \times 5^3 = 15^3 \qquad\qquad x^8 \times y^8 = (xy)^8$$

And for division:

$$33^2 \div 3^2 = 11^2 \qquad\qquad x^{20} \div y^{20} = \left(\frac{x}{y}\right)^{20}$$

If exponential terms have different bases and different exponents, then there's no way to combine them by adding, subtracting, dividing, or multiplying.

Adding and Subtracting When *Bases* and *Exponents* Are the Same

Terms with exponents can be added or subtracted only when they have the same base and exponent.

$$2a^3 + a^3 = 3a^3 \qquad\qquad 5x^2 - 4x^2 = x^2$$

If they don't have the same base and exponent, exponential terms can never be combined by addition or subtraction.

Raising Powers to Powers

When an exponential term is raised to another power, the exponents are multiplied.

$$(x^2)^8 = x^{2 \times 8} = x^{16} \qquad\qquad (7^5)^4 = 7^{5 \times 4} = 7^{20}$$

If there is a coefficient included in the term, then the coefficient is also raised to that power.

$$(3c^4)^3 = 27c^{12} \qquad\qquad (5g^3)^2 = 25g^6$$

Using these rules, you should be able to manipulate exponents wherever you find them.

More Important Exponent Stuff

There are a few important things to remember about the effects of exponents on various numbers:

- A positive number raised to any power remains positive. No exponent can make a positive number negative.
- A negative number raised to an odd power remains negative.
- A negative number raised to an even power becomes positive.

In other words, anything raised to an odd power keeps its sign. If a^3 is negative, then a is negative; if a^3 is positive, then a is positive. A term with an odd exponent has only one root. For example, if $a^3 = -27$, there's only one value of a that makes it true: $a = -3$.

On the other hand, anything raised to an even power becomes positive, regardless of its original sign. This means that an equation with an even exponent has two roots. For example, if $b^2 = 25$, then b has two possible values: 5 and -5. It's important to remember that two roots exist for any equation with an even exponent (the only exception is when $b^2 = 0$, in which case b can equal only 0, and b^2 has only one root).

One last thing to remember—since any real number becomes positive when raised to an even exponent, certain equations will have no real roots. For example, the equation $x^2 = -9$ has no real roots. There's no integer or fraction, positive or negative, that can be squared to produce a negative number. In this equation, x is said to be an imaginary number. The equation is considered to have no real solution.

But Watch Out For...

Exponents are shorthand for multiplication, so the rules apply only when you multiply or divide the same base.

$$\text{Does } x^2 + x^3 = x^5? \text{ NO!}$$

$$\text{Does } x^4 - x^2 = x^2? \text{ NO!}$$

$$\text{Does } \frac{x^2 + y^3 + z^4}{x^2 + y^3} = z^4? \text{ NO!}$$

You would expect that raising a number to a power would increase that number, and usually it does, but there are exceptions.

- If you raise a positive fraction of less than 1 to a power, it gets smaller.

$$\left(\frac{1}{2}\right)^2 = \frac{1^2}{2^2} = \frac{1}{4}$$

- If you raise a negative number to an odd power, the number gets smaller (unless it is between 0 and −1).

$$(-3)^3 = (-3)(-3)(-3) = -27$$

(Remember: −27 is smaller than −3.)

- If you raise a negative number to an even power, the number becomes positive.
$$(-3)^2 = (-3)(-3) = 9$$

Roots

Roots are exponents in reverse. For example, $4 \times 4 = 16$. That means that $4^2 = 16$. It also means that $\sqrt{16} = 4$. Square roots are by far the most common roots on the PCAT. The square root of a number is simply whatever you would square to get that number.

You may also encounter other roots: cube roots, fourth roots, fifth roots, and so on. Each of these roots is represented by a radical with a number attached, like $\sqrt[3]{x}$, which means the cube root of x. Roots of higher degrees work just as square roots do. The expression $\sqrt[4]{81}$, for example, equals 3—the number that you'd raise to the 4th power to get 81. Similarly, $\sqrt[5]{32}$ is the number that, raised to the 5th power, equals 32—in this case, 2.

When the number under a radical has a factor whose root is an integer, then the radical can be *simplified*. This means that the root can be pulled out. For example, $\sqrt{48}$ is equal to $\sqrt{16 \times 3}$. Because 16 is a perfect square, its root can be pulled out, leaving the 3 under the radical sign, as $4\sqrt{3}$. That's the simplified version of $\sqrt{48}$.

Working with Roots

The rules for manipulating roots when they appear in equations are the same as the rules for manipulating exponents. Roots can be combined by addition and subtraction only when they are roots of the same order and roots of the same number.

$$3\sqrt{5} - \sqrt{5} = 2\sqrt{5} \qquad\qquad 3\sqrt[3]{x} + 2\sqrt[3]{x} = 5\sqrt[3]{x}$$

Roots can be multiplied and divided freely as long as all the roots are of the same order—all square roots, or all cube roots, and so on. The answer must also be kept under the radical.

$$\sqrt{a} \times \sqrt{b} = \sqrt{ab} \qquad\qquad \sqrt[3]{24} \div \sqrt[3]{3} = \sqrt[3]{8} = 2$$

$$\sqrt{18} \times \sqrt{2} = \sqrt{36} = 6 \qquad\qquad \sqrt[4]{5} \div \sqrt[4]{2} = \sqrt[4]{\frac{5}{2}}$$

Be sure to memorize these rules before working with roots.

Fractional Exponents

A fractional exponent is a way of raising a number to a power and taking a root of the number at the same time. The number on top is the normal exponent. The number on the bottom is the root—you can think of it as being in the "root cellar."

So, in order to raise a number to the $\frac{2}{3}$ power, you would square the number and then take the cube root of your result. You could also take the cube root first and then square the result—it doesn't matter which one you do first, as long as you realize that 2 is the exponent and 3 is the order of the root.

Remember that an exponent of 1 means the number itself, so $x^{\frac{1}{2}}$ is equal to $\sqrt{x}$, the square root of x to the first power.

The Principal Idea

Remember how both 2 and –2 raised to the 4th power equal 16? Well, for the PCAT, a radical refers only to the *principal* root of an expression. When there is only one root, that's the principal root. An example of this is $\sqrt[3]{27}$. The only root of this expression is 3. When you have both a positive *and* a negative root, the positive root is considered to be the principal root and is the only root symbolized by the radical sign. So, even though $2^4 = 16$ and $(-2)^4 = 16$, $\sqrt[4]{16}$ means 2 only, and not –2.

$$27^{\frac{1}{3}} = \sqrt[3]{27} = 3 \qquad\qquad b^{\frac{5}{2}} = \sqrt{b^5}$$

$$8^{\frac{2}{3}} = \sqrt[3]{8^2} = \sqrt[3]{64} = 4 \qquad\qquad x^{\frac{4}{3}} = \sqrt[3]{x^4}$$

Rules to Remember About Roots

- $\sqrt{x} + \sqrt{x} = 2\sqrt{x}$

For example, $2\sqrt{5} + 20\sqrt{5} = 22\sqrt{5}$

- $\sqrt{x} \bullet \sqrt{y} = \sqrt{xy}$

For example, $\left(\sqrt{12}\right)\left(\sqrt{3}\right) = \sqrt{36}$, or 6.

$$3\sqrt{5} \bullet 6\sqrt{2} = 18\sqrt{10}$$

- $\sqrt{\dfrac{x}{y}} = \dfrac{\sqrt{x}}{\sqrt{y}}$

For example, $\sqrt{\dfrac{3}{16}} = \dfrac{\sqrt{3}}{\sqrt{16}} = \dfrac{\sqrt{3}}{4}$

- To simplify a radical, try factoring. Look for a perfect square to factor out.

$$\sqrt{32} = \sqrt{16}\sqrt{2} = 4\sqrt{2}$$

$$2\sqrt{5} + 4\sqrt{125} = 2\sqrt{5} + 4\left(\sqrt{25}\right)\left(\sqrt{5}\right) =$$

$$2\sqrt{5} + (4)(5)\left(\sqrt{5}\right) = 22\sqrt{5}$$

- The square root of a positive fraction less than 1 is actually larger than the original fraction.

For example, $\sqrt{\dfrac{1}{4}} = \dfrac{1}{2}$

- Always try to have a ballpark idea of how large the number you are dealing with actually is. $\sqrt{63}$ is a bit less than $\sqrt{64}$ or 8. $\sqrt[3]{9}$ is a bit more than $\sqrt[3]{8}$ or 2. Some good approximations to memorize and helpful hints to remember them are as follows:

$\sqrt{2} \approx 1.4$ (Valentine's Day is 2/14.)

$\sqrt{3} \approx 1.7$ (St. Patrick's Day is 3/17.)

Scientific Notation

Scientific notation is a way of expressing numbers that are too large to be written out easily. To write the number 1,204 in scientific notation, you would move the decimal point three places to the left and multiply by 10 to the third power, 1.204×10^3. Five million (5,000,000) written in scientific notation would look like 5.0×10^6. So you divide the number by 10 until there is only one digit to the left of the decimal point. Then you have to multiply it by the power of 10 that equals the number of 10s you took out originally.

The purpose of scientific notation is to express very large numbers or very small numbers without endless strings of zeros.

$$3.24 \times 10^2$$

To simplify this expression, move the decimal point over to the right by the same number as the power of 10—in this case, two places. If the power of 10 is negative, move the decimal point to the left instead.

$$3.24 \times 10^3 = 3,240$$

$$3.24 \times 10^2 = 324$$

$$3.24 \times 10^{-1} = 0.324$$

$$3.24 \times 10^{-2} = 0.0324$$

The Dance of the Decimal
Remember that dividing a number by a power of 10 is the same as moving the decimal to the left and that multiplying a number by a power of 10 is the same as moving the decimal to the right. The number of places you move the decimal is the same as the exponent (or power) of 10 being divided or multiplied.

Scientists are examining the reaction that occurs between two substances that has an expected reaction rate of 2.76×10^{-5} seconds. If the reaction lasted 1,000 times longer than expected, how long did the reaction last, in seconds?

    A. 2.76×10^{-15}
    B. 2.76×10^{-9}
    C. 2.76×10^{-8}
    D. 2.76×10^{-2}

First, let's write out 2.76×10^{-5}. Since we are working with negative exponents, we will move five spaces to the left, which will give us 0.0000276.

Next, since we are told the reaction lasted 1,000 times longer than expected, we would multiply the decimal by 1,000, moving the decimal place three spaces to the right: $0.0000276 \times 1,000 = 0.0276$

To rewrite this in scientific notation, we would then move the decimal two spaces to the right, giving a negative exponent of 2; 2.76×10^{-2}. Thus, the answer is (D).

Alternatively, if you recall your laws of exponents, you could solve the question by writing the question as $2.76 \times 10^{-5} \times 10^3 = 2.76 \times 10^{-2}$.

MATH BASICS DRILL

1. The marked price of an item is x. A dealer raises the marked price and then gives a discount of 15% on the item such that there is no loss on the sale of the item. By how much does the dealer raise the marked price of the item?

   A. $0.15x$

   B. $\dfrac{17}{20x}$

   C. $\dfrac{3}{17x}$

   D. $x + \dfrac{15}{100}$

2. A shop decides to conduct a survey to find out the most popular organic food among buyers. After the end of a particular month, the shop takes a count of the different types of organic foods sold in that month. The table below shows the result of the survey.

Food	Percent (%)
Fresh vegetables	29
Fruits	20
Eggs	19
Milk/dairy	17
Poultry	15

   If 24,800 shoppers were surveyed, then how many shoppers voted for fruits?

   A. 4,712
   B. 4,860
   C. 4,960
   D. 5,000

3. A coffee shop lists the numbers of sandwiches sold on a particular day, in a table as shown below.

Variety of Sandwich	Numbers sold
Roast Beef	40
Turkey	27
Ham	36
Veggie	24
Meatloaf	30
Super Sub	12

   Just before closing shop for the day, an additional eight roast beef sandwiches are sold. Which variety of sandwich amounts to exactly three-fourths the number of roast beef sandwiches sold?

   A. Ham
   B. Meatloaf
   C. Veggie
   D. Super Sub

4. A 5-gallon can of paint is required to paint 1,500 square feet of a surface. What is the rate of coverage of paint in square feet, per gallon?

   A. 30
   B. 150
   C. 300
   D. 1,500

5. Hannah needs 24 light bulbs for her new apartment. A package of 24 light bulbs costs $5.98, a package of 12 light bulbs costs $2.64, a package of 6 light bulbs costs $1.38, and a package of 4 light bulbs costs $1.04. Which package is the least expensive to buy for 24 bulbs?

   A. The package of 4
   B. The package of 6
   C. The package of 12
   D. The package of 24

6. Leon buys a tablet that has an online price of $900, before the 8% sales tax. If he uses a 10% discount coupon to buy the tablet, how much has he saved?

    A. $64.80
    B. $79.20
    C. $90.00
    D. $97.20

7. A canoe rental company charges two people $26 per canoe for a short trip of 2–4 hours. Each canoe can accommodate a maximum of three people. There is an additional charge of $8 for an extra rider. How much does the company charge five riders for a trip of two hours?

    A.   40
    B.   50
    C.   52
    D.   60

8. A local club sells packets of candy for a charity fundraiser. It charges $3.75 for each packet of candy. On a particular day, the club sells 52 packets of candy. How much does the club raise for charity that day?

    A. $185
    B. $195
    C. $200
    D. $208

9. Joel buys a car for $22,000. Its value depreciates at a rate of 14% per annum. What will be the value of the car after 2 years?

    A. $431.20
    B. $3,080.00
    C. $16,271.20
    D. $18,920.00

10. A student scores an average of 26 on four quizzes. He scores exactly 29 in each of the next several successive attempts. How many quizzes does he take for an average score of 28?

    A.   2
    B.   4
    C.   8
    D.   12

11. A pack of 12 cartons of milk costs $24. Each carton holds 8 ounces of milk. What is the cost per quart?

    A. $3
    B. $4
    C. $6
    D. $8

12. A coffee machine takes 1 minute to fill a 60 ml cup (1 ounce = 29.57 ml). How long does it approximately take to fill an 11-ounce mug?

    A.   1 min 11 sec
    B.   10 min
    C.   5 min 30 sec
    D.   11 min

13. A bookstore has five branches in a city. The following bar graph shows the number of books (in thousands) sold at each branch in the years 2001 and 2002.

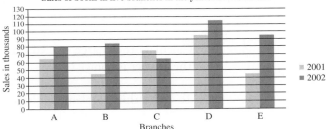

Sales of books in five branches in the years 2001 and 2002

What is the ratio (to the nearest tenth) of the total sales at Branch B to those at Branch E for both years?

    A.   17.6
    B.   61.9
    C.   92.9
    D.   107.7

Want More Practice?

Register your book online for more drill questions!

Answers and Explanations

1. **C** If the original price is x and is to be increased by some unknown amount, y, such that 15% off of $x + y = x$, then focus on the amount that will remain after the reduction: 85%. $\frac{85}{100}(x + y) = x$. The question asks how much the original price, x, was increased, so solve for y. The answer is choice (C).

2. **C** To solve this problem, calculate 20% of 24,800, $\frac{20}{100} \times 24{,}800 = 4{,}960$. The answer is choice (C).

3. **A** Calculate three fourths of 48. Therefore, $48 \times \frac{3}{4} = 36$. The answer is choice (A).

4. **C** To determine the coverage for one gallon, you must divide 1,500 by 5, the number of gallons required. $1{,}500 \div 5 = 300$. The answer is choice (C).

5. **C** Calculate the price of a single light bulb in each deal, $5.98 \div 24 = 0.249$, $2.64 \div 12 = 0.22$, $1.38 \div 6 = 0.23$, and $1.04 \div 4 = 0.26$. Choose the cheapest of all, which is choice (C).

6. **D** He'll save 10%, or $90, off the online price and the 8% sales tax, or $7.20, that he would have paid on the $90. The answer is choice (D).

7. **D** Calculate the charge of two canoes and a charge for an additional rider $26 + 26 + 8 = 60$. The answer is choice (D).

8. **B** To solve this problem, multiply the cost of each packet by the number of packets sold. $\$3.75 \times 52 = \$195.00$. The answer is choice (B).

9. **C** Unless you're familiar with the depreciation formula, you'll have to complete this solution in two steps. First, find the value of the car after one year. $\$22{,}000 \times .14 = \$3{,}080$ (the dollar amount of depreciation in the first year). $\$22{,}000 - \$3{,}080 = \$18{,}920$ (the value of the car after one year). Next, find the value of the car after the second year. $\$18{,}920 \times 0.14 = \$2{,}648.80$ (the dollar amount of depreciation in the second year). $\$18{,}920 - \$2{,}648.80 = \$16{,}271.20$ (the value of the car after two years). The correct answer is (C).

10. **C** Solve this problem by forming the equation $\frac{(26)4 + 29x}{4 + x} = 28$ and solve for x. Therefore, $104 + 29x = 112 + 28x \Rightarrow x = 8$. The answer is choice (C).

11. **D** Here's one way to solve this problem. First, determine the cost of each carton. To do this, divide the cost by the number of cartons $\$24 \div 12 = \$2$. Next to determine how many cartons are in a quart, divide the number of ounces in a quart (32) by the number of ounces in each carton (8). $32 \div 8 = 4$. Now you know there are four cartons in a quart. To determine the cost of a quart, multiply the cost per carton ($2) by the number of cartons in a quart (4). $\$2 \times 4 = \$8$. The correct answer is choice (D).

12. **C** Convert 11 ounces to 325 ml and then divide by 60. The answer is (C).

13. **C** The required ratio is $\left(\frac{45 + 85}{45 + 95}\right) = \left(\frac{130}{140}\right) = 92.9\%$. The answer is (C).

13.2 ALGEBRA

Algebra: Operations with Numbers

Algebra is simply a way of performing operations without numbers; in algebraic expressions, a variable stands in for the missing number or numbers. While the quantitative section of the PCAT is not by and large an algebra test, you should be comfortable with the basics of working with equations.

Algebra on the PCAT

Many algebra questions are best answered by using the simple algebra rules outlined in this chapter. Others can be shortcut with our techniques.

Review of Definitions

Here are some algebraic terms that will probably appear on the PCAT. Make sure you're familiar with them. If the meaning of any of these vocabulary words keeps slipping your mind, add those words to your flash cards.

> It seems like a small thing, but memorizing your times tables will really help you on test day.

Variable	An unknown quantity in an equation represented by a letter (usually from the end of the alphabet), for example, x, y, or z.
Constant	An unchanging numerical quantity—either a number or a letter that represents a number (usually from the beginning of the alphabet), for example, 5, 7.31, a, b, or k.
Term	An algebraic unit consisting of constants and variables multiplied together, such as $5x$ or $9x^2$.
Coefficient	In a term, the constant before the variable. In ax^2, a is the coefficient. In $7x$, 7 is the coefficient.
Polynomial	An algebraic expression consisting of more than one term joined by addition or subtraction. For example, $x^2 - 3x^2 + 4x - 5$ is a polynomial with four terms.
Binomial	A polynomial with exactly two terms, such as $(x - 5)$.
Quadratic	A quadratic expression is a polynomial with one variable whose largest exponent is a 2, for example, $x^2 - 5x + 6$ or $y = x^2 + 4$.
Root	A root of a polynomial is a value of the variable that makes the polynomial equal to zero. More generally, the roots of an equation are the values that make the equation true. Roots are also known as zeros, solutions, and x-intercepts.

A Few Laws

These two basic laws are not necessary for success on the PCAT, so if you have trouble with them, don't worry too much. However, if you're comfortable with these two laws, you'll be able to simplify problems using them, so it's definitely worth it to use them.

13.2

A linear equation
is an equation of
two variables that
gives a straight
line when plotted
on a graph.

Equations and Inequalities

Although you can often avoid algebra on the PCAT by using Plugging In and PITA, you will still need to know how to manipulate equations. When working with equations, the goal is often to solve for a variable, but sometimes you simply need to shift terms around.

To solve a **linear equation** (one without exponents), you need to get all the variables on one side and all the numbers on the other.

Manipulating Equations

When working with equations, you can do pretty much anything you want to them as long as you follow the golden rule:

Don't assume
you'll always
need to solve for
the variable on the
PCAT; sometimes
you'll simply have
to manipulate the
equation to get
the answer.

> Whatever you do on one side of the equals sign you must also do on the other side.

Solving for One Variable

You can solve equations that have just one variable. In these cases, you start by isolating the variable on one side of the equation and the numbers on the other side. You can do this by adding, subtracting, multiplying, or dividing both sides of the equation by the same number. Just remember that anything you do to one side of an equation, you must do to the other side. Be sure to write down every step. Let's look at a simple example:

$$3x - 4 = 5$$

Here's How to Crack It

In this case, you can collect all the constants on the right side of the equation by adding 4 to both sides of the equation. (If for some reason you wanted to move the 5 to the left side of the equation, you would have to subtract 5 from both sides. That's just how it works.) In general, you can eliminate negative numbers by adding them to both sides of the equation, just as you can eliminate positives by subtracting them from both sides of the equation.

$$
\begin{aligned}
3x - 4 &= 5 \\
+ 4 &= + 4 \\
\hline
3x &= 9
\end{aligned}
$$

The above rule also applies to numbers in the equation that are divided or multiplied. So in this case, in order to get rid of the 3 that's multiplied by the variable, x, we would need to divide both sides of the equation by 3 to solve for x.

$$\frac{3x}{3} = \frac{9}{3}$$

$$x = 3$$

Let's try another one:

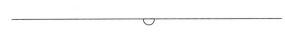

$$5x - 13 = 12 - 20x$$

Here's How to Crack It

Again, we want to get all the x values on the same side of the equation:

$$
\begin{array}{r}
5x - 13 = 12 - 20x \\
+\,20x \qquad\qquad +\,20x \\
\hline
25x - 13 = 12
\end{array}
$$

Now let's get rid of that negative 13:

$$
\begin{array}{r}
25x - 13 = 12 \\
+\,13 + 13 \\
\hline
25x = 25
\end{array}
$$

It might be pretty obvious that x is 1, but let's just finish it:

$$25x = 25$$

$$\frac{25x}{25} = \frac{25}{25}$$

$$x = 1$$

Let's try another one:

$$5x + \frac{3}{2} = 7x$$

Here's How to Crack It

First multiply both sides by 2 to get rid of the fraction. Remember to multiply all of the members of the equation!

$$10x + 3 = 14x$$

Now collect the x's on the same side:

$$\begin{array}{r} 10x + 3 = 14x \\ -10x \qquad -10x \\ \hline 3 = 4x \end{array}$$

You must always do the same thing to both sides of an equation.

Now finish it up:

$$3 = 4x$$

$$\frac{3}{4} = \frac{4x}{4}$$

$$\frac{3}{4} = x$$

Factoring and Distributing

When manipulating algebraic equations, you'll need to use the tools of factoring and distributing. These are simply ways of rearranging equations to make them easier to work with.

Factoring

Factoring simply means finding some factor that is in every term of an expression and "pulling it out." By "pulling it out," we mean dividing each individual term by that factor, and then placing the whole expression in parentheses with that factor on the outside. Here's an example:

$$x^3 - 5x^2 + 6x = 0$$

On the left side of this equation, every term contains at least one x—that is, x is a factor of every term in the expression. That means you can factor out an x:

$$x^3 - 5x^2 + 6x = 0$$

$$x(x^2 - 5x + 6) = 0$$

The new expression has exactly the same value as the old one; it's just written differently, in a way that might make your calculations easier. Numbers as well as variables can be factored out, as seen in the example below.

$$17c - 51 = 0$$

On the left side of this equation, every term is a multiple of 17. Because 17 is a factor of each term, you can pull it out.

$$17c - 51 = 0$$

$$17(c - 3) = 0$$

$$c - 3 = 0$$

$$c = 3$$

As you can see, factoring can make equations easier to solve.

Distributing

Distributing is factoring in reverse. When an entire expression in parentheses is being multiplied by some factor, you can "distribute" the factor into each term, and get rid of the parentheses. For example,

$$3x(4 + 2x) = 6x^2 + 36$$

On the left side of this equation, the parentheses make it difficult to combine terms and simplify the equation. You can get rid of the parentheses by distributing.

$$3x(4 + 2x) = 6x^2 + 36$$

$$12x + 6x^2 = 6x^2 + 36$$

And suddenly, the equation is much easier to solve.

$$12x + 6x^2 = 6x^2 + 36$$

$$-6x^2 \quad -6x^2$$

$$12x = 36$$

$$x = 3$$

Cross Multiplication

Whenever you have an equals sign between two fractions, you can solve by cross multiplying. Thus,

$$\frac{3}{2y} = \frac{2}{5}$$

becomes

$$4y = 15 \text{ and } y = \frac{15}{4}$$

Note that you can cross multiply only when you have an equals sign between two fractions. You cannot cross-multiply across an addition, subtraction, or multiplication sign.

Inequalities

The point of the inequality sign always points to the smaller value.

In an equation, one side is always equals to another. In an **inequality**, one side of the equation does *not* equal the other. Equations contain equal signs, while inequalities contain one of the following symbols:

$\neq$	is not equal to
$>$	is greater than
$<$	is less than
$\geq$	is greater than or equal to
$\leq$	is less than or equal to

You can manipulate any inequality in the same way you can an equation, with one important difference. When you multiply or divide both sides of an inequality by a negative number, the direction of the inequality symbol must change. That is, if $x > y$, then $-x < -y$.

To see what we mean, take a look at this simple inequality:

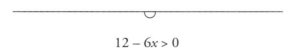

$$12 - 6x > 0$$

Here's How to Crack It

You could manipulate this inequality without ever multiplying or dividing by a negative number by just adding $6x$ to both sides. The inequality sign stays the same. Then divide both sides by positive 6. Again, the sign stays the same.

$$
\begin{aligned}
12 - 6x &> 0 \\
+ 6x &> + 6x \\
\hline
12 &> 6x \\
\frac{12}{6} &> \frac{6x}{6} \\
2 &> x
\end{aligned}
$$

But suppose you subtract 12 from both sides at first:

$$12 - 6x > 0$$
$$\underline{-12 \qquad\; > -12}$$
$$-6x \;> -12$$
$$\frac{-6x}{-6} < \frac{-12}{-6}$$
$$x < 2$$

Notice that the sign flipped because you divided both sides by a negative number. But the answer means the same thing: the first answer says that the number 2 is greater than x, and the second says that x is less than the number 2!

Flip the sign! When you multiply or divide both sides of an inequality by a negative number, the greater than/less than sign points the opposite way.

Sometimes, the question will give you a range for two variables and then combine them in some way. It looks something like this:

If $0 < x < 10$, and $-10 < y < -1$, then what is the range for $x - y$?

Here's How to Crack It.

First, treat the inequality sign like an equals sign. You need all possible combinations of $x - y$, which means that you need the biggest x minus the biggest y, the biggest x minus the smallest y, the smallest x minus the biggest y, and the smallest x minus the smallest y. There is a simple setup to do this.

On your whiteboard write:

Now just solve for $x - y$. When you're done, the biggest and smallest numbers are your answers.

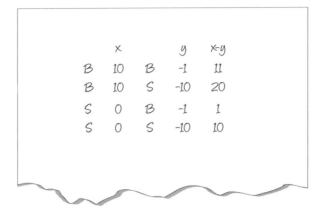

The range for $x - y$, therefore, is $1 < x - y < 20$. Check your answer choices and eliminate.

Working With Two Variables

So far we've dealt only with simple equations that involve one variable. But you may have to deal with equations with two variables. Here's an example:

$$3x + 10y = 64$$

Here's How to Crack It

You can't solve an equation with two variables unless you have a second equation.

The important thing to note about this situation is that we cannot solve this equation. Why, you ask? The problem is that since there are two variables, there are many possible solutions to this equation and we have no way of knowing which solutions are correct. For example, the values $x = 8$ and $y = 4$ satisfy the equation. But so do the values $x = 10$ and $y = 3.4$. Which solutions are correct? We just don't know. In order to solve equations with two variables, we need two equations. Having two equations allows us to find definitive values for our variables.

$$3x + 10y = 64$$
$$6x - 10y = 8$$

When we're given two equations, we can combine them by adding or subtracting them. We do this so that we can cancel out one of the variables, leaving us with a simple equation with one variable. In this case, it's easier to add the two equations together:

$$\begin{array}{r} 3x + 10y = 64 \\ \underline{6x - 10y = 8} \\ 9x \quad\quad = 72 \end{array}$$

When we add these two equations we get $9x = 72$. This is a simple equation which we can solve to find $x = 8$. Once we've done that, we plug that value back into one of the equations and solve for the other variable. Substituting $x = 8$ into either equation gives us $y = 4$.

Simultaneous Equations

It's possible to have a set of equations that can't be solved individually but can be solved in combination. Here's a good example of such a set of equations:

In the system of equations below, what is the value of $10x + 6y$?

$$4x + 2y = 18$$

$$x + y = 5$$

You can't solve either equation by itself. But you can if you put them together. It's called simultaneous equations. All you do is stack them and then add or subtract them to find what you're looking for. Often, what you're looking for is another equation. For example, the question above wants to know what the value of $10x + 6y$ is. Do you need to know x or y? No! You just need to know $10x + 6y$. Let's try adding the two equations:

$$
\begin{array}{r}
4x + 2y = 18 \\
+x + y = 5 \\
\hline
5x + 3y = 23
\end{array}
$$

Did adding help? It did! Even though we didn't get what they were asking for, we did get half of what they were asking for. So just multiply the entire equation by 2 and you have your answer: $10x + 6y = 46$.

Here's another example of a system of simultaneous equations as they might appear on a PCAT question. Try it.

If x and y are real numbers such that $3x + 4y = 10$ and $2x - 4y = 5$, then what is the value of x ?

$$
\begin{array}{r}
3x + 4y = 10 \\
+ 2x - 4y = 5 \\
\hline
5x = 15 \\
x = 3
\end{array}
$$

Add It Up
Do you notice how adding brings you close to what the question is asking for?

In the question above, instead of solving to find a third equation, you need to find one of the variables. Your job doesn't change: stack 'em; then add or subtract. This will be the case with every simultaneous equations question. Every once in a while you may want to multiply or divide one equation by a number before you add or subtract.

13.2

Try another one. Solve it yourself before checking the explanation.

If $12a - 3b = 131$ and $5a - 10b = 61$, then what is the value of $a + b$?

This time adding didn't work, did it? Let's go through and see what subtraction does:

Avoid Subtraction Mistakes

If adding doesn't work and you want to try subtracting, wait! Multiply one of the equations by –1 and add instead. That way you ensure that you don't make any calculation errors along the way.

$$
\begin{array}{r}
12a - 3b = 131 \\
-1(5a - 10b) = 61 \\
\hline
12a - 3b = 131 \\
-5a + 10b = -61 \\
\hline
7a + 7b = 70 \\
7(a + b) = 70 \\
a + b = 10
\end{array}
$$

A little practice will enable you to see quickly whether adding or subtracting will be more helpful. Sometimes it may be necessary to multiply one of the equations by a convenient factor to make terms that will cancel out properly. Here's an example:

If $4n - 8m = 6$, and $-5n + 4m = 3$, then $n =$

$$
\begin{array}{l}
4n - 8m = 6 \\
-5n + 4m = 3
\end{array}
$$

Here, it quickly becomes apparent that neither adding nor subtracting will combine these two equations very usefully. However, things look a little brighter when the second equation is multiplied by 2.

# of Equations = # of Variables

We've been talking about two equations, two variables. But the PCAT doesn't stop there. A good rule of thumb is, if the number of equations is equal to the number of variables, you can solve the equations. So count 'em and don't get discouraged! They're always easier than they look!

$$
2(-5n + 4m = 3)
$$

$$
\begin{array}{r}
4n - 8m = 6 \\
-10n + 8m = 6 \\
\hline
-6n = 12 \\
n = -2
\end{array}
$$

Occasionally, a simultaneous equation can be solved only by *multiplying* all of the pieces together. This will generally be the case only when the equations themselves involve multiplication alone, not the kind of addition and subtraction that the previous equations contained.

Take a look at this example:

$$ab = 3 \qquad bc = \frac{5}{9} \qquad ac = 15$$

If the above statements are true, what is one possible value of *abc*?

A. 5.0
B. 8.33
C. 9.28
D. 25.0

Here's How to Crack It

This is a tough one. No single one of the three small equations can be solved by itself. In fact, no two of them together can be solved. It takes all three to solve the system, and here's how it's done:

$$ab \times bc \times ac = 3 \times \frac{5}{9} \times 15$$

$$aabbcc = 25$$

$$a^2 b^2 c^2 = 25$$

Once you've multiplied all three equations together, all you have to do is take the square roots of both sides, and you've got a value for *abc*.

$$a^2 b^2 c^2 = 25$$

$$abc = 5, -5$$

And so (A) is the correct answer.

Solving Equations with Absolute Value

The rules for solving equations with absolute value are the same. The only difference is that, because what's inside the absolute value signs can be positive or negative, you're solving for two different results.

Let's look at an example:

$$|x - 2| = 17$$

Now, we know that either $(x - 2)$ is a negative number or a non-negative number. When a number is negative, the absolute value makes it the inverse, or multiplies it by -1 to yield a positive result. If the

13.2

number is positive, it remains the same after being sent through the absolute value machine. So when we remove the absolute value bars, we're left with two different equations:

$$x - 2 = 17 \qquad \text{or} \qquad -(x - 2) = 17$$

Now simply solve both equations:

$$
\begin{array}{llll}
x - 2 = 17 & \text{or} & -(x - 2) = 17 \\
\underline{+ 2 \ + 2} & & x - 2 \ = -17 \\
& & \underline{+ 2 \ = + 2} \\
x \quad = 19 & \text{or} & x \qquad = -15
\end{array}
$$

And that's all there is to it!

Quadratics

An expression like $x^2 + 3x + 10$ is a quadratic polynomial. A quadratic is an expression that fits into the general form $ax^2 + bx + c$, with a, b, and c as constants. An equation in general quadratic form looks like this:

> **General Form of a Quadratic Equation**
>
> $$ax^2 + bx + c = 0$$

Unlike simple linear equations, quadratic equations have exponents. On the PCAT, the key to working with quadratic equations is converting them to their other form by **foiling** or **factoring**.

FOIL

A **binomial** is an algebraic expression that has two terms (pieces connected by addition or subtraction). FOIL is the method used to multiply two binomials together.

The letters of FOIL stand for First, Outside, Inside, Last. Suppose you want to multiply the two binomials $(x - 3)$ and $(x + 2)$.

First

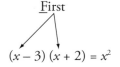

$(x - 3)(x + 2) = x^2$

Outside

$(x - 3)(x + 2) = x^2 + 2x$

Inside

$(x - 3)(x + 2) = x^2 + 2x - 3x$

Last

$(x - 3)(x + 2) = x^2 + 2x - 3x - 6$

Here's another example. Suppose you wanted to do the following multiplication:

$$(x + 5)(x - 2)$$

You would multiply the two *first* terms together, $(x)(x) = x^2$.
And then the *outside* terms, $(x)(-2) = -2x$.
And then the *inside* terms, $(5)(x) = 5x$.
And finally the two *last* terms, $(5)(-2) = -10$.

String the four products together and simplify them to produce an answer.

$$x^2 - 2x + 5x - 10$$

$$x^2 + 3x - 10$$

And that's the product of $(x + 5)$ and $(x - 2)$.

Factor

Often, the best way to solve a quadratic equation is to factor it into two binomials—basically FOIL in reverse. Let's take a look at the quadratic you just worked with and the binomials that are its factors.

$$x^2 + 3x - 10 = (x + 5)(x - 2)$$

Notice that the coefficient of the quadratic's middle term (3) is the sum of the constants in the binomials (5 and -2), and that the third term of the quadratic (-10) is the product of those constants. That relationship between a quadratic expression and its factors will always be true. To factor a quadratic, look for a pair of constants whose sum equals the coefficient of the middle term, and whose product equals the last term of the quadratic. Suppose you had to solve this equation:

$$x^2 - 6x + 8 = 0$$

First, set up the parentheses.

$$x^2 - 6x + 8 = 0 \quad (\quad)(\quad)$$

Next, find the first part. To get x^2, the F in FOIL must be multiplied by x.

$$x^2 - 6x + 8 = 0 \quad (x\quad)(x\quad)$$

Then look for a pair of numbers that add up to -6 and multiply to 8. Because their sum is negative but their product is positive, you know that the numbers are both negative. And as always, there's only one pair of numbers that fits the bill—in this case, -2 and -4.

$$x^2 - 6x + 8 = 0$$

$$(x - 2)(x - 4) = 0$$

Since zero multiplied by anything is equal to zero, this equation will be true if $(x - 2) = 0$ or if $(x - 4) = 0$. Therefore,

$$x = \{2, 4\}$$

Two and four are therefore called the zeros of the equation. They are also known as the **roots** or solutions of the equation.

13.2

Once a quadratic is factored, it's easy to solve for x. The product of the binomials can be zero only if one of the binomials is equal to zero—and there are only two values of x that will make one of the binomials equal to zero (2 and 4). The equation is solved.

Finding Roots

Let's look at another example of finding the roots, or solutions, of a quadratic equation. The roots are values of x that make the equation true. If a quadratic is set equal to 0, you can factor it, and solve for x to find the roots.

Find the roots of this quadratic.

$$x^2 - 8x = -15$$

First add 15 from both sides so that the equation is set equal to 0.

$$x^2 - 8x + 15 = 0$$

Now, factor the quadratic.

$$x^2 - 8x + 15 = 0 = (x - 5)(x - 3)$$

Now set each term equal to 0 and solve.

$$\text{If } (x - 5) = 0, \text{ then } x = 5$$
$$\text{If } (x - 3) = 0, \text{ then } x = 3$$

Therefore, the roots of this equation are 5 and 3.

Common Quadratics

There are certain quadratics that the test-writers love to test repeatedly. You will save yourself a lot of time on the test if you memorize them.

> 1. Factored form: $x^2 - y^2$ (the difference between two squares)
>   Unfactored form: $(x + y)(x - y)$
>
> 2. Factored form: $(x + y)^2$
>   Unfactored form: $x^2 + 2xy + y^2$
>
> 3. Factored form: $(x - y)^2$
>   Unfactored form: $x^2 - 2xy + y^2$

Here are some examples of these quadratic identities in action.

1. $n^2 + 10n + 25 = (n + 5)(n + 5) = (n + 5)^2$
2. $r^2 - 16 = (r + 4)(r - 4)$
3. $n^2 - 4n + 4 = (n - 2)(n - 2) = (n - 2)^2$

But knowing the quadratic identities will do more for you than just allow you to factor some expressions quickly. Such questions are easy to solve if you remember these equations and use them, and quite tricky (or even impossible) if you don't.

Here's an example.

If $a + b = 7$, and $a^2 + b^2 = 37$, then what is the value of ab ?

A. 6
B. 12
C. 15
D. 22

Here's How to Crack It

Algebraically, this is a tough problem to crack. You can't divide $a^2 + b^2$ by $a + b$ and get anything useful. In fact, most of the usual algebraic approaches to questions like these don't work here. Even plugging the answer choices back into the question (PITA) isn't very helpful. What you can do is recognize that the question is giving you all of the pieces you need to build the quadratic identity: $(x + y)^2 = x^2 + 2xy + y^2$. To solve the problem, just rearrange the identity a little and plug in the values given by the question.

$$(a + b)^2 = a^2 + b^2 + 2ab$$
$$(7)^2 = 37 + 2ab$$
$$49 = 37 + 2ab$$
$$12 = 2ab$$
$$6 = ab$$

And presto, the answer appears. It's not easy to figure out what a or b is specifically—and you don't need to. Just find the value asked for in the question. If you remember the quadratic identities, solving the problem is easy.

The Quadratic Formula

Unfortunately, not all quadratic equations can be factored by the reverse-FOIL method. The reverse-FOIL method is practical only when the roots of the equation are integers. Sometimes, however, the roots of a quadratic equation will be non-integer decimal numbers, and sometimes a quadratic equation will have no real roots at all. Consider the following quadratic equation:

$$x^2 - 7x + 8 = 0$$

There are no integers that add up to –7 and multiply to 8. This quadratic cannot be factored in the usual way. To solve this equation, it's necessary to use the quadratic formula—a formula that produces the root or roots of any equation in the general quadratic form $ax^2 + bx + c = 0$.

The Quadratic Formula

$$x = \frac{-b \pm \sqrt{b^2 - 4ac}}{2a}$$

The a, b, and c in the formula refer to the coefficients of an expression in the form $ax^2 + bx + c$. For the equation $x^2 - 7x + 8 = 0$, $a = 1$, $b = -7$, and $c = 8$. Plug these values into the quadratic formula and you get the roots of the equation.

In Case You Were Worried...

The quadratic formula is necessary only on difficult questions. You may be able to skip over tough quadratic equation questions and avoid having to use the quadratic formula altogether.

$$x = \frac{-(-7) + \sqrt{(-7)^2 - 4(1)(8)}}{2(1)}$$

$$x = \frac{7 + \sqrt{49 - 32}}{2}$$

$$x = \frac{7 + \sqrt{17}}{2}$$

$$x = 5.56$$

$$x = \frac{-(-7) - \sqrt{(-7)^2 - 4(1)(8)}}{2(1)}$$

$$x = \frac{7 - \sqrt{49 - 32}}{2}$$

$$x = \frac{7 - \sqrt{17}}{2}$$

$$x = 1.44$$

So the equation $x^2 - 7x + 8 = 0$ has two real roots, 5.56 and 1.44.

It's possible to tell quickly, without going all the way through the quadratic formula, how many roots an equation has. The part of the quadratic formula under the radical, $b^2 - 4ac$, is called the **discriminant**. The value of the discriminant gives you the following information about a quadratic equation:

- If $b^2 - 4ac > 0$, then the equation has two distinct real roots.
- If $b^2 - 4ac = 0$, then the equation has one distinct real root and is a perfect square. Actually, it has two identical real roots, which you might see called a "double root."
- If $b^2 - 4ac < 0$, then the equation has no real roots. Both of its roots are imaginary.

Don't Forget Those Strategies

Don't Forget to Plug In

Plugging In is a technique for short-cutting algebra questions. It works on a certain class of algebra questions in which relationships are defined, but no real numbers are introduced. Here's an example:

Speedy RX prescription delivery service costs d dollars for a membership and c cents for each prescription sent. If a membership sends the first four prescriptions for free, which of the following reflects the cost, in dollars, of getting a membership with Speedy RX and having p prescriptions sent, if p is greater than four?

A. $100d + cp - 4c$

B. $d + 100pq - 25c$

C. $d + cp - \dfrac{p}{25}$

D. $n + \dfrac{pq}{100} - \dfrac{p}{25}$

To Number or Not to Number?

Let's say you walk into a candy store. The store is selling certain pieces of candy for 5 cents and 10 cents each. You want to get 3 pieces of the 5 cent candy and 6 pieces of the 10 cent candy. You give the cashier a $5 bill. What's your change?

Ok, now let's say you walk into a candy store. This store is selling certain pieces of candy for x cents and y cents each. You want to get m pieces of the x cent candy and n pieces of the y cent candy. You give the cashier a $$z$ bill. What's your change?

Which problem would be easier to solve? The one with the numbers! Numbers make everything easier. So why bother with variables when you don't have to?

Here's How to Crack It

In this problem you see a lot of variables in the question and in the answer choices. That's a big clue!

When you see variables in the answer choices, PLUG IN!

Let's Plug In! We'll start with d, the membership fee to Speedy RX.

Plug in an easy number like 5, so that a membership costs $5.00.

Then, plug in a number for c, the charge per prescription. Since this number is in cents, and we'll need to convert it to dollars in the answers, choose a number that can be converted easily to dollars, like 100. Let's make $c = 100$, so a prescription costs $1.00.

Finally, let's say that p, the number of prescriptions, is 5. So, with 4 free prescriptions, you're paying for only 1.

13.2

Then, work out the answer to the question using your numbers. How much does it cost for a membership and 5 prescriptions? Well, that's $5.00 for a membership, 4 prescriptions free, and 1 prescription for $1.00. The total is $6.00. Accordingly, if you plug your numbers into the answer choices, the right answer should give you 6. We call that your target number—the number you are looking for in the answer choices. Put a double circle around your target number, so that it stands out from all the other numbers you've written down. It looks like a bull's-eye that you're trying to hit:

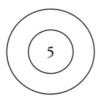

When you plug in $d = 5$, $c = 100$, and $p = 6$ into the answer choices, the only answer choice that gives you 6 is (D). That means you've hit your target number, and you're done.

Take a look at one more:

Not Sure When to Plug In? Here Are Some Hints:

- The answer choices contain variables, percentages, fractions, or ratios.
- There are unknown quantities or variables in the question.
- The question seems to call for an algebraic equation.
- You see the phrase "in terms of" followed by a variable (for example "in terms of *p*"). Cross off the phrase "in terms of *p*," because you don't need it to solve the problem.

The size of an art collection is tripled, and then 70 percent of the collection is sold. Acquisitions then increase the size of the collection by 10 percent. The size of the art collection is then what percent of its size before these three changes?

A. 240%
B. 210%
C. 111%
D. 99%

Here's How to Crack It

Here's another question in which you aren't given numbers. In this case, you don't know the original size of the art collection. Instead of variables, though, the question and answers contain percents. This is another sign that you can plug in whatever numbers you like. Because you're working with percentages, 100 is a good number to plug in—it'll make your math easier.

You start with a collection of 100 items. It's tripled, meaning it increases to 300. Then it's decreased by 70%. That's a decrease of 210, so the collection's size decreases to 90. Then, finally, it increases by 10%. That's an increase of 9, for a final collection size of 99. Since the collection began at 100, it's now at 99% of its original size. The answer is (D). It doesn't matter what number you choose for the original size of the collection—you'll always get the right answer. The trick to choosing numbers is picking ones that make your math easier.

The idea behind Plugging In is that if these relationships are true, then it doesn't matter what numbers you put into the question; you'll always arrive at the same answer choice. So the easiest way to get through the question is to plug in easy numbers, follow them through the question, and see which answer choice they lead you to.

Occasionally, more than one answer choice will produce the correct answer. When that happens, eliminate the answer choices that didn't work out, and plug in some different kinds of numbers. Some numbers you might try are odd and even integers, positive and negative numbers, fractions, zero, positive or negative one, and really big or really small numbers, like 1,000 or –1,000. The new numbers will produce a new target number. Use this new target number to eliminate the remaining incorrect answer choices. You will rarely have to plug in more than two sets of numbers.

> When using Plugging In, keep a few simple rules in mind:
>
> - Avoid plugging in 1 or 0, which often makes more than one answer choice produce the same number. For the same reason, avoid plugging in numbers that appear in the answer choices— they're more likely to cause several answer choices to produce your target number.
> - Plug in numbers that make your math easy—2, 3, and 5 are good choices in ordinary algebra. Multiples of 100 are good in percentage questions, and multiples of 60 are good in questions dealing with seconds, minutes, and hours.

Plugging In can be an incredibly useful technique. By plugging in numbers, you're checking your math as you do the problem. When you use algebra, it takes an extra step to check your work with numbers. Also, there are fewer chances to mess up when you plug in. And you can plug in even when you don't know how to set up an algebraic equation.

Plugging In is often safer because the answer choices are designed so that, if you mess up the algebra, your result will be one of the wrong answers. When your answer matches one of the choices, you think it must be right. Very tempting. Furthermore, all of the answer choices look very similar, algebraically. But when you plug in, the answers often look very different. Often you'll be able to approximate to eliminate numbers that are obviously too big or too small, without doing a lot of calculation, and that will save you lots of time!

Plugging In the Answers (PITA)

Plugging In the Answers (PITA) is another approach to solving algebra questions. It uses numbers instead of algebra to find the answer. As you've just seen, Plugging In is useful on questions whose answer choices contain variables, percentages, fractions, or ratios—not actual numbers. PITA, on the other hand, is useful on questions whose answer choices do contain actual numbers.

Answers are always organized in numerical order—usually from least to greatest. You can use this to your advantage by combining PITA and POE.

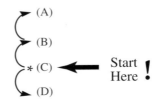

To use PITA on an algebra question, start with (C) and stick it back into the problem. If it makes all of the statements in the question true, then it's the right answer. If it doesn't, eliminate (C) and try another answer choice. Usually, you'll know from your experience with (C) whether you want to try a smaller or larger answer choice. If (C) is too small, you can eliminate any smaller choices and try again with any larger ones.

Like Plugging In, PITA can open doors for you when you're unsure how to approach a question with algebra. Also, like Plugging In, it checks your answers as you pick them, eliminating careless errors. Particularly at the tough end of a long day of testing, Plugging In and PITA can enable you to solve problems that would otherwise stump you.

Let's take a look at a PITA example.

A nurse must go to the hospital pharmacy to fill a prescription for a patient. If she runs 20% of the way, walks 35% of the way, and is given a ride by the security guards for the final 5 minutes, for how many total minutes did the nurse travel?

A. 10.5
B. 11.1
C. 11.7
D. 12

Here's How to Crack It

To use PITA on this question, you'd start with (C). The answer choices represent the quantity asked for in the question—in this case, the total number of minutes traveled by the nurse. Always know what question you're answering. Choice (C), therefore, means that the nurse traveled for 11.7 minutes. Follow this information through the problem.

The nurse spends 20% of the time running to the pharmacy. 20% of 11.7 minutes is 2.34 minutes.

The nurse spends 35% of the time walking to the pharmacy. 35% of 11.7 minutes is 4.09 minutes.

Thus, the first two forms of travel take the nurse 6.43 minutes. But, since the nurse spends the final 5 minutes riding with the security guard, the nurse would spend 2.33 + 4.08 + 5 = 11.43 minutes traveling. BUT that doesn't match choice (C).

That means that (C) isn't the right answer. It also tells you that the trip took fewer minutes. Eliminate (D) and move to (B).

The nurse spends 20% of the time running to the pharmacy. 20% of 11.1 minutes is 2.22 minutes.

The nurse spends 35% of the time walking to the pharmacy. 35% of 11.1 minutes is 3.89 minutes.

Accordingly, the first two forms of travel take the nurse 6.41 minutes. But, since the nurse spends the final 5 minutes riding with the security guard, the nurse would spend 2.22 + 3.88 + 5 = 11.1 minutes traveling. That's the answer!

Generally, you'll never have to try more than two answer choices when using PITA thanks to POE—and sometimes, the first answer you try, (C), will be correct. Keep your eyes open for PITA opportunities on the PCAT, particularly when you run into an algebra question that you're not sure how to solve. You might even want to go back through the problems in the last drill and see if there are any that could have been solved more easily using PITA.

> **You Should Try PITA Whenever**
> - there is an unknown or variable in the question, the question asks for an actual value, and the answer choices are all numbers arranged in increasing or decreasing order
> - you have the bizarre urge to translate a word problem into a complicated algebraic equation
> - you find yourself reading a long, convoluted story about some number, and you don't even know what the number is
> - you have no idea how to solve the problem

If, after you plug in (C), you're not sure which way to go in the answer choices, don't haggle for too long. Just eliminate (C), pick a direction, and go! If you go the wrong way, you'll know pretty quickly, and then you can head the other way.

ALGEBRA DRILL

1. If $7(q - r) = 10$, what is q in terms of r?

   A. $r + \dfrac{10}{7}$

   B. $r - \dfrac{10}{7}$

   C. $7r + 10$

   D. $10 - 7r$

2. Keisha, Toni, and Sumit decide to split up the work in filling a set of prescriptions. Sumit fills twice the number of prescriptions as Toni fills, and Keisha fills 3 fewer prescriptions than Sumit does. If Keisha fills k prescriptions, then, in terms of k, how many prescriptions does Toni fill?

   A. $\dfrac{r - 7}{2}$

   B. $\dfrac{r - 2}{2}$

   C. $2k + 3$

   D. $2k + 6$

3. At a crafts supply store, the price of a type of decorative string is c cents per foot. At this rate, what would be the price, in dollars, of y yards of this string?

   A. $\dfrac{cy}{300}$

   B. $\dfrac{100}{3cy}$

   C. $\dfrac{3y}{100c}$

   D. $\dfrac{3cy}{100}$

$$x - 2y + 3z = 9$$
$$-x + 3y = -4$$
$$2x - 5y + 5z = 17$$

4. What is the value of x in the system of equations shown above?

   A. 1
   B. 2
   C. 5
   D. 16

5. Aaron purchases some books for $60 at a book store. He gets 2 books free because of a sale, along with the purchased books. If he gets 10 books in all, then what is the average cost of the books he purchased?

   A. $5.00
   B. $6.00
   C. $6.50
   D. $7.50

6. The average shank length of screwdrivers manufactured by a company is 25 cm. The shank is rejected if its length deviates from the average by 3.5 mm either way. Which of the following equations gives the **least** and the **greatest** acceptable length of the screwdriver shank?

   A. $|x - 25| \geq 3.5$
   B. $|x - 0.35| \leq 25$
   C. $|x - 25| \leq .35$
   D. $|x - 35| \geq 25$

7. Adam plans to build a pathway of uniform width around the rectangular garden in front of his house. The garden is 24 feet long and 18 feet wide. If the area of the pathway is 184 square feet, then what is its width?

A. 2 feet
B. 3 feet
C. 4 feet
D. 6 feet

8. Which of the following inequalities represents the solution of $|2x + 5| > 9$?

A. $-7 > x > 2$
B. $-7 < x < 2$
C. $x < -7$ or $x > 2$
D. $x > -7$ or $x < 2$

9. A pharmacist wants to increase the concentration of 4 quarts of 60% solution of boric acid by adding x quarts of 75% solution of boric acid. The equation $P(x) = \dfrac{240 + 75x}{4 + x}$ describes the percentage of boric acid concentration. How many quarts of 75% solution of boric acid does he add to get 70% solution of boric acid?

A. $\dfrac{1}{8}$

B. $\dfrac{1}{4}$

C. 4

D. 8

10. Brian spent $\dfrac{1}{4}$ of his paycheck to repair his car, and then paid the registration and insurance, which each cost $\dfrac{1}{3}$ of the remainder of his paycheck. If Brian had \$0 before he was paid, and he now has \$231 left, what was the amount of his paycheck?

A. \$2,772
B. \$1,622
C. \$924
D. \$870

Want More Practice?
Register your book online for more drill questions!

Answers and Explanations

1. **A** It's a little difficult to plug in on this one because you have to pick numbers that make $7(q - r) = 10$ true. First, divide both sides by 7 to find $q - r = \frac{10}{7}$. Then, add r to both sides to find $q = \frac{10}{7} + r$ or $q = r + \frac{10}{7}$. The answer is choice (A).

2. **B** Plugging In is the best approach to this question. Start with a value for k and build from there. Let $k = 5$. If Keisha fills 5 prescriptions and that is 3 fewer prescriptions than Sumit fills, Sumit fills 8 prescriptions. If Sumit fills 8 prescriptions, and that is twice the number that Toni filled, Toni would have filled 8 / 2 = 4 prescriptions; 4 is your target. Now, plug in $k =$ into the answer choices to find that only choice (B) equals 4.

3. **D** If the string costs c cents per foot, then it costs $3c$ cents per yard (because 1 yard = 3 feet). So the price of y yards of the string will be $3cy$ cents. Dividing this by 100 (to convert from cents per dollars), the cost of the string will be $\frac{3cy}{100}$ dollars, choice (D). Alternatively, you can plug in values for the variables. For example, let $c = 100$ and $y = 2$. Then the price of the string is 100 cents (or 1 dollar) per foot. It follows that the string is 3 dollars per yard, so the price of 2 yards would be 6 dollars. If you now plug in $c = 100$ and $y = 2$ into the answer choices, the only one that equals 6 is choice (D).

4. **A** Solve the first and the second equations to eliminate x. Eliminate x by solving the first and the third equations. After solving two equations obtained in y and z, you get $z = 2$ and $y = -1$. Plugging these values in one of the equations, find the value of x as 1. The answer is choice (A).

5. **D** Form the equation $\frac{60}{x} + 2 = 10$ and solve for x. Therefore, the average cost of the book is $x = \frac{60}{8} = 7.50$. The answer is choice (D). Alternatively, you could PITA.

6. **C** Convert 3.5 mm to 0.35 cm and then write the inequality as the difference in length, $|x - 25|$ must be less than 0.35 cm. The answer is choice (C).

7. **A** To solve this problem, form the equation as $\{(24 + 2x)(18 + 2x)\} - 432 = 184$ and solve for x. Therefore, $x^2 + 21x - 46 = 0 \Rightarrow (x + 23)(x - 2) = 0 \Rightarrow x = 2$. The answer is choice (A).

8. **C** Solve the inequality as

$2x + 5 < -9$ or $2x + 5 > 9$

$\Rightarrow x < -7$ or $x > 2$

The answer is choice (C).

9. **D** Substitute 70 for $P(x)$ in the equation and solve for x. $70 = \dfrac{240 + 75x}{4 + x} \Rightarrow 280 + 70x = 240 + 75x \Rightarrow 40 = 5x \Rightarrow x = 8$. The answer is choice (D).

10. **C** It's an algebra question with numbers for answer choices, so set up your whiteboard to plug in the answers. Start with choice (C). If Brian's paycheck was $924, and he spent $\dfrac{1}{4}$ on the repair, then he spent $231, leaving him with $693; the insurance and registration each cost $\dfrac{1}{3}$ of the balance, or $231, so he spends another $462, leaving him with $693 − $462 = $231. This matches the information in the question, so choice (C) is correct.

13.3 PROBABILITY, RATIOS, PROPORTIONS, AND STATISTICS

13.3

Probability

Words referring to probability or chance are commonly used in conversation. For example, we often come across statements like these:

- It is likely to rain today, so please take your umbrella with you.
- It was an easy test. I'll probably get an A on it.
- The Yankees have a much better chance of winning than the Mets.

Words like "probably," "likely," and "chance" carry similar meanings in conversation. They all convey uncertainty. By using probability, we can also make a numerical statement about uncertainty. For example, bank managers can never know exactly when their depositors will make a withdrawal or exactly how much they'll withdraw. Managers also know that though most loans they've granted will be paid back, some of them will result in defaults—but they can't know exactly which ones. In other words, a variety of outcomes is possible, and therefore bank managers can never know exactly how much money the bank will have at any given moment in the future. However, the bankers can use the rules of probability and their past experience to make a reasonable estimation, and then use that estimation when making business decisions.

What Is "Probability"?

Probability is a mathematical expression of the likelihood of an event. The basis of probability is simple. The likelihood of any event is discussed in terms of all of the possible outcomes. To express the probability of a given event, x, you would count the number of possible outcomes, count the number of outcomes that give you what you want, and arrange them in a fraction, like this:

$$\text{Probability of } x = \frac{\text{number of outcomes that are } x}{\text{total number of possible outcomes}}$$

Not!
You can find the probability that something WILL NOT happen by subtracting the probability that it WILL happen from 1. For example, if the weatherperson tells you that there is a 0.3 probability of rain today, then there must be a 0.7 probability that it won't rain, because $1 - 0.3 = 0.7$.

Every probability is a fraction. The largest a probability can be is 1. A probability of 1 indicates total certainty. The smallest a probability can be is 0, meaning that it's something that cannot happen.

Single-Event Probability

Figuring out the probability of any single event is usually simple. When you flip a coin, there are only two possible outcomes, heads and tails. The probability of getting heads is therefore 1 out of 2, or $\frac{1}{2}$. When you roll a die, there are six possible outcomes, 1 through 6; the odds of getting a 6 are therefore $\frac{1}{6}$. The odds of getting an even result when rolling a die are $\frac{1}{2}$ since there are three even results in six possible outcomes.

> AND Probability = Multiply events
>
> OR Probability = Add events

Probability of Multiple Events

Some advanced probability questions require you to calculate the probability of more than one event. When calculating consecutive events that are dependent upon one another, multiply the individual probabilities together. When calculating the probability of events that are independent of one another, add the individual probabilities together.

Here's a typical example:

If a fair coin is flipped three times, what is the probability that the result will be tails exactly twice?

A. $\frac{1}{8}$

B. $\frac{1}{5}$

C. $\frac{3}{8}$

D. $\frac{5}{8}$

Here's How to Crack It

When the number of possibilities involved is small enough, the easiest and safest way to do a probability question like this is to write out all of the possibilities and count the ones that give you what you want. Here are all the possible outcomes of flipping a coin three times.

heads, heads, heads	tails, tails, tails
heads, heads, tails	tails, tails, heads
heads, tails, heads	tails, heads, tails
heads, tails, tails	tails, heads, heads

As you can see by counting, only three of the eight possible outcomes produce tails exactly twice. The chance of getting exactly two tails is therefore $\frac{3}{8}$. The correct answer is (C).

Sometimes, however, you'll be asked to calculate probabilities for multiple events when there are too many outcomes to write out easily.

Try this one.

A bag contains 7 blue pills and 14 red pills. What is the probability that the first three pills drawn at random from this bag will be blue?

A. $\dfrac{1}{3}$

B. $\dfrac{1}{9}$

C. $\dfrac{1}{21}$

D. $\dfrac{1}{38}$

Here's How to Crack It

Three random drawings from a bag of 21 pills produce a huge number of possible outcomes. It's not practical to write them all out. To calculate the likelihood of three events combined, you need to take advantage of a basic rule of probability.

In order to calculate the probability of a series of events, calculate the odds of each event happening separately and multiply them together. This is especially important in processes like drawings, because each event affects the odds of following events. This is how you'd calculate the probability of those three pill drawings.

The first drawing is just like the simple question you did earlier; there are 7 blue pills out of 21 total—a probability of $\dfrac{1}{3}$.

For the second drawing, the numbers are different. There are now 6 blue pills out of a total of 20, making the probability of drawing another blue pill $\dfrac{6}{20}$, or $\dfrac{3}{10}$.

For the third drawing, there are now 5 blue pills remaining out of a total of 19. The odds of getting a blue pill this time are $\dfrac{5}{19}$.

To calculate the odds of getting blue pills on the first three random drawings, just multiply these numbers together.

$$\frac{1}{3} \times \frac{3}{10} \times \frac{5}{19} = \frac{1}{38}$$

The odds of getting three blue marbles is therefore $\frac{1}{38}$, and the answer is (D). This can also be expressed as a decimal, as 0.026.

———————◯———————

Let's try a question!

———————◯———————

A pill bottle contains 4 Vitamin A pills, 12 Vitamin B pills, 6 Vitamin C pills, and 8 Vitamin D pills. What is the probability of randomly selecting either a Vitamin A or Vitamin D pill?

A. $\dfrac{8}{225}$

B. $\dfrac{8}{210}$

C. $\dfrac{178}{435}$

D. $\dfrac{3}{5}$

Here's How to Crack It

This question requires you to find the probability of selecting either a Vitamin A or Vitamin D pill when randomly selecting a single pill. Since we are unable to select both a Vitamin A and Vitamin D pill from a single selection, we must calculate the likelihood of selecting a Vitamin A pill *or* selecting a Vitamin D pill.

First, find that the total number of pills in the bottle is 4 + 12 + 6 + 8 = 30. Therefore, the probability of randomly selecting a Vitamin A pill is $\frac{4}{30} = \frac{2}{15}$ and the probability of randomly selecting a Vitamin D pill is $\frac{8}{30} = \frac{4}{15}$.

Finally, add the two mutually exclusive events together to find that the probability of randomly selecting either a Vitamin A or Vitamin D pill is $\frac{2}{15} + \frac{4}{15} = \frac{6}{15} = \frac{3}{5}$.

———————◯———————

Proportions

Unit conversion relates to proportional relationships; e.g., there are 12 inches in a foot, 3 feet in a yard, and 60 minutes in an hour. You will have to convert between units on the PCAT, especially in complex word problems. In essence, whenever you are converting between units, you are setting up a proportion. A proportion simply shows that two ratios are equal. The following are examples of some simple proportions:

$$\frac{10}{30} = \frac{1}{3} \qquad\qquad \frac{52}{4} = \frac{13}{2} \qquad\qquad \frac{2}{4} = \frac{1}{2}$$

In all of these examples, the quantity on the left is equal to the quantity on the right.

When converting between units, you can set up proportions in order to ensure that you use the proper units.

For example, let's say that you need to determine the amount of sodium, in milligrams, in 15 bottles of medicine, where each bottle contains 500 milligrams of sodium. Your proportion is going to use what you know to determine an unknown. Set up what you know:

$$\frac{1 \text{ bottle}}{500 \text{ milligrams}} \times \frac{15 \text{ bottles}}{x \text{ milligrams}}$$

Cross-multiply and divide:

$$x \text{ milligrams} = \frac{7{,}500 \text{ (bottles) (milligrams)}}{1 \text{ bottle}}$$

$$x \text{ milligrams} = 7{,}500 \text{ milligrams}$$

You will find that x milligrams = 7,500 milligrams.

Let's try a question!

Every 5 ml of CoughEZ cough syrup contains 80 mg of Guaifenesin. How many milliliters of CoughEZ cough syrup would be needed to obtain a dosage of 380mg of Guaifenesin?

A. 22.25
B. 23.75
C. 400
D. 6,080

Here's How to Crack It

This question asks you to find how many milliliters of CoughEZ cough syrup is needed to obtain a dosage of 380 mg of Guaifenesin. Set up what you know:

$$\frac{5 \text{ ml EZ}}{80 \text{ mg Guaifenasin}} = \frac{x \text{ ml EZ}}{380 \text{ mg Guaifenasin}}$$

Cross-multiply and divide:

$$\frac{1{,}900 \text{ ml EZ}}{80} = x \text{ ml EZ}$$

You will find that x ml EZ = 23.75 ml, or choice (B).

Let's try one more question!

If a tablet of Tquilz contains 250 milligrams of acetaminophen, and a bottle of Tquilz contains 40 tablets, how many grams of acetaminophen are in 12 bottles of Tquilz?

A.   12
B.   120
C.   12,000
D.   120,000

Here's How to Crack It

This question requires you to perform multiple operations, so break the question down into bite-sized pieces. First, you are told that a tablet of Tquilz contains 250 milligrams of acetaminophen and a bottle of Tquilz contains 40 tablets. Accordingly, set up what you know, and let's solve for the total number of milligrams of acetaminophen in a bottle of Tquilz.

$$\frac{1 \text{ tablet}}{250 \text{ milligrams}} = \frac{40 \text{ tablets}}{x \text{ milligrams}}$$

Cross-multiply and divide:

$$x \text{ milligrams} = \frac{(40 \text{ tablets})(250 \text{ milligrams})}{1 \text{ tablet}}$$

$$x \text{ milligrams} = 10,000 \text{ milligrams}$$

Therefore, there are 10,000 milligrams of acetaminophen in one bottle of Tquilz. Next, solve for the number of milligrams of acetaminophen in 12 bottles of Tquilz.

$$\frac{1 \text{ bottle}}{10,000 \text{ milligrams}} = \frac{12 \text{ bottles}}{y \text{ milligrams}}$$

Cross-multiply and divide:

$$y \text{ milligrams} = \frac{\left(12 \text{ bottles}\right)\left(10,000 \text{ milligrams}\right)}{1 \text{ bottle}}$$

$$y \text{ milligrams} = 120,000 \text{ milligrams}$$

Accordingly, there are 120,000 milligrams of acetaminophen in 12 bottles of Tquilz. Finally, the question asks you to provide the answer in grams, so you need to convert 120,000 milligrams to grams.

$$\frac{1 \text{ gram}}{1,000 \text{ milligrams}} = \frac{z \text{ grams}}{120,000 \text{ milligrams}}$$

Cross-multiply and divide:

$$\frac{\left(1 \text{ gram}\right)\left(120,000 \text{ milligrams}\right)}{1,000 \text{ milligrams}} = z \text{ grams}$$

$$120 \text{ grams} = z \text{ grams}.$$

Thus, the correct answer is (B).

Ratios

Ratios—another way to show the relationship between two quantities—can be expressed in numerous forms, such as "one cup of water for every four cups of vinegar," "a ratio of 1 to 4," or mathematically as either 1:4 or $\frac{1}{4}$. While $\frac{1}{4}$ looks like a fraction, this form relates part:part, not part:whole.

Ratios are always given in their most reduced form and you may be asked to use a ratio to calculate the actual values in a situation. In this case, use a **Ratio Box**.

- When using the Ratio Box, always add the ratio parts to find the ratio whole.

- All the ratio numbers are multiplied by the *same* factor to convert ratios to actual numbers; your job is to find the factor that connects a ratio number to the actual number.

Let's see how the Ratio Box works on a question!

Of the pharmacy's 84 prescriptions filled on Monday, the ratio of prescriptions filled for women to men was 5:7. What was the total number of prescriptions filled for men on Monday?

A. 7
B. 12
C. 35
D. 49

Here's How to Crack It

This question asks you to find the total number of prescriptions filled for men on Monday. First, fill in the information you know: the pharmacy filled 84 prescriptions on Monday. Accordingly, the *Actual Number* for the *Whole* is 84.

	Women	Men	Whole
Ratio			
Multiply By			
Actual Number			84

You are also told that the *Ratio* of prescriptions filled for *Women* to *Men* was 5:7; fill in the *Ratio* row for Men and Women.

	Women	Men	Whole
Ratio	5	7	
Multiply By			
Actual Number			84

Next, add together the ratio parts, *Men* and *Women*, to find the *Ratio Whole*: 5 + 7 = 12.

	Women	Men	Whole
Ratio	5	7	12
Multiply By			
Actual Number			84

Then, find the factor that links the *Ratio Whole* to the *Actual Whole*; $12 \times m = 84$ and $m = 7$. Therefore, the multiplier is 7 and the *Multiply By* row can be filled in accordingly.

	Women	Men	Whole
Ratio	5	7	12
Multiply By	7	7	7
Actual Number			84

Finally, multiply the *Ratio Women* and *Ratio Men* by the multiplier to find the *Actual Number* of *Women* and *Men*.

	Women	Men	Whole
Ratio	5	7	12
Multiply By	7	7	7
Actual Number	35	49	84

Accordingly, of the 84 prescriptions filled on Monday, 35 of them were for women and 49 of them were for men. Thus, the correct answer is (D).

If you have more parts to the whole than two, simply add an extra column. Let's try it out!

A certain drug contains one part glycerin to three parts water to four parts paracetamol. What is the total number of units of paracetamol dispensed in 72 pills?

A. 8
B. 9
C. 27
D. 36

Here's How to Crack It

This question asks you to find the total number of units of paracetamol dispensed in 72 pills. First, fill in the information you know: the ratio of glycerin to water to paracetamol is 1:3:4 and the total number of pills dispensed was 72.

	Glycerin	Water	Paracetamol	Whole
Ratio	1	3	4	
Multiply By				
Actual Number				72

Next, add together the ratio parts, *glycerin, water,* and *paracetamol,* to find the *Ratio Whole*: 1 + 3 + 4 = 8.

	Glycerin	Water	Paracetamol	Whole
Ratio	1	3	4	8
Multiply By				
Actual Number				72

Then, find the factor that links the *Ratio Whole* to the *Actual Whole*; $8 \times m = 72$ and $m = 9$. Therefore, the multiplier is 9 and the *Multiply By* row can be filled in accordingly.

	Glycerin	Water	Paracetamol	Whole
Ratio	1	3	4	8
Multiply By	9	9	9	9
Actual Number				72

Finally, multiply the *Ratios* of *glycerin, water,* and *paracetamol* by the multiplier to find the *Actual Numbers*

	Glycerin	Water	Paracetamol	Whole
Ratio	1	3	4	8
Multiply By	9	9	9	9
Actual Number	9	27	36	72

Accordingly, of the 72 pills filled, the total units of paracetamol dispensed was 36. The correct answer is 36, or choice (D).

Statistics

Statistics is a science of data. We all use data to estimate unknown quantities, to make decisions, and to develop and implement policies. To draw any sensible conclusions from collected data, we need to summarize the data or examine the patterns that it forms. The most commonly tested statistical measures are measures of central tendency and measures of variability.

Definitions

Here are some terms dealing with sets and statistics that appear on the PCAT. Make sure you're familiar with them. If the meaning of any of these vocabulary words keeps slipping your mind, add that word to your flash cards.

Mean	An average—also called an arithmetic mean.
Median	The middle value in a list of numbers when the numbers are arranged in order. When there is an even number of values in the list, the median is the average of the two middle values.
Mode	The value that occurs most often in a list.
Range	The result when you subtract the smallest value from the largest value in a list.
Standard Deviation	A measure of the variation of the values in a list.

Measures of Central Tendency

Measures of central tendency determine the central point of a variable or the point around which all the measurements are scattered. The three measures of central tendency are the mean, median, and mode.

Mean: The arithmetic mean (often called the **average**) is the most commonly used measure of the center of a set of data. The mean can be described as a data set's center of gravity, the point at which the whole group of data balances. Unlike the median, the mean is affected by extreme or outlier measurements. One very large or very small measurement can pull the mean up or down. We say that the mean is not resistant; it is not resistant to changes caused by outliers.

Median: The median is another commonly used measure of central tendency. The median is the point that divides the measurements in half. That is, half of the values are at or below the median, and half are at or above the median. The median is *not* affected by outliers. Therefore, for skewed data sets or data sets containing outliers, it's better to use the median rather than the mean to measure the center of the data. The median is resistant; it resists changes caused by outliers.

Note that if the data set contains an odd number of measurements, then the median belongs to the data set. But if the data set contains an even number of measurements, then the median may not belong to the data set. It is instead the mean of the middle two measurements. For example, if a data set contains five measurements, then the median is the third smallest (or third largest) measurement. But if the data set contains six measurements, then the median is the mean of the third smallest and the fourth smallest measurements.

Mode: The mode of a set is simply the value that occurs most often in that list.

Range is the difference between the largest and the smallest measurement in a data set.

Let's try a couple questions based on the following information!

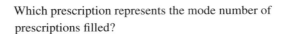

Prescriptions Dispensed on June 8, 2020		
Prescription Name	Number of Prescriptions Filled	Total Pills Dispersed
Lisinopril	15	675
Zithromax	8	720
Atorvastatin	12	960
Hydralazine	13	1,000
Verapamil	4	240

Which is the range of prescriptions filled?

A.   2
B.   11
C.   13
D.   15

Here's How to Crack It

This question requires you to find the range of prescriptions filled based on the data. The Range = Largest Measurement – Smallest Measurement, so the range of prescriptions filled is 15 – 4 = 11. The correct answer (B).

Which prescription represents the mode number of prescriptions filled?

A.   Lisinopril
B.   Atorvastatin
C.   Hydralazine
D.   Zithromax

Here's How to Crack It

This question requires you to identify the prescription that represents the mode number of prescriptions filled. Recall that the mode of the data is the value that occurs most frequently in a data set. Here we see that there were 15 prescriptions of Lisinopril dispensed, which is more than any other prescription, indicating that the correct answer is (A).

The average number of pills in a Verapamil prescription is how much greater than the average number of pills in a Lisinopril prescription?

A.   11
B.   15
C.   60
D.   435

Here's How to Crack It

This question requires you to identify the difference between the average number of pills in a Verapamil prescription and those in a Lisinopril prescription. Whenever you see the word *average*, remember to draw an average pie and fill in what you know. Here, you can draw two average pies, representing the Verapamil and Lisinopril prescriptions with the information provided in the table.

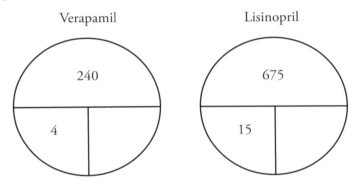

The table tells us that 4 prescriptions of Verapamil were filled with a total of 240 pills. Therefore, the average number of Verapamil pills filled is 240 ÷ 4 = 60. The table also tells us that 15 prescriptions of Lisinopril were filled with a total of 675 pills. Therefore, the average number of Lisinopril pills filled is 675 ÷ 15 = 45.

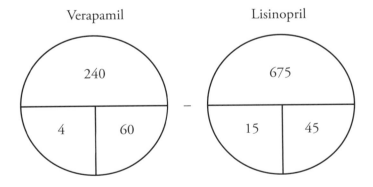

Finally, find the difference between the average number of pills to see that 60 − 45 = 15. Thus, the correct answer is (B).

Standard Deviation

The **standard deviation** of a set is a measure of the set's variation from its mean. A set composed of 10 identical values (having a range of 0) could have the same mean as a set with widely scattered values. The first list would have a much smaller standard deviation than the second. Remember that the standard deviation is a measure of how far the typical value in a set is from the set's average. The bigger the standard deviation, the more widely dispersed the values are. The smaller the standard deviation, the more closely grouped the values in a set are around the mean.

Let's try a question!

Which of the followings sets of data has the greatest standard deviation?

A. (−500, 0, 500}
B. {−10, 0, 10, 20}
C. {0, 1, 2, 3, 4, 5}
D. {1000,1010,1020,1030}

Here's How to Crack It

This question requires you to identify the set that has the greatest standard deviation. Remember that the more widely dispersed the numbers in a set are, the greater the standard deviation is. Accordingly, the standard deviation of choice (A) is 500, choice (B) is 10, choice (C) is 1, and choice (D) is 10. Thus, the correct answer is (A).

Let's try one more question!

A pharmacist fills orders for 5 different individuals who receive 1, 4, 10, 13, and 7 prescriptions, respectively. If the pharmacist then adds 2 prescriptions to each order, how much greater is the new median number of prescriptions per order than the standard deviation of the original 5 orders?

A. 1
B. 4
C. 6
D. 9

Here's How to Crack It

This question requires you to first identify two key pieces of information: the standard deviation of the original five orders and the median number of prescriptions per order *after* the pharmacist adds 2 prescriptions to each order. Recall that the standard deviation is the spread between numbers; here, the constant difference between the numbers, and thus the standard deviation of the original five orders is 3.

Next, you need to find the median number of prescriptions per order *after* the pharmacist adds 2 prescriptions to each order. First, add 2 prescriptions to each of the original orders to find the new list is 3, 6, 12, 15, 9. Order the list and identify the middle number, or the median. The ordered list is 3, 6, 9, 12, 15 and the median is 9.

Finally, find the difference between the new median and the standard deviation. You will see that 9 − 3 = 6, so the answer is (C).

Charts and Graphs

In an attempt to make the PCAT better reflect what students learn and people need to understand in the real world, they use Charts and Graphs to present data for test-takers to analyze. The situations will typically include real-life applications, such as finance and business situations, social science issues, and, of course, scientific matter.

Always read the titles of all graphs, look for a key if there is one, and notice the units before answering any questions. Let's take a look at some of the charts and graphs you will encounter on the PCAT!

Bar Graphs

A **bar graph** is another way to represent data. Instead of providing points, each value for the variable at the bottom of the graph is represented by a bar. The height of the bar corresponds to a value on the left side of the graph. If the bars in a graph represent ranges of data, rather than distinct categories, the graph is a **histogram**. Regardless of whether you are dealing with a bar graph or a histogram, always read the title, key or legend, variables, and units before tackling the questions. And, remember, use POE to your advantage!

The bar graph below shows the number of men and women assigned to each experimental group.

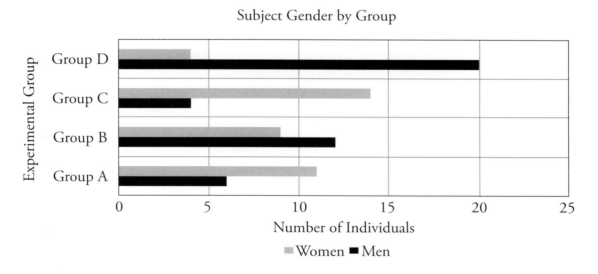

Let's try a couple questions based on this data.

According to the data in the bar graph provided, the probability of randomly selecting a female subject from Group D is

A. $\dfrac{1}{6}$

B. $\dfrac{1}{5}$

C. $\dfrac{1}{4}$

D. $\dfrac{11}{17}$

Here's How to Crack It

This question requires you to find the probability of randomly selecting a female subject from Group D. Recall that probability is $\dfrac{What\ you\ want}{Total}$. Here, we want a female subject from Group D, and there are 4 female subjects and 24 total subjects in Group D. Thus, the probability of randomly selecting a female subject from Group D is $\dfrac{4}{24} = \dfrac{1}{6}$, or choice (A).

Let's try one more!

Approximately what percent of the total number of men in all experimental groups are in Groups A and B?

A. 43
B. 47
C. 57
D. 53

Here's How to Crack It

When working with percentages, translate the English words to their math equivalents. Recall that *what* is represented by the variable (*x, y, z*), *percent* is represented by $\overline{100}$, *of* is represented by $\times$, and *is, are, were, did,* or *does* is represented by =. Use the data in the graph to find that the total number of men in all experimental groups is equal to 20 + 4 + 12 + 6 = 42 and the number of men in Groups A and B is equal to 6 + 12 = 18. Put the equation together to find $\dfrac{x}{100} \times 42 = 18$, $42x = 1,800$, and $x = 42.85$. 42.85 is approximately 43, so the correct answer is (A).

Scatterplot Graph

In a **scatterplot**, each dot represents one data point. Sometimes, a **trend line** or curve "of best fit" will be drawn to represent the equation that most closely matches the data. Read the titles of all graphs, look for a key if there is one, and notice the units before answering any questions.

The scatterplot below shows the weekly earnings for 22 selected pharmacists at HappyDrugs Inc. during a one-week period in June of 2020.

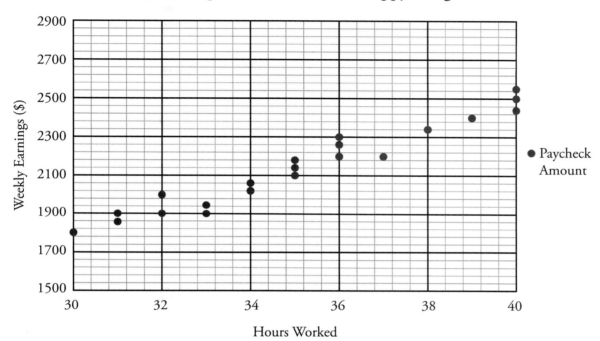

Weekly Earnings for Pharmacists at Happy Drugs Inc.

When working with a scatterplot in which the trend line is not provided, identify the trend line; this will help with many questions that require you to predict a given trend.

Let's try a couple questions based on this data.

According to the scatterplot above, which of the following is closest to the average weekly earnings for the pharmacists working 32 hours or fewer at HappyDrugs Inc. during the one-week period in question?

A. $1,800
B. $1,850
C. $1,900
D. $1,950

Here's How to Crack It

Here, the question asks you to find the average weekly earnings for pharmacists working. We've already tackled averages, so identify the information you need and set up your average pie. There are 5 pharmacists working 32 hours or fewer and their total earnings equals $1,800 + $1,850 + $1,900 + $1,900 + $2,000 = $9,450. Fill in your average pie accordingly.

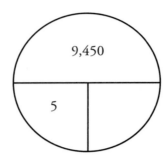

In order to find the average weekly earnings, divide the total earnings by the five pharmacists; $9,450 ÷ 5 = $1,890. Since the question asks you to find the closest to the weekly average, the best option is $1,900, or choice (C).

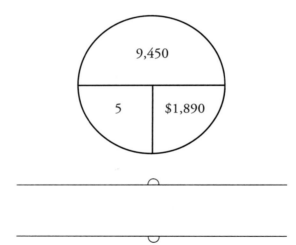

Let's try one more!

If the trend in the relationship between the number of hours worked and weekly earnings remains consistent with the data provided for employees who worked fewer than 30 hours a week during the week in question, then which of the following would most likely be the weekly earnings of a pharmacist who worked 28 hours that week?

A. $1,550
B. $1,600
C. $1,650
D. $1,700

Here's How to Crack It

Let's take a look at the scatterplot and identify the trend line. This scatterplot exhibits a direct relationship between hours worked and weekly earnings; draw in the trend line accordingly.

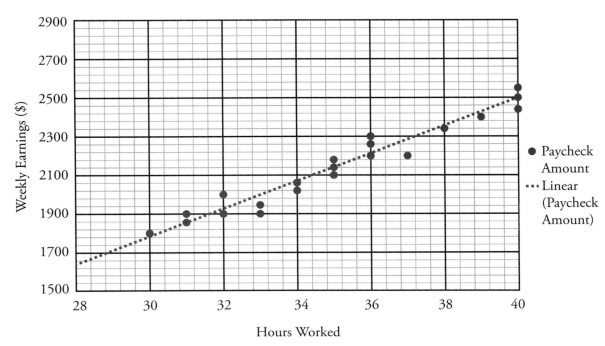

Now, the question asks you to identify the most likely weekly earnings of a pharmacist who worked 28 hours in a given week. Continue the trend of best fit beyond the axes initially provided. Extend both your *x*-axis to mark the 28 hour work period and the trend line to find that the most likely weekly earnings of a pharmacist who worked 28 hours a week would be $1,650.

Box-and-Whisker Plots

Another method of data display is the **box-and-whisker plot**, which presents information from a **five-number summary**—(1) the minimum value, (2) the lower quartile, (3) the median value, (4) the upper quartile, and (5) the maximum value—of the data set. Depicting the five-number summary graphically is particularly useful for determining whether the distribution is skewed and whether there are any **outliers**, or unusual observations that skew the data, in a data set.

As an example, let's construct a box-and-whisker plot from a data set concerning the number of grams of sodium utilized by a given lab for the month of August. Imagine that we were given the following data set that includes 31 data points, all in grams: 65, 62, 60, 64, 70, 71, 68, 65, 72, 73, 67, 62, 61, 62, 59, 43, 56, 60, 62, 63, 65, 70, 70, 71, 69, 81, 68, 65, 74, 75, 70. Based on this data, a box plot like the following could be created.

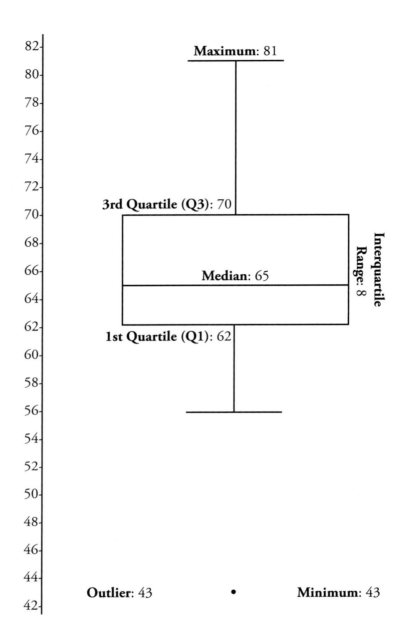

You'll notice that there are a bunch of labels on this box-and-whisker plot that reflect the five-number summary referred to previously. So, how did we get these numbers and what do they mean? Let's start with the basics.

The **minimum** value shown in a box plot is equal to the data point with the least value in a data set. In our data set, the fewest grams of sodium disbursed was 43 grams and, therefore, is the minimum. Conversely, the **maximum** value shown in a box plot is equal to the data point with the greatest value in a data set. In our data set, the greatest number of grams of sodium disbursed was 81 and is therefore the maximum. The **median** value shown in the box plot is the middle value of an ordered data set. When we order the 31 data points, the median of our data set is 65 grams, as shown as follows: 43, 56, 59, 60, 60, 61, 62, 62, 62, 62, 63, 64, 65, 65, 65, **65**, 67, 68, 68, 69, 70, 70, 70, 70, 71, 71, 72, 73, 74, 75, 81.

618 | For more free content, visit PrincetonReview.com

Now let's discuss quartiles and the interquartile range. **Quartiles** divide a data set into four equal parts. You will notice in the box plot that the there is a box that stretches from the 1st Quartile (Q1) to the 3rd Quartile (Q3). Q1 is the median value in the first half of an ordered data set, Q2 is the median value of the data set, and Q3 is the median value of the second half of an ordered data set. The **interquartile range** is the difference between Q3 and Q1 and represents the middle 50% of the data. In our data set, the middle 50% of data points occurs between 62 grams and 70 grams, so our interquartile range is 8.

Extending out from the box are **whiskers**. The bottom whisker extends from the bottom of the box to the smallest non-outlier in the data set, while the top whisker extends from the top of the box to the largest non-outlier in the data set. Notice that in this box plot, the first whisker extends from Q1, 62, to the point 56. However, we have an **outlier** in our data set, the data point representing 43 grams, which is a data point more than 1.5 interquartile ranges away from either Q1 or Q3. Since the value of our interquartile range is 8, and Q1 is at 62, any value below 50 would be considered an outlier.

Let's try a question based on the box-and-whisker plot above!

What is the range of the data set?

A. 8
B. 19
C. 25
D. 38

Here's How to Crack It

This question asks you to identify the range of the data. The range of a data set can be found by using the following formula: *Range* = Largest Measurement − Smallest Measurement. Accordingly, the range of this data set is *Range* = 81 − 43 = 38, or choice (D).

You may also be asked to determine how data is distributed in a box plot. This is one place where box plots shine: they depict the spread of data quite effectively. Note that box plots can be drawn either horizontally or vertically. Here, we've shown the box plots and distributions horizontally so that you are familiar with both styles.

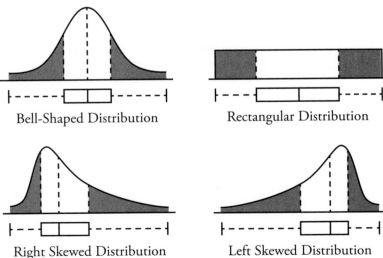

Bell-Shaped Distribution

Rectangular Distribution

Right Skewed Distribution

Left Skewed Distribution

13.3

Once your data is graphed in a box-and-whisker plot, you can interpret the boxplot and figure out all sorts of fun facts regarding the variability and the spread of data.

Let's see how we can tackle some questions using a box plot.

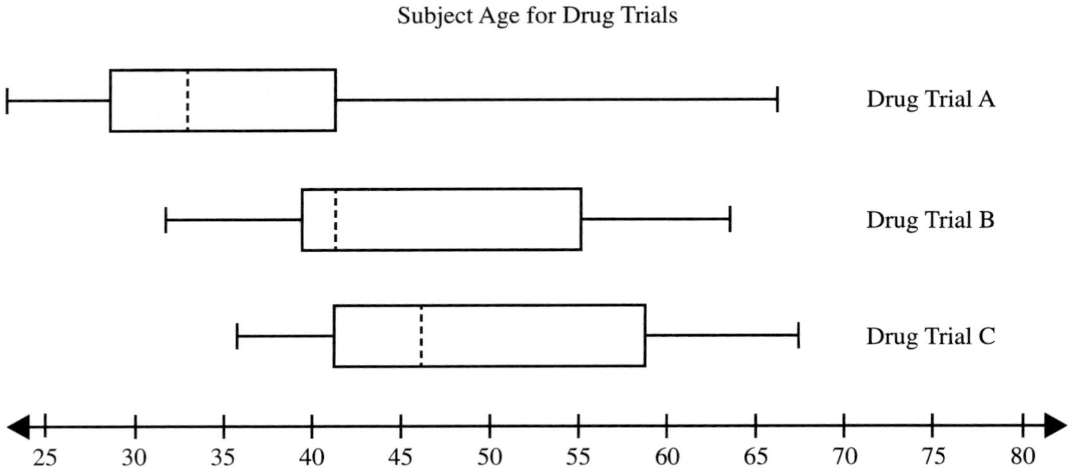

Subject Age for Drug Trials

Based on the box-and-whisker plot above, the drug trial that has the greatest standard deviation among subject age is

A. Drug A
B. Drug B
C. Drug C
D. Information cannot be determined

Here's How to Crack It

This question requires you to analyze the three drug trials in order to determine the drug trial that has the greatest standard deviation among subject age. Remember that a high standard deviation leads to greater data spread from the median, while a low standard deviation leads to data clustering around the median. Accordingly, the drug trial with the greatest standard deviation is Drug Trial A, or choice (A).

Let's try one more question!

Based on the box-and-whisker plot above, the median age of participants in Drug Trial C is approximately how much greater than the median age of participants in Drug Trial A?

A. 5
B. 8
C. 13
D. 30

Here's How to Crack It

Here you need to identify the median age of the participants in both Drug Trials A and C and calculate the difference. Recall that the median is the line within the box in your graph. Accordingly, the median age of participants in Drug Trial A is approximately 33 and the median age of participants in Drug Trial C is approximately 46. Therefore, the median age of participants in Drug Trial C is approximately 13 years greater than the median age of participants in Drug Trial A; 46 – 33 = 13. The correct answer is (C).

PROBABILITY, RATIOS, PROPORTIONS, AND STATISTICS DRILL

1. John buys a house with a mortgage. The mortgage interest rates for a period of five months are listed in the table below.

Mortgage Interest Rate	
Months	Interest Rate (%)
September	4.68
October	4.85
November	5.16
December	4.46
January	4.39

What was the median mortgage interest rate, in percent, for the five-month period?

A. 4.680
B. 4.708
C. 4.775
D. 5.160

2. The median of the following set of data is 63.

39 41 48 52 x $x+2$ 72 78 84 95

What is the value of x ?

A. 61
B. 62
C. 63
D. 64

3. The following data shows the scores of 12 students in a class test.

14, 15, 11, 13, 13, 15, 15, 14, 12, 13, 14, 15

Which statement about the distribution of the above data is true?

A. The distribution is not skewed as Median = Mode.
B. The distribution is positively skewed as Mean < Median < Mode.
C. The distribution is symmetric as Mean = Median = Mode
D. The distribution is negatively skewed as Mean < Median < Mode.

4. The spinner shown in the picture below decides the cost of the ticket for a game.

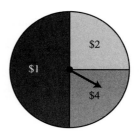

What is the expected value of the ticket to play this game?

A. $1.00
B. $2.00
C. $2.75
D. $3.50

5. Out of 50 pills in a bag, 25 are blue, 15 are yellow, and 10 are white. What is the probability of randomly selecting a white pill or a yellow pill?

A. $\dfrac{1}{10}$

B. $\dfrac{1}{5}$

C. $\dfrac{3}{10}$

D. $\dfrac{1}{2}$

6. The table below lists the following Vax4You vaccines:

Vax4You Vaccines	
Vaccine	Number of Doses Available
PusBGone	12
NoMoreMoles	11
AnxietyAway	7

Three vaccines are randomly picked from the Vax4You inventory without replacement. What is the probability of selecting a PusBGone, an AnxietyAway, and another PusBGone vaccine in order?

A. $\dfrac{33}{1,015}$

B. $\dfrac{14}{375}$

C. $\dfrac{11}{290}$

D. $\dfrac{6}{145}$

7. The graph below shows the rough breakup of the average annual expenditure of a person.

Expenditure

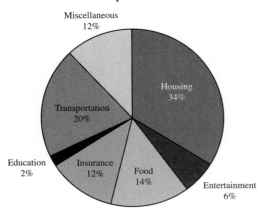

The actual annual amount spent on housing by the person is $11,900. How much does the person roughly spend on food each year?

A. $ 350
B. $1,666
C. $4,046
D. $4,900

8. The mean, median, and mode of the data given below is x.

74, 27, 48, 17, 69, x, 44, 72, 33

What is the value of x?

A. 44
B. 46
C. 48
D. 57

9. The table shows the sales of television sets in a store in a two-week period.

	Sun	Mon	Tue	Wed	Thur	Fri	Sat
Week 1	24	22	19	14	29	34	12
Week 2	26	10	24	27	19	18	23

Which statement **correctly** compares the two data sets?

A. The mean and standard deviation are both higher in Week 1.
B. The mean and standard deviation are both higher in Week 2.
C. The mean is higher in Week 1, but the standard deviation is higher in Week 2.
D. The mean is higher in Week 2, but the standard deviation is higher in Week 1.

10. A survey was conducted on the time spent assessing patients by a group a physician assistants. The physician assistants were divided into four different age groups and four random members were chosen from each group. The table below shows the results of the survey.

Group	Time (minutes)
Group A	40, 60, 120, 45, 50
Group B	50, 55, 60, 60, 40
Group C	75, 60, 45, 50, 55
Group D	60, 70, 120, 100, 80

Which group has the **greatest** standard deviation?

A. Group A
B. Group B
C. Group C
D. Group D

11. The graph below shows the weights (in pounds) of 10 crates of tomatoes.

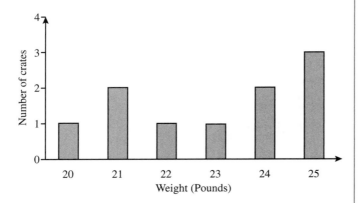

What is the mean weight of the crates of tomatoes?

A. 22.5 lb
B. 23 lb
C. 23.5 lb
D. 25 lb

12. The shelf life of a particular type of cookie is normally distributed with a mean of 20 days and a standard deviation of 2.5 days. What is the probability that the product lasts between 20 to 25 days?

A. 0.340
B. 0.475
C. 0.500
D. 0.680

13. The number of passengers using the city bus service over a week is shown in the table below.

Passengers	Frequency
0–4	2
5–9	4
10–14	10
15–19	16
20–24	11
25–29	7

What is the mean number of passengers per trip?

A. 8.3
B. 15.1
C. 17.1
D. 19.1

14. The following table shows the parking times logged by a car in a parking lot over 6 days.

Day	Time (min)
1	17
2	23
3	35
4	25
5	11
6	33

What is the standard deviation of the data to the nearest tenth?

A. 2.6
B. 7.0
C. 8.4
D. 20.5

Want More Practice?
Register your book online for more drill questions!

Answers and Explanations

1. **A** Arrange the data from the smallest to the largest, 4.39, 4.46, 4.68, 4.85, and 5.16. Hence, the median of the data is the middle value. The answer is choice (A).

2. **B** The number of data is 10, which is even, so the median of the set of data is the average of the middle two values: $\dfrac{x + x + 2}{2} = 63$. The answer is choice (B).

3. **D** In a negatively skewed distribution, the mean is less than the median and the median is less than the mode. The answer is (D).

4. **B** Calculate the average value as $\dfrac{1}{2}(1) + \dfrac{1}{4}(2) + \dfrac{1}{4}(4) = 2$. The answer is choice (B).

5. **D** Find the probability of selecting either a yellow or white pill on a single draw. Since there are 15 yellow pills and 10 white pills, the probability can be calculated as $P(x) = \dfrac{15}{50} + \dfrac{10}{50} = \dfrac{1}{2}$. The answer is choice (D).

6. **C** This question is testing AND probability, so you need to find the probability of choosing a PusBGone vaccine, followed by an AnxietyAway vaccine, followed by another PusBGone vaccine in order. Calculate the probability as $\dfrac{12}{30} \times \dfrac{7}{29} \times \dfrac{11}{28}$. Simplify the fractions to get $\dfrac{1}{5} \times \dfrac{1}{29} \times \dfrac{11}{2}$. The answer is choice (C).

7. **D** If 11,900 is 34%, then $\dfrac{11,900}{34}$ is 1%. Multiply that by 14 to find the cost of the food. Calculate the value as $14 \times \dfrac{11,900}{34} = 4,900$. The answer is choice (D).

8. **C** Arranging the data in ascending order shows that x could be any number between 44 and 48. As x is the mode and the numbers 44 and 48 are already there in the list, the possibilities are narrowed down to either 44 or 48. Finally, find that the average of the given numbers is 48. Hence, the value of x is 48. The answer is choice (C).

9. **A** Calculate the mean of Week 1 as 22 and the mean of Week 2 as 21 and the standard deviation of Week 1 as 7.27 and the standard deviation of Week 2 as 5.45. The answer is choice (A).

10. **A** Recall that the more dispersed the values in a set, the greater the standard deviation of that set. As the data values of Group A are widely spread, this group has the greatest standard deviation. The answer is choice (A).

11. **B** Calculate the mean as $\bar{x} = \dfrac{20(1) + 21(2) + 22(1) + 23(1) + 24(2) + 25(3)}{10} = 23$. The answer is choice (B).

12. **B** Calculate the probability as

$$P\left(20 \le x \le 25\right) = P\left(20 \le x \le 22.5\right) + P\left(22.5 \le x \le 25\right) = 0.340 + 0.135 = 0.475.$$

The answer is choice (B).

13. **C** The midpoints of the classes are 2, 7, 12, 17, 22, 27. So, the mean is

$$\text{mean} = \frac{2(2) + 7(4) + 12(10) + 17(16) + 22(11) + 27(7)}{50}$$
$$= \frac{4 + 28 + 120 + 272 + 242 + 189}{50} = 17.1$$

The answer is choice (C).

14. **C** The mean of the given data is 24. Hence, the standard deviation of the data is

$$\sqrt{\frac{(17-24)^2 + (23-24)^2 + (35-24)^2 + (25-24)^2 + (11-24)^2 + (33-24)^2}{6}}$$
$$= \sqrt{\frac{49 + 1 + 121 + 1 + 169 + 81}{6}} = \sqrt{70.3} \approx 8.4$$

The answer is choice (C).

13.4 PRECALCULUS

Introduction

In this section we'll review topics such as functions, graphs, polynomial equations, logarithms, and trigonometry, which are commonly tested on the PCAT. We will assume that you're comfortable with the laws of exponents and radicals as well as with basic arithmetic operations involving real numbers, complex numbers, and general algebraic expressions.

Functions

Functions constitute a very important notion in mathematics, and the definition of a function becomes increasingly sophisticated as your mathematical education progresses. Basically, a **function** is a rule that assigns to each element of one set (the **domain**) exactly one element of another set (the **range**). You can think of a function as a machine: you put raw materials into a machine and the machine will provide you with a finished product. For functions, you will put in an x-value and the result will be the corresponding y-value. The y-value is usually referred to as $f(x)$. Keep in mind that the f in $f(x)$ is not a variable, but simply the name of the function.

Let's try a few questions!

1. If $f(x) = x^3 + 3x - 3$, what is the value of $f(2)$?

   A. 7
   B. 9
   C. 11
   D. 14

Here's How to Crack It

In order to evaluate this function, you need to replace the x-values with 2. Accordingly, $f(2) = 2^3 + 3(2) - 3$, $f(2) = 8 + 6 - 3$, and $f(2) = 11$. Thus, the correct answer is (C).

Let's try another question!

13.4

2. The function z is define by $z(x) = 14x - 6$. If $6 \times z(p) = 132$, what is the value of p ?

    A. 2
    B. 4
    C. 22
    D. 28

Here's How to Crack It

There is a lot happening here, so break the question down into bite-sized pieces. First, you are told that $6 \times z(p) = 132$, so solve for $z(p)$: $z(p) = 132/6$, and $z(p) = 22$. Next, you can tackle the function by substituting 22 for $z(p)$: $22 = 14x - 6$. Finally, solve for p: $14p = 28$ and $p = 2$. Thus, the correct answer is (A).

You may also be asked to identify an x-value that can be put into a function in order to obtain a certain y-value. These questions may ask you to identify x-values that fall within a certain range.

Let's take a look at a question that exemplifies this concept!

3. If $f(x) = \left(\dfrac{1}{x}\right)^4$, what is one possible value for x for which $\dfrac{1}{625} < f(x) < \dfrac{1}{81}$?

    A. 2
    B. 3
    C. 4
    D. 5

Here's How to Crack It

This question requires you to find the x-value for the function that will yield a result between the given extremes $\dfrac{1}{625}$ and $\dfrac{1}{81}$. You can utilize the PITA technique we discussed earlier and plug in the answer choices to the function to find the correct answer. If you start with (B), you will find that $f(3) = \left(\dfrac{1}{3}\right)^4$ and $f(3) = \dfrac{1}{81}$; since this is the lower end of our inequality, we need a greater value and can eliminate both choices (A) and (B). If we plug in 4 to the function, we will find that $f(4) = \left(\dfrac{1}{4}\right)^4$ and $f(4) = \dfrac{1}{256}$; since $\dfrac{1}{625} < \dfrac{1}{256} < \dfrac{1}{81}$ is a true statement, the correct answer is (C).

You can also evaluate functions graphically by using a process similar to the one you use for evaluating functions numerically. Let's take a look at a couple questions that exemplify this concept!

Questions 4 and 5 are based upon the graph of $k(x)$, shown below.

13.4

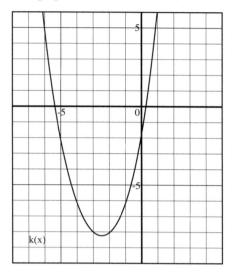

4. In the graph of $k(x)$, what is the value of $k(-5)$?

    A. −5.75
    B. −2
    C. −0.75
    D. 0

Here's How to Crack It

This question requires you to evaluate the value of $k(-5)$, given the graph of $k(x)$. Since you are given the input value, $x = -5$, your goal is to find the associated output value, or y-value, of the function. Based on the graph of $k(x)$, $k(-5) = -2$, as shown in the following graph. Thus, the correct answer is (B).

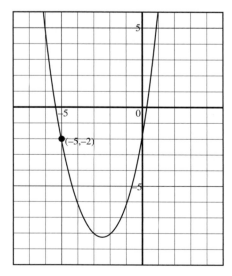

5. In the graph of $k(x)$, if $k(x) = -8.25$, what is the value of x ?

    A.   −5
    B.   −2.5
    C.   0
    D.   15

Here's How to Crack It

Like the previous question, you are asked to find a value based upon the graph of $k(x)$. However, here you are given the output value, $k(x) = -8.25$, and you need to find the associated input value, or x-value, of the function. Based on the graph of $k(x)$, when the graph has a y-value of −8.25, it has an x-value of −2.5, and the correct answer is (B).

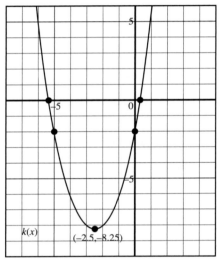

A major difference between functions and equations is that each input is related to exactly one output in a function. Note that each input must relate to a single output, but multiple inputs can result in a single output. Furthermore, unlike the method used to write equations, function notation provides more flexibility; rather than using "$y =$" for every equation, you can effectively and efficiently use informative, descriptive variables.

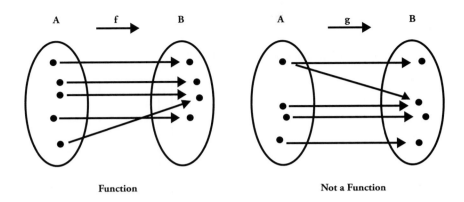

Function   **Not a Function**

> In order to be a function, each input (*x*-value) must correspond to only one output (*y*-value).

One way to visually assess whether or not you are dealing with a function is through the **vertical line test**. If you were to draw a vertical line through any part of a given graph and the vertical line does not intersect with the graph at more than one point, you are dealing with a function. If your vertical line passes through more than one point on a graph, you are not dealing with a function.

For example, if we were to look at the following graph of $x = y^2$, and draw a vertical line at $x = 2$, we would see that the vertical line passes through two *x*-values. Here, when $x = 2$, $y = 1.414$ and $y = -1.414$. Therefore, $x = y^2$ is not a function.

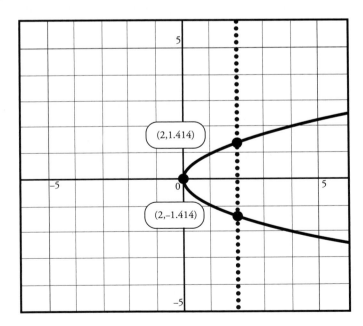

Based on this information, let's take a look at a couple questions and see if we can identify functions!

13.4

6. All of the following are functions EXCEPT:

A.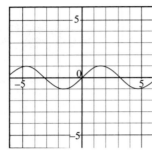

B.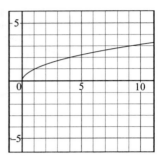

C.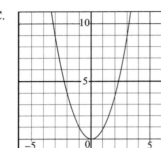

D.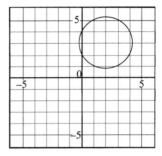

Here's How to Crack It

Use the vertical line test on each graph in order to determine the number of y-values associated with each x-value. All of the graphs pass the vertical line test except for the graph of the circle, or choice (D).

7. Which of the following relations is NOT a function?

A.

x	y
2	1
4	2
6	3
8	4
10	5

B.

x	y
1	1
2	2
3	1
4	2
5	1

C.

x	y
2	3
4	6
6	9
2	12
10	15

D.

x	y
1	10
3	6
6	9
8	7
10	8

Here's How to Crack It

This question is concerned with the definition of a function, a relation in which each input is related to exactly one output. In the first set shown in (A), each x-value is related to a single y-value; $2\rightarrow 1$, $4\rightarrow 2$, $6\rightarrow 3$, $8\rightarrow 4$, and $10\rightarrow 5$. Therefore, (A) is a function and can be eliminated.

In the second set shown in (B), each x-value is related to a single y-value; $1\rightarrow 1$, $2\rightarrow 2$, $3\rightarrow 1$, $4\rightarrow 2$, and $5\rightarrow 1$. Keep in mind that, while each input must relate to a single output, more than one input can relate to a single output; thus, (B) is a function and can be eliminated.

In the third set shown in (C), the input value of 2 is related to output values of 3 and 12; $2\rightarrow 3$ and $2\rightarrow 12$. Since a single input is related to more than one output, (C) is not a function and should be kept.

In the final set shown in (D), each x-value is related to a single y-value; $1\rightarrow 10$, $3\rightarrow 6$, $6\rightarrow 9$, $8\rightarrow 7$, and $10\rightarrow 8$. Therefore, (D) is a function and can be eliminated. Thus, all of the sets are functions except for (C), which is the answer.

Domain, Range, and Interval Notation

You will also encounter questions that ask you to determine the domain and range of a function. In a function, the set of input values, or x-values, is known as the **domain**. The set of output elements, or y-values, is known as the **range**. When determining the domains and ranges of a function, we must consider what is mathematically sound. For example, we cannot include any values in the domain that would cause us to divide by zero or take the root of a negative number.

Often the domain and range of a function will be written using interval notation. An interval is a set of real numbers between, and at times including, two numbers. Consider the following examples that express the domain of a function using interval notation:

Interval from *a* to *b*	
Notation	Meaning
[*a*, *b*]	$a < x < b$
(*a*, *b*)	$a < x < b$
[*a*, *b*)	$a < x < b$
(*a*, *b*]	$a < x < b$

Interval from −4 to 3	
Notation	Meaning
[−4, 3]	$-4 < x < 3$
(−4, 3)	$-4 < x < 3$
[−4, 3)	$-4 < x < 3$
(−4, 3]	$-4 < x < 3$

The use of brackets ([ ]) in interval notation indicates that the value of the endpoint is included in the interval; graphically, the endpoints will be filled circles. Conversely, the use of parentheses (( )) in interval notation indicates that the value of the endpoint is not included in the interval; graphically, the endpoints will be unfilled circles.

Consider the graph of $g(x)$, below. In this function, the least x-value is −4 and the greatest x-value is 3. Therefore, the domain of $g(x)$ includes all real numbers between −4 and 3, including both −4 and 3, and is written in interval notation as [−4, 3]. You can also use interval notation to express the range, or all possible y-values, of a function.

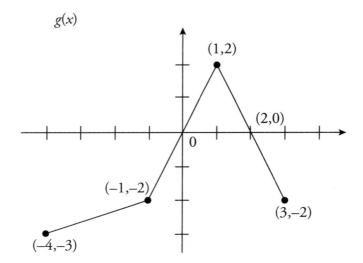

But what if the function is discontinuous at various points? How would it be represented in interval notation? To express a domain that is true over multiple intervals, you use the **union symbol: ∪**. To understand how this works, let's take a look at the graph of $m(x)$ below.

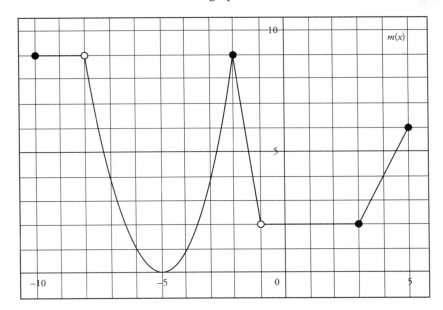

Based on the graph, you can determine that $m(x)$ is has x-values that range from $x = -10$ to $x = -8$, where $x = -8$ is not included in the domain. Therefore, you would express this interval as $[-10, -8)$. Then find the next interval, which exists from $x = -8$ to $x = -2$; again, $x = -8$ is not included. Thus, this interval is expressed as $(-8, -2]$. Repeat the process for the next interval, which goes from $x = -2$ to $x = -1$, where -1 is not included. This interval is expressed as $[-2, -1)$. Finally, find the last interval, which goes from $x = -1$ to $x = 5$, where $x = -1$ is not included. This interval is expressed as $(-1, 5]$. Now, you need to join all of the intervals together with the union symbol to express the domain of $m(x)$. Therefore, the domain of $m(x)$ is $[-10, -8) \cup (-8, -2] \cup [-2, -1) \cup (-1, 5]$.

But what if the function goes on forever? Is that even possible? Of course it is! In these instances, the domain and range can be expressed as going from negative infinity to positive infinity.

Interval from $-\infty$ to ∞	
Notation	Meaning
$(-\infty, \infty)$	$-\infty < x < \infty$

Notice that the infinity sign is not associated with brackets. Since the infinity symbol does not represent a specific number, it will always be accompanied by parentheses.

13.4

Consider the linear function $f(x) = x + 6$:

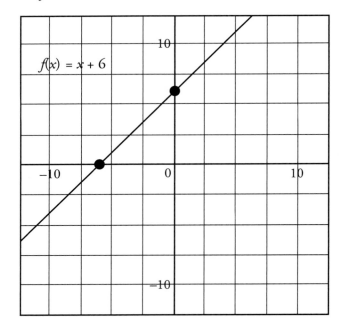

$f(x) = x + 6$

Unlike the previous graphs, $g(x)$ and $m(x)$, the graph of $f(x)$ doesn't have any endpoints. No worries—you can still define the domain and range of $f(x)$ using the infinity sign (∞) in your interval notation to represent intervals that extend indefinitely in one or both directions. Since the function $f(x) = x + 6$ extends infinitely in both directions, across all x- and y-values, both the domain and range of $f(x)$ would be represented by the interval $(-\infty, \infty)$.

Let's tackle some more questions and make sure we understand this material!

Let's try a couple questions that focus on finding the domain and range and expressing it in interval notation.

Questions 8 and 9 are based upon the following graph of $g(x)$.

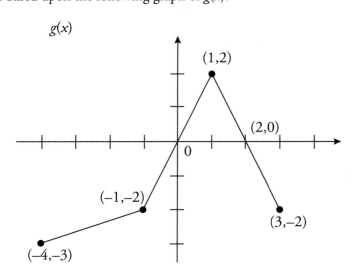

8. What is the domain of $g(x)$?

    A. [–4, 3]
    B. (–4, 3]
    C. (–3, 2]
    D. (–4, 1]

Here's How to Crack It

Recall that the domain of a function is equal to all of the possible x-values of the function. Since $g(x)$ has x-values that range from –4 to 3, but point (–4, –3) has an unfilled endpoint and is therefore not included in the domain, the domain of $g(x)$ is (–4, 3] and the correct answer is (B).

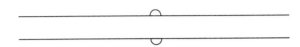

9. What is the range of $g(x)$?

    A. (–4, 3]
    B. [–3, –2]
    C. (–3, 2]
    D. [–3, 2]

Here's How to Crack It

In the graph of $g(x)$, the lowest y–value is –3, which occurs at point (–4, –3), and the greatest y value is 2, which occurs at point (1, 2). Point (3, –2) has a filled endpoint and will be included in the range, but since point (–4, –3) has an unfilled endpoint, it will not be included in the range. Therefore, the function $g(x)$ has a range of (–3, 2] and the correct answer is (C).

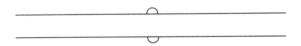

10. What is the domain of the function $b(x) = \dfrac{x+1}{-x+3}$?

    A. $(-\infty, -3) \cup (-3, \infty)$
    B. $[-\infty, -3) \cup (-3, \infty]$
    C. $(-\infty, 3) \cup (3, \infty)$
    D. $[-\infty, 3) \cup (3, \infty]$

Here's How to Crack It

You may not always be given a graph when finding the domain of a function. Recall that the domain of a function is equal to all of the possible x-values of the function, and we can include only x-values that do not force the denominator to be zero. Accordingly, set the denominator equal to zero and solve for x; $-x + 3 = 0$ and $x = 3$. Therefore, we must exclude 3 from the domain, but include all other real numbers where $x > 3$ or $x < 3$. Thus, the domain of $b(x)$ is $(-\infty, 3) \cup (3, \infty)$, and the correct answer is (C).

13.4

11. What is the domain of the function $f(x) = \sqrt{x+6}$?

    A. $(-\infty, -6]$
    B. $[-6, \infty)$
    C. $(\infty, -6]$
    D. $[6, \infty)$

Here's How to Crack It

If you are faced with a function that has an even root in the formula, you want to exclude any numbers that will result in the square root of a negative number, as this would be imaginary. Here, you will set the radicand greater than or equal to zero and solve for x: $x + 6 \geq 0$ and $x \geq -6$. Accordingly, the domain will exclude any number less than -6 from the domain. Thus, the domain is $[-6, \infty)$, or choice (B).

12. What is the range of the function $f(x) = \sqrt{x+6}$?

    A. $(-\infty, \infty]$
    B. $(-\infty, 0]$
    C. $[0, \infty)$
    D. $[-6, \infty)$

Here's How to Crack It

We just tackled the domain of this function, so now we need to find the range, or all possible y-values of the function. Since we know that $f(-6) = 0$, and the function value increases as x increases to infinity, we can conclude that the range of $f(x) = \sqrt{x+6}$ is $[0, \infty)$. The correct answer is (C).

Zeros of a Function

Functions can be graphed just like equations. When graphed, the horizontal axis of a function represents the domain, and the vertical axis of a function represents the range. In the same way that a linear equation is an equation for a straight line, a linear function will also lead to a graph of a straight line. Take a look at the following examples:

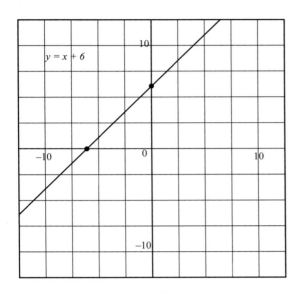

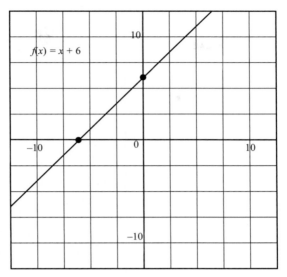

The graph on the left is a linear equation, while the graph on the right is a linear function that we had looked at previously. So, what's the difference? Not much! Both of these graphs are equivalent and represent straight lines. Furthermore, in the same way that you are able to find the x- and y-intercepts of an equation, you can find the find x- and y-intercepts of a function. In fact, the process for finding intercepts in functions is extremely similar to the process you use for equations.

For example, imagine that you need to find the y-intercept of the function above, $f(x) = x + 6$. Simply set $x = 0$ and solve: $f(0) = 0 + 6 = 6$. Thus, the y-intercept of $f(x) = x + 6$ is the point $(0, 6)$, which is shown on the graph above.

You may also need to find the zeroes of a function, which are similar to the x-intercepts found in equations; a **zero of a function** is an x-value that makes the function equal to zero. Likewise, in order to find the zeros of $f(x) = x + 6$, simply set $f(x) = 0$ and solve: $f(x) = x + 6$, $0 = x + 6$, and $x = -6$. The zeros of $f(x) = x + 6$ is the point $(-6, 0)$, which is also shown on the previous graph.

Let's try a question that tackles the zeros of a function!

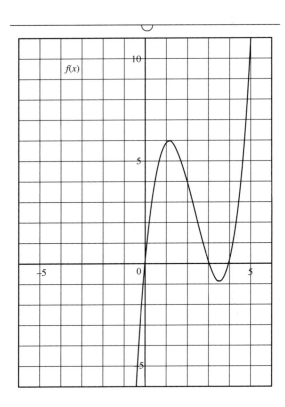

13. The graph of $f(x)$ is shown above. Which of the following accurately represents the function $f(x)$?

    A. $f(x) = x(x + 3)(x + 4)$
    B. $f(x) = x(x - 3)(x + 4)$
    C. $f(x) = x(x + 3)(x - 4)$
    D. $f(x) = x(x - 3)(x - 4)$

Here's How to Crack It

Every time the graph of $f(x)$ crosses the x-axis, there is an x-intercept of the function, or a zero of the function, at that point. Based on the graph, the function $f(x)$ goes through points (0, 0), (0, 3), and (0, 4), and, therefore, must have three x factors. Since the function crosses the x-axis at (3, 0) and (4, 0), we need a function formula that has the factors $(x - 3)$ and $(x - 4)$. Therefore, $f(x) = x(x - 3)(x - 4)$, and the correct answer is (D).

If you don't remember how the zeros of a function are represented in factored form, you can use Plugging In. Since the graph of $f(x)$ includes the points (0, 0), (3, 0), and (4, 0), we would expect $f(x) = 0$ when we set $x = 0$, 3, or 4. If you set $x = 3$, the output for (A) is 126, the output for (B) is 0, the output for (C) is −18, and the output for (D) is 0; eliminate (A) and (D). If you set $x = 4$, the output for (B) is 32 and the output for (C) is 0; eliminate (B). Therefore, the only choice that gives $f(x) = 0$ when we set $x = 0$, 3, or 4, is (D).

Quadratic Functions

We previously discussed quadratic equations—equations with a degree of 2 that are written in standard form as $ax^2 + bx + c = 0$. Quadratic equations are used to find the specific value of a variable and, therefore, are always equal to a number. A quadratic equation may be factored in the form $(x + m)(x + n)$, which allows us to determine that the roots, zeros, or solutions, of the quadratic equation are $x = -m$ or $x = -n$.

Now, we are going to expand upon our knowledge of quadratics by discussing the purpose and characteristics of quadratic functions. Unlike quadratic equations, **quadratic functions** are written in standard form as $f(x) = ax^2 + bx + c$ and are always set equal to $f(x)$ or y. A quadratic function is the algebraic representation of the path of a **parabola**, the symmetrical curve produced by a quadratic equation. The main difference between quadratic equations and quadratic functions is that a quadratic function is set equal to $f(x)$, or y, which means that you are not solving for a single value. Rather, a function allows you to determine the output for a number of inputs, where the output is dependent upon the input.

Unlike quadratic equations, which could have complex solutions, or solutions that include imaginary numbers, you may need to determine the number of real solutions a quadratic function has by finding the **discriminant**, or the value of $b^2 - 4ac$.

- If the discriminant is positive, the quadratic function will have two real solutions.
- If the discriminant is zero, the quadratic function will have one real solution.
- If the discriminant is negative, the quadratic function will have two complex solutions, or solutions that include the imaginary number i.

Let's take a look at a scenario in which quadratic functions could be helpful!

Imagine that you have decided to sell vitamins. Being the entrepreneur that you are, you would like to know how much profit you can expect to make after a certain period of time. Your amazing accountant tells you that the profit you will make can be found using the function $p(x) = -0.005x^2 + 20x - 400$, which accounts for the number of vitamins sold, the amount earned in sales, and the costs of running your business. Using this information, you can find your profit for any number of vitamins sold, and you can view the graph of your projected profit, as shown on the graph on the following page:

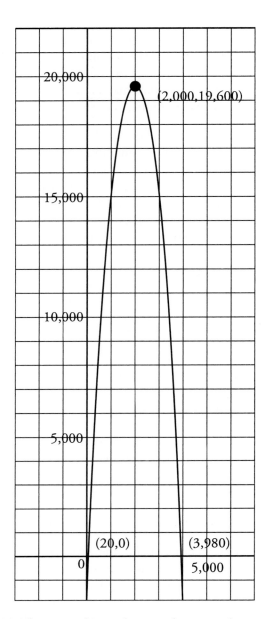

Using the function $p(x) = -0.005x^2 + 20x - 400$ and its graph we can determine the profit of your business for all prices of vitamins. First, let's find out how many real solutions this function has by calculating the discriminant, or $b^2 - 4ac$; $400 - 4(.005)(-400) = 400 - 8 = 392$. Thus, this function has two real solutions, which represent the bounds of profit for your vitamin company.

Based on the graph, we can see that your profit would be 0 at $p(20)$ and $p(3,980)$, or a sale price of \$20 and \$3,980. Conversely, you would achieve a maximum profit of \$19,600 at $p(2,000)$, which, due to the symmetrical nature of parabolas, can be found when x is halfway between the zeros: $(20 + 3,980)/2 = 2,000$. Furthermore, we can also find your profit for any sale price in between—which is the real power of functions.

So, let's analyze a quadratic function and discuss some key features that you may be asked about on the PCAT. Let's consider the function $f(x) = x^2 - 5x + 6$. First, let's graph the function by creating a table of inputs and outputs for the function:

$f(x) = x^2 - 5x + 6$	
Input (x)	Output $f(x)$
0	6
1	2
2	0
3	0
4	2

You can now graph the function in the coordinate plane:

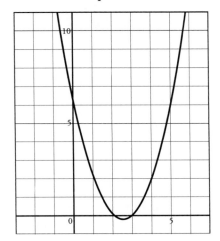

You can also find the x- and y-intercepts of the quadratic. To find the x-intercepts, or zeros, of the quadratic, set $x^2 - 5x + 6$ equal to zero and factor. Based on the rules for factoring quadratics in the standard form $x^2 - 5x + 6$, if the value of the c-term is positive and the value of the b-term is negative, the factors m and n, whose product is c, will both be negative. The only factors of the c-term, 6, that add up to the b term, -5, are -2 and -3. Accordingly, we can factor the quadratic as follows: $x^2 - 5x + 6 = (x - 2)(x - 3)$. Therefore, the zeros of $f(x) = x^2 - 5x + 6$ occur at $x = 2$ and $x = 3$.

Next, you can find the y-intercept of the function by setting $x = 0$ and solving for $f(x)$ in $f(x) = x^2 - 5x + 6$. Therefore, $f(x) = 0 - 0 + 6$ and $f(x) = 6$. Accordingly, the y-intercept of the graph is $(0, 6)$.

13.4

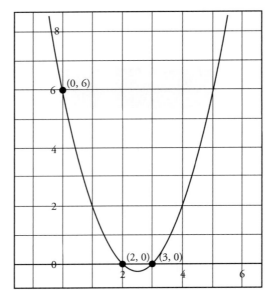

You will also need to know how to find the vertex and axis of symmetry of a quadratic function. Both the vertex and axis of symmetry are found by using portions of the quadratic formula. Let's refresh our memory and review these concepts.

- The quadratic formula is $x = \dfrac{-b \pm \sqrt{b^2 - 4ac}}{2a}$
- The vertex (h, k) for any quadratic $ax^2 + bx + c$ can be determined with $(h, k) = \left(-\dfrac{b}{2a}, \dfrac{4ac - b^2}{4a} \right)$
- The axis of symmetry for any quadratic $ax^2 + bx + c$ can be determined with $x = -\dfrac{b}{2a}$

Now that we've reviewed these concepts, let's find the vertex of our quadratic function $f(x) = x^2 - 5x + 6$, where $a = 1$, $b = -5$, and $c = 6$. Solve to find:

$$(h, k) = \left(-\frac{b}{2a}, \frac{4ac - b^2}{4a} \right)$$

$$(h, k) = \left(-\frac{-5}{2(1)}, \frac{4(1)(6) - (-5)^2}{4(1)} \right)$$

$$(h, k) = (-\frac{-5}{2}, \frac{24 - 25}{4})$$

$$(h, k) = (\frac{5}{2}, \frac{-1}{4}) \text{ or } (2.5, -0.25)$$

Accordingly, the vertex of $f(x) = x^2 - 5x + 6$ is (2.5, −0.25)

Now let's find the axis of symmetry, which is determined with $x = -\frac{b}{2a}$. Note that you had already solved

for the axis of symmetry when finding the h-value of the vertex; $x = -\frac{b}{2a} = 2.5$. Accordingly, the axis of symmetry is found at $x = 2.5$.

You will also be asked to find the minimum or the maximum of a quadratic function, which is closely related to both the vertex and the axis of symmetry.

Given a quadratic function in standard form, $f(x) = ax^2 + bx + c$:

- If $a > 0$, the function will have a minimum value at $x = -\frac{b}{2a}$

- If $a < 0$, the function will have a maximum value at $x = -\frac{b}{2a}$

Let's take a look at our function now. In our function, $f(x) = x^2 - 5x + 6$; since $a > 0$ and $x = -\frac{b}{2a} = 2.5$, the minimum value occurs at $x = 2.5$.

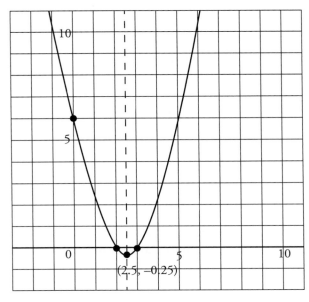

(2.5, −0.25)

Let's bring in some of the functions concepts we discussed earlier, domain and range, and discuss how we can determine those with a quadratic function. Looking at the graph of $f(x) = x^2 - 5x + 6$, the function continues to both the left and right indefinitely. Therefore, the domain would be expressed in interval notation as $(-\infty, \infty)$.

Now look at the possible y-values for the function and determine the range. The minimum y-value occurs at -0.25, and the graph continues upward indefinitely. Thus, the range of the function would be expressed in interval notation as $[-0.25, \infty)$.

Phew! That was a lot of information! Let's tackle a question that deals with all of the new knowledge that we've gained!

Questions 13 and 14 are based upon the function $f(x) = 4x\left(\dfrac{x+1}{2}\right) - 72$.

14. Use the discriminant to determine the number of real solutions in the function $f(x) = 4x\left(\dfrac{x+1}{2}\right) - 72$. If real solutions exist, find the zeros of the function.

   A. $x = -9$ and $x = -8$
   B. $x = -8$ and $x = 9$
   C. $x = -9$ and $x = 8$
   D. $x = 9$ and $x = 8$

Here's How to Crack It

Recall that the discriminant of a function in standard form, $f(x) = ax^2 + bx + c$, is equal to $b^2 - 4ac$. The function we are given, however, is not in standard form, so we must expand the function and put it into standard form as follows:

$$f(x) = 4x\left(\frac{x+1}{4}\right) - 72$$

$$f(x) = \frac{4x^2 + 4x}{4} - 72$$

$$f(x) = \frac{4x^2}{4} + \frac{4x}{4} - 72$$

$$f(x) = x^2 + x - 72$$

Accordingly, $a = 1$, $b = 1$, and $c = -72$, and we can plug these values into the discriminant $b^2 - 4ac$ to find that $b^2 - 4ac = 1 - 4(1)(-72) = 1 + 288 = 289$. Since the value of the discriminant is positive, we know the quadratic function has two real solutions.

Since the function has two real solutions, we can now find the zeros of the function by factoring the quadratic. Recall that when factoring quadratics in the form $ax^2 + bx + c = (x + m)(x + n)$, where m and n are factors of ac and $m + n = b$, if the value of c is negative and the value of b is positive, m and n will have opposite signs, and the larger factor will be positive. In the case of our function, which is written as $f(x) = x^2 + x - 72$ in standard form, the only factors that fit the conditions necessary are $f(x) = x^2 + x - 72 = (x + 9)(x - 8)$. Therefore, the zeros of the function $f(x) = x^2 + x - 72$ occur at $(-9, 0)$ and $(8, 0)$, and the correct answer is (C).

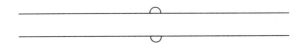

15. Identify the vertex and minimum value of the function

$$f(x) = 4x\left(\frac{x+1}{2}\right) - 72.$$

    A. $(h, k) = (-0.5, 72.75)$ and $x = -0.5$
    B. $(h, k) = (-0.5, 72.75)$ and $x = 0.5$
    C. $(h, k) = (0.5, -72.75)$ and $x = -0.5$
    D. $(h, k) = (0.5, 72.75)$ and $x = 0.5$

Here's How to Crack It

Start by using the information you found in the previous question to represent the function in standard form: $f(x) = x^2 + x - 72$. Next, recall that the vertex (h, k) for any quadratic function $ax^2 + bx + c$ can be determined with $(h, k) = (-\frac{b}{2a}, \frac{4ac - b^2}{4a})$. In this function, $a = 1$, $b = 1$, and $c = -72$. Plug these values into the vertex formula to find that

$$(h, k) = (-\frac{b}{2a}, \frac{4ac - b^2}{4a})$$

$$(h, k) = (-\frac{1}{2(1)}, \frac{4(1)(-72) - (1)^2}{4(1)})$$

$$(h, k) = (-\frac{1}{2}, \frac{-288 - 1}{4})$$

$$(h, k) = (-\frac{1}{2}, \frac{-289}{4})$$

$$(h, k) = (-0.5, 72.75)$$

Therefore, the vertex of the function $f(x) = 4x\left(\frac{x+1}{2}\right) - 72$ is $(h, k) = (-0.5, 72.75)$, and you can eliminate choices (C) and (D).

Next, let's find the minimum value of the function; recall that the minimum of a function occurs at $x = -\dfrac{b}{2a}$. Accordingly, the minimum of this function occurs at $x = -\dfrac{b}{2a} = -\dfrac{1}{2}$ or -0.5. Therefore, the minimum value of the function occurs at $x = -0.5$, and the correct answer is (A).

Manipulating Functions

We've now covered a whole bunch of information related to functions, but we haven't discussed function manipulation. Let's consider the graph of the most basic quadratic function, $f(x) = x^2$:

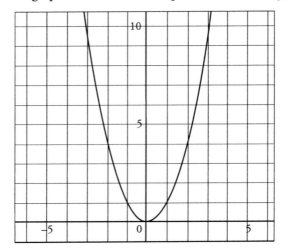

While we've looked at and graphed many functions by this point, each one of them has been a transformation of the function $f(x) = x^2$. A **transformation** is the result of changing the shape or scale of a point, line, or shape. Often, textbooks will refer to the original graph as the **pre-image** and the transformed graph as the **image**. Let's take a look at three types of transformations: **vertical** and **horizontal translations**, **reflections**, and **vertical** and **horizontal scaling**.

Since you're basically a function guru at this point, you know that the standard form of a quadratic function is $f(x) = ax^2 + bx + c$. The values of the constants play a huge role in how a function is graphed. Consider again the most basic function, $f(x) = x^2$. Here, the value of $a = 1$, $b = 0$, and $c = 0$.

But what would happen if you altered the value of the constant, which we will represent as k from here forward? If you change the value of k, the image will experience horizontal or vertical shifts that change the location, but not the size, of the figure. So how does the value of k hold so much power? Take a look at the following examples.

Consider our original function, $f(x) = x^2$, and a second function, $f(x) = x^2 + 2$, in which $a = 1$, $b = 0$, and $k = 2$. Here, the function experiences a vertical shift *up* by 2:

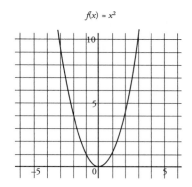

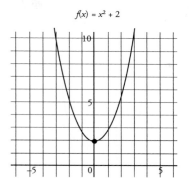

Conversely, if $k = -2$, the function $f(x) = x^2$ becomes $f(x) = x^2 - 2$, and the function will experience a vertical shift *down* by 2.

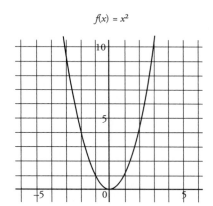

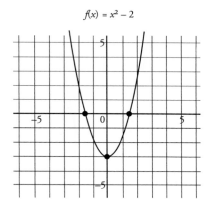

Regardless of the function, if the k-term is not equal to zero, you will have a vertical translation that has a resulting graph with the same x-coordinates, but different y-coordinates.

Given the function $f(x) = x^2 + k$:

If $k > 0$, the function shifts upward by k units.

If $k < 0$, the function shifts downward by k units.

But that's not the only transformation possible! Let's again consider the vertex form of the quadratic function $f(x) = (x - h)^2 + k$. If the value of h is grouped with the x-term, the resulting graph will be shifted either left or right. For example, the function $f(x) = (x + 2)^2$ would result in a shift of two units to the left, while the function $f(x) = (x - 2)^2$ would result in a shift of two units to the right.

$f(x) = x^2$

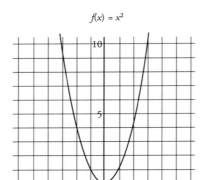

$f(x) = (x + 2)^2$

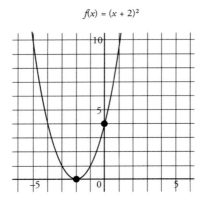

$f(x) = x^2$

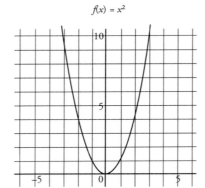

$f(x) = (x - 2)^2$

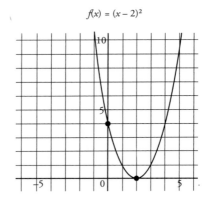

Given the function $f(x) = (x + h)^2$:

If $h > 0$, the function shifts to the left by h units.

If $h < 0$, the function shifts to the right by h units.

Let's try a couple questions that deal with function translations!

16. If $f(x) = x^2 + 6$ and $s(x) = f(x) - 2$, which of the following graphs represents $s(x)$?

A.
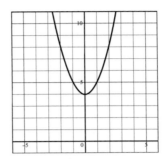

B.
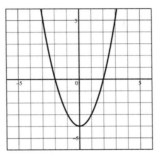

C.
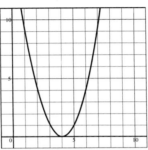

D.
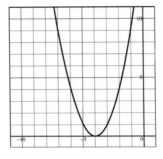

Here's How to Crack It

First, we have to find the value of $s(x)$, given $f(x)$. If $f(x) = x^2 + 6$ and $s(x) = f(x) - 2$, then $s(x) = x^2 + 6 - 2$ and $s(x) = x^2 + 4$. Recall that if you are given the function $f(x) = x^2 + k$, and $k > 0$, the function shifts upward by k units. In the function $s(x) = x^2 + 4$, $k = 4$, which means that the graph of x^2 is shifted upward by four units. Accordingly, the correct answer is (A).

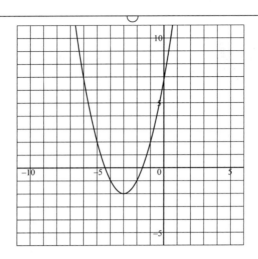

17. Which of the following expressions represents the graph of $g(x)$ above?

    A. $g(x) = (x + 3)^2 - 2$
    B. $g(x) = (x - 3)^2 - 2$
    C. $g(x) = (x + 2)^2 - 3$
    D. $g(x) = (x + 3)^2 + 2$

Here's How to Crack It

In order to identify the accurate representation of this function, recall that if you are given a function $f(x) = (x + h)^2$ that the function shifts to the left by h units if $h > 0$ and the function shifts to the right by h units if $h < 0$. Since our vertex shifts three units to the left, $h < 0$, and $h = -3$. If $h = -3$, the first part of our expression will be $(h + 3)^2$. Thus, the first part of our function will be $g(x) = (x + 3)^2$. Eliminate choices (B) and (C). Next, recall that if you are given the function $f(x) = x^2 + k$, the function shifts upward by k unit if $k > 0$ and the function shifts downward by k units if $k < 0$. Here, our graph is shifted downward by 2 units, so $k = -2$. Therefore, $g(x) = (x + 3)^2 - 2$, and the correct answer is (A).

A **reflection** is a graph that results from flipping the original graph over the x- or y-axis. The function $f(x) = x^2$ reflected across the x-axis as $-f(x)$ results in the following graphs:

$f(x) = x^2$ $-f(x)$

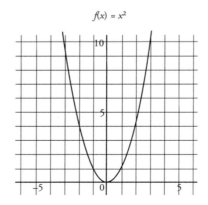
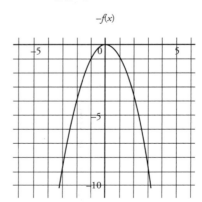

Now, here's where it gets a little crazy. If we were to then reflect the graph of $-f(x)$ about the x-axis, the resulting graph would be the original graph of $f(x)$; a reflection of a reflection is the original image.

Given the function $f(x) = x^2$, the image of $f(-x)$ would be identical to the pre-image when reflected over the y-axis, due to the symmetrical nature of the parabola and its location on the y-axis.

Let's take a look at a reflection about the y-axis. Consider the following graph of $h(x) = x^3 + 4$ and its reflection about the y-axis, $h(-x)$.

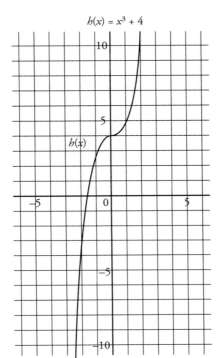

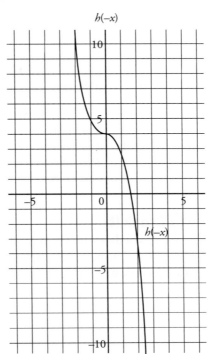

> $-f(x)$ reflects $f(x)$ about the x-axis.
>
> $f(-x)$ reflects $f(x)$ about the y-axis.

The fact that $f(x) = f(-x)$ is no small thing. In fact, you may encounter questions that ask you to determine whether a function is even or odd. But what does that mean? Whenever you have a function where $f(x) = f(-x)$, the function is considered even; this means that the function is symmetrical about the y-axis. If you find that $f(x) = -f(x)$, the function is considered odd. And if neither $f(x) = f(-x)$ nor $f(x) = -f(x)$, the function is considered neither even nor odd.

> For any function $f(x)$, if $f(x) = f(-x)$, the function is **even**.
>
> For any function $f(x)$, if $f(x) = -f(x)$, the function is **odd**.
>
> If neither $f(x) = f(-x)$ nor $f(x) = -f(x)$, the function is considered neither even nor odd.

Let's try a couple questions that deal with function reflections and odd and even functions!

18. Given the function $z(x) = 4x^2 + 3$, which of the following is true?

    A. The function is even.
    B. The function is odd.
    C. The function is neither even nor odd.
    D. There is not enough information to determine.

Here's How to Crack It

In order to determine whether a function is even, odd, or neither, plug in $-x$ to the function, $z(x) = 4x^2 + 3$. Therefore, $z(-x) = 4(-x)^2 + 3$ and $z(-x) = 4x^2 + 3$. That's all there is to it! Since $z(x) = z(-x)$, the function $z(x)$ is even, and the correct answer is (A).

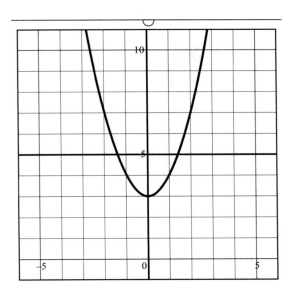

19. The graph above shows the function $f(x) = x^2 + 3$. Which of the following graphs represents $r(x) = f(-x) + 1$?

A.

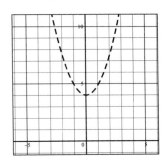

B.

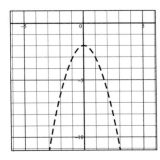

C.

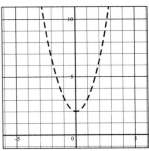

D.

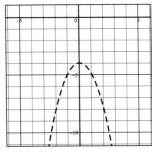

Here's How to Crack It

In order to find the graph of $r(x) = f(-x) + 1$, we need to tackle each part of the function. First, recall that $f(-x)$ reflects $f(x)$ about the y-axis. Accordingly, if we were to reflect $f(x) = x^2 + 3$ about the y-axis, due to the symmetry of parabolas, we would end up with an identical graph as the original. Since there is no reflection about the x-axis, eliminate choices (B) and (D). Next, let's tackle the k value of our function. Since $r(x) = f(-x) + 1$, we must account for a vertical shift of one unit upward; eliminate choice (C) since it shows a vertical shift of one unit downward. Accordingly, the graph that represents $r(x)$ is (A).

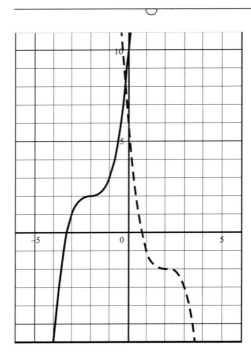

20. The graph above shows the functions $p(x) = (x + 2)^3 + 2$ and $q(x)$, represented as a solid and dashed line, respectively. Which of the following functions could represent $q(x)$?

    A. $q(x) = (x + 2)^3 + 2$
    B. $q(x) = (x + 2)^3 - 2$
    C. $q(x) = -(x - 2)^3 + 2$
    D. $q(x) = -(x - 2)^3 - 2$

Here's How to Crack It

There's a lot happening in this question, so break it into bite-sized pieces. Rather than trying to develop the function yourself, use POE on the answer choices to determine which equation matches $q(x)$. First, let's take a look at choice (A), which states that $q(x) = (x + 2)^3 + 2$; this function indicates that $q(x)$ would be identical to $p(x)$, but with a vertical shift of $k = 2$ units upward. In the graph of $q(x)$ provided, there is a reflection about the x-axis, so we can eliminate choice (A). Let's take a look at choice (B), which states that $q(x) = (x + 2)^3 - 2$; as with choice (A), this function indicates that $q(x)$ would be identical to $p(x)$, but with a vertical shift of $k = 2$ units downward. Eliminate choice (B). Choice (C) states that $q(x) = -(x - 2)^3 + 2$. Without getting too caught up in the minutia, note that the negative preceding the $(x - 2)^3$ indicates a reflection of the function $p(x)$ about the x-axis, which is evident in the provided graph. However, the k-value here of $k = 2$ would indicate a vertical shift of 2 units upward. The graph of $q(x)$ indicates a vertical shift downward, so eliminate choice (C). Thus, the correct answer is (D), $q(x) = -(x - 2)^3 - 2$, in which the original function $p(x)$ is reflected over the x-axis, shifted four units to the right, and shifted two units downward.

So far, we've transformed functions in a way that preserves the size of the image, but you can also transform a function by altering the **scale** of an image by stretching or compressing a figure.

You can resize transformations by changing the value of a in the function $f(x) = ax^2 + bx + c$. When the value of $a > 1$, the image will have a vertical stretch in the y-direction, appearing taller and thinner than the pre-image. Conversely, if $0 < a < 1$, the image will have a vertical compression in the y-direction, appearing shorter and wider than the pre-image. In short, the value of a determines the stretching or shrinking of an image. Take a look at how this works in the following graphs:

13.4

$\frac{1}{2}f(x)$ $f(x) = x^2$ $2f(x)$

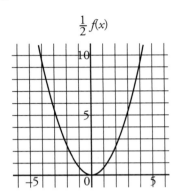 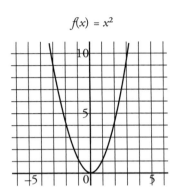 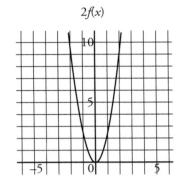

You can also stretch or compress the scale of an image by changing the value of b within the argument of any function $f(bx) = y$. If $b > 1$, the image will have a horizontal compression in the x-direction, appearing taller and thinner than the original function. On the other hand, if $0 < b < 1$, the image will have a horizontal stretch in the x-direction, appearing shorter and wider than the pre-image.

$f(\frac{1}{2}x)$ $f(x) = x^2$ $f(2x)$

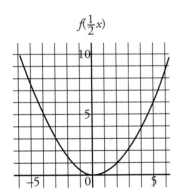 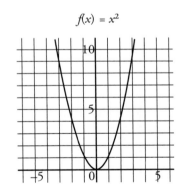 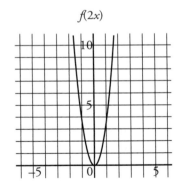

Now let's try a question that deals with horizontal and vertical scaling!

13.4

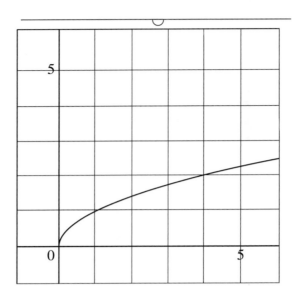

21. The graph above depicts the function $f(x) = \sqrt{x}$. Which of the following graphs depicts the function $f(-8x)$?

A.

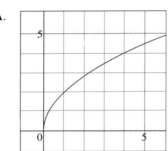

B.

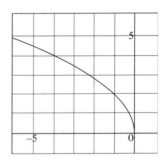

C.

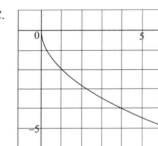

D.

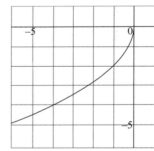

Here's How to Crack It

Here, we are provided a graph of the function $f(x) = \sqrt{x}$ and we need to identify the graph that depicts function $f(-4x)$. Two things are changing in our original graph when we look for $f(-4x)$. First, we are introducing a negative sign within the argument of the function, and we are changing the scale of the function. Recall that introducing a negative within a function's argument will cause the original function to be reflected about the y-axis. Accordingly, eliminate both choices (A), and (C), as they represent a reflection about the x-axis.

Awesome! Now you know how to manipulate functions in multiple ways. Just as a quick review, let's look at all our rules one last time.

$$af[b(x + c) + d$$

- a affects both up-down orientation and vertical stretching and shrinking
  - $|a| > 1$ stretches image
  - $|a| < 1$ shrinks image
  - If a is negative, the graph is reflected across the x-axis
- b affects horizontal stretching and shrinking
  - $|b| > 1$ shrinks image
  - $|b| < 1$ stretches image
  - If b is negative, the graph is reflected across the y-axis
- c affects horizontal shifts
  - $c > 0$ shifts image to the left
  - $c < 0$ shifts image to the right
- d affects vertical shifts
  - $d > 0$ shifts image upward
  - $d < 0$ shift image downward

Composite Functions

Function composition is the application of one function to the result of another function. So, for any function $f(g(x))$, sometimes written as $(f \circ g)(x)$, the result of $g(x)$ becomes the input for the function $f(x)$.

Let's look at an example:

Given the functions $f(x) = x^2 + 4x + 6$ and $g(x) = 2x^3 - 4$, what is the value of $(f \circ g)(2)$?

First, let's rewrite the function $(f \circ g)(2)$ as $f(g(2))$.

Next, let's solve for $g(2)$:

$g(x) = 2(2)^3 - 4$
$g(x) = 2(8) - 4$
$g(x) = 16 - 4$
$g(x) = 12$

Now that we know the value of $g(2) = 12$, we can solve for $f(12)$:

$f(x) = x^2 + 4x + 6$
$f(12) = (12)^2 + 4(12) + 6$
$f(12) = 144 + 48 + 6$
$f(12) = 198$

Thus, the value of $(f \circ g)(2) = 198$. That's all there is to it!

There are three steps for solving composite functions:

1) If written as $(f \circ g)(x)$, rewrite as $(f(g(x))$.

2) Replace each occurrence of x in $f(x)$ with the value of $g(x)$.

3) Simplify and solve.

Let's try a couple practice questions out!

---

22. Given the functions $p(x) = x^3 - 5x + 1$ and $q(x) = -2x^2 + 45$, what is the value of $(p \circ q)(-5)$?

    A.   126
    B.   101
    C.   −99
    D.   −101

Here's How to Crack It

First, let's rewrite the function $(p \circ q)(-5)$ as $p(q(-5))$. Next, let's solve for $q(-5)$:

$$q(x) = -2x^2 + 45$$
$$q(-5) = -2(-5)^2 + 45$$
$$q(-5) = -2(25) + 45$$
$$q(-5) = -50 + 45$$
$$q(-5) = -5$$

Now that we know the value of $q(-5) = -5$, we can solve for $p(-5)$:

$$p(x) = x^3 - 5x + 1$$
$$p(-5) = (-5)^3 - 5(-5) + 1$$
$$p(-5) = -125 + 25 + 1$$
$$p(-5) = -99$$

Thus, the value of $(p \circ q)(-5) = -99$, and the correct answer is (C).

---

23. Given the functions $f(x) = \sqrt{x}$ and $g(x) = 4\sqrt{x-1}$, what is the value of $f(g(x))$?

 A. $2\sqrt[4]{x-1}$

 B. $4\sqrt[4]{x-1}$

 C. $2\sqrt{x-1}$

 D. $4x-1$

13.4

Here's How to Crack It

Here, you don't have a numbers to use, so you will just substitute the entire $g(x)$ function into your $f(x)$) function:

$$f(x) = \sqrt{x} \text{ and } g(x) = 4\sqrt{x-1}$$

$$f(g(x)) = \sqrt{4\sqrt{x-1}}$$

You can now separate this into two expressions:

$$f(g(x)) = \sqrt{4\sqrt{x-1}}$$

$$f(g(x)) = \sqrt{4} \times \sqrt{\sqrt{x-1}}$$

$$f(g(x)) = 2 \times \sqrt{\sqrt{x-1}}$$

Now, we don't see any answer choices that use a double radical, and to be honest, you probably never will, but you can now implement the rules of exponents that you learned earlier in this book!

$$f(g(x)) = 2 \times \sqrt{\sqrt{x-1}}$$

$$f(g(x)) = 2 \times \left[(x-1)^{\frac{1}{2}}\right]^{\frac{1}{2}}$$

$$f(g(x)) = 2(x-1)^{\frac{1}{4}}$$

However, we don't see any answers with exponents, so now convert your exponent back to a radical to find the answer.

$$f(g(x)) = 2(x-1)^{\frac{1}{4}}$$

$$f(g(x)) = 2\sqrt[4]{x-1}$$

Therefore, the correct answer is (A).

Inverse Functions

If you were wondering if there were more fun things to learn about functions, you're in luck! You may be asked to find the inverse function when given a function. So, what is an inverse function?

Let's imagine that you want to find a person's number in your phone. Here, you would input the person's name and the output would be the person's number. The inverse of this process would be if you were to input a person's number in your phone and the output received would be the person's name.

In the math world, an **inverse function**, represented by the notation $f^{-1}(x)$, is a function that undoes the action of a function and replaces the dependent and independent variables of the original function. In short, if a function takes an input value and exports an output value, an inverse function will take the output value and produce the original input value.

When you are asked to solve for the inverse of a function, follow a few simple steps.

Solving for Inverse Functions

1) Given a function, replace the term $f(x)$ with y.

2) Switch the x- and y- terms.

3) Solve for y.

4) Replace y for $f^{-1}(x)$.

To see how this works, find $f^{-1}(x)$ of the function $f(x) = x^2 + 4$.

The first step in solving for $f^{-1}(x)$ is to replace $f(x)$ with y in the original function.

$$f(x) = x^2 + 4$$

$$y = x^2 + 4$$

Next, switch x and y in the equation and solve for y.

$$y = x^2 + 4$$

$$x = y^2 + 4$$

$$x - 4 = y^2$$

$$y = \sqrt{x - 4}$$

Finally, replace the y with $f^{-1}(x)$ to find that $f^{-1}(x) = \sqrt{x - 4}$.

Let's try a couple practice questions out!

24. Given the function $d(x) = 6x - 2$, which of the following represents $d^{-1}(x)$?

    A. $d^{-1}(x) = 6y - 2$

    B. $d^{-1}(x) = 6x + 2$

    C. $d^{-1}(x) = \dfrac{x - 2}{6}$

    D. $d^{-1}(x) = \dfrac{x + 2}{6}$

Here's How to Crack It

Here, you need to identify $d^{-1}(x)$ given that $d(x) = 6x - 2$. The first step in solving for $d^{-1}(x)$ is to replace $d(x)$ with y in the original function.

$d(x) = 6x - 2$

$y = 6x - 2$

Next, switch x and y in the equation and solve for y.

$y = 6x - 2$

$x = 6y - 2$

$x + 2 = 6y$

$y = \dfrac{x + 2}{6}$

Finally, replace the y with $d^{-1}(x)$ to find that $d^{-1}(x) = \dfrac{x + 2}{6}$, so the correct answer is (D).

25. Given the function $f(x) = (x + 3)^3 + 1$, which of the following represents $f^{-1}(x)$?

    A. $f^{-1}(x) = 3\sqrt{y - 1} + 3$

    B. $f^{-1}(x) = 3\sqrt{y - 1} - 3$

    C. $f^{-1}(x) = 3\sqrt{y + 1} + 3$

    D. $f^{-1}(x) = 3\sqrt{y + 1} - 3$

Here's How to Crack It

Here, you need to identify the inverse of $f(x) = (x + 3)^3 + 1$, or $f^{-1}(x)$. The first step in solving for $f^{-1}(x)$ is to replace $f(x)$ with y in the original function.

$$f(x) = (x + 3)^3 + 1$$

$$y = (x + 3)^3 + 1$$

Next, switch x and y in the equation and solve for y.

$$y = (x + 3)^3 + 1$$

$$x = (y + 3)^3 + 1$$

$$x - 1 = (y + 3)^3$$

$$\sqrt[3]{x - 1} = y + 3$$

$$y = \sqrt[3]{x - 1} - 3$$

Finally, replace the y with $f^{-1}(x)$ to find that $f^{-1}(x) = \sqrt[3]{x - 1} - 3$ and the correct answer is (B).

The compositions $g \circ f$ and $f \circ g$ are rarely the same. For example, if $f(x) = x^2$ and $g(x) = x + 7$, then

$$(g \circ f)(x) = g(x^2) = x^2 + 7 \qquad \text{but} \qquad (f \circ g)(x) = f(x + 7) = (x + 7)^2$$

It's also important to remember to work from right to left when applying the functions in a composition; the notation $g \circ f$ tells you to apply f first, then g.

Example: Define f by the equation $f(x) = x^3 + x - 4$. Given that this function has a well-defined inverse, determine the value of $f^{-1}(-2)$.

Solution: If $a = f^{-1}(-2)$, then by definition, $f(a) = -2$. So we simply need to find the value of a such that $f(a) = -2$:

$$f(a) = -2 \quad \Rightarrow \quad a^3 + a - 4 = -2 \quad \Rightarrow \quad a^3 + a = 2$$

By inspection, we can see that $a = 1$, so $f^{-1}(-2) = 1$.

Graphs in the xy-Plane

If the domain and range of a function are subsets of the real numbers, then the function can be graphed in the xy-plane. The **graph** of f consists of all points (x, y) in the plane such that $y = f(x)$. A graph is said to be **symmetric with respect to the y-axis** if, whenever (x, y) is on the graph, $(-x, y)$ is also. A graph is said to be **symmetric with respect to the origin** if, whenever (x, y) is on the graph, $(-x, -y)$ is also. The graph of $y = f(x)$ and the graph of its inverse function $y = f^{-1}(x)$ are **symmetric with respect to the line $y = x$**, since if (x, y) lies on one of the graphs, then (y, x) lies on the other.

Any equation that involves two variables can be sketched in the plane: the graph simply consists of all points (x, y) that satisfy the equation. In some cases, the resulting graph may not be the graph of a function. The **vertical-line test** says that a given graph is not the graph of a function if there are two (or more) points that lie on the same vertical line; this would be a violation of the definition of a function, which says that for every value of the **independent variable** (from the domain), a function assigns *exactly one* value to the **dependent variable** (from the range). A graph is said to be **symmetric with respect to the x-axis** if, whenever (x, y) is on the graph, $(x, -y)$ is also. The x-coordinate (**abscissa**) of a point at which a graph crosses the x-axis is called an **x-intercept**, and the y-coordinate (**ordinate**) of a point at which a graph crosses the y-axis is called a **y-intercept**.

Analytic Geometry

Analytic geometry centers on the interplay between algebra and geometry. In this section, we'll review lines, parabolas, circles, ellipses, and hyperbolas in the xy-plane. All of these curves fall under a common heading: they are **conic sections** and have as their universal equation the general second-degree equation in x and y:

$$Ax^2 + Bxy + Cy^2 + Dx + Ey + F = 0$$

The identity of the graph depends on the values of the coefficients. If the curve is not a straight line or circle, then its symmetry axis (or axes) will not be parallel to one of the coordinate axes if $B \neq 0$, but the coordinate axes can be rotated to simplify the equation of the curve and place the axis of the conic parallel to one of the coordinate axes.

Lines

The equation for a straight line in the xy-plane is

$$ax + by + c = 0$$

in which a and b are not both 0. If the line is not vertical, then the equation of the line with slope m passing through the point (x_1, y_1) can be written as

$$y - y_1 = m(x - x_1)$$

This is called the **point-slope form**. If (x_1, y_1) and (x_2, y_2) are any two points on a nonvertical line, then the **slope** is defined as

$$m = \frac{\Delta y}{\Delta x} = \frac{y_2 - y_1}{x_2 - x_1}$$

We do not define the slope of a vertical line. If two nonvertical lines have the same slope, then they're parallel (or overlapping), and if the product of the slopes of two nonvertical lines is equal to -1, then they're perpendicular.

For example, let's consider the equations $y = 2x + 12$ and $z = 2x - 6$. While these equations will never intersect, they both have a slope equal to 2, and will be parallel to one another.

Conversely, consider the equations $y = 3x - 2$ and $z = -\dfrac{1}{3}x + 4$. These equations have slopes that are negative reciprocals of one another and are therefore perpendicular to one another.

Let's try a couple questions that deal with our knowledge of lines!

1. If points $(4, -1)$ and $(2, 5)$ exist on line y, the slope of line y is

    A.   3

    B.   2

    C. $-\dfrac{1}{2}$

    D. $-\dfrac{1}{3}$

Here's How to Crack It

Here you need to find the slope of line y given points $(4, -1)$ and $(2, 5)$ with the point-slope formula, $m = \dfrac{y_2 - y_1}{x_2 - x_1}$. Accordingly,

$$m = \frac{5 - (-1)}{2 - 4}$$

$$m = \frac{6}{2}$$

$$m = 3$$

Thus, the slope of the line containing points $(4, -1)$ and $(2, 5)$ is 3 and the correct answer is (A).

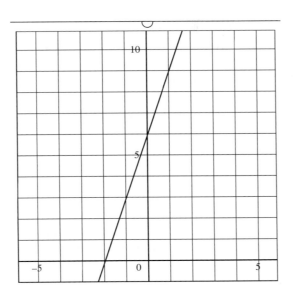

2. Given the graph of line p above, all of the following are true EXCEPT:

    A. The slope of line p is 3.
    B. $2y = 6x - 4$ is parallel to line p.
    C. $(0, 6)$ is the y-intercept of line p.
    D. $3y = -6x + 12$ is perpendicular to line p.

Here's How to Crack It

In order to identify the false statement, fact check each statement. Choice (A) states that the slope of line p is 3. Based on the graph, we see that line p crosses through the x-axis at point $(-2, 0)$ and the y-axis at point $(0, 6)$. Use the point-slope formula, $m = \dfrac{y_2 - y_1}{x_2 - x_1}$ to find that

$$m = \frac{6 - 0}{0 - (-2)}$$

$$m = \frac{6}{2}$$

$$m = 3$$

Accordingly, choice (A) is true and can be eliminated. Choice (B) states that $2y = 6x - 4$ is parallel to line p. Isolate y to find that $y = 3x - 2$. The equation is now in standard $y = mx + b$ form, where m represents the slope, indicating that the slope of this line is 3. Since the slope of this line equals the slope of the line in the graph, these two lines are parallel; eliminate (B). Choice (C) states that $(0, 6)$ is the y-intercept of line p; we found this to be true when finding the slope previously, so choice (C) can be eliminated. Choice (D) states that $3y = -6x + 12$ is perpendicular to line p. Isolate y to find that $y = -2x + 4$ and the slope of this line is -2. Perpendicular lines have slopes that are negative reciprocals of one another, so choice (D) is false and the correct answer.

Parabolas

Let F be a given fixed point and D a given fixed line that doesn't contain F. By definition, a **parabola** is the set of points in the plane containing F and D that are equidistant from the point F (the **focus**) and the line D (the **directrix**). The **axis** of a parabola is the line through the focus and perpendicular to the directrix. The **vertex** of a parabola is the turning point, the point on the parabola's axis that's midway between the focus and the directrix. The standard equations of the parabolas with vertex at the origin and axis either the x- or y-axis are

$$y = \pm \frac{1}{4p}x^2 \quad \text{or} \quad x = \pm \frac{1}{4p}y^2$$

The following diagrams summarize the basic characteristics of these standard parabolas. The axis of the top two parabolas is the y-axis; the bottom two parabolas have the x-axis as their axis.

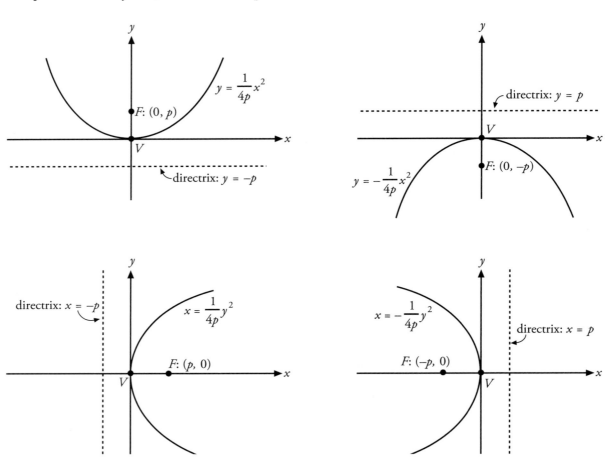

Let's try a question that deals with parabolas!

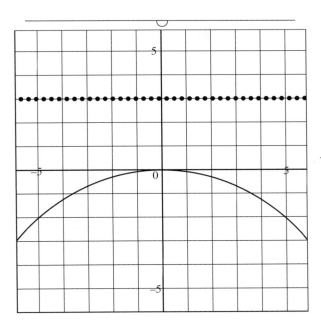

1. Given the graph of the parabola above, in which the dotted line represents the directrix, the focus is located at

    A. (0, –3)
    B. (0, 3)
    C. (3, 0)
    D. (–3, 0)

Here's How to Crack It

Recall that the focus of a parabola opening downward is located at point $(0, -p)$, where the directrix tells us that $y = p$. The directrix in this graph is the dotted line, which exists at $y = 3$; if $y = p$, we know that $p = 3$. Accordingly, the focus of this parabola is located at point $(0, -p)$ or $(0, -3)$, and the correct answer is (A).

Circles

A **circle** is the set of points in the plane that are all at a constant, positive distance from a given fixed point. This constant distance is called the **radius**, and the given fixed point is the **center**. The standard equation of the circle with radius a, centered at the origin, is

$$x^2 + y^2 = a^2$$

or, equivalently,

$$\frac{x^2}{a^2} + \frac{y^2}{a^2} = 1$$

If the center is at the point (h, k), then we can replace x by $x - h$ and y by $y - k$ and write

$$(x - h)^2 + (y - k)^2 = a^2 \quad \text{or} \quad \frac{(x - h)^2}{a^2} + \frac{(y - k)^2}{a^2} = 1$$

13.4

Let's see how this looks graphically given the equation $x^2 + (y + 2)^2 = 4$. Recall that the formula for a circle is $(x - h)^2 + (y - k)^2 = a^2$, where the center exists at point (h, k) and a is the radius. Accordingly, a circle represented by the equation $x^2 + (y + 2)^2 = 4$ would have a center at point $(0, -2)$ and a radius of 2. You could plot these points out on the coordinate plane to find that the graph of $x^2 + (y + 2)^2 = 4$ would look as follows:

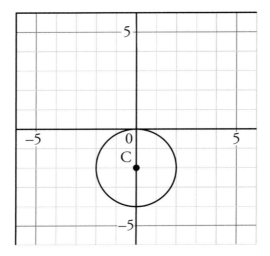

Now let's try a question that deals with circles!

1. Which of the following equations represents a circle with a center at point $(2, -4)$ and a radius of 5?

    A. $(x - 2)^2 + (y + 4)^2 = 5$
    B. $(x + 2)^2 + (y - 4)^2 = 5$
    C. $(x - 2)^2 + (y + 4)^2 = 25$
    D. $(x + 2)^2 + (y - 4)^2 = 25$

Here's How to Crack It

Recall that the formula for a circle is $(x - h)^2 + (y - k)^2 = a^2$, where the center exists at point (h, k) and a is the radius. The question states that the radius of the circle is 5, so we can eliminate choices (A) and (B), since the radius of these circles is $\sqrt{5}$. Next, let's look find the center of choice (C). The center of the circle in the equation $(x - 2)^2 + (y + 4)^2 = 25$ is located at point $(2, -4)$; keep choice (C) and check choice (D). The center of the circle in the equation $(x + 2)^2 + (y - 4)^2 = 25$ is located at point $(-2, 4)$; eliminate choice (D). Therefore, the correct answer is (C).

Ellipses

By definition, an **ellipse** is the set of points in the plane such that the sum of the distances from every point on the ellipse to two given fixed points (the **foci**) is a constant. (And to avoid a degenerate case, the constant sum must be greater than the distance between the foci.) The standard equation of an ellipse centered at the origin—with axes parallel to the coordinate axes—is

$$\frac{x^2}{a^2} + \frac{y^2}{b^2} = 1$$

The longer symmetry axis of the ellipse is called the **major axis** (on which the foci are located), and the shorter one is the **minor axis**. The endpoints of the major axis are called the **vertices**. The **eccentricity** of an ellipse is a number (denoted e) between 0 and 1 that measures its "flatness." The closer e is to zero, the more the ellipse resembles a perfect circle; as e increases to 1, the ellipse flattens out.

By comparing the standard equations for the circle and the ellipse, we notice that the only difference is that while the x^2- and y^2-terms always have identical positive coefficients for a circle, these terms have different positive coefficients for an ellipse. Therefore, a circle can be transformed into an ellipse (or vice versa) by changing the scale on one of the axes. For example, we can turn the circle $\frac{x^2}{a^2} + \frac{y^2}{a^2} = 1$ into the ellipse $\frac{x^2}{a^2} + \frac{y^2}{b^2} = 1$ by replacing every point (x, y) on the circle by the point $(x, \frac{by}{a})$.

The following diagrams summarize the basic characteristics of the ellipse, where the cases $a > b$ and $a < b$ are considered separately.

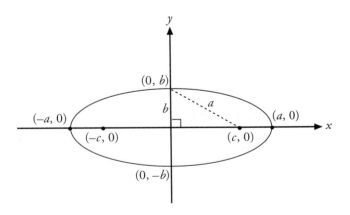

$\frac{x^2}{a^2} + \frac{y^2}{b^2} = 1$, $a > b$

foci: $(-c, 0)$, where $c = \sqrt{a^2 - b^2}$

vertices: $(-a, 0)$

major axis length = $2a$

minor axis length = $2b$

eccentricity: $e = \frac{c}{a}$

13.4

$$\frac{x^2}{a^2} + \frac{y^2}{b^2} = 1, \ a < b$$

foci: $(0, -c)$, where $c = \sqrt{b^2 - a^2}$

vertices: $(0, -b)$

major axis length = $2b$

minor axis length = $2a$

eccentricity: $e = \dfrac{c}{b}$

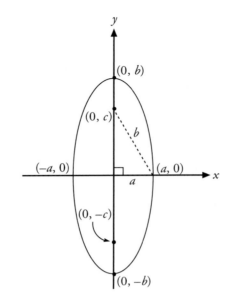

Let's try a question that deals with ellipses!

1. Given the equation $\dfrac{x^2}{9} + \dfrac{y^2}{16} = 1$, what is the eccentricity of the ellipse?

   A. $\dfrac{\sqrt{7}}{4}$

   B. $\dfrac{\sqrt{7}}{3}$

   C. $\dfrac{1}{3}$

   D. $\dfrac{1}{4}$

Here's How to Crack It

Recall that the standard form of an ellipse is $\dfrac{x^2}{a^2} + \dfrac{y^2}{b^2} = 1$, where $a < b$, $c = \sqrt{b^2 - a^2}$. In the equation

$\dfrac{x^2}{9} + \dfrac{y^2}{16} = 1$, we know that $a^2 = 9$ and $b^2 = 16$. Therefore, $c = \sqrt{16 - 9}$ and $c = \sqrt{7}$. Next, recall that the

eccentricity of an ellipse can be found with the formula $e = \dfrac{c}{b}$. Since $b^2 = 16$, $b = 4$, and the eccentricity of

the ellipse is $e = \dfrac{\sqrt{7}}{4}$. Therefore, the correct answer is (A).

Hyperbolas

By definition, a **hyperbola** is the set of points in the plane such that the difference between the distances from every point on the hyperbola to two fixed points (the **foci**) is a constant. (And to avoid a degenerate case, the constant difference must be smaller than the distance between the foci.) Unlike a parabola, circle, or ellipse, a hyperbola is not a single curve; instead, it consists of two separate curves called **branches**. A hyperbola is also different from these other curves in that it has **asymptotes**, which are lines that its branches approach but never touch, as the magnitudes of x and y increase.

13.4

The line that contains the foci is called the **focal axis**; the midpoint of the segment joining the foci is the **center** of the hyperbola; and the points at which the branches of the hyperbola intersect the focal axis are called the **vertices**. The standard equations of the hyperbolas centered at the origin with either the x- or the y-axis as their focal axis are

$$\frac{x^2}{a^2} - \frac{y^2}{b^2} = 1 \quad \text{or} \quad \frac{y^2}{b^2} - \frac{x^2}{a^2} = 1$$

The diagrams below summarize the basic characteristics of these standard hyperbolas. Notice that the hyperbolas of the first family do not intersect the y-axis, and those of the second family do not intersect the x-axis.

$$\frac{x^2}{a^2} - \frac{y^2}{b^2} = 1$$

foci: $(\pm c, 0)$, where $c = \sqrt{a^2 + b^2}$

vertices: $(\pm a, 0)$

asymptotes: $y = \pm \frac{b}{a} x$

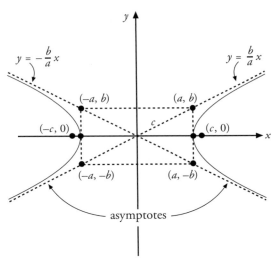

13.4

$$\frac{y^2}{b^2} - \frac{x^2}{a^2} = 1$$

foci: $(0, \pm c)$, where $c = \sqrt{a^2 + b^2}$

vertices: $(0, \pm b)$

asymptotes: $y = \pm \frac{b}{a} x$

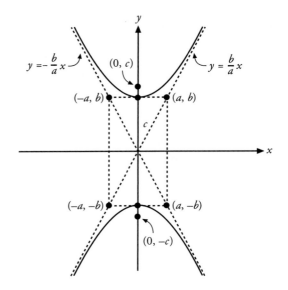

Now let's try a question that deals with hyperbolas!

1. Given the equation $\dfrac{x^2}{64} - \dfrac{y^2}{36} = 1$, the foci of the hyperbola are located at

    A. $(0, \pm 10)$
    B. $(0, \pm 2\sqrt{7})$
    C. $(\pm 10, 0)$
    D. $(\pm 2\sqrt{7}, 0)$

Here's How to Crack It

Recall that a hyperbola that is expressed in the form $\dfrac{x^2}{a^2} - \dfrac{y^2}{b^2} = 1$ will never cross the y-axis, the foci are located at $(\pm c, 0)$, and $c = \sqrt{a^2 + b^2}$. Since choices (A) and (B) are points on the y-axis, they can be eliminated.

In the equation $\dfrac{x^2}{64} - \dfrac{y^2}{36} = 1$, we know that $a^2 = 64$ and $b^2 = 36$. Therefore, $c = \sqrt{64 + 36}$, $c = \sqrt{100}$, and $c = 10$. Since the foci of a hyperbola are located at $(\pm c, 0)$, we know that the foci of $\dfrac{x^2}{64} - \dfrac{y^2}{36} = 1$ are located at $(\pm 10, 0)$. Accordingly, the correct answer is (C).

Logarithms

Logarithms are exponents. Given the equation $b^y = x$, the exponent is y, which means that the logarithm is y. More precisely, we'd say that y is the **logarithm** base b of x, and write $y = \log_b x$. The laws of logarithms follow directly from the corresponding laws of exponents. In the equations below, b is a positive number that's not equal to 1.

- $\log_b x = y$ means $b^y = x$
- The function $y = \log_b x$ is the inverse of the exponential function $y = b^x$. The domain of the function $f(x) = \log_b x$ is $x > 0$, and the range is the set of all real numbers. If $b > 1$, the function is increasing (see the diagram below); if $0 < b < 1$, the function is decreasing.

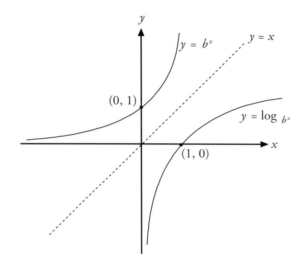

- $\log_b(x_1 x_2) = \log_b x_1 + \log_b x_2$

- $\log_b \dfrac{x_1}{x_2} = \log_b x_1 - \log_b x_2$

- $\log_b (x^a) = a \log_b x$

- $b^{\log_b x} = x$

- $(\log_b a)(\log_a x) = \log_b x$ (this is the **change-of-base formula,** with $a \neq 1$)

The two most important bases for logarithms are $b = 10$ [because we use a base-10 (decimal) number system] and $b = e$, where e is an irrational constant, approximately equal to 2.718. The selection of this seemingly unusual number is based on considerations in calculus and is so important that the function $f(x) = \log_e x$ is called the **natural logarithm function**.

> On the PCAT, the "e" is understood, so log x means $\log_e x$. It's important to be aware of this, since in many precalculus and calculus texts, log x denotes $\log_{10} x$ and the abbreviation for $\log_e x$ is ln x.

13.4

Let's try some questions!

1. If $\log y = 5$, what is the value of y ?

   A. 2
   B. 50
   C. 10,000
   D. 100,000

Here's How to Crack It

If no base is provided, assume it is the common base of 10. Accordingly, $\log y = 5$ means $10^5 = y$. Therefore, $y = 100,000$ and the correct answer is (D).

Let's try another question!

2. If $\log_x 8 = 3$, what is the value of $4x$?

   A. 2
   B. 4
   C. 8
   D. 24

Here's How to Crack It

Recall that $\log_b n = x$ =means $b^x = n$. Therefore, $\log_x 8 = 3$ is equivalent to $x^3 = 8$. Solve the equation to find that $x = \sqrt[3]{8}$ and $x = 2$. The question asks you to find the value of $4x$, so the correct answer is $(4)(2) = 8$, or choice (C).

Let's try one more!

3. If $\log 0.2 = p$, then $p = $?

   A. −10
   B. −2
   C. 0.2
   D. 2

Here's How to Crack It

If no base is provided, assume it is the common base of 10. Accordingly, $\log_{10} 0.01 = p$, $10^p = 0.01$, $10^p = 10^{-2}$, and $p = -2$. The correct answer is (B).

Let's try another question!

---

4. For which of the following values of z is $\log_{(z-6)}(z^2 + 12) = 2$?

    A. -2
    B. 2
    C. 4
    D. 8

Here's How to Crack It

Recall that $\log_b n = x$ means $b^x = n$. Therefore, $\log_{(z-6)}(z^2 + 12) = 2$ is equivalent to $(z-6)^2 = z^2 + 12$, which equates to $z^2 - 12z + 36 = z^2 + 12$. Simplify the equation to find that $12z = 24$ and $z = 2$. The correct answer is (B). Alternatively, you can use PITA on the answer choices and POE away any choice that leads to an incorrect equation.

Let's try one last question!

---

5. What is the value of $(\log_5 10 - \log_5 2) + \log_5 5$?

    A. $\log_5 40$
    B. $2 \log_5 5$
    C. $5 \log_5 5$
    D. $13 \log_5 5$

Here's How to Crack It

Follow order of operations and handle the information within the parentheses first. Recall that $\log_b x - \log_b y = \log_b \frac{x}{y}$. Accordingly, $\log_5 10 - \log_5 2 = \log_5 \frac{10}{2} = \log_5 5$. Next, remember that $\log_b x + \log_b y = \log_b xy$. Therefore, $\log_5 5 + \log_5 5 = \log_5 25 = \log_5 5^2$. Finally, recall that $\log_b x^y = y \log_b x$. Thus, $\log_5 5^2 = 2 \log_5 5$, and the correct answer is (B).

Trigonometry

Although trigonometry began as the study of triangles, the usefulness of the trigonometric functions now extends far beyond this simple geometric form. We'll begin our study by reviewing the definitions of the trig functions, first with acute angles in right triangles and then with arbitrary angles and real numbers.

Trig Functions of Acute Angles

The classical definitions of the six trig functions—sine, cosine, tangent, cosecant, secant, and cotangent—use the lengths of the sides of a right triangle. In the figure below, triangle ABC is a right triangle with its right angle at C. The lengths of the legs BC and AC are denoted a and b, respectively, and the length of the hypotenuse AB is denoted c.

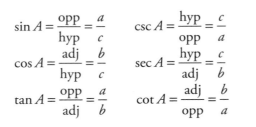
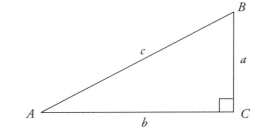

$$\sin A = \frac{\text{opp}}{\text{hyp}} = \frac{a}{c} \qquad \csc A = \frac{\text{hyp}}{\text{opp}} = \frac{c}{a}$$

$$\cos A = \frac{\text{adj}}{\text{hyp}} = \frac{b}{c} \qquad \sec A = \frac{\text{hyp}}{\text{adj}} = \frac{c}{b}$$

$$\tan A = \frac{\text{opp}}{\text{adj}} = \frac{a}{b} \qquad \cot A = \frac{\text{adj}}{\text{opp}} = \frac{b}{a}$$

Angles A and B are complementary (that is, the sum of their measures is 90°), and notice that $\sin A = \cos B$. That is, the sine of B's complement (namely, A) is $\cos B$, which is where the name "cosine" comes from (<u>complement's</u> <u>sine</u>). The same is true for the other pairs of cofunctions—tangent and cotangent, secant and cosecant. You'll also notice certain reciprocal relationships among the functions. Cosecant is the reciprocal of sine, secant is the reciprocal of cosine, and cotangent is the reciprocal of tangent. Finally, all of the trig functions can be written in terms of sine and cosine: the reciprocal relationships take care of secant and cosecant, and it's easy to see that tangent is the ratio of sine to cosine, and cotangent is the ratio of cosine to sine.

Two special right triangles allow us to determine the numerical values of the trig functions of the angles 30°, 45°, and 60°.

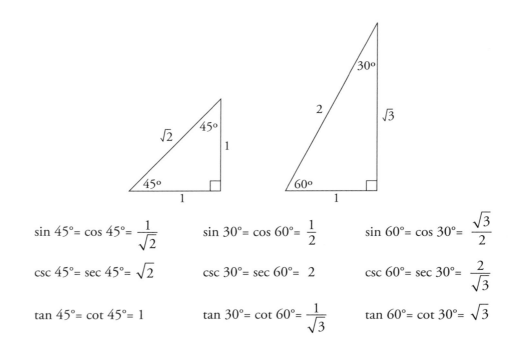

$$\sin 45° = \cos 45° = \frac{1}{\sqrt{2}} \qquad \sin 30° = \cos 60° = \frac{1}{2} \qquad \sin 60° = \cos 30° = \frac{\sqrt{3}}{2}$$

$$\csc 45° = \sec 45° = \sqrt{2} \qquad \csc 30° = \sec 60° = 2 \qquad \csc 60° = \sec 30° = \frac{2}{\sqrt{3}}$$

$$\tan 45° = \cot 45° = 1 \qquad \tan 30° = \cot 60° = \frac{1}{\sqrt{3}} \qquad \tan 60° = \cot 30° = \sqrt{3}$$

Let's try some questions!

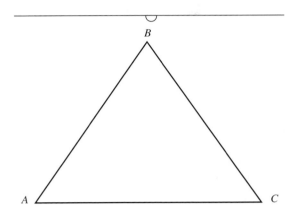

1. Equilateral triangle *ABC,* shown above, has a perimeter of 6. If point *D* is the midpoint of segment *AC,* what is the value of tan ∠*ABD* ?

A. 1

B. $\dfrac{\sqrt{3}}{3}$

C. $\dfrac{\sqrt{3}}{2}$

D. $\sqrt{3}$

Here's How to Crack It

First, fill in the information you know: the perimeter of triangle *ABC* is 6, which means each side is 2, and point *D* is the midpoint of segments *AC*. Now, you can drop the vertical height from point *B* to point *D* to create two 30°:60°:90° triangles. Recall that the 30°:60°:90° angles have proportions equivalent to 1:2:$\sqrt{3}$.

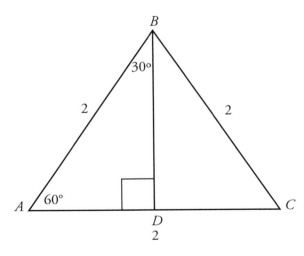
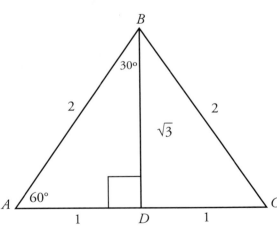

Finally, the question asks you to identify the value of tan $\angle ABD$. Remember that tan $= \dfrac{opp}{adj}$, so tan

$\angle ABD = \dfrac{1}{\sqrt{3}}$. However, you can't keep a radical in the denominator so multiply by 1, or $\dfrac{\sqrt{3}}{\sqrt{3}}$, to find that

tan $\angle ABD = \dfrac{1}{\sqrt{3}} \times \dfrac{\sqrt{3}}{\sqrt{3}} = \dfrac{\sqrt{3}}{3}$. The correct answer is (B).

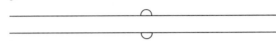

2. Triangle *DEF* is shown below. If segment *DE = EF*, and the area of triangle *DEF* = 8, what is the value of sin $\angle FDE$?

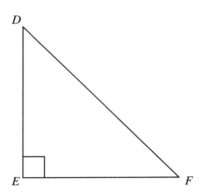

A. $\dfrac{\sqrt{2}}{2}$

B. 1

C. $\sqrt{2}$

D. 2

Here's How to Crack It

First, work with what you know. You are told that segment *DE = EF*, which means that triangle *DEF* is a 45°:45°90° triangle with proportions of $x{:}x{:}x\sqrt{2}$. Furthermore, you are told that the area of triangle *DEF* is 8. Recall that the formula for the area of a triangle is $A_{\triangle} = \dfrac{1}{2}(base)(height)$. Fill in what you know: the area is 16 and the base and height are equal, so $8 = \dfrac{1}{2}(base)(base)$, $8 = \dfrac{base^2}{2}$, $16 = base^2$, and $4 = base$. Accordingly, segment *DE = EF* = 4 and segment *DF* = $4\sqrt{2}$.

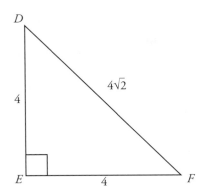

13.4

Finally, the question asks you to identify the value of sin $\angle FDE$. Remember that sin = $\dfrac{opp}{hyp}$, so sin $\angle FDE$ = $\dfrac{4}{4\sqrt{2}} = \dfrac{1}{\sqrt{2}}$. However, you can't keep a radical in the denominator so multiply by 1, or $\dfrac{\sqrt{2}}{\sqrt{2}}$, to find that sin $\angle FDE$ = $\dfrac{1}{\sqrt{2}} \times \dfrac{\sqrt{2}}{\sqrt{2}} = \dfrac{\sqrt{2}}{2}$. The correct answer is (A).

Trig Functions of Real Numbers

An alternate but equivalent definition of the trig functions utilizes the unit circle in the xy-plane. This circle has a radius of 1, is centered at the origin, and has the equation $x^2 + y^2 = 1$. Let θ be any real number and measure the arc of length θ along the circle, starting at the point A: (1, 0). If θ is positive, travel along the circle in the counterclockwise direction; if θ is negative, measure a length θ clockwise. If P: (x, y) denotes the endpoint of the arc, then the trig functions of θ are defined as follows.

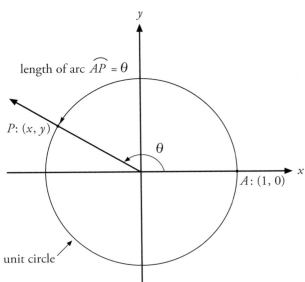

$$\sin\theta = y \qquad \csc\theta = \frac{1}{y}$$
$$\cos\theta = x \qquad \sec\theta = \frac{1}{x}$$
$$\tan\theta = \frac{y}{x} \qquad \cot\theta = \frac{x}{y}$$

13.4

These definitions are the same as those preceding if we interpret θ as the radian measure of the central angle. Recall that if the central angle in a circle of radius r subtends an arc of length s, then the radian measure of the angle is defined as $\dfrac{s}{r}$. In particular, if the central angle measures 180°, it subtends half the circle, and its arc length is $s = \dfrac{1}{2}(2\pi r) = \pi r$; thus, the radian measure of this angle is $\theta = \dfrac{s}{r} = \dfrac{\pi r}{r} = \pi$.

This gives the conversion between radian measure and degree measure:

$$\pi \text{ radians} = 180°$$

Using this equation, we have the following correspondences for some special small angles:

$$\frac{\pi}{6} \leftrightarrow 30° \qquad \frac{\pi}{4} \leftrightarrow 45° \qquad \frac{\pi}{3} \leftrightarrow 60° \qquad \frac{\pi}{2} \leftrightarrow 90°$$

Memorizing these four correspondences makes it easier to determine the radian measure of larger special angles; for example, the radian measure of a 150° angle is $\dfrac{5\pi}{6}$, since $150° = 5(30°)$.

Graphs of the Trig Functions

From the definitions, we can determine the domain and range of each of the six trig functions.

- The functions $\sin x$ and $\cos x$ are defined for every real x, and the range of each of these functions is the set of y such that $|y| \ge 1$, that is, the closed interval $[-1, 1]$.

- The function $\csc x$ is defined for all values of x for which $\sin x \ne 0$, that is, for all x except multiples of π; the range of this function consists of all y such that $|y| \ge 1$.

- The function $\sec x$ is defined for all values of x for which $\cos x \ne 0$, that is, for all x except odd multiples of $\dfrac{1}{2}\pi$; the range of this function consists of all y such that $|y| \ge 1$.

- The function $\tan x$ is defined for all values of x for which $\cos x \ne 0$, that is, for all x except odd multiples of $\dfrac{1}{2}\pi$; the range of this function consists of all real numbers y.

- The function $\cot x$ is defined for all values of x for which $\sin x \ne 0$, that is, for all x except multiples of π; the range of this function also consists of all real y.

Using this information, we can sketch the graphs of the six trig functions in the xy-plane:

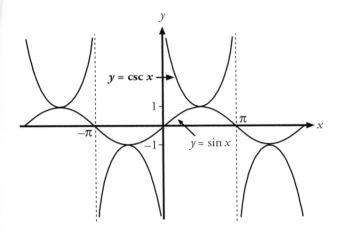

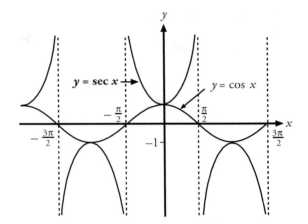

13.4

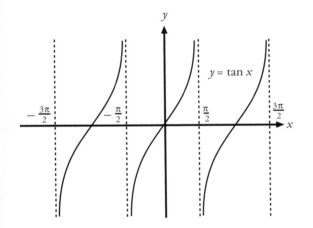

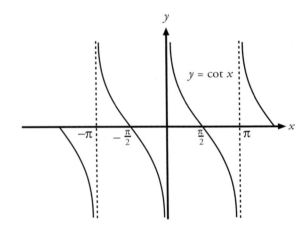

Memorize These

You must be able to work in radians and know that $2\pi = 360°$.

You should know the following:

$\sin 0 = 0$	$\cos 0 = 1$	$\tan 0 = 0$
$\sin 30° = \dfrac{1}{2}$	$\cos 30° = \dfrac{\sqrt{3}}{2}$	$\tan 30° = \dfrac{1}{\sqrt{3}}$
$\sin 45° = \dfrac{1}{\sqrt{2}}$	$\cos 45° = \dfrac{1}{\sqrt{2}}$	$\tan 45° = 1$
$\sin 60° = \dfrac{\sqrt{3}}{2}$	$\cos 60° = \dfrac{1}{2}$	$\tan 60° = \sqrt{3}$
$\sin 90° = 1$	$\cos 90° = 0$	$\tan 90° = \infty$
$\sin 180° = 0$	$\cos 180° = -1$	$\tan 180° = 0$
$\sin 270° = 1$	$\cos 270° = 0$	$\tan 270° = \infty$
$\sin 360° = 0$	$\cos 360° = 1$	$\tan 360° = 0$

Imaginary Numbers

The only numbers that aren't real are *imaginary*—a negative number under an even root. $\sqrt{-1}$ is defined as the imaginary number, i. All other imaginary numbers are something multiplied by i.

You should memorize the following powers of i:

$$i = \sqrt{-1}$$

$$i^2 = -1$$

$$i^3 = -i$$

$$i^4 = 1$$

Note that the powers of i repeat every four terms, so

$$i^5 = \sqrt{-1}$$

$$i^6 = -1$$

$$i^7 = -i$$

$$i^8 = 1$$

$$\dots$$

The pattern continues ad infinitum, so if you're faced with a power larger than 4, simply divide by 4 to find the remainder, which will align with the power of i you need.

For example, if you are asked to find the value of i^7, you would find that $7 \div 4$ yields 1 with a remainder of 3; thus, $i^7 = i^3 = -i$.

Let's see how we can use i in action. What if you were told that $y = 2i^4 + 12i^2$ and asked to find the value of y?

Recall that $i^2 = -1$ and $i^4 = 1$. Plug these values of i into the expression provided to find that

$$y = 2i^4 + 12i^2$$

$$y = 2(1) + 12(-1)$$

$$y = 2 - 10 - 4$$

$$y = -8$$

If you end up dividing by a complex number, you will have to multiply by the **complex conjugates** to remove the imaginary numbers from the denominator. A conjugate is an expression in which the sign in the middle of two terms is changed. For complex numbers, an expression written in the form $a + bi$ has a complex conjugate of $a - bi$; i.e., the complex conjugate of $2i + 4$ is $2i - 4$.

Let's see how complex conjugates come into play if we were asked to simplify the expression $\dfrac{3 + 2i}{5 - 4i}$.

In order to eliminate the imaginary numbers in the denominator, we must multiply both the top and bottom of the expression by the complex conjugate of $5 - 4i$, which is $5 + 4i$.

$$\frac{3 + 2i}{5 - 4i} \times \frac{5 + 4i}{5 + 4i} =$$

$$\frac{15 + 12i + 10i + 8i^2}{25 + 20i - 20i - 16i^2} =$$

$$\frac{15 + 22i + 8i^2}{25 - 16i^2}$$

Next, recall that $i^2 = -1$, and substitute that into your expression.

$$\frac{15 + 22i + 8i^2}{25 - 16i^2} =$$

$$\frac{15 + 22i + 8(-1)}{25 - 16(-1)} =$$

$$\frac{7 + 22i}{41}$$

Finally, put the expression back into $a + bi$ form to find the answer is $\dfrac{7}{41} + \dfrac{22i}{41}$.

It's that simple! Now let's try a couple questions that deal imaginary numbers!

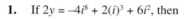

1. If $2y = -4i^8 + 2(i)^3 + 6i^2$, then

    A. $y = 5 - i$
    B. $y = -10 - 2i$
    C. $y = 2 - 2i$
    D. $y = 1 - i$

Here's How to Crack It

Given the equation $2y = -4i^8 + 2(i)^3 - 6i^2$, we must solve for y. Recall that $i^8 = 1$, $i^3 = -i$, and $i^2 = -1$. Plug these values of i into the expression provided to find that

$$2y = -4i^8 + 2(i)^3 - 6i^2$$

$$2y = -4(1) + 2(-i) - 6(-1)$$

$$2y = -4 - 2i + 6$$

$$2y = 2 - 2i$$

Finally, divide by 2 on both sides to solve for y.

$$y = \frac{2 - 2i}{2}$$

$$y = \frac{2(1 - i)}{2}$$
$$y = 1 - i$$

Therefore, the correct answer is (D).

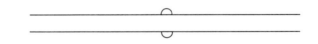

2. What is the value of $\dfrac{4 - 2i}{6 - 3i}$?

A. $\dfrac{2}{3} - \dfrac{24i}{45}$

B. $\dfrac{2}{3} + \dfrac{24i}{45}$

C. $\dfrac{2}{3} + \dfrac{2}{3}i$

D. $\dfrac{2}{3}$

Here's How to Crack It

Recall that you must multiply both the top and bottom of the expression by the complex conjugate of $6 - 3i$, which is $6 + 3i$, in order to clear the denominator of imaginary numbers.

$$\frac{4 - 2i}{6 - 3i} \times \frac{6 + 3i}{6 + 3i} =$$

$$\frac{24 + 12i - 12i - 6i^2}{36 + 18i - 18i - 9i^2} =$$

$$\frac{24 - 6i^2}{36 - 9i^2}$$

Now, substitute $i^2 = -1$ into your expression.

$$\frac{24 - 6i^2}{36 - 9i^2} =$$

$$\frac{24 - 6(-1)}{36 - 9(-1)} =$$

$$\frac{24 + 6}{36 + 9} = \frac{30}{45} = \frac{2}{3}$$

Therefore, the correct answer is (D).

Vectors

Some physical quantities that are represented as vectors are displacement, velocity, acceleration, force, momentum, and electric and magnetic fields. Since vectors play such a recurring role, it's important to become comfortable working with them. In this section, we restrict our study to two-dimensional vectors (that is, ones that lie flat in a plane).

Definition

A **vector** is a quantity that involves both magnitude and direction and obeys the **commutative law for addition,** which we'll explain in a moment. A quantity that does not involve direction is a **scalar**. For example, the quantity *55 miles per hour* is a scalar, while the quantity *55 miles per hour to the north* is a vector. Other examples of scalars include mass, work, energy, power, temperature, and electric charge.

Vectors can be denoted in several ways, including

$$\mathbf{A}, \mathit{A}, \vec{\mathrm{A}}, \bar{\mathrm{A}}$$

In textbooks, you'll usually see one of the first two, but when it's handwritten, you'll see one of the last two.

Displacement (which is net distance traveled plus direction) is the prototypical example of a vector:

$$\underbrace{\mathbf{A}}_{\text{displacement}} = \underbrace{\text{4 miles}}_{\text{magnitude}} \underbrace{\text{to the north}}_{\text{direction}}$$

When we say that vectors obey the commutative law for addition, we mean that if we have two vectors of the same type, for example, another displacement,

$$\mathbf{B} = \underbrace{\text{3 miles}}_{\text{magnitude}} \underbrace{\text{to the east}}_{\text{direction}}$$

then **A** + **B** must equal **B** + **A**. The vector sum **A** + **B** means *the vector A followed by B*, while the vector sum **B** + **A** means *the vector B followed by A*. That these two sums are indeed identical is shown in the following figure:

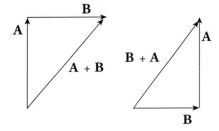

Two vectors are equal if they have the same magnitude and the same direction.

Vector Addition (Geometric)

The figure above illustrates how vectors are added to each other geometrically. Place the tail (the initial point) of one vector at the tip of the other vector and then connect the exposed tail to the exposed tip. It is essential that the original magnitude and direction of each vector be preserved. The vector formed is the sum of the first two. This is called the **tip-to-tail method** of vector addition.

Example: Add the following two vectors:

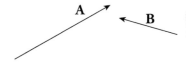

Solution: Place the tail of **B** at the tip of **A** and connect them:

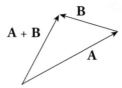

Scalar Multiplication

A vector can be multiplied by a scalar (that is, by a number), and the result is a vector. If the original vector is **A** and the scalar is k, then the scalar multiple k**A** is as follows:

$$\text{magnitude of } k\mathbf{A} = |k| \times (\text{magnitude of } \mathbf{A})$$

$$\text{direction of } k\mathbf{A} = \begin{cases} \text{the same as } \mathbf{A} \text{ if } k \text{ is positive} \\ \text{the opposite of } \mathbf{A} \text{ if } k \text{ is negative} \end{cases}$$

Vector Subtraction (Geometric)

To subtract one vector from another, for example, to get **A** − **B**, simply form the vector −**B**, which is the scalar multiple (−1)**B**, and add it to **A**:

$$\mathbf{A} - \mathbf{B} = \mathbf{A} + (-\mathbf{B})$$

Standard Basis Vectors

Two-dimensional vectors, that is, vectors that lie flat in a plane, can be written as the sum of a horizontal vector and a vertical vector. For example, in the following diagram, the vector **A** is equal to the horizontal vector **B** plus the vertical vector **C**:

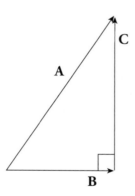

The horizontal vector is always considered a scalar multiple of what's called the **horizontal basis vector, i**, and the vertical vector is a scalar multiple of the **vertical basis vector, j**. Both of these special vectors have a magnitude of 1, and for this reason, they're called **unit vectors.** Unit vectors are often represented by placing a hat (caret) over the vector; for example, the unit **vectors i** and **j** are sometimes denoted $\hat{i}$ and $\hat{j}$.

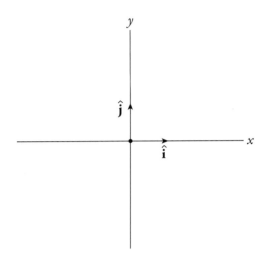

For instance, the vector **A** in the figure below is the sum of the horizontal vector $\mathbf{B} = 3\hat{i}$ and the vertical vector $\mathbf{C} = 4\hat{j}$.

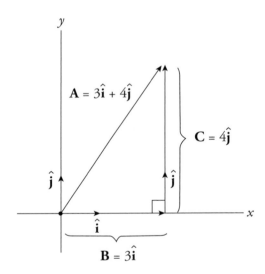

The vectors **B** and **C** are called the **vector components** of **A**, and the scalar multiples of $\hat{i}$ and $\hat{j}$ which give **A**—in this case, 3 and 4—are called the **scalar components** of **A**. So vector **A** can be written as the sum $A_x\hat{i} + A_y\hat{j}$, where A_x and A_y are the scalar components of **A**. The component A_x is called the **horizontal** scalar component of **A**, and A_y is called the **vertical** scalar component of **A**.

Vector Operations Using Components

The use of components makes the vector operations of addition, subtraction, and scalar multiplication pretty straightforward:

Vector addition: *Add the respective components.*
$$\mathbf{A} + \mathbf{B} = (A_x + B_x)\hat{\mathbf{i}} + (A_y + B_y)\hat{\mathbf{j}}$$

Vector subtraction: *Subtract the respective components.*
$$\mathbf{A} - \mathbf{B} = (A_x - B_x)\hat{\mathbf{i}} + (A_y - B_y)\hat{\mathbf{j}}$$

Scalar multiplication: *Multiply each component by k.*
$$k\mathbf{A} = (kA_x)\hat{\mathbf{i}} + (kA_y)\hat{\mathbf{j}}$$

Magnitude of a Vector

The magnitude of a vector can be computed with the Pythagorean Theorem. The magnitude of vector $\mathbf{A}$ can be denoted in several ways: A or $|\mathbf{A}|$ or $\|\mathbf{A}\|$. In terms of its components, the magnitude of $\mathbf{A} = A_x\hat{\mathbf{i}} + A_y\hat{\mathbf{j}}$ is given by the equation

$$A = \sqrt{\left(A_x\right)^2 + \left(A_y\right)^2}$$

which is the formula for the length of the hypotenuse of a right triangle with sides of lengths A_x and A_y.

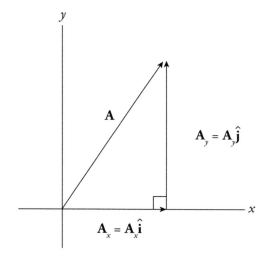

Direction of a Vector

The direction of a vector can be specified by the angle it makes with the positive *x* axis. You can sketch the vector and use its components (and an inverse trig function) to determine the angle. For example, if θ denotes the angle that the vector $\mathbf{A} = 3\hat{\mathbf{i}} + 4\hat{\mathbf{j}}$ makes with the +*x* axis, then $\tan \theta = 4/3$, so $\theta = \tan^{-1}(4/3) = 53.1°$.

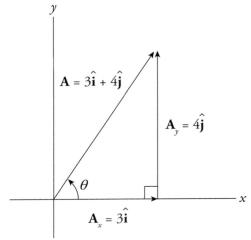

If $\mathbf{A}$ makes the angle θ with the +*x* axis, then its *x*- and *y*-components are $A \cos \theta$ and $A \sin \theta$, respectively (where A is the magnitude of $\mathbf{A}$).

$$\mathbf{A} = \underbrace{\left(A\cos\theta\right)\hat{\mathbf{i}}}_{A_x} + \underbrace{\left(A\sin\theta\right)\hat{\mathbf{j}}}_{A_y}$$

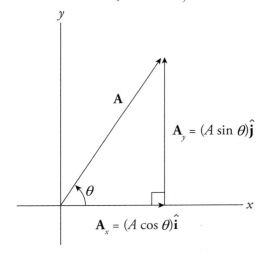

In general, any vector in the plane can be written in terms of two perpendicular component vectors. For example, vector **W** (shown below) is the sum of two component vectors whose magnitudes are $W \cos \theta$ and $W \sin \theta$:

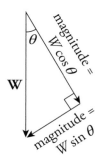

13.4

Let's try a few questions!

Questions 1–3 are based upon the following graph.

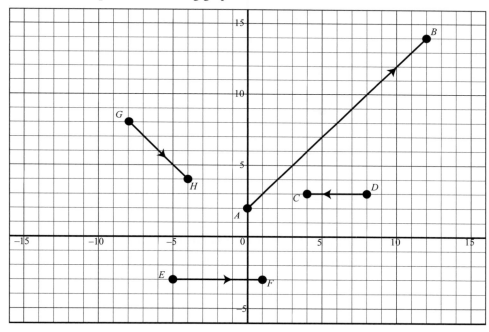

1. What is the magnitude of $\overrightarrow{GH}$?

    A. $2\sqrt{2}$
    B. 4
    C. $4\sqrt{2}$
    D. 6

Here's How to Crack It

Recall that the magnitude of a vector can be found using the formula $GH = \sqrt{\left(GH_x\right)^2 + \left(GH_y\right)^2}$.

Create a right triangle with $\overrightarrow{GH}$ as the hypotenuse to find that $GH_x = 4$ and $GH_y = 4$. Thus, the magnitude of $GH = \sqrt{\left(4\right)^2 + \left(4\right)^2} = \sqrt{32} = 4\sqrt{2}$. The correct answer is (C).

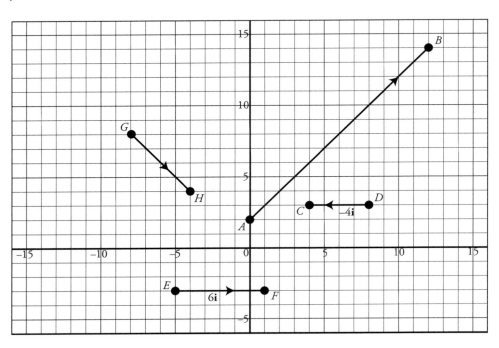

2. Vectors $\overrightarrow{AB}$, $\overleftarrow{DC}$, $\overrightarrow{EF}$, and $\overrightarrow{GH}$ are shown in the standard (x, y) coordinate plane. What is the unit vector notation of $\overrightarrow{AB} + \overrightarrow{EF}$?

    A. 18i + 12j
    B. 12i + 18j
    C. 6i + 12j
    D. 12i + 6j

Here's How to Crack It

In order to solve this question, you need to find the horizontal and vertical components of $\overrightarrow{AB}$ and add it to the horizontal component of $\overrightarrow{EF}$. Create a right triangle with vector $\overrightarrow{AB}$ to find that $\overrightarrow{AX}$ = 12**i** and $\overrightarrow{BX}$ = 12**j**. Accordingly, vector $\overrightarrow{AB}$ = 12**i** + 12**j**. Since vector $\overrightarrow{EF}$ is horizontal, the value is just 6**i** with no **j** value. Therefore, $\overrightarrow{AB}$ + $\overrightarrow{EF}$ = 12**i** + 12**j** + 6**i** = 18**i** + 12**j**, or choice (A).

13.4

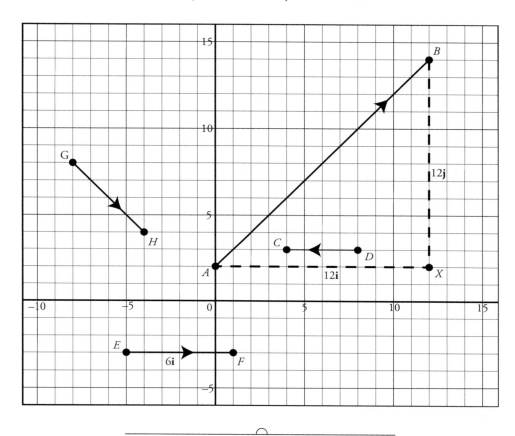

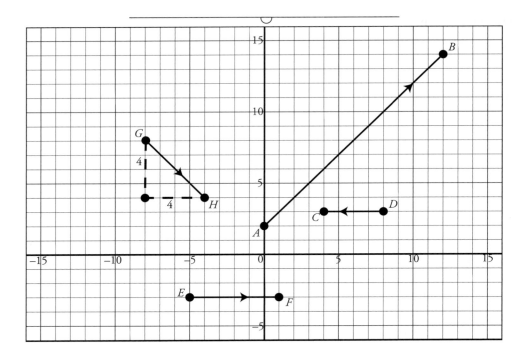

3.   Vectors $\overrightarrow{AB}$, $\overleftarrow{DC}$, $\overrightarrow{EF}$, and $\overrightarrow{GH}$ are shown in the standard (x, y) coordinate plane. What is the unit vector notation of $\overrightarrow{EF} - \overleftarrow{DC}$?

   A.   −2**i**
   B.   2**i**
   C.   8**i**
   D.   10**i**

Here's How to Crack It

In order to solve this question, you need to subtract the horizontal components of $\overleftarrow{DC}$, and from the horizontal component of $\overrightarrow{EF}$. $\overrightarrow{EF}$ has a horizontal component of 6**i**. In addition, $\overleftarrow{DC}$, which is heading in a negative direction, has a value of −4**i**. Therefore, the value of $\overrightarrow{EF} - \overleftarrow{DC}$ is 6**i** − (−4**i**) = 10**i**.

Let's try another question!

—————————————○—————————————

4. Using unit vector notation, $u = x\mathbf{i} + 3\mathbf{j}$, $v = -4\mathbf{i} + y\mathbf{j}$, and $u + v = -8\mathbf{i} + 2\mathbf{j}$. Which of the following is the ordered pair (x, y)?

   A. $(-12, -1)$
   B. $(-3, 4)$
   C. $(-4, -1)$
   D. $(-4, 1)$

13.4

Here's How to Crack It

There is a lot happening in this question, so break it down into bite-sized pieces. You are told that $\mathbf{u} + \mathbf{v} = -8\mathbf{i} + 2\mathbf{j}$. First solve for x using the $\mathbf{u}$ parts of the vector. Therefore, $(x - 4)\mathbf{i} = -8\mathbf{i}$, $x - 4 = -8$, and $x = -4$. Repeat this process to solve for y; $(3 + y)\mathbf{j} = 2\mathbf{j}$, $3 + y = 2$, and $y = -1$. Accordingly, the ordered pair (x, y) is $(-4, -1)$, or choice (C).

—————————————○—————————————

PRECALCULUS DRILL

1. If $\log x^2 + \log 100 = 10$, then what is the value of x ?

    A. 10^3
    B. 10^4
    C. 10^5
    D. 10^6

2. An 81-foot mobile tower is supported by a guy wire. The length of the guy wire is $54\sqrt{3}$ feet. What is the angle made by the guy wire with the ground?

    A. $30°$
    B. $45°$
    C. $60°$
    D. $90°$

3. The pH of a solution is defined by the equation $\text{pH} = -\log x$, where x is the hydrogen ion concentration of the solution in moles per liter. What is the concentration of the hydrogen ion in a cup of coffee with a pH of 5.5 ?

    A. 3.16×10^{-5}
    B. 4.08×10^{-3}
    C. 4.08×10^{3}
    D. 3.16×10^{5}

4. A biologist studies the growth of bacteria in a certain environment created in the laboratory. The biologist starts with an initial bacterial sample of approximately 5,000 bacteria and observes that the population gets doubled after every 1 hour. If the rate of growth of the bacterial population is proportional to the size of the population present at any given time, what would be the population of bacteria after 9 hours?

    A.   405,000
    B.   1,280,000
    C.   2,560,000
    D.   5,120,000

5. Which of the following values is equivalent to the expression $\log_6 2 + \log_6 54 - \log_6 3$?

    A.   2
    B.   6
    C. $4 \log_6 3$
    D. $2 \log_6 18$

6. If $f(x) = x + 2$, $g(x) = \dfrac{5x^2}{x+3}$, and $h(x) = \dfrac{x^3 - 6}{3}$, then

$(f + g - h)(3) =$

    A.   2
    B.   4
    C.   6
    D.   18

7. If $f(x) = 2x^2 + 11x + 15$ and $g(x) = 2x^2 - 3x - 20$, then which of the following expressions is equivalent to $\left(\dfrac{f}{g}\right)(y + 3)$?

    A. $\dfrac{(y+6)}{(y-1)}$

    B. $\dfrac{(y+6)}{(y+7)}$

    C. $\dfrac{(y+6)}{(y+3)}$

    D. $\dfrac{(y+6)}{(y-2)}$

8. Which of the following expressions is equivalent to the expression $\dfrac{1}{2}\left[\log_3 y + 2\log_3(y+4)\right] - \log_3(y-2)$?

    A. $\left[\log_3 \dfrac{y(y+4)}{(y-2)}\right]$

    B. $\left[\log_3 \dfrac{\sqrt{y}(y+4)^2}{(y-2)}\right]$

    C. $\left[\log_3 \dfrac{y(y+4)^2}{(y-2)}\right]$

    D. $\left[\log_3 \dfrac{\sqrt{y}(y+4)}{(y-2)}\right]$

9. If $f(x) = x^2 + 4$ and $g(x) = x - 1$, then which of the following expressions is equivalent to $(f + g)(t - 2)$?

A. $[t^2 - 5t + 5]$
B. $[t^2 + t - 3]$
C. $[t^2 - 3t + 5]$
D. $[t^2 + 5t - 3]$

10. If $f(x) = \dfrac{x}{x+1}$ and $g(x) = x^3$, then $(f \cdot g)(2) + \dfrac{f}{g}(3) =$

A. $\dfrac{11}{12}$

B. $\dfrac{193}{36}$

C. $\dfrac{61}{3}$

D. $\dfrac{307}{12}$.

11. Which of the following expressions is equivalent to $\left(\sqrt{(-3)}\right)^6$?

A. -27
B. $-27i$
C. 27
D. $27i$

12. Which statement describes the characteristics of the exponential function shown below?

$$y = a^{-x}$$

A. The domain is the set of all positive real numbers.
B. The graph is increasing for $a > 1$.
C. The graph does not have a y-intercept.
D. The x-intercept of the graph is at 1.

13. The time, T, in minutes, taken by an airplane to climb to an altitude of h feet is given by $T(h) = 50 \log \dfrac{20,000}{20,000 - h}$, where 20,000 is the maximum height the airplane can reach. What is the equation of the height (h) of the plane as a function of T ?

A. $\dfrac{T}{50}$

B. $20,000 \left(\dfrac{10^{\frac{T}{50}} - 1}{10^{\frac{T}{50}}} \right)$

C. $10^{\frac{T}{50}}$

D. $20,000 \left(10^{\frac{T}{50}} - 1 \right)$

Want More Practice?
Register your book online for more drill questions!

Answers and Explanations

1. **B** Solve the equation as $\log x^2 + \log (10^2) = 10 \Rightarrow 2 \log x + 2 = 10 \Rightarrow 2 \log x = 8 \Rightarrow \log x = 4 \Rightarrow x = 10^4$. The answer is choice (B).

2. **C** Calculate: $\sin\theta = \dfrac{81}{54\sqrt{3}} \Rightarrow \theta = \sin^{-1}\left(\dfrac{81}{54\sqrt{3}}\right) \Rightarrow \theta = 60°$. The answer is choice (C).

3. **A** Substitute 5.5 for pH in the equation and solve for x. Therefore, $5.5 = -\log x \Rightarrow x = 3.16 \times 10^{-5}$. The answer is choice (A).

4. **C** Form the equation as $A(x) = 5{,}000 \times 2^x$ and substitute 9 for x. The answer is choice (C).

5. **A** Simplify the expression: $\log_6 2 + \log_6 54 - \log_6 3 = \log_6\left(\dfrac{2\times54}{3}\right) = \log_6\left(6^2\right) = 2$. The answer is choice (A).

6. **B** Simplify the expression: $(f + g - h)(3) = (3+2) + \left(\dfrac{4\cdot3^2}{3+3}\right) - \left(\dfrac{3^3-6}{3}\right) = 4$. The answer is choice (B).

7. **A** Simplify the expression: $\left(\dfrac{f}{g}\right)(x) = \dfrac{2x^2+11x+15}{2x^2-3x-20} = \dfrac{(x+3)(2x+5)}{(2x+5)(x-4)} = \dfrac{(x+3)}{(x-4)}$

   $\left(\dfrac{f}{g}\right)(y+3) = \dfrac{(y+3+3)}{(y+3-4)} = \dfrac{(y+6)}{(y-1)}$. The answer is choice (A).

8. **D** To solve this problem, calculate as follows:

   $$\frac{1}{2}\left[\log_3 y + 2\log_3(y+4)\right] - \log_3(y-2)$$
   $$= \frac{1}{2}\left[\log_3 y + \log_3(y+4)^2\right] - \log_3(y-2)$$
   $$= \frac{1}{2}\left[\log_3 y(y+4)^2\right] - \log_3(y-2)$$
   $$= \left[\log_3 \frac{y^{\frac{1}{2}}(y+4)^{2\left(\frac{1}{2}\right)}}{(y-2)}\right]$$
   $$= \left[\log_3 \frac{\sqrt{y}(y+4)}{(y-2)}\right]$$

   The answer is choice (D).

9. **C** To solve this problem, calculate as follows: $f(x) = x^2 + 4$, $g(x) = x - 1$. So $(f + g)(x) = (x^2 + 4 + x - 1) = (x^2 + x + 3)$ and $(f+g)(t-2) = [(t-2)^2 + (t-2) + 3] = [t^2 - 4t + 4 + t - 2 + 3] = [t^2 - 3t + 5]$. The answer is choice (C).

10. **B** Evaluate the functions as follows:

$$(f \cdot g)(2) + \frac{f}{g}(3)$$

$$f.g(2) = \frac{2^4}{2+1} = \frac{16}{3}$$

and

$$\frac{f}{g}(3) = \frac{\frac{3}{3+1}}{3^3} = \frac{3}{4} \times \frac{1}{27} = \frac{1}{36}$$

$$\therefore f.g(2) + \frac{f}{g}(3) = \frac{16}{3} + \frac{1}{36} = \frac{192+1}{36} = \frac{193}{36}$$

The answer is choice (B).

11. **A** Solve the expression as follows:

$$\left(\sqrt{(-3)}\right)^6 = \left(\sqrt{3i^2}\right)^6$$
$$= \left(i\sqrt{3}\right)^6$$
$$= \left(i\sqrt{3}\right) \times \left(i\sqrt{3}\right) \times \left(i\sqrt{3}\right) \times \left(i\sqrt{3}\right) \times \left(i\sqrt{3}\right) \times \left(i\sqrt{3}\right)$$
$$= i^6 \times 27$$
$$= (i^2)^3 \times 27$$
$$= -27$$

The answer is (A).

12. **D** The graph intercepts at the point (0, 1). Hence, the x-intercept of the graph is at 1. The answer is choice (D).

13. **B** Calculate as follows:

$$\frac{T}{50} = \log \frac{20,000}{20,000 - h} \text{ gives } 10^{\frac{T}{50}} = \frac{20,000}{20,000 - h}$$

Therefore, $10^{\frac{T}{50}}(20,000 - h) = 20,000$.

$$h = 20,000 \left(1 - \frac{1}{10^{\frac{T}{50}}} \right)$$

$$h = 20,000 \left(\frac{10^{\frac{T}{50}} - 1}{10^{\frac{T}{50}}} \right)$$

The answer is choice (B).

13.5 CALCULUS

Limits of Functions

In order to understand calculus, you need to know what a "limit" is. A limit is the value a function (which usually is written "$f(x)$" on the PCAT) approaches as the variable within that function (usually "x") gets nearer and nearer to a particular value. In other words, when x is very close to a certain number, what is $f(x)$ very close to?

Let's look at an example of a limit. What is the limit of the function $f(x) = x^2$ as x approaches 2? In limit notation, the expression "the limit of $f(x)$ as x approaches 2" is written like this: $\lim_{x \to 2} f(x)$. In order to evaluate the limit, let's check out some values of $\lim_{x \to 2} f(x)$ as x increases and gets closer to 2 (without ever exactly getting there).

> When $x = 1.9$, $f(x) = 3.61$.
> When $x = 1.99$, $f(x) = 3.9601$.
> When $x = 1.999$, $f(x) = 3.996001$.
> When $x = 1.9999$, $f(x) = 3.99960001$.

As x increases and approaches 2, $f(x)$ gets closer and closer to 4. This is called the **left-hand limit** and is written like this: $\lim_{x \to 2^-} f(x)$. Notice the little minus sign!

What about when x is bigger than 2?

> When $x = 2.1$, $f(x) = 4.41$.
> When $x = 2.01$, $f(x) = 4.0401$.
> When $x = 2.001$, $f(x) = 4.004001$.
> When $x = 2.0001$, $f(x) = 4.00040001$.

As x decreases and approaches 2, $f(x)$ still approaches 4. This is called the **right-hand limit** and is written like this: $\lim_{x \to 2^+} f(x)$. Notice the little plus sign!

We got the same answer when evaluating both the left- and right-hand limits, because when x is 2, $f(x)$ is 4. You should always check both sides of the independent variable because, as you'll see shortly, sometimes you don't get the same answer. Therefore, we write that $\lim_{x \to 2} x^2 = 4$.

We didn't really need to look at all of these decimal values to know what was going to happen when x got really close to 2. But it's important to go through the exercise because, typically, the answers get a lot more complicated. Let's do a few examples.

Example 1: Find $\lim_{x \to 5} x^2$.

The approach is simple: plug in 5 for x, and you get 25.

Example 2: Find $\lim_{x \to 3} x^3$.

Here, the answer is 27.

There are some simple algebraic rules of limits that you should know.

$$\lim_{x \to a} kf(x) = k \lim_{x \to a} f(x)$$

Example: $\lim_{x \to 5} 3x^2 = 3 \lim_{x \to 5} x^2 = 75$

$$\text{If } \lim_{x \to a} f(x) = L_1 \text{ and } \lim_{x \to a} g(x) = L_2 \text{, then}$$

$$\lim_{x \to a} [f(x) + g(x)] = L_1 + L_2$$

Example: $\lim_{x \to 5} \left[x^2 + x^3 \right] = \lim_{x \to 5} x^2 + \lim_{x \to 5} x^3 = 150$

$$\text{If } \lim_{x \to a} f(x) = L_1 \text{ and } \lim_{x \to a} g(x) = L_2 \text{, then}$$

$$\lim_{x \to a} [f(x) \cdot g(x)] = L_1 \cdot L_2$$

Example: $\lim_{x \to 5} \left[(x^2 + 1)\sqrt{x-1} \right] = \lim_{x \to 5} (x^2 + 1) \lim_{x \to 5} \sqrt{x-1} = 52$

Example 3: Find $\lim_{x \to 0} (x^2 + 5x)$.

Plug in 0, and you get 0.

So far, so good. All you do to find the limit of a simple polynomial is plug in the number that the variable is approaching and see what the answer is. Naturally, the process can get messier—especially if x approaches zero.

Example 4: Find $\lim_{x \to 0} \dfrac{1}{x^2}$.

If you plug in some very small values for x, you'll see that this function approaches ∞. And it doesn't matter whether x is positive or negative, you still get ∞. Look at the graph of $y = \dfrac{1}{x^2}$:

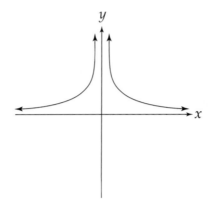

On either side of $x = 0$ (the y-axis), the curve approaches ∞.

Example 5: Find $\lim_{x \to 0} \dfrac{1}{x}$.

Here you have a problem. If you plug in some very small positive values for x (0.1, 0.01, 0.001, and so on), you approach ∞. In other words, $\lim_{x \to 0^+} \dfrac{1}{x} = \infty$. But, if you plug in some very small negative values for x (−0.1, −0.01, −0.001, and so on), you approach $-\infty$. That is, $\lim_{x \to 0^-} \dfrac{1}{x} = -\infty$. Because the right-hand limit is not equal to the left-hand limit, the limit does not exist.

Look at the graph of $\dfrac{1}{x}$.

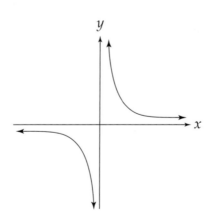

You can see that on the left side of $x = 0$, the curve approaches $-\infty$, and on the right side of $x = 0$, the curve approaches ∞. There are some very important points that we need to emphasize from the last two examples.

Why do we state the limit in Example 4 but not for Example 5? Because when we have $\dfrac{k}{x^2}$, the function is always positive no matter what the sign of x is and thus the function has the same limit from the left and the right. But when we have $\dfrac{k}{x}$, the function's sign depends on the sign of x, and you get a different limit from each side.

13.5

Let's look at an example. Consider the function g given as follows:

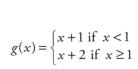

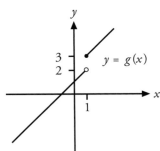

$y = g(x)$

Then, as its graph shows,

$$\lim_{x \to 1-} g(x) = 2 \qquad \text{but} \qquad \lim_{x \to 1+} g(x) = 3$$

Since the left-hand limit at 1 is not equal to the right-hand limit at 1, the limit of $g(x)$ as x approaches 1 does not exist.

Let's look at a few examples in which the independent variable approaches infinity.

Example 6: Find $\lim\limits_{x \to \infty} \dfrac{1}{x}$.

As x gets bigger and bigger, the value of the function gets smaller and smaller. Therefore, $\lim\limits_{x \to \infty} \dfrac{1}{x} = 0$.

Example 7: Find $\lim\limits_{x \to -\infty} \dfrac{1}{x}$.

It's the same situation as the one in Example 6; as x decreases (approaches negative infinity), the value of the function increases (approaches zero). We write the following:

$$\lim_{x \to -\infty} \dfrac{1}{x} = 0$$

---

(1) If the left-hand limit of a function is not equal to the right-hand limit of the function, then the limit does not exist.

(2) A limit equal to infinity is not the same as a limit that does not exist, but sometimes you will see the expression "no limit," which serves both purposes. If $\lim\limits_{x \to a} f(x) = \infty$, the limit, technically, does not exist.

(3) If k is a positive constant, then $\lim\limits_{x \to 0^+} \dfrac{k}{x} = \infty$, $\lim\limits_{x \to 0^-} \dfrac{k}{x} = -\infty$, and $\lim\limits_{x \to 0} \dfrac{k}{x}$ does not exist.

(4) If k is a positive constant, then

$$\lim_{x \to 0^+} \dfrac{k}{x^2} = \infty, \ \lim_{x \to 0^-} \dfrac{k}{x^2} = \infty, \ \text{and}$$

$$\lim_{x \to 0} \dfrac{k}{x^2} = \infty.$$

We don't have the same problem here that we did when x approached zero because "positive zero" is the same thing as "negative zero," whereas positive infinity is different from negative infinity.

Here's another rule:

> If k and n are constants, $|x| > 1$, and $n > 0$, then $\lim\limits_{x \to \infty} \dfrac{k}{x^n} = 0$, and $\lim\limits_{x \to -\infty} \dfrac{k}{x^n} = 0$.

Example 8: Find $\lim\limits_{x \to \infty} \dfrac{3x + 5}{7x - 2}$.

When you have variables in both the top and the bottom, you can't just plug ∞ into the expression. You'll get $\dfrac{\infty}{\infty}$. We solve this by using the following technique:

> When an expression consists of a polynomial divided by another polynomial, divide each term of the numerator and the denominator by the highest power of x that appears in the expression.

The highest power of x in this case is x^1, so we divide every term in the expression (both top and bottom) by x, like so:

$$\lim_{x \to \infty} \frac{3x + 5}{7x - 2} = \lim_{x \to \infty} \frac{\dfrac{3x}{x} + \dfrac{5}{x}}{\dfrac{7x}{x} - \dfrac{2}{x}} = \lim_{x \to \infty} \frac{3 + \dfrac{5}{x}}{7 - \dfrac{2}{x}}$$

Now when we take the limit, the two terms containing x approach zero. We're left with $\dfrac{3}{7}$.

Example 9: Find $\lim\limits_{x \to \infty} \dfrac{8x^2 - 4x + 1}{16x^2 + 7x - 2}$.

Remember to focus your attention on the highest power of x.

Divide each term by x^2. You get

$$\lim_{x \to \infty} \frac{8 - \dfrac{4}{x} + \dfrac{1}{x^2}}{16 + \dfrac{7}{x} - \dfrac{2}{x^2}} = \frac{8}{16} = \frac{1}{2}$$

Example 10: Find $\displaystyle\lim_{x\to\infty} \frac{-3x^{10} - 70x^5 + x^3}{33x^{10} + 200x^8 - 1,000x^4}$.

Divide each term by x^{10} .

$$\lim_{x\to\infty} \frac{-3x^{10} - 70x^5 + x^3}{33x^{10} + 200x^8 - 1,000x^4} = \lim_{x\to\infty} \frac{-3 - \dfrac{70}{x^5} + \dfrac{1}{x^7}}{33 + \dfrac{200}{x^2} - \dfrac{1,000}{x^6}} = -\frac{3}{33} = -\frac{1}{11}$$

The other powers don't matter because they're all going to disappear. Now we have three new rules for evaluating the limit of a rational expression as x approaches infinity.

> (1)　If the highest power of x in a rational expression is in the numerator, then the limit as x approaches infinity is infinity.

Example: $\displaystyle\lim_{x\to\infty} \frac{5x^7 - 3x}{16x^6 - 3x^2} = \infty$

> (2)　If the highest power of x in a rational expression is in the denominator, then the limit as x approaches infinity is zero.

Example: $\displaystyle\lim_{x\to\infty} \frac{5x^6 - 3x}{16x^7 - 3x^2} = 0$

> (3)　If the highest power of x in a rational expression is the same in both the numerator and denominator, then the limit as x approaches infinity is the coefficient of the highest term in the numerator divided by the coefficient of the highest term in the denominator.

Example: $\displaystyle\lim_{x\to\infty} \frac{5x^7 - 3x}{16x^7 - 3x^2} = \frac{5}{16}$

Continuous Functions

In order for a function $f(x)$ to be continuous at a point $x = c$, it must fulfill *all three* of the following conditions:

Condition 1: $f(c)$ exists.

Condition 2: $\lim\limits_{x \to c} f(x)$ exists.

Condition 3: $\lim\limits_{x \to c} f(x) = f(c)$

Let's look at a simple example of a continuous function.

Example 1: Is the function $f(x) = \begin{cases} x + 1, & x < 2 \\ 2x - 1, & x \geq 2 \end{cases}$ continuous at the point $x = 2$?

Condition 1: Does $f(2)$ exist?

Yes. It's equal to $2(2) - 1 = 3$.

Condition 2: Does $\lim\limits_{x \to 2} f(x)$ exist?

You need to look at the limit from both sides of 2. The left-hand limit is $\lim\limits_{x \to 2^-} f(x) = 2 + 1 = 3$. The right-hand limit is $\lim\limits_{x \to 2^+} f(x) = 2(2) - 1 = 3$.

Because the two limits are the same, the limit exists.

Condition 3: Does $\lim\limits_{x \to 2} f(x) = f(2)$?

The two equal each other, so yes; the function is continuous at $x = 2$.

A simple and important way to check whether a function is continuous is to sketch the function. If you can't sketch the function without lifting your pencil from the paper at some point, then the function is not continuous.

Now let's look at some examples of functions that are not continuous.

Polynomials are continuous for all reals in their domains.

Example 2: Is the function $f(x) = \begin{cases} x + 1, & x < 2 \\ 2x - 1, & x > 2 \end{cases}$ continuous at $x = 2$?

Condition 1: Does $f(2)$ exist?

Nope. The function of x is defined if x is greater than or less than 2, but not if x is equal to 2. Therefore, the function is not continuous at $x = 2$. Notice that we don't have to bother with the other two conditions. Once you find a problem, the function is automatically not continuous, and you can stop.

Example 3: Is the function $f(x) = \begin{cases} x+1, & x < 2 \\ 2x+1, & x \geq 2 \end{cases}$ continuous at $x = 2$?

Condition 1: Does $f(x)$ exist?

Yes. It is equal to $2(2) + 1 = 5$.

Condition 2: Does $\lim_{x \to 2} f(x)$ exist?

The left-hand limit is $\lim_{x \to 2^-} f(x) = 2 + 1 = 3$.

The right-hand limit is $\lim_{x \to 2^+} f(x) = 2(2) + 1 = 5$.

The two limits don't match, so the limit doesn't exist and the function is not continuous at $x = 2$.

13.5

Example 4: Is the function $f(x) = \begin{cases} x+1, & x < 2 \\ x^2, & x = 2 \\ 2x-1, & x > 2 \end{cases}$ continuous at $x = 2$?

Condition 1: Does $f(2)$ exist?

Yes. It's equal to $2^2 = 4$.

Condition 2: Does $\lim_{x \to 2} f(x)$ exist?

The left-hand limit is $\lim_{x \to 2^-} f(x) = 2 + 1 = 3$.

The right-hand limit is $\lim_{x \to 2^+} f(x) = 2(2) - 1 = 3$.

Because the two limits are the same, the limit exists.

Condition 3: Does $\lim_{x \to 2} f(x) = f(2)$?

The $\lim_{x \to 2} f(x) = 3$, but $f(2) = 4$. Because these aren't equal, the answer is "no" and the function is not continuous at $x = 2$.

Discontinuities

There are four types of discontinuities you have to know: jump, point, essential, and removable.

> A **jump** discontinuity occurs when the curve "breaks" at a particular place and starts somewhere else. In other words, $\lim_{x \to a^-} f(x) \neq \lim_{x \to a^+} f(x)$.

An example of jump discontinuity looks like this.

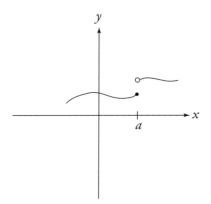

Intermediate Learning

The Intermediate Value Theorem says that if a function is continuous on the interval [a, b], then for any value c in the interval [a, b], there exists a value f(c) between f(a) and f(b) inclusive. In other words, if the function is continuous in some interval, then all of the possible values of f between the two end values of f exist in that interval.

A **point** discontinuity occurs when the curve has a "hole" in it from a missing point because the function has a value at that point that is "off the curve." In other words, $\lim_{x \to a} f(x) \neq f(a)$.

Here's what a point discontinuity looks like.

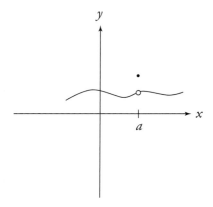

An **essential** discontinuity occurs when the curve has a vertical asymptote.

This is an example of an essential discontinuity.

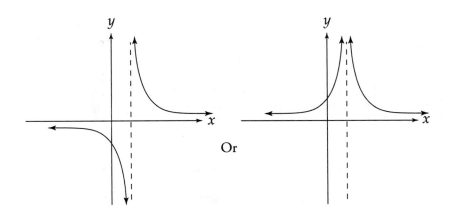

Or

> A **removable** discontinuity occurs when you have a rational expression with common factors in the numerator and denominator. Because these factors can be canceled, the discontinuity is "removable."

Here's an example of a removable discontinuity.

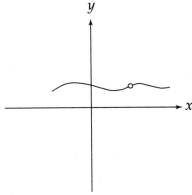

Now that you know what these four types of discontinuities look like, let's see what types of functions are not everywhere continuous.

Example 5: Consider the following function:

$$f(x) = \begin{cases} x + 3, & x \le 2 \\ x^2, & x > 2 \end{cases}$$

The left-hand limit is 5 as x approaches 2, and the right-hand limit is 4 as x approaches 2. Because the curve has different values on each side of 2, the curve is discontinuous at $x = 2$. We say that the curve "jumps" at $x = 2$ from the left-hand curve to the right-hand curve because the left- and right-hand limits differ. It looks like the following:

> This curve looks very similar to a point discontinuity, but notice that with a removable discontinuity, $f(x)$ is not defined at the point, whereas with a point discontinuity, $f(x)$ is defined there.

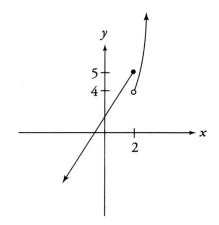

This is an example of a jump discontinuity.

Example 6: Consider the following function:

$$f(x) = \begin{cases} x^2, & x \ne 2 \\ 5, & x = 2 \end{cases}$$

Because $\lim\limits_{x \to 2} f(x) \ne f(2)$, the function is discontinuous at $x = 2$. The curve is continuous everywhere except at the point $x = 2$. It looks like the following:

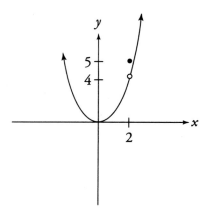

This is an example of a point discontinuity.

Example 7: Consider the following function: $f(x) = \dfrac{5}{x-2}$.

The function is discontinuous because it's possible for the denominator to equal zero (at $x = 2$). This means that $f(2)$ doesn't exist, and the function has an asymptote at $x = 2$. In addition, $\lim\limits_{x \to 2^-} f(x) = -\infty$ and $\lim\limits_{x \to 2^+} f(x) = \infty$.

The graph looks like the following:

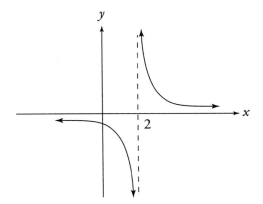

This is an example of an essential discontinuity.

Example 8: Consider the following function:

$$f(x) = \frac{x^2 - 8x + 15}{x^2 - 6x + 5}$$

If you factor the top and bottom, you can see where the discontinuities are.

$$f(x) = \frac{x^2 - 8x + 15}{x^2 - 6x + 5} = \frac{(x-3)(x-5)}{(x-1)(x-5)}$$

The function has a zero in the denominator when $x = 1$ or $x = 5$, so the function is discontinuous at those two points. But you can cancel the term $(x - 5)$ from both the numerator and the denominator, leaving you with

$$f(x) = \frac{x-3}{x-1}$$

Now the reduced function *is* continuous at $x = 5$. Thus, the original function has a removable discontinuity at $x = 5$. Furthermore, if you now plug $x = 5$ into the reduced function, you get

$$f(5) = \frac{2}{4} = \frac{1}{2}$$

The discontinuity is at $x = 5$, and there's a hole at $\left(5, \dfrac{1}{2}\right)$. In other words, if the original function were continuous at $x = 5$, it would have the value $\dfrac{1}{2}$. Notice that this is the same as $\lim\limits_{x \to 5} f(x)$.

These are the types of discontinuities that you can expect to encounter on the PCAT. Here are some sample problems and their solutions. Cover the answers as you work; then check your results.

PROBLEM 1. Is the function $f(x) = \begin{cases} 2x^3 - 1, & x < 2 \\ 6x - 3, & x \geq 2 \end{cases}$ continuous at $x = 2$?

Answer: Test the conditions necessary for continuity.

Condition 1: $f(2) = 9$, so we're okay so far.

Condition 2: The $\lim\limits_{x \to 2^-} f(x) = 15$ and the $\lim\limits_{x \to 2^+} f(x) = 9$. These two limits don't agree, so the $\lim\limits_{x \to 2} f(x)$ doesn't exist and the function is not continuous at $x = 2$.

PROBLEM 2. Is the function $f(x) = \begin{cases} x^2 + 3x + 5, & x < 1 \\ 6x + 3, & x \geq 1 \end{cases}$ continuous at $x = 1$?

Answer: Condition 1: $f(1) = 9$.

Condition 2: The $\lim\limits_{x \to 1^-} f(x) = 9$ and the $\lim\limits_{x \to 1^+} f(x) = 9$.

Therefore, the $\lim\limits_{x \to 1} f(x)$ exists and is equal to 9.

Condition 3: $\lim\limits_{x \to 1} f(x) = f(1) = 9$.

The function satisfies all three conditions, so it is continuous at $x = 1$.

PROBLEM 3. For what value of a is the function $f(x) = \begin{cases} ax + 5, & x < 4 \\ x^2 - x, & x \geq 4 \end{cases}$ continuous at $x = 4$?

Answer: Because $f(4) = 12$, the function passes the first condition.

For Condition 2 to be satisfied, the $\lim\limits_{x \to 4^-} f(x) = 4a + 5$ must equal the $\lim\limits_{x \to 4^+} f(x) = 12$. So set $4a + 5 = 12$. If $a = \dfrac{7}{4}$, the limit will exist at $x = 4$ and the other two conditions will also be fulfilled. Therefore, the value $a = \dfrac{7}{4}$ makes the function continuous at $x = 4$.

PROBLEM 4. Where does the function $f(x) = \dfrac{2x^2 - 7x - 15}{x^2 - x - 20}$ have (a) an essential discontinuity and (b) a removable discontinuity?

Answer: If you factor the top and bottom of this fraction, you get

$$f(x) = \frac{2x^2 - 7x - 15}{x^2 - x - 20} = \frac{(2x + 3)(x - 5)}{(x + 4)(x - 5)}$$

Thus, the function has an essential discontinuity at $x = -4$. If we then cancel the term $(x - 5)$, and substitute $x = 5$ into the reduced expression, we get $f(5) = \dfrac{13}{9}$. Therefore, the function has a removable discontinuity at $\left(5, \dfrac{13}{9}\right)$.

Let's look at some examples. The functions whose graphs are shown below are continuous at all points except at $x = 1$, but the reason that f fails to be continuous at $x = 1$ is different in each case.

13.5

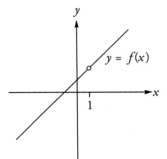

$$f(x) = \frac{x^2 - 1}{x - 1}$$

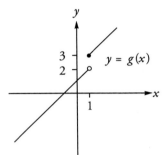

$$g(x) = \begin{cases} x + 1 & \text{if } x < 1 \\ x + 2 & \text{if } x \geq 1 \end{cases}$$

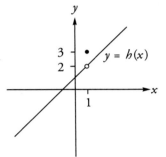

$$h(x) = \begin{cases} x + 1 & \text{if } x \neq 1 \\ 3 & \text{if } x = 1 \end{cases}$$

The function f is discontinuous at $x = 1$ because f is not defined at this point. The function g is discontinuous at $x = 1$ because, even though g is defined at $x = 1$, $\lim_{x \to 1} g(x)$ does not exist (since the left-hand limit at 1 is not equal to the right-hand limit at 1, as we saw above). Finally, the function h is discontinuous at $x = 1$ because, although h is defined at $x = 1$ and $\lim_{x \to 1} h(x)$ exists (it's equal to 2), the value of h at $x = 1$ is 3, so $\lim_{x \to 1} h(x) \neq h(1)$.

Note: Don't confuse coordinate parentheses with interval notation. In interval notation, square brackets include endpoints and parentheses do not. For example, the interval $2 \leq x \leq 4$ is written $[2, 4]$ and the interval $2 < x < 4$ is written $(2, 4)$.

13.5

The list below summarizes some important properties of continuous functions.

1. The following functions are continuous everywhere:
   Every constant function, $f(x) = k$
   Every polynomial function, $f(x) = a_n x^n + a_{n-1} x^{n-1} + \cdots + a_1 x + a_0$
   Every exponential function, $f(x) = k^x$ (with $k > 0$)
2. The following functions are continuous everywhere they're defined:
   Every function of the form $f(x) = x^r$, where r is a rational number
   The logarithm function, $f(x) = \log x$
3. If the functions f and g are both continuous at a, then each of the following functions is also continuous at a:
   $f + g$
   $f - g$
   fg
   $\dfrac{f}{g}$ (provided that $g(a) \neq 0$)
4. If f is continuous at a and g is continuous at $f(a)$, then the composite function $g \circ f$ is continuous at $x = a$.

The Derivative

The best way to understand the definition of the derivative is to start by looking at the simplest continuous function: a line. As you should recall, you can determine the slope of a line by taking two points on that line and plugging them into the slope formula.

$$m = \frac{y_2 - y_1}{x_2 - x_1}$$
m stands for slope.

For example, suppose a line goes through the points (3, 7) and (8, 22). First, you subtract the y-coordinates

$(22 - 7) = 15$. Next, subtract the corresponding x-coordinates $(8 - 3) = 5$. Finally, divide the first number by the

second: $\dfrac{15}{5} = 3$. The result is the slope of the line: $m = 3$.

Let's look at the graph of that line. The slope measures the steepness of the line, which looks like the following:

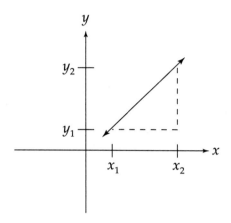

Notice that you can use the coordinates in reverse order and still get the same result. It doesn't matter in which order you do the subtraction as long as you're consistent.

You probably remember your teachers referring to the slope as the "rise" over the "run." The rise is the difference between the y-coordinates, and the run is the difference between the x-coordinates. The slope is the ratio of the two.

Now for a few changes in notation. Instead of calling the x-coordinates x_1 and x_2, we're going to call them x_1 and $x_1 + h$, where h is the difference between the two x-coordinates. Second, instead of using y_1 and y_2, we use $f(x_1)$ and $f(x_1 + h)$. So now the graph looks like the following:

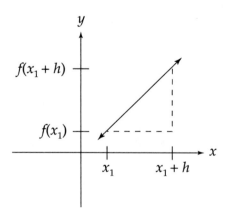

The picture is exactly the same—only the notation has changed.

The Slope of a Curve

Suppose that instead of finding the slope of a line, we wanted to find the slope of a curve. Here, the slope formula no longer works because the distance from one point to the other is along a curve, not a straight line. But we could find the approximate slope if we took the slope of the line between the two points. This is called the **secant line**.

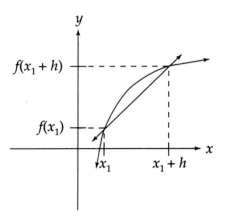

The formula for the slope of the secant line is

$$\frac{f(x_1 + h) - f(x_1)}{h}$$

Remember this formula! This is called the **Difference Quotient**.

The Secant and the Tangent

As you can see, the farther apart the two points are, the less the slope of the line corresponds to the slope of the curve.

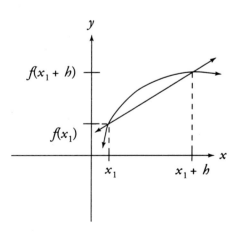

Conversely, the closer the two points are, the more accurate the approximation is.

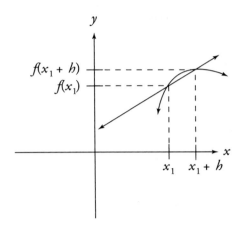

In fact, there is one line, called the **tangent line**, that touches the curve at exactly one point. The slope of the tangent line is equal to the slope of the curve at exactly this point. The object of using the above formula, therefore, is to shrink h down to an infinitesimally small amount. If we could do that, then the difference between $(x_1 + h)$ and x_1 would be a point.

Keep in mind that there are infinitely many tangents for any curve because there are infinitely many points on the curve.

Graphically, it looks like the following:

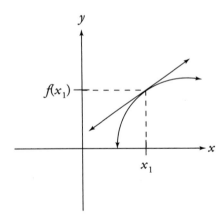

How do we perform this shrinking act? We set up a limit during which h approaches zero, like the following:

$$\lim_{h \to 0} \frac{f(x_1 + h) - f(x_1)}{h}$$

This is the **definition of the derivative**, and we call it $f'(x)$.

Notice that the equation is just a slightly modified version of the difference quotient, with different notation. The only difference is that we're finding the slope between two points that are infinitesimally close to each other.

Example 1: Find the slope of the curve $f(x) = x^2$ at the point $(2, 4)$.

This means that $x_1 = 2$ and $f(2) = 2^2 = 4$. If we can figure out $f(x_1 + h)$, then we can find the slope. Well, how did we find the value of $f(x)$? We plugged x_1 into the equation $f(x) = x^2$. To find $f(x_1 + h)$, we plug $x_1 + h$ into the equation, which now looks like this

$$f(x_1 + h) = (2 + h)^2 = 4 + 4h + h^2$$

Now plug this into the slope formula.

$$\lim_{h \to 0} \frac{f(x_1 + h) - f(x_1)}{h} = \lim_{h \to 0} \frac{4 + 4h + h^2 - 4}{h} = \lim_{h \to 0} \frac{4h + h^2}{h}$$

Next, simplify by factoring h out of the top.

$$\lim_{h \to 0} \frac{4h + h^2}{h} = \lim_{h \to 0} \frac{h(4 + h)}{h} = \lim_{h \to 0}(4 + h)$$

Taking the limit as h approaches 0, we get 4. Therefore, the slope of the curve $y = x^2$ at the point $(2, 4)$ is 4. Now we've found the slope of a curve at a certain point, and the notation looks like this: $f'(2) = 4$. Remember this notation!

Example 2: Find the derivative of the equation in Example 1 at the point $(5, 25)$. This means that $x_1 = 5$ and $f(x) = 25$. This time,

$$(x_1 + h)^2 = (5 + h)^2 = 25 + 10h + h^2$$

Now plug this into the formula for the derivative.

$$\lim_{h \to 0} \frac{f(x_1 + h) - f(x_1)}{h} = \lim_{h \to 0} \frac{25 + 10h + h^2 - 25}{h} = \lim_{h \to 0} \frac{10h + h^2}{h}$$

Once again, simplify by factoring h out of the top.

$$\lim_{h \to 0} \frac{10h + h^2}{h} = \lim_{h \to 0} \frac{h(10 + h)}{h} = \lim_{h \to 0}(10 + h)$$

Taking the limit as h goes to 0, you get 10. Therefore, the slope of the curve $y = x^2$ at the point (5, 25) is 10, or: $f'(5) = 10$.

Using this pattern, let's forget about the arithmetic for a second and derive a formula.

Example 3: Find the slope of the equation $f(x) = x^2$ at the point $\left(x_1, x_1^2\right)$.

Follow the steps in the last two problems, but instead of using a number, use x_1. This means that $f(x_1) = x_1^2$ and $(x_1 + h)^2 = x_1^2 + 2x_1h + h^2$. Then the derivative is

$$\lim_{h \to 0} \frac{x_1^2 + 2x_1h + h^2 - x_1^2}{h} = \lim_{h \to 0} \frac{2x_1h + h^2}{h}$$

13.5

Factor h out of the top.

$$\lim_{h \to 0} \frac{h(2x_1 + h)}{h} = \lim_{h \to 0}(2x_1 + h)$$

Now take the limit as h goes to 0: you get $2x_1$. Therefore, $f'(x_1) = 2x_1$.

This example gives us a general formula for the derivative of this curve. Now we can pick any point, plug it into the formula, and determine the slope at that point. For example, the derivative at the point $x = 7$ is 14. At the point $x = \dfrac{7}{3}$, the derivative is $\dfrac{14}{3}$.

Differentiability

One of the important requirements for the differentiability of a function is that the function be continuous. But, even if a function is continuous at a point, the function is not necessarily differentiable there. Check out the graph below.

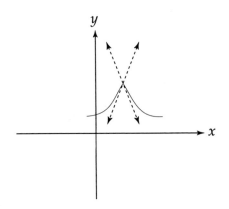

If a function has a "sharp corner," you can draw more than one tangent line at that point, and because the slopes of these tangent lines are not equal, the function is not differentiable there.

Another possible problem occurs when the tangent line is vertical (which can occur at a cusp, or point on a continuous function where the derivative function does not exist) because a vertical line has an infinite slope. For example, if the derivative of a function is $\dfrac{1}{x+1}$, it doesn't have a derivative at $x = -1$.

13.5

Try these problems on your own; then check your work against the answers immediately beneath each problem.

PROBLEM 1. Find the derivative of $f(x) = 3x^2$ at $(4, 48)$.

Answer: $f(4 + h) = 3(4 + h)^2 = 48 + 24h + 3h^2$. Use the definition of the derivative.

$$f'(4) = \lim_{h \to 0} \frac{48 + 24h + 3h^2 - 48}{h}$$

Simplify.

$$\lim_{h \to 0} \frac{24h + 3h^2}{h} = \lim_{h \to 0}(24 + 3h) = 24$$

The slope of the curve at the point $(4, 48)$ is 24.

PROBLEM 2. Find the derivative of $f(x) = 3x^2$.

Answer: $f(x + h) = 3(x + h)^2 = 3x^2 + 6xh + 3h^2$. Use the definition of the derivative.

$$f'(x) = \lim_{h \to 0} \frac{3x^2 + 6xh + 3h^2 - 3x^2}{h}$$

Simplify.

$$\lim_{h \to 0} \frac{6xh + 3h^2}{h} = \lim_{h \to 0}(6x + 3h) = 6x$$

The derivative is $6x$.

PROBLEM 3. Find the derivative of $f(x) = x^3$.

Answer: $f(x + h) = (x + h)^3 = x^3 + 3x^2h + 3xh^2 + h^3$. First, use the definition of the derivative.

$$f'(x) = \lim_{h \to 0} \frac{x^3 + 3x^2h + 3xh^2 + h^3 - x^3}{h}$$

And simplify.

$$\lim_{h \to 0} \frac{3x^2 h + 3xh^2 + h^3}{h} = \lim_{h \to 0} \left(3x^2 + 3xh + h^2\right) = 3x^2$$

The derivative is $3x^2$.

This next one will test your algebraic skills. Don't say we didn't warn you!

PROBLEM 4. Find the derivative of $f(x) = \sqrt{x}$.

Answer: $f(x + h) = \sqrt{x + h}$.

Use the definition of the derivative.

$$f'(x) = \lim_{h \to 0} \frac{\sqrt{x + h} - \sqrt{x}}{h}$$

Notice that this one doesn't cancel as conveniently as the other problems did. In order to simplify this expression, we have to multiply both the top and the bottom of the expression by $\sqrt{x + h} + \sqrt{x}$ (the conjugate of the numerator).

$$f'(x) = \lim_{h \to 0} \frac{\sqrt{x + h} - \sqrt{x}}{h}\left(\frac{\sqrt{x + h} + \sqrt{x}}{\sqrt{x + h} + \sqrt{x}}\right) = \lim_{h \to 0} \frac{x + h - x}{h\left(\sqrt{x + h} + \sqrt{x}\right)} = \lim_{h \to 0} \frac{h}{h\left(\sqrt{x + h} + \sqrt{x}\right)}$$

Simplify.

$$\lim_{h \to 0} \frac{1}{\left(\sqrt{x + h} + \sqrt{x}\right)} = \frac{1}{2\sqrt{x}}$$

The derivative is $\dfrac{1}{2\sqrt{x}}$.

We've used a prime symbol (′) to denote the derivative of a function. Another very common notation for derivatives of functions is called **Leibniz notation**. The difference quotient used in the definition of the derivative is a change in f divided by a change in x; that is, we can write

$$f'(x) = \lim_{\Delta x \to 0} \frac{f(x + \Delta x) - f(x)}{\Delta x} = \lim_{\Delta x \to 0} \frac{\Delta f}{\Delta x} = \frac{df}{dx}$$

There are several different notations for derivatives in calculus. We'll use two different types interchangeably throughout this book, so get used to them now.

13.5

We'll refer to functions three different ways: $f(x)$, u or v, and y. For example, we might write $f(x) = x^3$, $g(x) = x^4$, $h(x) = x^5$. We'll also use notation like $u = \sin x$ and $v = \cos x$. Or we might use $y = \sqrt{x}$. Usually, we pick the notation that causes the least confusion.

The derivatives of the functions will use notation that depends on the function, as shown in the following table:

Function	First Derivative	Second Derivative
$f(x)$	$f'(x)$	$f''(x)$
$g(x)$	$g'(x)$	$g''(x)$
y	y' or $\dfrac{dy}{dx}$	y'' or $\dfrac{d^2y}{dx^2}$

In addition, if we refer to a derivative of a function in general (for example, $ax^2 + bx + c$), we might enclose the expression in parentheses and use either of the following notations:

$$\left(ax^2 + bx + c\right)', \text{ or } \frac{d}{dx}\left(ax^2 + bx + c\right)$$

Sometimes math books refer to a derivative using either D_x or f_x. We're not going to use either of them.

When we want to find the derivative of a function, we usually use a table of standard derivatives and rules that make the computation easy, rather than going back to the definition every time. Following is a list of rules, all of which can be proved directly from the definition of a derivative. You should memorize these rules for the PCAT.

Rules of Derivatives

1. *Derivative of a sum*
   The derivative of a sum is the sum of the derivatives: $(f+g)'(x) = f'(x) + g'(x)$

2. *Derivative of a constant times a function:* $(kf)'(x) = kf'(x)$

3. *Derivative of a product*
   The **product rule** says that $(fg)'(x) = f(x)g'(x) + f'(x)g(x)$

4. *Derivative of a quotient*
   The **quotient rule** says that $\left(\dfrac{f}{g}\right)'(x) = \dfrac{g(x)f'(x) - f(x)g'(x)}{[g(x)]^2}$

5. *Derivative of a composite function*
   The **chain rule** says that $(f \circ u)'(x) = f'(u(x)) \bullet u'(x)$

6. *Derivative of an inverse function*

   The **inverse-function rule** says that if f^{-1} is the inverse of f, and f

   has a nonzero derivative at x_0, then f^{-1} has a derivative at

   $y_0 = f(x_0)$, and $(f^{-1})'(y_0) = \dfrac{1}{f'(x_0)}$.

In the list below, k is any constant, a is any positive constant, and u is any differentiable function.

There are also a bunch of specialized derivative rules that you should also memorize!

$$d(k) = 0$$
$$d(u^k) = ku^{k-1}\,du$$
$$d(e^u) = e^u\,du$$
$$d(a^u) = (\log a)\,a^u\,du$$
$$d(\log u) = \frac{1}{u}\,du$$
$$d(\log_a u) = \frac{1}{(u \log a)}\,du \ (a \neq 1)$$
$$d(\sin u) = \cos u\,du$$

$$d(\cos u) = -\sin u\,du$$
$$d(\tan u) = \sec^2 u\,du$$
$$d(\cot u) = -\csc^2 u\,du$$
$$d(\sec u) = \sec u \tan u\,du$$
$$d(\csc u) = -\csc u \cot u\,du$$
$$d(\arcsin u) = \frac{du}{\sqrt{1-u^2}}$$
$$d(\arctan u) = \frac{du}{1+u^2}$$

The Power Rule

In the previous section, you learned how to find a derivative using the definition of the derivative, a process that is very time-consuming and sometimes involves a lot of complex algebra. Fortunately, there's a shortcut to taking derivatives, so you'll never have to use the definition again—except when it's a question on an exam!

The basic technique for taking a derivative is called the **Power Rule**.

13.5

> Rule No. 1: If $y = x^n$, then $\dfrac{dy}{dx} = nx^{n-1}$

Notice that when the power of the function is negative, the power of the derivative is more negative.

That's it. Wasn't that simple? Of course, this and all of the following rules can be derived easily from the definition of the derivative. Look at these next few examples of the Power Rule in action.

Example 1: If $y = x^5$, then $\dfrac{dy}{dx} = 5x^4$.

Example 2: If $y = x^{20}$, then $\dfrac{dy}{dx} = 20x^{19}$.

Example 3: If $f(x) = x^{-5}$, then $f'(x) = -5x^{-6}$.

When the power is a fraction, you should be careful to get the subtraction right [you'll see the powers 1/2, 1/3, 3/2, –1/2, and –1/3 often, so be comfortable with subtracting 1 from them].

Example 4: If $u = x^{\frac{1}{2}}$, then $\dfrac{du}{dx} = \dfrac{1}{2}x^{-\frac{1}{2}}$.

Example 5: If $y = x^1$, then $\dfrac{dy}{dx} = 1x^0 = 1$. (Because x^0 is 1!)

Example 6: If $y = x^0$, then $\dfrac{dy}{dx} = 0$.

This leads to the next three rules.

When the power is 1, the derivative is just a constant. When the power is 0, the derivative is 0.

> Rule No. 2: If $y = x$, then $\dfrac{dy}{dx} = 1$
>
> Rule No. 3: If $y = kx$, then $\dfrac{dy}{dx} = k$ (where k is a constant)
>
> Rule No. 4: If $y = k$, then $\dfrac{dy}{dx} = 0$ (where k is a constant)

Note: For future reference, a, b, c, n, and k always stand for constants.

Example 7: If $y = 8x^4$, then $\dfrac{dy}{dx} = 32x^3$.

Example 8: If $y = 5x^{100}$, then $y' = 500x^{99}$.

Example 9: If $y = -3x^{-5}$, then $\dfrac{dy}{dx} = 15x^{-6}$.

Example 10: If $f(x) = 7x^{\frac{1}{2}}$, then $f'(x) = \dfrac{7}{2}x^{-\frac{1}{2}}$.

Example 11: If $y = x\sqrt{15}$, then $\dfrac{dy}{dx} = \sqrt{15}$.

Example 12: If $y = 12$, then $\dfrac{dy}{dx} = 0$.

If you have any questions about any of these 12 examples (especially the last two), review the rules. Now for one last rule.

The Addition Rule

> If $y = ax^n + bx^m$, where a and b are constants, then
> $$\frac{dy}{dx} = a\left(nx^{n-1}\right) + b\left(mx^{m-1}\right)$$

Example 1: If $y = 3x^4 + 8x^{10}$, then $\dfrac{dy}{dx} = 12x^3 + 80x^9$.

Example 2: If $y = 7x^{-4} + 5x^{-\frac{1}{2}}$, then $\dfrac{dy}{dx} = -28x^{-5} - \dfrac{5}{2}x^{-\frac{3}{2}}$.

Example 3: If $y = 5x^4(2 - x^3)$, then $\dfrac{dy}{dx} = 40x^3 - 35x^6$.

Example 4: If $y = (3x^2 + 5)(x - 1)$, then

$$y = 3x^3 - 3x^2 + 5x - 5 \text{ and } \frac{dy}{dx} = 9x^2 - 6x + 5$$

Example 5: If $y = ax^3 + bx^2 + cx + d$, then $\dfrac{dy}{dx} = 3ax^2 + 2bx + c$.

After you've worked through all 17 of these examples, you should be able to take the derivative of any polynomial with ease.

As you may have noticed from the examples above, in calculus, you are often asked to convert from fractions and radicals to negative powers and fractional powers. In addition, don't freak out if your answer doesn't match any of the answer choices. Because answers to problems are often presented in simplified form, your answer may not be simplified enough.

This first
formula is also
known as the
Reciprocal Rule.

13.5

There are two basic expressions that you'll often be asked to differentiate. You can make your life easier by memorizing the following derivatives:

$$\text{If } y = \frac{k}{x}, \text{ then } \frac{dy}{dx} = -\frac{k}{x^2}.$$

$$\text{If } y = k\sqrt{x}, \text{ then } \frac{dy}{dx} = \frac{k}{2\sqrt{x}}.$$

Higher Order Derivatives

This may sound like a big deal, but it isn't. The term higher order derivatives refers only to taking the derivative of a function more than once. You don't have to stop at the first derivative of a function; you can keep taking derivatives. The derivative of a first derivative is called the second derivative. The derivative of the second derivative is called the third derivative, and so on.

Generally, you'll have to take only first and second derivatives.

Notice how we
simplified the
derivatives
in the latter
example? You
should be able
to do this
mentally.

Function	First Derivative	Second Derivative
x^6	$6x^5$	$30x^4$
$8\sqrt{x}$	$\dfrac{4}{\sqrt{x}}$	$-2x^{-\frac{3}{2}}$

Here are some sample problems involving the rules we discussed above. As you work, cover the answers with an index card, and then check your work after you're done. By the time you finish them, you should know the rules by heart.

PROBLEM 1. If $y = 50x^5 + \dfrac{3}{x} - 7x^{-\frac{5}{3}}$, then $\dfrac{dy}{dx} =$

Answer: $\dfrac{dy}{dx} = 50\left(5x^4\right) + \left(-\dfrac{3}{x^2}\right) - 7\left(-\dfrac{5}{3}\right)x^{-\frac{8}{3}} = 250x^4 - \dfrac{3}{x^2} + \dfrac{35}{3}x^{-\frac{8}{3}}$

This handy rule
works for
subtraction too.

PROBLEM 2. If $y = 9x^4 + 6x^2 - 7x + 11$, then $\dfrac{dy}{dx} =$

Answer: $\dfrac{dy}{dx} = 9\left(4x^3\right) + 6\left(2x\right) - 7\left(1\right) + 0 = 36x^3 + 12x - 7$

PROBLEM 3. If $f(x) = 6x^{\frac{3}{2}} - 12\sqrt{x} - \dfrac{8}{\sqrt{x}} + 24x^{-\frac{3}{2}}$, then $f'(x) =$

Answer: $f'(x) = 6\left(\dfrac{3}{2}x^{\frac{1}{2}}\right) - \left(\dfrac{12}{2\sqrt{x}}\right) - 8\left(-\dfrac{1}{2}x^{-\frac{3}{2}}\right) + 24\left(-\dfrac{3}{2}x^{-\frac{5}{2}}\right) = 9\sqrt{x} - \dfrac{6}{\sqrt{x}} + 4x^{-\frac{3}{2}} - 36x^{-\frac{5}{2}}$

How'd you do? Did you notice the changes in notation? How about the fractional powers, radical signs, and x's in denominators? You should be able to switch back and forth between notations, between fractional powers and radical signs, and between negative powers in a numerator and positive powers in a denominator.

The Product Rule

Now that you know how to find derivatives of simple polynomials, it's time to get more complicated. What if you had to find the derivative of this?

$$f(x) = (x^3 + 5x^2 - 4x + 1)(x^5 - 7x^4 + x)$$

You could multiply out the expression and take the derivative of each term, like

$$f(x) = x^8 - 2x^7 - 39x^6 + 29x^5 - 6x^4 + 5x^3 - 4x^2 + x$$

And the derivative is

$$f'(x) = 8x^7 - 14x^6 - 234x^5 + 145x^4 - 24x^3 + 15x^2 - 8x + 1$$

Needless to say, this process is messy. Naturally, there's an easier way. When a function involves two terms multiplied by each other, use the **Product Rule**.

$$\text{The Product Rule: If } f(x) = uv, \text{ then } f'(x) = u\frac{dv}{dx} + v\frac{du}{dx}$$

To find the derivative of two things multiplied by each other, you multiply the first function by the derivative of the second, and add that to the second function multiplied by the derivative of the first.

Let's use the Product Rule to find the derivative of our example.

$$f'(x) = (x^3 + 5x^2 - 4x + 1)(5x^4 - 28x^3 + 1) + (x^5 - 7x^4 + x)(3x^2 + 10x - 4)$$

If we were to simplify this, we'd get the same answer as before. But here's the best part: we're not going to simplify it. One of the great things about the PCAT is that when it's difficult to simplify an expression, you almost never have to. Nonetheless, you'll often need to simplify expressions when you're taking second derivatives, or when you use the derivative in some other equation. Practice simplifying whenever possible.

Example 1: $f(x) = (9x^2 + 4x)(x^3 - 5x^2)$

$$f'(x) = (9x^2 + 4x)(3x^2 - 10x) + (x^3 - 5x^2)(18x + 4)$$

Example 2: $y = \left(\sqrt{x} + 4\sqrt[3]{x}\right)\left(x^5 - 11x^8\right)$

$$y' = \left(\sqrt{x} + 4\sqrt[3]{x}\right)\left(5x^4 - 88x^7\right) + \left(x^5 - 11x^8\right)\left(\frac{1}{2\sqrt{x}} + \frac{4}{3\sqrt[3]{x^2}}\right)$$

Example 3: $y = \left(\dfrac{1}{x} + \dfrac{1}{x^2} - \dfrac{1}{x^3}\right)\left(\dfrac{1}{x} - \dfrac{1}{x^3} + \dfrac{1}{x^5}\right)$

$$y' = \left(\frac{1}{x} + \frac{1}{x^2} - \frac{1}{x^3}\right)\left(-\frac{1}{x^2} + \frac{3}{x^4} - \frac{5}{x^6}\right) + \left(\frac{1}{x} - \frac{1}{x^3} + \frac{1}{x^5}\right)\left(-\frac{1}{x^2} - \frac{2}{x^3} + \frac{3}{x^4}\right)$$

The Chain Rule

The most important rule in this section (and sometimes the most difficult one) is called the **Chain Rule**. It's used when you're given composite functions—that is, a function inside of another function. You'll always see one of these on the PCAT, so it's important to know the Chain Rule cold.

A composite function is usually written as $f(g(x))$.

For example, if $f(x) = \dfrac{1}{x}$ and $g(x) = \sqrt{3x}$, then $f\left(g(x)\right) = \dfrac{1}{\sqrt{3x}}$.

We could also find $g\left(f(x)\right) = \sqrt{\dfrac{3}{x}}$.

When finding the derivative of a composite function, we take the derivative of the "outside" function, with the inside function g considered as the variable, leaving the "inside" function alone. Then, we multiply this by the derivative of the "inside" function, with respect to its variable x.

Here is another way to write the Chain Rule.

> The Chain Rule: If $y = f\left(g(x)\right)$, then $y' = \left(\dfrac{df\left(g(x)\right)}{dg}\right)\left(\dfrac{dg}{dx}\right)$

This rule is tricky, so here are several examples. The last couple incorporate the Product Rule and the Quotient Rule.

Example 1: If $y = (5x^3 + 3x)^5$, then $\frac{dy}{dx} = 5(5x^3 + 3x)^4(15x^2 + 3)$.

We just dealt with the derivative of something to the fifth power, like this:

$$y = (g)^5, \text{ so } \frac{dy}{dg} = 5(g)^4, \text{ where } g = 5x^3 + 3x$$

Then we multiplied by the derivative of g: $(15x^2 + 3)$.

13.5

Always do it this way. The process has several successive steps, like peeling away the layers of an onion until you reach the center.

Example 2: If $y = \sqrt{x^3 - 4x}$, then $\frac{dy}{dx} = \frac{1}{2}(x^3 - 4x)^{-\frac{1}{2}}(3x^2 - 4)$.

Again, we took the derivative of the outside function, leaving the inside alone. Then we multiplied by the derivative of the inside.

Chain Rule—always work from the outside in, kind of like Russian dolls or peeling an onion.

Example 3: If $y = \sqrt{(x^5 - 8x^3)(x^2 + 6x)}$, then

$$\frac{dy}{dx} = \frac{1}{2}\left[(x^5 - 8x^3)(x^2 + 6x)\right]^{-\frac{1}{2}}\left[(x^5 - 8x^3)(2x + 6) + (x^2 + 6x)(5x^4 - 24x^2)\right]$$

Messy, isn't it? That's because we used the Chain Rule and the Product Rule. Now for one with the Chain Rule and the Quotient Rule.

Example 4: If $y = \left(\frac{2x + 8}{x^2 - 10x}\right)^5$, then

$$\frac{dy}{dx} = 5\left[\frac{2x + 8}{x^2 - 10x}\right]^4\left[\frac{(x^2 - 10x)(2) - (2x + 8)(2x - 10)}{(x^2 - 10x)^2}\right]$$

Example 5: If $y = \sqrt{5x^3 + x}$, then $\frac{dy}{dx} = \frac{1}{2}(5x^3 + x)^{-\frac{1}{2}}(15x^2 + 1)$.

Now we use the Product Rule and the Chain Rule to find the second derivative.

$$\frac{d^2 y}{dx^2} = \frac{1}{2}(5x^3 + x)^{-\frac{1}{2}}(30x) + (15x^2 + 1)\left[-\frac{1}{4}(5x^3 + x)^{-\frac{3}{2}}(15x^2 + 1)\right]$$

You can also simplify this further, if necessary.

There's another representation of the Chain Rule that you need to learn.

$$\text{If } y = y(v) \text{ and } v = v(x), \text{ then } \frac{dy}{dx} = \frac{dy}{dv}\frac{dv}{dx}.$$

13.5

Example 6: If $y = 8v^2 - 6v$ and $v = 5x^3 - 11x$, then

$$\frac{dy}{dx} = (16v - 6)(15x^2 - 11)$$

Then substitute for v.

$$\frac{dy}{dx} = \left(16\left(5x^3 - 11x\right) - 6\right)\left(15x^2 - 11\right) = \left(80x^3 - 176x - 6\right)\left(15x^2 - 11\right)$$

Here are some solved problems. Cover the answers first; then check your work.

PROBLEM 1. Find $\frac{dy}{dx}$ if $y = \left(5x^4 + 3x^7\right)\left(x^{10} - 8x\right)$.

Answer: $\frac{dy}{dx} = \left(5x^4 + 3x^7\right)\left(10x^9 - 8\right) + \left(x^{10} - 8x\right)\left(20x^3 + 21x^6\right)$

PROBLEM 2. Find $\frac{dy}{dx}$ if $y = \left(x^3 + 3x^2 + 3x + 1\right)\left(x^2 + 2x + 1\right)$.

Answer: $\frac{dy}{dx} = \left(x^3 + 3x^2 + 3x + 1\right)\left(2x + 2\right) + \left(x^2 + 2x + 1\right)\left(3x^2 + 6x + 3\right)$

PROBLEM 3. Find $\frac{dy}{dx}$ if $y = \left(\sqrt{x} + \frac{1}{x}\right)\left(\sqrt[3]{x^2} - \frac{1}{x^3}\right)$.

Answer: $\frac{dy}{dx} = \left(\sqrt{x} + \frac{1}{x}\right)\left(\frac{2}{3}x^{-\frac{1}{3}} + \frac{3}{x^4}\right) + \left(\sqrt[3]{x^2} - \frac{1}{x^3}\right)\left(\frac{1}{2\sqrt{x}} - \frac{1}{x^2}\right)$

PROBLEM 4. Find $\frac{dy}{dx}$ if $y = \left(x^3 + 1\right)\left(x^2 + 5x - \frac{1}{x^5}\right)$.

Answer: $\frac{dy}{dx} = \left(x^3 + 1\right)\left(2x + 5 + \frac{5}{x^6}\right) + \left(x^2 + 5x - \frac{1}{x^5}\right)\left(3x^2\right)$

PROBLEM 5. Find $\dfrac{dy}{dx}$ if $y = \dfrac{2x - 4}{x^2 - 6}$.

Answer: $\dfrac{dy}{dx} = \dfrac{\left(x^2 - 6\right)(2) - (2x - 4)(2x)}{\left(x^2 - 6\right)^2} = \dfrac{-2x^2 + 8x - 12}{\left(x^2 - 6\right)^2}$

13.5

PROBLEM 6. Find $\dfrac{dy}{dx}$ if $y = \dfrac{x^2 + 1}{x^2 + x + 4}$.

Answer: $\dfrac{dy}{dx} = \dfrac{\left(x^2 + x + 4\right)(2x) - \left(x^2 + 1\right)(2x + 1)}{\left(x^2 + x + 4\right)^2} = \dfrac{x^2 + 6x - 1}{\left(x^2 + x + 4\right)^2}$

PROBLEM 7. Find $\dfrac{dy}{dx}$ if $y = \dfrac{x + 5}{x - 5}$.

Answer: $\dfrac{dy}{dx} = \dfrac{(x - 5)(1) - (x + 5)(1)}{(x - 5)^2} = \dfrac{-10}{(x - 5)^2}$

PROBLEM 8. Find $\dfrac{dy}{dx}$ if $y = (x^4 + x)^2$.

Answer: $\dfrac{dy}{dx} = 2\left(x^4 + x\right)\left(4x^3 + 1\right)$

PROBLEM 9. Find $\dfrac{dy}{dx}$ if $y = \left(\dfrac{x + 3}{x - 3}\right)^3$.

Answer: $\dfrac{dy}{dx} = 3\left(\dfrac{x + 3}{x - 3}\right)^2\left(\dfrac{(x - 3)(1) - (x + 3)(1)}{(x - 3)^2}\right) = -18\left(\dfrac{(x + 3)^2}{(x - 3)^4}\right)$

As you can see, these grow quite complex, so we simplify these only as a last resort. If you must simplify, the PCAT will have only a very simple Chain Rule problem.

PROBLEM 10. Find $\dfrac{dy}{dx}$ at $x = 1$ if $y = \left[\left(x^3 + x\right)\left(x^4 - x^2\right)\right]^2$.

Answer: $\dfrac{dy}{dx} = 2\left[\left(x^3 + x\right)\left(x^4 - x^2\right)\right]\left[\left(x^3 + x\right)\left(4x^3 - 2x\right) + \left(x^4 - x^2\right)\left(3x^2 + 1\right)\right]$

Once again, plug in right away. Never simplify until after you've substituted.

At $x = 1$, $\dfrac{dy}{dx} = 0$.

Derivatives of Trig Functions

There are a lot of trigonometry problems in calculus and on the PCAT. You'll need to remember your trig formulas, the values of the special angles, and the trig ratios, among other stuff.

In addition, angles are *always* referred to in radians. You can forget all about using degrees.

You should know the derivatives of all six trig functions. The good news is that the derivatives are pretty easy, and all you have to do is memorize them. Because the PCAT might ask you about this, though, let's use the definition of the derivative to figure out the derivative of sin x.

13.5

$$\text{If } f(x) = \sin x, \text{ then } f(x + h) = \sin(x + h).$$

Substitute this into the definition of the derivative.

$$\lim_{h \to 0} \frac{f(x+h) - f(x)}{h} = \lim_{h \to 0} \frac{\sin(x+h) - \sin x}{h}$$

Remember that $\sin(x + h) = \sin x \cos h + \cos x \sin h$. Now simplify it.

$$\lim_{h \to 0} \frac{\sin x \cos h + \cos x \sin h - \sin x}{h}$$

Next, rewrite this as

$$\lim_{h \to 0} \frac{\sin x (\cos h - 1) + \cos x \sin h}{h} = \lim_{h \to 0} \frac{\sin x (\cos h - 1)}{h} + \lim_{h \to 0} \frac{\cos x \sin h}{h}$$

These formulas can also be found online in your Student Tools.

Next, use some of the trigonometric limits. Specifically,

$$\lim_{h \to 0} \frac{(\cos h - 1)}{h} = 0 \text{ and } \lim_{h \to 0} \frac{\sin h}{h} = 1$$

This gives you

$$\lim_{h \to 0} \frac{\sin x (\cos h - 1)}{h} + \lim_{h \to 0} \frac{\cos x \sin h}{h} = \sin x (0) + \cos x (1) = \cos x$$

$$\frac{d}{dx} \sin x = \cos x$$

Example 1: Find the derivative of $\sin\left(\dfrac{\pi}{2} - x\right)$.

$$\frac{d}{dx}\sin\left(\frac{\pi}{2} - x\right) = \cos\left(\frac{\pi}{2} - x\right)(-1) = -\cos\left(\frac{\pi}{2} - x\right)$$

Use some of the rules of trigonometry you remember from last year. Because

$$\sin\left(\frac{\pi}{2} - x\right) = \cos x \text{ and } \cos\left(\frac{\pi}{2} - x\right) = \sin x,$$

you can substitute into the above expression and get

$$\frac{d}{dx}\cos x = -\sin x$$

Now, let's derive the derivatives of the other four trigonometric functions.

Example 2: Find the derivative of $\dfrac{\sin x}{\cos x}$.

Use the Quotient Rule.

$$\frac{d}{dx}\frac{\sin x}{\cos x} = \frac{(\cos x)(\cos x) - (\sin x)(-\sin x)}{(\cos x)^2} = \frac{\cos^2 x + \sin^2 x}{\cos^2 x} = \frac{1}{\cos^2 x} = \sec^2 x$$

Because $\dfrac{\sin x}{\cos x} = \tan x$, you should get

$$\frac{d}{dx}\tan x = \sec^2 x$$

Example 3: Find the derivative of $\dfrac{\cos x}{\sin x}$.

Use the Quotient Rule.

$$\frac{d}{dx}\frac{\cos x}{\sin x} = \frac{(\sin x)(-\sin x) - (\cos x)(\cos x)}{(\sin x)^2} = \frac{-(\cos^2 x + \sin^2 x)}{\sin^2 x} = -\frac{1}{\sin^2 x} = -\csc^2 x$$

Because $\dfrac{\cos x}{\sin x} = \cot x$, you get $\dfrac{d}{dx}\cot x = -\csc^2 x$.

Example 4: Find the derivative of $\dfrac{1}{\cos x}$.

Use the Reciprocal Rule.

$$\frac{d}{dx}\frac{1}{\cos x} = \frac{-1}{(\cos x)^2}(-\sin x) = \frac{\sin x}{\cos^2 x} = \frac{1}{\cos x}\frac{\sin x}{\cos x} = \sec x \tan x$$

Because $\dfrac{1}{\cos x} = \sec x$, you get

$$\frac{d}{dx}\sec x = \sec x \tan x$$

Example 5: Find the derivative of $\dfrac{1}{\sin x}$.

You get the idea by now.

$$\frac{d}{dx}\frac{1}{\sin x} = \frac{-1}{(\sin x)^2}(\cos x) = \frac{-\cos x}{\sin^2 x} = \frac{-1}{\sin x}\frac{\cos x}{\sin x} = -\csc x \cot x$$

Because $\dfrac{1}{\sin x} = \csc x$, you get

$$\frac{d}{dx}\csc x = -\csc x \cot x$$

There you go. We have now found the derivatives of all six of the trigonometric functions. (These appear in the Formula Appendix in your Student Tools.) Now memorize them. You'll thank us later.

Let's do some more examples.

Example 6: Find the derivative of sin(5x).

$$\frac{d}{dx}\sin(5x) = \cos(5x)(5) = 5\cos(5x)$$

Example 7: Find the derivative of sec(x²).

$$\frac{d}{dx}\sec(x^2) = \sec(x^2)\tan(x^2)(2x)$$

Example 8: Find the derivative of csc(x³ − 5x).

$$\frac{d}{dx}\csc(x^3 - 5x) = -\csc(x^3 - 5x)\cot(x^3 - 5x)(3x^2 - 5)$$

These derivatives are almost like formulas. You just follow the pattern and use the Chain Rule when appropriate.

Here are some solved problems. Do each problem, covering the answer first and then checking your answer.

PROBLEM 1. Find $f'(x)$ if $f(x) = \sin(2x^3)$.

Answer: Follow the rule: $f'(x) = \cos(2x^3)6x^2$

PROBLEM 2. Find $f'(x)$ if $f(x) = \cos\left(\sqrt{3x}\right)$.

Answer: $f'(x) = -\sin\left(\sqrt{3x}\right)\left[\frac{1}{2}(3x)^{-\frac{1}{2}}(3)\right] = \frac{-3\sin\left(\sqrt{3x}\right)}{2\sqrt{3x}}$

PROBLEM 3. Find $f'(x)$ if $f(x) = \tan\left(\frac{x}{x+1}\right)$.

Answer: $f'(x) = \sec^2\left(\frac{x}{x+1}\right)\left[\frac{(x+1)-x}{(x+1)^2}\right] = \left(\frac{1}{(x+1)^2}\right)\sec^2\left(\frac{x}{x+1}\right)$

PROBLEM 4. Find $f'(x)$ if $f(x) = \csc(x^3 + x + 1)$.

Answer: Follow the rule: $f'(x) = -\csc(x^3 + x + 1)\cot(x^3 + x + 1)(3x^2 + 1)$

Graphical Derivatives

Sometimes, we are given the graph of a function and we are asked to graph the derivative. We do this by analyzing the sign of derivative at various places on the graph and then sketching a graph of the derivative from that information. Let's start with something simple. Suppose we have the graph of $y = f(x)$ below and we are asked to sketch the graph of its derivative.

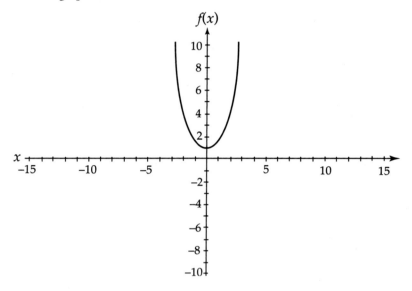

First, note that the derivative is zero at the point (0, 1) because the tangent line is horizontal there. Next, the derivative is negative for all $x < 0$ because the tangent lines to the curve have negative slopes everywhere on the interval $(-\infty, 0)$. Finally, the derivative is positive for all $x > 0$ because the tangent lines to the curve have positive slopes everywhere on the interval $(0, \infty)$. Now we can make a graph of the derivative. It will go through the origin (because the derivative is 0 at $x = 0$), it will be negative on the interval $(-\infty, 0)$, and it will be positive on the interval $(0, \infty)$. The graph looks something like the following:

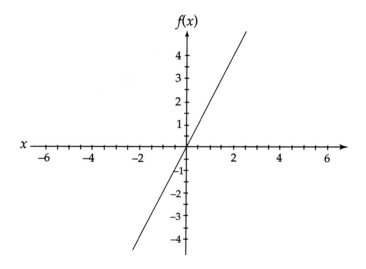

Now let's try something a little harder. Suppose we have the following graph and we are asked to sketch the graph of the derivative:

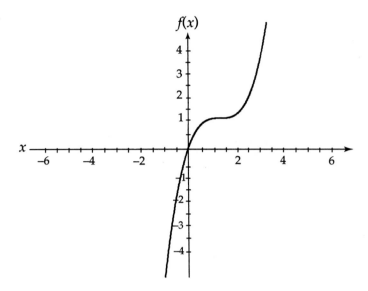

Notice that the tangent line looks as if it's horizontal at $x = 1$. This means that the graph of the derivative is zero there. Next, the curve is increasing for all other values of x, so the graph of the derivative will be positive. As we go from left to right on the graph, notice that the slope starts out very steep, so the derivatives are large positive numbers. As we approach $x = 1$, the curve starts to flatten out, so the derivatives will approach zero but will still be positive. Then, the slope is zero at $x = 1$. Then the curve gets steep again. If we sketch the derivative, we get something like the following:

Note that it's not important for your graph to be exact. All we are doing here is sketching the derivative. The important parts of the graph are where the derivative is positive, negative, and zero.

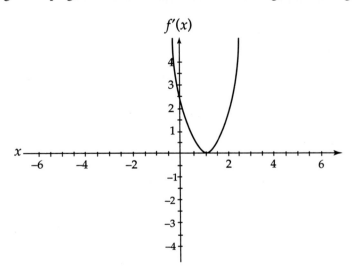

Maxima and minima on the graph of f become zeroes on the graph of f'.

Here is an important one to understand. Suppose we have the graph of $y = \sin x$.

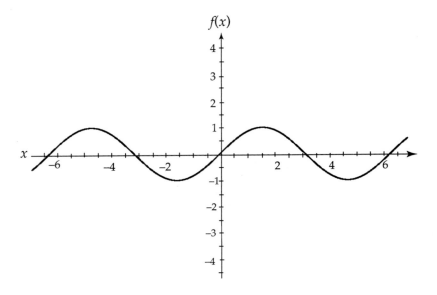

Notice that the slope of the tangent line will be horizontal at all of the maxima and minima of the graph. Because the slope of a horizontal line is zero, this means that the derivative will be zero at those values ($\pm\dfrac{\pi}{2}, \dfrac{3\pi}{2}, \cdots$). Next, notice that the slope of the curve is about 1 as the curve goes through the origin. This should make sense if you recall that $\lim\limits_{x \to 0} \dfrac{\sin x}{x} = 1$. The slope of the curve is about -1 as the curve goes through $x = \pi$, and so on. If we now sketch the derivative, it looks something like the following:

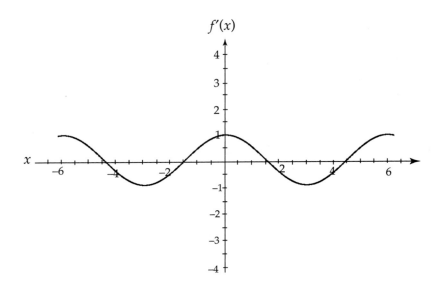

Notice that this is the graph of $y = \cos x$. This should be obvious because the derivative of $\sin x$ is $\cos x$.

Now let's do a hard one. Suppose we have the following graph:

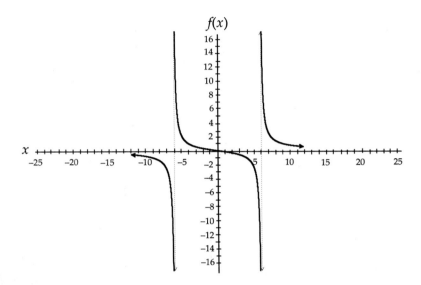

First, notice that we have two vertical asymptotes at $x = 6$ and $x = -6$. This means that the graph of the derivative will also have vertical asymptotes at $x = 6$ and $x = -6$. Next, notice that the curve is always decreasing. This means that the graph of the derivative will always be negative. Moving from left to right, the graph starts out close to flat, so the derivative will be close to zero. Then, the graph gets very steep and points downward, so the graph of the derivative will be negative and getting more negative. Then, we have the asymptote $x = -6$. Next, the graph begins very steep and negative and starts to flatten out as we approach the origin. At the origin, the slope of the graph is approximately $-\frac{1}{2}$. This means that the graph of the derivative will increase until it reaches $\left(0, -\frac{1}{2}\right)$. Then, the graph starts to get steep again as we approach the other asymptote $x = 6$. Thus, the graph will get more negative again. Finally, to the right of the asymptote $x = 6$, the graph starts out steep and negative and flattens out, approaching zero. This means that the graph of the derivative will start out very negative and will approach zero. If we now sketch the derivative, it looks something like the following:

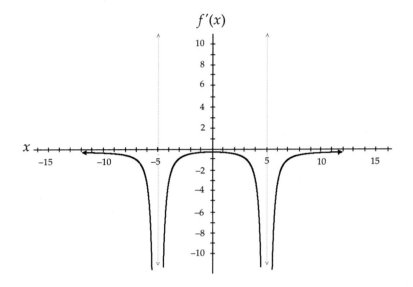

Implicit Differentiation

By now, it should be easy for you to take the derivative of an equation, such as $y = 3x^5 - 7x$. If you're given an equation such as $y^2 = 3x^5 - 7x$, you can still figure out the derivative by taking the square root of both sides, which gives you y in terms of x. This is known as finding the derivative **explicitly**. It's messy, but possible.

If you have to find the derivative of $y^2 + y = 3x^5 - 7x$, you don't have an easy way to get y in terms of x, so you can't differentiate this equation using any of the techniques you've learned so far. That's because each of those previous techniques needs to be used on an equation in which y is in terms of x. When you can't isolate y in terms of x (or if isolating y makes taking the derivative a nightmare), it's time to take the derivative **implicitly**.

Implicit differentiation is one of the simpler techniques you need to learn to do in calculus, but for some reason it gives many students trouble. Suppose you have the equation $y^2 = 3x^5 - 7x$. This means that the value of y is a function of the value of x. When we take the derivative, $\dfrac{dy}{dx}$, we're looking at the rate at which y changes as x changes. Thus, given $y = x^2 + x$, when we write

$$\frac{dy}{dx} = 2x + 1$$

we're saying that "the rate" at which y changes, with respect to how x changes, is $2x + 1$.

Now, suppose you want to find $\dfrac{dx}{dy}$. As you might imagine,

$$\frac{dx}{dy} = \frac{1}{\dfrac{dy}{dx}}$$

So here, $\dfrac{dx}{dy} = \dfrac{1}{2x+1}$. But notice that this derivative is in terms of x, not y, and you need to find the derivative with respect to y. This derivative is an **implicit** one. When you can't isolate the variables of an equation, you often end up with a derivative that is in terms of both variables.

Another way to think of this is that there is a hidden term in the derivative, $\dfrac{dx}{dx}$, and when we take the derivative, what we really get is

$$\frac{dy}{dx} = 2x\left(\frac{dx}{dx}\right) + 1\left(\frac{dx}{dx}\right)$$

A fraction that has the same term in its numerator and denominator is equal to 1, so we write

$$\frac{dy}{dx} = 2x(1) + 1(1) = 2x + 1$$

Every time we take a derivative of a term with x in it, we multiply by the term $\dfrac{dx}{dx}$, but because this is 1, we ignore it. Suppose however, that we wanted to find out how y changes with respect to t (for time). Then we would have

$$\frac{dy}{dt} = 2x\left(\frac{dx}{dt}\right) + 1\left(\frac{dx}{dt}\right)$$

If we wanted to find out how y changes with respect to r, we would have

$$\frac{dy}{dr} = 2x\left(\frac{dx}{dr}\right) + 1\left(\frac{dx}{dr}\right)$$

and if we wanted to find out how y changes with respect to y, we would have

$$\frac{dy}{dy} = 2x\left(\frac{dx}{dy}\right) + 1\left(\frac{dx}{dy}\right) \quad \text{or} \quad 1 = 2x\frac{dx}{dy} + \frac{dx}{dy}$$

This is how we really do differentiation. Remember the following:

$$\frac{dx}{dy} = \frac{1}{\frac{dy}{dx}}$$

When you have an equation of x in terms of y, and you want to find the derivative with respect to y, simply differentiate. But if the equation is of y in terms of x, find $\frac{dy}{dx}$ and take its reciprocal to find $\frac{dx}{dy}$. Go back to our original example.

$$y^2 + y = 3x^5 - 7x$$

To take the derivative according to the information in the last paragraph, you get

$$2y\left(\frac{dy}{dx}\right) + 1\left(\frac{dy}{dx}\right) = 15x^4\left(\frac{dx}{dx}\right) - 7\left(\frac{dx}{dx}\right)$$

Notice how each variable is multiplied by its appropriate $\frac{d}{dx}$. Now, remembering that $\frac{dx}{dx} = 1$, rewrite the expression this way: $2y\left(\frac{dy}{dx}\right) + 1\left(\frac{dy}{dx}\right) = 15x^4 - 7$.

Next, factor $\frac{dy}{dx}$ out of the left-hand side: $\frac{dy}{dx}(2y+1) = 15x^4 - 7$.

Isolating $\frac{dy}{dx}$ gives you $\frac{dy}{dx} = \frac{15x^4 - 7}{(2y+1)}$.

This is the derivative you're looking for. Notice how the derivative is defined in terms of y **and** x. Up until now, $\frac{dy}{dx}$ has been strictly in terms of x. This is why the differentiation is "implicit."

Confused? Let's do a few examples and you will get the hang of it.

You should use implicit differentiation any time you can't write a function explicitly in terms of the variable that you want the derivative for.

Example 1: Find $\frac{dy}{dx}$ if $y^3 - 4y^2 = x^5 + 3x^4$.

Using implicit differentiation, you get

$$3y^2\left(\frac{dy}{dx}\right) - 8y\left(\frac{dy}{dx}\right) = 5x^4\left(\frac{dx}{dx}\right) + 12x^3\left(\frac{dx}{dx}\right)$$

Remember that $\dfrac{dx}{dx} = 1$: $\dfrac{dy}{dx}\left(3y^2 - 8y\right) = 5x^4 + 12x^3$.

After you factor out $\dfrac{dy}{dx}$, divide both sides by $3y^2 - 8y$.

$$\frac{dy}{dx} = \frac{5x^4 + 12x^3}{\left(3y^2 - 8y\right)}$$

Note: Now that you understand that the derivative of an x term with respect to x will always be multiplied by $\dfrac{dx}{dx}$, and that $\dfrac{dx}{dx} = 1$, we won't write $\dfrac{dx}{dx}$ anymore. You should understand that the term is implied.

Example 2: Find $\dfrac{dy}{dx}$ if $\sin y^2 - \cos x^2 = \cos y^2 + \sin x^2$.

Use implicit differentiation.

$$\cos y^2 \left(2y\frac{dy}{dx}\right) + \sin x^2 \left(2x\right) = -\sin y^2 \left(2y\frac{dy}{dx}\right) + \cos x^2 \left(2x\right)$$

Then simplify.

$$2y\cos y^2 \left(\frac{dy}{dx}\right) + 2x\sin x^2 = -2y\sin y^2 \left(\frac{dy}{dx}\right) + 2x\cos x^2$$

Next, put all of the terms containing $\dfrac{dy}{dx}$ on the left and all of the other terms on the right.

$$2y\cos y^2 \left(\frac{dy}{dx}\right) + 2y\sin y^2 \left(\frac{dy}{dx}\right) = -2x\sin x^2 + 2x\cos x^2$$

Next, factor out $\dfrac{dy}{dx}$.

$$\frac{dy}{dx}\left(2y\cos y^2 + 2y\sin y^2\right) = -2x\sin x^2 + 2x\cos x^2$$

And isolate $\dfrac{dy}{dx}$.

$$\frac{dy}{dx} = \frac{-2x\sin x^2 + 2x\cos x^2}{\left(2y\cos y^2 + 2y\sin y^2\right)}$$

This can be simplified further to the following:

$$\frac{dy}{dx} = \frac{-x\left(\sin x^2 - \cos x^2\right)}{y\left(\cos y^2 + \sin y^2\right)}$$

Example 3: Find $\dfrac{dy}{dx}$ if $3x^2 + 5xy^2 - 4y^3 = 8$.

Implicit differentiation should result in the following:

$$6x + \left[5x\left(2y\dfrac{dy}{dx}\right)+(5)\,y^2\right]-12y^2\left(\dfrac{dy}{dx}\right)=0$$

You can simplify this to

$$6x + 10xy\dfrac{dy}{dx}+5y^2-12y^2\dfrac{dy}{dx}=0$$

Next, put all of the terms containing $\dfrac{dy}{dx}$ on the left and all of the other terms on the right.

$$10xy\dfrac{dy}{dx}-12y^2\dfrac{dy}{dx}=-6x-5y^2$$

Next, factor out $\dfrac{dy}{dx}$.

$$\left(10xy-12y^2\right)\dfrac{dy}{dx}=-6x-5y^2$$

Then, isolate $\dfrac{dy}{dx}$.

$$\dfrac{dy}{dx}=\dfrac{-6x-5y^2}{\left(10xy-12y^2\right)}$$

Example 4: Find the derivative of $3x^2 - 4y^2 + y = 9$ at $(2, 1)$.

You need to use implicit differentiation to find $\dfrac{dy}{dx}$.

$$6x-8y\left(\dfrac{dy}{dx}\right)+\left(\dfrac{dy}{dx}\right)=0$$

Now, instead of rearranging to isolate $\dfrac{dy}{dx}$, plug in $(2, 1)$ immediately and solve for the derivative.

$$6(2)-8(1)\left(\dfrac{dy}{dx}\right)+\left(\dfrac{dy}{dx}\right)=0$$

Simplify: $12-7\left(\dfrac{dy}{dx}\right)=0$, so $\dfrac{dy}{dx}=\dfrac{12}{7}$.

Applied Maxima and Minima Problems

One of the most common applications of the derivative is to find a maximum or minimum value of a function. These values can be called extreme values, optimal values, or critical points. Each of these problems involves the same, very simple principle.

> A maximum or a minimum of a function occurs at a point where the derivative of a function is zero, or where the derivative fails to exist.

At a point where the first derivative equals zero, the curve has a horizontal tangent line, at which point it could be reaching either a "peak" (maximum) or a "valley" (minimum).

There are a few exceptions to every rule. This rule is no different.

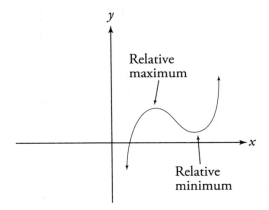

> An **absolute** maximum or minimum occurs either at an artificial point or an end point. In the figure below, the two indicated points are absolute maxima/minima. A relative maximum can also be an absolute maximum.

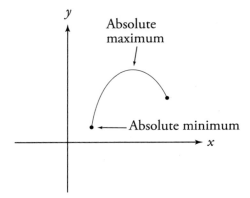

A typical word problem will ask you to find a maximum or a minimum value of a function, as it pertains to a certain situation. Sometimes you're given the equation; other times, you have to figure it out for yourself. Once you have the equation, you find its derivative and set it equal to zero. The values you get are called critical values. That is, if $f'(c) = 0$ or $f'(c)$ does not exist, then c is a critical value. Then, test these values to determine whether each value is a maximum or a minimum. The simplest way to do this is with the second derivative test.

> If a function has a critical value at $x = c$, then that value is a relative maximum if $f''(c) < 0$ and it is a relative minimum if $f''(c) > 0$.

If the second derivative is also zero at $x = c$, then the point is neither a maximum nor a minimum but a point of inflection. More about that later.

It's time to do some examples.

Example 1: Find the minimum value on the curve $y = ax^2$, if $a > 0$.

Take the derivative and set it equal to zero.

$$\frac{dy}{dx} = 2ax = 0$$

The first derivative is equal to zero at $x = 0$. By plugging 0 back into the original equation, we can solve for the y-coordinate of the minimum (the y-coordinate is also 0, so the point is at the origin).

In order to determine if this is a maximum or a minimum, take the second derivative.

$$\frac{d^2y}{dx^2} = 2a$$

Because a is positive, the second derivative is positive and the critical point we obtained from the first derivative is a minimum point. Had a been negative, the second derivative would have been negative and a maximum would have occurred at the critical point.

Example 2: A manufacturing company has determined that the total cost of producing an item can be determined from the equation $C = 8x^2 - 176x + 1,800$, where x is the number of units that the company makes. How many units should the company manufacture in order to minimize the cost?

Once again, take the derivative of the cost equation and set it equal to zero.

$$\frac{dC}{dx} = 16x - 176 = 0$$

$$x = 11$$

This tells us that 11 is a critical point of the equation. Now we need to figure out if this is a maximum or a minimum using the second derivative.

$$\frac{d^2C}{dx^2} = 16$$

Because 16 is always positive, any critical value is going to be a minimum. Therefore, the company should manufacture 11 units in order to minimize its cost.

Example 3: A rocket is fired into the air, and its height in meters at any given time t can be calculated using the formula $h(t) = 1,600 + 196t - 4.9t^2$. Find the maximum height of the rocket and the time at which it occurs.

Take the derivative and set it equal to zero.

$$\frac{dh}{dt} = 196 - 9.8t$$

$$t = 20$$

Now that we know 20 is a critical point of the equation, use the second derivative test.

$$\frac{d^2h}{dt^2} = -9.8$$

This is always negative, so any critical value is a maximum. To determine the maximum height of the rocket, plug $t = 20$ into the equation.

$$h(20) = 1,600 + 196(20) - 4.9(20^2) = 3,560 \text{ meters}$$

13.5

> The technique is always the same: (a) take the derivative of the equation; (b) set it equal to zero; and (c) use the second derivative test.

13.5

The hardest part of these word problems is when you have to set up the equation yourself. The following is a classic PCAT problem.

Example 4: Max wants to make a box with no lid from a rectangular sheet of cardboard that is 18 inches by 24 inches. The box is to be made by cutting a square of side x from each corner of the sheet and folding up the sides (see figure below). Find the value of x that maximizes the volume of the box.

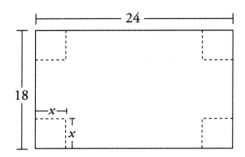

After we cut out the squares of side x and fold up the sides, the dimensions of the box will be

width: $18 - 2x$
length: $24 - 2x$
depth: x

Using the formula for the volume of a rectangular prism, we can get an equation for the volume in terms of x.

$$V = x(18 - 2x)(24 - 2x)$$

Multiply the terms together (and be careful with your algebra).

$$V = x(18 - 2x)(24 - 2x) = 4x^3 - 84x^2 + 432x$$

Now take the derivative.

$$\frac{dV}{dx} = 12x^2 - 168x + 432$$

Set the derivative equal to zero, and solve for x.

$$12x^2 - 168x + 432 = 0$$

$$x^2 - 14x + 36 = 0$$

$$x = \frac{14 \pm \sqrt{196 - 144}}{2} = 7 \pm \sqrt{13} \approx 3.4, 10.6$$

Common sense tells us that you can't cut out two square pieces that measure 10.6 inches to a side (the sheet's only 18 inches wide!), so the maximizing value has to be 3.4 inches. Here's the second derivative test, just to be sure.

$$\frac{d^2V}{dx^2} = 24x - 168$$

At $x = 3.4$,

$$\frac{d^2V}{dx^2} = -86.4$$

So, the volume of the box will be maximized when $x = 3.4$.

Therefore, the dimensions of the box that maximize the volume are approximately: 11.2 in. × 17.2 in. × 3.4 in.

Sometimes, particularly when the domain of a function is restricted, you have to test the endpoints of the interval as well. This is because the highest or lowest value of a function may be at an endpoint of that interval; the critical value you obtained from the derivative might be just a local maximum or minimum. For the purposes of the PCAT, however, endpoints are considered separate from critical values.

Example 5: Find the absolute maximum and minimum values of $y = x^3 - x$ on the interval $[-3, 3]$.

Take the derivative and set it equal to zero.

$$\frac{dy}{dx} = 3x^2 - 1 = 0$$

Solve for x.

$$x = \pm \frac{1}{\sqrt{3}}$$

Test the critical points.

$$\frac{d^2y}{dx^2} = 6x$$

At $x = \frac{1}{\sqrt{3}}$, we have a minimum. At $x = -\frac{1}{\sqrt{3}}$, we have a maximum.

$$\text{At } x = -\frac{1}{\sqrt{3}}, \, y = -\frac{1}{3\sqrt{3}} + \frac{1}{\sqrt{3}} = \frac{2}{3\sqrt{3}} \approx 0.385$$

$$\text{At } x = \frac{1}{\sqrt{3}}, \, y = \frac{1}{3\sqrt{3}} - \frac{1}{\sqrt{3}} = -\frac{2}{3\sqrt{3}} \approx -0.385$$

Now it's time to check the endpoints of the interval.

$$At\ x = -3,\ y = -24$$

$$At\ x = 3,\ y = 24$$

We can see that the function actually has a *lower* value at $x = -3$ than at its "minimum" when $x = \dfrac{1}{\sqrt{3}}$. Similarly, the function has a *higher* value at $x = 3$ than at its "maximum" of $x = -\dfrac{1}{\sqrt{3}}$. This means that the function has a "local minimum" at $x = \dfrac{1}{\sqrt{3}}$ and an "absolute minimum" when $x = -3$.

And, the function has a "local maximum" at $x = -\dfrac{1}{\sqrt{3}}$ and an "absolute maximum" at $x = 3$.

Example 6: A rectangle is to be inscribed in a semicircle with radius 4, with one side on the semicircle's diameter. What is the largest area this rectangle can have?

Let's look at this on the coordinate axes. The equation for a circle of radius 4, centered at the origin, is $x^2 + y^2 = 16$; a semicircle has the equation $y = \sqrt{16 - x^2}$. Our rectangle can then be expressed as a function of x, where the height is $\sqrt{16 - x^2}$ and the base is $2x$. See the following figure:

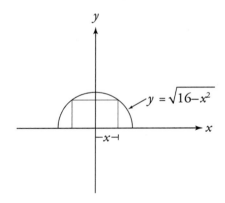

The area of the rectangle is $A = 2x\sqrt{16 - x^2}$. Let's take the derivative of the area.

$$\frac{dA}{dx} = 2\sqrt{16 - x^2} - \frac{2x^2}{\sqrt{16 - x^2}}$$

The derivative is not defined at $x = \pm 4$. Setting the derivative equal to zero, we get

$$2\sqrt{16 - x^2} - \frac{2x^2}{\sqrt{16 - x^2}} = 0$$

$$2\sqrt{16 - x^2} = \frac{2x^2}{\sqrt{16 - x^2}}$$

$$2\left(16 - x^2\right) = 2x^2$$

$$32 - 2x^2 = 2x^2$$

$$32 = 4x^2$$

$$x = \pm\sqrt{8}$$

Note that the domain of this function is $-4 \le x \le 4$, so these numbers serve as endpoints of the interval. Let's compare the critical values and the endpoints.

When $x = -4$, $y = 0$ and the area is 0.

When $x = 4$, $y = 0$ and the area is 0.

When $x = \sqrt{8}$, $y = \sqrt{8}$ and the area is 16.

Thus, the maximum area occurs when $x = \sqrt{8}$ and the area equals 16.

Related Rates

The derivative of a function $f(x)$ gives the rate of change of f with respect to x. So, if the variable t represents time, the derivative of a function $f(t)$ tells us how f changes with time. For example, consider a spherical balloon that's being inflated. How fast does its volume change? Let's see. The volume of a sphere of radius r is given by the formula $V(r) = \frac{4}{3}\pi r^3$; differentiating this equation with respect to time, we find that, using Leibniz notation,

$$\frac{dV}{dt} = 4\pi r^2 \frac{dr}{dt}$$

So, the rate at which V changes depends on the sphere's radius and how fast the radius is changing. This equation illustrates the concept of **related rates**: V depends on r, and the rate at which V changes is related to the rate at which r changes.

The idea behind these problems is very simple. In a typical problem, you'll be given an equation relating two or more variables. These variables will change with respect to time, and you'll use derivatives to determine how the rates of change are related. (Hence the name: related rates.) Sounds easy, doesn't it?

Example 1: A circular pool of water is expanding at the rate of 16π in.²/sec. At what rate is the radius expanding when the radius is 4 inches?

Note: The pool is expanding in square inches per second. We've been given the rate that the area is changing, and we need to find the rate of change of the radius. What equation relates the area of a circle to its radius? $A = \pi r^2$.

Step 1: Set up the equation and take the derivative of this equation with respect to t (time).

$$\frac{dA}{dt} = 2\pi r \frac{dr}{dt}$$

In this equation, $\frac{dA}{dt}$ represents the rate at which the area is changing, and $\frac{dr}{dt}$ is the rate at which the radius is changing. The simplest way to explain this is that whenever you have a variable in an equation (r, for example), the derivative with respect to time $\left(\frac{dr}{dt}\right)$ represents the rate at which that variable is increasing or decreasing.

Step 2: Now we can plug in the values for the rate of change of the area and for the radius. (Never plug in the values until after you have taken the derivative or you will get nonsense!)

$$16\pi = 2\pi(4)\frac{dr}{dt}$$

Solving for $\frac{dr}{dt}$, we get

$$16\pi = 8\pi\frac{dr}{dt} \text{ and } \frac{dr}{dt} = 2$$

The radius is changing at a rate of 2 in./sec. It's important to note that this is the rate only when the radius is 4 inches. As the circle gets bigger and bigger, the radius will expand at a slower and slower rate.

Example 2: A 25-foot long ladder is leaning against a wall and sliding toward the floor. If the foot of the ladder is sliding away from the base of the wall at a rate of 15 ft/sec, how fast is the top of the ladder sliding down the wall when the top of the ladder is 7 feet from the ground?

Here's another classic related rates problem. As always, a picture is worth 1,000 words.

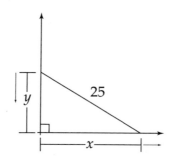

You can see that the ladder forms a right triangle with the wall. Let x stand for the distance from the foot of the ladder to the base of the wall, and let y represent the distance from the top of the ladder to the ground. What's our favorite theorem that deals with right triangles? The Pythagorean Theorem tells us here that $x^2 + y^2 = 25^2$. Now we have an equation that relates the variables to each other.

Now take the derivative of the equation with respect to t.

$$2x\frac{dx}{dt} + 2y\frac{dy}{dt} = 0$$

Just plug in what you know and solve. Because we're looking for the rate at which the vertical distance is changing, we're going to solve for $\frac{dy}{dt}$.

Let's see what we know. We're given the rate at which the ladder is sliding away from the wall: $\frac{dx}{dt} = 15$. The distance from the ladder to the top of the wall is 7 feet ($y = 7$). To find x, use the Pythagorean Theorem. If we plug in $y = 7$ to the equation $x^2 + y^2 = 25^2$, $x = 24$.

Now plug all this information into the derivative equation.

$$2(24)(15) + 2(7)\frac{dy}{dt} = 0$$

$$\frac{dy}{dt} = -\frac{360}{7}\frac{\text{feet}}{\text{sec}}$$

Example 3: A spherical balloon is expanding at a rate of 60π in.³/sec. How fast is the surface area of the balloon expanding when the radius of the balloon is 4 inches?

Step 1: You're given the rate at which the volume's expanding, and you know the equation that relates volume to radius. But you have to relate radius to surface area as well, because you have to find the surface area's rate of change. This means that you'll need the equations for volume and surface area of a sphere.

$$V = \frac{4}{3}\pi r^3$$

$$A = 4\pi r^2$$

You're trying to find $\dfrac{dA}{dt}$, but A is given in terms of r, so you have to get $\dfrac{dr}{dt}$ first. Because we know the volume, if we work with the equation that gives us volume in terms of radius, we can find $\dfrac{dr}{dt}$. From there, work with the other equation to find $\dfrac{dA}{dt}$. If we take the derivative of the equation with respect to t, we get $\dfrac{dV}{dt} = 4\pi r^2 \dfrac{dr}{dt}$. Plugging in for $\dfrac{dV}{dt}$ and for r, we get $60\pi = 4\pi(4)^2 \dfrac{dr}{dt}$. Solving for $\dfrac{dr}{dt}$, we get

$$\frac{dr}{dt} = \frac{15}{16} \text{ in./sec}$$

Step 2: Now we take the derivative of the other equation with respect to t.

$$\frac{dA}{dt} = 8\pi r \frac{dr}{dt}$$

We can plug in for r and $\dfrac{dr}{dt}$ from the previous step to get

$$\frac{dA}{dt} = 8\pi(4)\frac{15}{16} = \frac{480\pi}{16}\frac{\text{in.}^2}{\text{sec}} = 30\pi \text{ in.}^2/\text{sec}$$

One final example.

Example 4: An underground conical tank, standing on its vertex, is being filled with water at the rate of 18π ft³/min. If the tank has a height of 30 feet and a radius of 15 feet, how fast is the water level rising when the water is 12 feet deep?

This "cone" problem is also typical. The key point to getting these right is knowing that the ratio of the height of a right circular cone to its radius is constant. By telling us that the height of the cone is 30 and the radius is 15, we know that at any level, the height of the water will be twice its radius, or $h = 2r$.

You must find the rate at which the water is rising (the height is changing), or $\dfrac{dh}{dt}$. Therefore, you want to eliminate the radius from the volume. By substituting $\dfrac{h}{2} = r$ into the equation for volume, we get

$$V = \frac{1}{3}\pi\left(\frac{h}{2}\right)^2 h = \frac{\pi h^3}{12}$$

Differentiate both sides with respect to t.

$$\frac{dV}{dt} = \frac{\pi}{12}3h^2\frac{dh}{dt}$$

Now we can plug in and solve for $\frac{dh}{dt}$.

$$18\pi = \frac{\pi}{12}3(12)^2\frac{dh}{dt}$$

$$\frac{dh}{dt} = \frac{1}{2} \text{ feet/min}$$

In order to solve related rates problems, you have to be good at determining relationships between variables. Once you figure that out, the rest is a piece of cake. Many of these problems involve geometric relationships, so review the formulas for the volumes and areas of cones, spheres, boxes, and other solids. Once you get the hang of setting up the problems, you'll see that these problems follow the same predictable patterns. Look through these sample problems.

PROBLEM 1. A circle is increasing in area at the rate of 16π in.²/s. How fast is the radius increasing when the radius is 2 in.?

Answer: Use the expression that relates the area of a circle to its radius: $A = \pi r^2$.

Next, take the derivative of the expression with respect to t.

$$\frac{dA}{dt} = 2\pi r\frac{dr}{dt}$$

Now, plug in $\frac{dA}{dt} = 16\pi$ and $r = 2$.

$$16\pi = 2\pi(2)\frac{dr}{dt}$$

When you solve for $\frac{dr}{dt}$, you'll get $\frac{dr}{dt} = 4$ in./sec.

PROBLEM 2. A rocket is rising vertically at a rate of 5,400 miles per hour. An observer on the ground is standing 20 miles from the rocket's launch point. How fast (in radians per second) is the angle of elevation between the ground and the observer's line of sight of the rocket increasing when the rocket is at an elevation of 40 miles?

Answer: First, draw a picture.

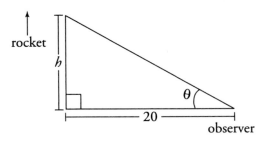

Now, find the equation that relates the angle of elevation to the rocket's altitude.

$$\tan\theta = \frac{h}{20}$$

If we take the derivative of both sides of this expression with respect to t, we get

$$\sec^2\theta\,\frac{d\theta}{dt} = \frac{1}{20}\frac{dh}{dt}$$

We know that $\frac{dh}{dt}$ = 5,400 miles per hour, but the problem asks for time in seconds, so we need to convert this number. There are 3,600 seconds in an hour, so $\frac{dh}{dt} = \frac{3}{2}$ miles per second. Next, we know that tan $\theta = \frac{h}{20}$, so when $h = 40$, $\tan\theta = 2$. Because $1 + \tan^2\theta = \sec^2\theta$, we get $\sec^2\theta = 5$.

Plug in the following information:

$$5\frac{d\theta}{dt} = \frac{1}{20}\left(\frac{3}{2}\right) \text{ and } \frac{d\theta}{dt} = \frac{3}{200} \text{ radians per second}$$

Position, Velocity, and Acceleration

If you have a function that gives you the position of an object (usually called a "particle") at a specified time, then the derivative of that function with respect to time is the velocity of the object, and the second derivative is the acceleration. These are usually represented by the following:

> Position: $x(t)$ or sometimes $s(t)$
> Velocity: $v(t)$, which is $x'(t)$
> Acceleration: $a(t)$, which is $x''(t)$ or $v'(t)$

By the way, speed is the absolute value of velocity.

Example 1: If the position of a particle at a time t is given by the equation $x(t) = t^3 - 11t^2 + 24t$, find the velocity and the acceleration of the particle at time $t = 5$.

First, take the derivative of $x(t)$.

$$x'(t) = 3t^2 - 22t + 24 = v(t)$$

Second, plug in $t = 5$ to find the velocity at that time.

$$v(5) = 3(5^2) - 22(5) + 24 = -11$$

Third, take the derivative of $v(t)$ to find $a(t)$.

$$v'(t) = 6t - 22 = a(t)$$

Finally, plug in $t = 5$ to find the acceleration at that time.

$$a(5) = 6(5) - 22 = 8$$

See the negative velocity? The sign of the velocity is important because it indicates the direction of the particle. Make sure that you know the following:

> When the velocity is negative, the particle is moving to the left.
>
> When the velocity is positive, the particle is moving to the right.
>
> When the velocity and acceleration of the particle have the same signs, the particle's speed is increasing.
>
> When the velocity and acceleration of the particle have opposite signs, the particle's speed is decreasing (or slowing down).
>
> When the velocity is zero and the acceleration is not zero, the particle is momentarily stopped and changing direction.

Example 2: If the position of a particle is given by $x(t) = t^3 - 12t^2 + 36t + 18$, where $t > 0$, find the point at which the particle changes direction.

The derivative is

$$x'(t) = v(t) = 3t^2 - 24t + 36$$

Set it equal to zero and solve for t.

$$x'(t) = 3t^2 - 24t + 36 = 0$$

$$t^2 - 8t + 12 = 0$$

$$(t - 2)(t - 6) = 0$$

So we know that $t = 2$ or $t = 6$.

You need to check that the acceleration is not 0: $x''(t) = 6t - 24$. This equals 0 at $t = 4$. Therefore, the particle is changing direction at $t = 2$ and $t = 6$.

Example 3: Given the same position function as in Example 2, find the interval of time during which the particle is slowing down.

When $0 < t < 2$ and $t > 6$, the particle's velocity is positive; when $2 < t < 6$, the particle's velocity is negative. You can verify this by graphing the function and seeing when it's above or below the x-axis. Or, try some points in the regions between the roots and outside the roots. Now, we need to determine the same information about the acceleration.

$$a(t) = v'(t) = 6t - 24$$

So the acceleration will be negative when $t < 4$, and positive when $t > 4$.

So we have

Time	Velocity	Acceleration
$0 < t < 2$	Positive	Negative
$2 < t < 4$	Negative	Negative
$4 < t < 6$	Negative	Positive
$t > 6$	Positive	Positive

Whenever the velocity and acceleration have opposite signs, the particle is slowing down. Here the particle is slowing down during the first two seconds ($0 < t < 2$) and between the fourth and sixth seconds ($4 < t < 6$).

Another typical question you'll be asked is to find the distance a particle has traveled from one time to another. This is the distance that the particle has covered without regard to the sign, not just the displacement. In other words, if the particle had an odometer on it, what would it read? Usually, all you have to do is plug the two times into the position function and find the difference.

Example 4: How far does a particle travel between the eighth and tenth seconds if its position function is $x(t) = t^2 - 6t$?

Find $x(10) - x(8) = (100 - 60) - (64 - 48) = 24$.

Be careful about one very important thing: **if the velocity changes sign during the problem's time interval**, you'll get the wrong answer if you simply follow the method in the paragraph above. For example, suppose we had the same position function as above but we wanted to find the distance that the particle travels from $t = 2$ to $t = 4$.

$$x(4) - x(2) = (-8) - (-8) = 0$$

This is wrong. The particle travels from –8 back to –8, but it hasn't stood still. To fix this problem, divide the time interval into the time when the velocity is negative and the time when the velocity is positive, and add the absolute values of each distance. Here the velocity is $v(t) = 2t - 6$. The velocity is negative when $t < 3$ and positive when $t > 3$. So we find the absolute value of the distance traveled from $t = 2$ to $t = 3$, and add to that the absolute value of the distance traveled from $t = 3$ to $t = 4$.

Because $x(t) = t^2 - 6t$,

$$\left|x(3) - x(2)\right| + \left|x(4) - x(3)\right| = \left|-9 + 8\right| + \left|-8 + 9\right| = 2$$

This is the distance that the particle traveled.

Example 5: Given the position function $x(t) = t^4 - 8t^2$, find the distance that the particle travels from $t = 0$ to $t = 4$.

First, find the first derivative ($v(t) = 4t^3 - 16t$) and set it equal to zero.

$$4t^3 - 16t = 0 \quad 4t(t^2 - 4) = 0 \quad t = 0, 2, -2$$

So we need to divide the time interval into $t = 0$ to $t = 2$ and $t = 2$ to $t = 4$.

$$\left|x(2) - x(0)\right| + \left|x(4) - x(2)\right| = 16 + 144 = 160$$

Here are some solved problems. Do each problem, covering the answer first; then check your answer.

Definite Integration

Welcome to the other half of calculus! This, unfortunately, is the more difficult half, but don't worry. We'll get you through it. In differential calculus, you learned all of the fun things that you can do with the derivative. Now you'll learn to do the reverse: how to take an integral. As you might imagine, there's a bunch of new fun things that you can do with integrals too.

It's also time for a new symbol, $\int$, which stands for integration. An integral actually serves several different purposes, but the first, and most basic, is that of the antiderivative.

The Antiderivative

An antiderivative is a derivative in reverse. Therefore, we're going to reverse some of the rules we learned with derivatives and apply them to integrals. For example, we know that the derivative of x^2 is $2x$. If we are given the derivative of a function and have to figure out the original function, we use antidifferentiation. Thus, the antiderivative of $2x$ is x^2. (Actually, the answer is slightly more complicated than that, but we'll get into that in a few moments.)

Now we need to add some info here to make sure that you get this absolutely correct. First, as far as notation goes, it is traditional to write the antiderivative of a function using its uppercase letter, so the antiderivative of $f(x)$ is $F(x)$, the antiderivative of $g(x)$ is $G(x)$, and so on.

The second idea is very important: each function has more than one antiderivative. In fact, there are an infinite number of antiderivatives of a function. Let's go back to our example to help illustrate this.

Remember that the antiderivative of $2x$ is x^2? Well, consider this. If you take the derivative of $x^2 + 1$, you get $2x$. The same is true for $x^2 + 2$, $x^2 - 1$, and so on. In fact, if *any* constant is added to x^2, the derivative is still $2x$ because the derivative of a constant is zero.

Because of this, we write the antiderivative of $2x$ as $x^2 + C$, where C stands for any constant.

Finally, whenever you take the integral (or antiderivative) of a function of x, you always add the term dx (or dy if it's a function of y, etc.) to the integrand (the thing inside the integral). You'll learn why later.

Here is the **Power Rule** for antiderivatives.

13.5

$$\text{If } f(x) = x^n, \text{ then } \int f(x)dx = \frac{x^{n+1}}{n+1} + C \text{ (except when } n = -1).$$

Example 1: Find $\int x^3 dx$.

Using the Power Rule, we get

$$\int x^3 dx = \frac{x^4}{4} + C$$

Don't forget the constant C!

Example 2: Find $\int x^{-3} dx$.

The Power Rule works with negative exponents too.

$$\int x^{-3} dx = \frac{x^{-2}}{-2} + C$$

Not terribly hard, is it? Now it's time for a few more rules that look remarkably similar to the rules for derivatives.

$$\int kf(x)dx = k\int f(x)dx$$

$$\int \left[f(x) + g(x)\right]dx = \int f(x)dx + \int g(x)dx$$

$$\int k\,dx = kx + C$$

Here are a few more examples to make you an expert.

Example 3: $\int 5\,dx = 5x + C$

Example 4: $\int 7x^3\,dx = \dfrac{7x^4}{4} + C$

Example 5: $\int \left(3x^2 + 2x\right)dx = x^3 + x^2 + C$

Example 6: $\int \sqrt{x}\,dx = \dfrac{x^{\frac{3}{2}}}{\frac{3}{2}} + C = \dfrac{2x^{\frac{3}{2}}}{3} + C$

Integrals of Trig Functions

The integrals of some trigonometric functions follow directly from the derivative formulas.

We didn't mention the integrals of tangent, cotangent, secant, and cosecant, because you need to know some rules about logarithms to figure them out. Notice also that each of the answers is divided by a constant. This is to account for the Chain Rule. Let's do some examples.

Example 1: Check the integral $\int \sin 5x\,dx = -\dfrac{\cos 5x}{5} + C$ by differentiating the answer.

$$\frac{d}{dx}\left[-\frac{\cos 5x}{5} + C\right] = -\frac{1}{5}(-\sin 5x)(5) = \sin 5x$$

Notice how the constant is accounted for in the answer?

Example 2: $\int \sec^2 3x\,dx = \dfrac{\tan 3x}{3} + C$

Example 3: $\int \cos \pi x\,dx = \dfrac{\sin \pi x}{\pi} + C$

Example 4: $\int \sec\left(\dfrac{x}{2}\right)\tan\left(\dfrac{x}{2}\right)dx = 2\sec\left(\dfrac{x}{2}\right) + C$

If you're not sure if you have the correct answer when you take an integral, you can always check by differentiating the answer to see if you get what you started with. Try to get into the habit of doing that at the beginning, because it'll help you build confidence in your ability to find integrals properly. You'll see that, although you can differentiate just about any expression that you'll normally encounter, you won't be able to integrate many of the functions you see.

Addition and Subtraction

By using the rules for addition and subtraction, we can integrate most polynomials.

Example 1: Find $\int \left(x^3 + x^2 - x\right) dx$.

We can break this into separate integrals, which gives us

$$\int x^3 dx + \int x^2 dx - \int x \, dx$$

Now you can integrate each of these individually.

$$\frac{x^4}{4} + C + \frac{x^3}{3} + C - \frac{x^2}{2} + C$$

You can combine the constants into one constant (it doesn't matter how many Cs we use, because their sum is one collective constant whose derivative is zero).

$$\frac{x^4}{4} + \frac{x^3}{3} - \frac{x^2}{2} + C$$

Sometimes you'll be given information about the function you're seeking that will enable you to solve for the constant. Often, this is an "initial value," which is the value of the function when the variable is zero. As we've seen, normally there are an infinite number of solutions for an integral, but when we solve for the constant, there's only one.

Example 2: Find the equation of y where $\dfrac{dy}{dx} = 3x + 5$ and $y = 6$ when $x = 0$.

Let's put this in integral form.

$$y = \int \left(3x + 5\right) dx$$

Integrating, we get

$$y = \frac{3x^2}{2} + 5x + C$$

Now we can solve for the constant because we know that $y = 6$ when $x = 0$.

$$6 = \frac{3(0)^2}{2} + 5(0) + C$$

Therefore, $C = 6$ and the equation is

$$y = \frac{3x^2}{2} + 5x + 6$$

Example 3: Find $f(x)$ if $f'(x) = \sin x - \cos x$ and $f(\pi) = 3$.

Integrate $f'(x)$.

$$f(x) = \int (\sin x - \cos x)\ dx = -\cos x - \sin x + C$$

Now solve for the constant.

$$3 = -\cos(\pi) - \sin(\pi) + C$$

$$C = 2$$

Therefore, the equation becomes

$$f(x) = -\cos x - \sin x + 2$$

Now we've covered the basics of integration. However, integration is a very sophisticated topic, and there are many types of integrals that will cause you trouble. We will need several techniques to learn how to evaluate these integrals. The first and most important is called *u*-substitution, which we will cover in the second half of this section.

In the meantime, here are some solved problems. Do each problem, covering the answer first; then check your answer.

PROBLEM 1. Evaluate $\int x^{\frac{3}{5}} dx$.

Answer: Here's the Power Rule again.

$$\int x^n dx = \frac{x^{n+1}}{n+1} + C$$

Using the rule,

$$\int x^{\frac{3}{5}} dx = \frac{x^{\frac{8}{5}}}{\frac{8}{5}} + C$$

You can rewrite it as $\dfrac{5x^{\frac{8}{5}}}{8} + C$.

The geometric motivation for the derivative is finding the slope of the line tangent to a curve. The motivation for the other principal idea of calculus, the integral, is finding the area *under* a curve. Following is a graph of the function $f(x) = 9 - x^2$, from $x = 0$ to $x = 3$. What's the area bounded by this curve and the *x*-axis?

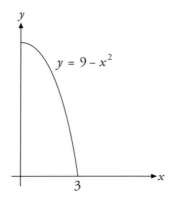

Well, we know the formulas for finding the areas of shapes like rectangles and triangles, whose sides are straight lines. But what about regions that have curved boundaries? One way to determine their areas is to approximate, using a collection of narrow rectangular strips:

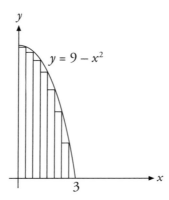

Let's imagine that we have n rectangular strips, each of which has a base of width of $\dfrac{3}{n}$. We'll take the height of each rectangle to be the value of $f(x)$ at the right-hand endpoint of the rectangle's base. Since the formula for the area of a rectangle is base × height, the sum of the areas of these rectangles is:

$$S_n = \frac{3}{n}\left[9 - \left(\frac{3}{n}\right)^2\right] + \frac{3}{n}\left[9 - \left(\frac{3 \cdot 2}{n}\right)^2\right] + \cdots + \frac{3}{n}\left[9 - \left(\frac{3(n-1)}{n}\right)^2\right] + \frac{3}{n}\left[9 - \left(\frac{3n}{n}\right)^2\right]$$

This sum, S_n, which is called a **Riemann sum**, is close to, but slightly less than, the area under the curve. But if we increase n, the little triangular-shaped wedges that the rectangles don't account for will get smaller and smaller, and in the limit as $n \to \infty$, the total area of these wedges decreases to zero. This means that the limit of the sum shown above will give us the exact area under the curve. Let's see what this limit is.

Simplifying the expression above, we find that

$$S_n = \frac{3}{n}\left[9 - \left(\frac{3}{n}\right)^2\right] + \frac{3}{n}\left[9 - \left(\frac{3 \cdot 2}{n}\right)^2\right] + \cdots + \frac{3}{n}\left[9 - \left(\frac{3(n-1)}{n}\right)^2\right] + \frac{3}{n}\left[9 - \left(\frac{3n}{n}\right)^2\right]$$

$$= n\left(\frac{3}{n} \cdot 9\right) - \frac{3}{n}\left(\frac{3}{n}\right)^2 [1^2 + 2^2 + \cdots + (n-1)^2 + n^2]$$

$$= 27 - \frac{27}{n^3}[1^2 + 2^2 + \cdots + (n-1)^2 + n^2]$$

$$= 27 - \frac{27}{n^3}\left[\frac{n(n+1)(2n+1)}{6}\right]$$

$$= 27 - \frac{27}{6}\left[\frac{2n^3 + 3n^2 + n}{n^3}\right]$$

where we've used the following formula

$$1^2 + 2^2 + \cdots + n^2 = \frac{n(n+1)(2n+1)}{6}$$

which may be proved by mathematical induction. We now take the limit:

$$\text{exact area under curve} = \lim_{n\to\infty} S_n = \lim_{n\to\infty}\left[27 - \frac{27}{6}\left(\frac{2n^3 + 3n^2 + n}{n^3}\right)\right]$$

$$= 27 - \frac{27}{6} \circ 2$$

$$= 18$$

Example 1: Approximate the area under the curve $y = x^3$ from $x = 2$ to $x = 3$ using four left-endpoint rectangles.

Draw four rectangles that look like the following:

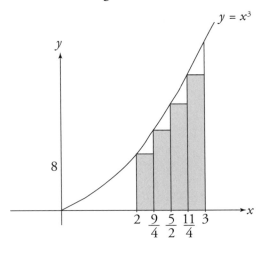

The width of each rectangle is $\frac{1}{4}$. The heights of the rectangles are

$$2^3, \left(\frac{9}{4}\right)^3, \left(\frac{5}{2}\right)^3, \text{ and } \left(\frac{11}{4}\right)^3$$

Therefore, the area is

$$\left(\frac{1}{4}\right)\left(2^3\right)+\left(\frac{1}{4}\right)\left(\frac{9}{4}\right)^3+\left(\frac{1}{4}\right)\left(\frac{5}{2}\right)^3+\left(\frac{1}{4}\right)\left(\frac{11}{4}\right)^3 = \frac{893}{64} \approx 13.953$$

Example 2: Repeat Example 1 using four right-endpoint rectangles.

Now draw four rectangles that look like the following:

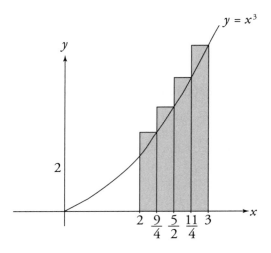

The width of each rectangle is still $\frac{1}{4}$, but the heights of the rectangles are now

$$\left(\frac{9}{4}\right)^3, \left(\frac{5}{2}\right)^3, \left(\frac{11}{4}\right)^3, \text{ and } \left(3^3\right)$$

The area is now

$$\left(\frac{1}{4}\right)\left(\frac{9}{4}\right)^3+\left(\frac{1}{4}\right)\left(\frac{5}{2}\right)^3+\left(\frac{1}{4}\right)\left(\frac{11}{4}\right)^3+\left(\frac{1}{4}\right)\left(3^3\right)=\frac{1,197}{64}\approx 18.703$$

Example 3: Repeat Example 1 using four midpoint rectangles.

Now draw four rectangles that look like the following:

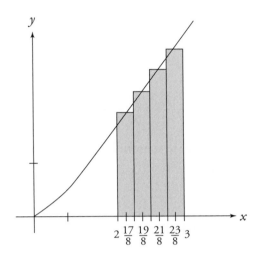

The width of each rectangle is still $\dfrac{1}{4}$, but the heights of the rectangles are now

$$\left(\frac{17}{8}\right)^3 , \left(\frac{19}{8}\right)^3 , \left(\frac{21}{8}\right)^3 , \text{ and } \left(\frac{23}{8}\right)^3$$

The area is now

$$\left(\frac{1}{4}\right)\left(\frac{17}{8}\right)^3 + \left(\frac{1}{4}\right)\left(\frac{19}{8}\right)^3 + \left(\frac{1}{4}\right)\left(\frac{21}{8}\right)^3 + \left(\frac{1}{4}\right)\left(\frac{23}{8}\right)^3 = \frac{2,075}{128} \approx 16.211$$

The Fundamental Theorem of Calculus

Before, we said that if you create an infinite number of infinitely thin rectangles, you'll get the area under the curve, which is an integral. For the example above, the integral is

$$\int_2^3 x^3 dx$$

There is a rule for evaluating an integral like this. The rule is called the **Fundamental Theorem of Calculus**, and it says

$$\int_a^b f(x)dx = F(b) - F(a); \text{ where } F(x) \text{ is the antiderivative of } f(x).$$

Using this rule, you can find $\int_2^3 x^3\,dx$ by integrating it, and we get $\dfrac{x^4}{4}$. Now all you do is plug in 3 and 2 and take the difference. We use the following notation to symbolize this:

$$\left.\frac{x^4}{4}\right|_2^3$$

Thus, we have

$$\frac{3^4}{4}-\frac{2^4}{4}=\frac{81}{4}-\frac{16}{4}=\frac{65}{4}$$

Because $\dfrac{65}{4}=16.25$, you can see how close we were with our three earlier approximations.

Example 1: Find $\int_1^3\left(x^2+2\right)dx$.

The Fundamental Theorem of Calculus yields the following:

$$\int_1^3\left(x^2+2\right)dx=\left.\left(\frac{x^3}{3}+2x\right)\right|_1^3$$

If we evaluate this, we get the following:

$$\left(\frac{3^3}{3}+2(3)\right)-\left(\frac{1^3}{3}+2(1)\right)=\frac{38}{3}$$

This is the first function for which we found the approximate area by using inscribed rectangles. Our final estimate, where we averaged the inscribed and circumscribed rectangles, was $\dfrac{51}{4}$, and as you can see, that was very close (off by $\dfrac{1}{12}$). When we used the midpoints, we were off by $\dfrac{1}{24}$.

We're going to do only a few approximations using rectangles, because it's not a big part of the PCAT. On the other hand, definite integrals are a huge part of the rest of this book.

Example 2: $\int_1^5\left(x^2-x\right)dx=\left.\left(\frac{x^3}{3}-\frac{x^2}{2}\right)\right|_1^5=\left(\frac{125}{3}-\frac{25}{2}\right)-\left(\frac{1}{3}-\frac{1}{2}\right)=\frac{88}{3}$

Example 3: $\int_0^{\frac{\pi}{2}}\sin x\,dx=\left.(-\cos x)\right|_0^{\frac{\pi}{2}}=\left(-\cos\frac{\pi}{2}\right)-(-\cos 0)=1$

Example 4: $\int_0^{\frac{\pi}{4}}\sec^2 x\,dx=\left.\tan x\right|_0^{\frac{\pi}{4}}=\tan\frac{\pi}{4}-\tan 0=1$

The Average Value of a Function

Let f be a function that's continuous on a closed interval $[a,b]$. Then, according to the **Mean-Value Theorem for Integrals**, there's at least one point c between a and b, such that

$$\int_a^b f(x)\,dx = f(c)(b-a)$$

13.5

What this says geometrically is that there's a point c such that the area of the rectangle whose base is $b-a$ and whose height is $f(c)$ is equal to the area under the curve from a to b.

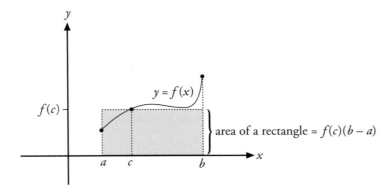

The value $f(c)$ is the **average value** of the function $f(x)$ on the interval $[a,b]$.

Finding the Area Between Two Curves

What's the area, A, of the region bounded by the curves $y = x^2$ and $y = \sqrt{x}$?

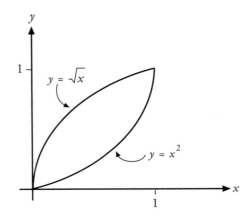

It's easy to see that this area is equal to the area under the curve $y = \sqrt{x}$ minus the area under the curve $y = x^2$, from $x = 0$ to $x = 1$; that is,

$$A = \int_0^1 (\sqrt{x})\,dx - \int_0^1 (x^2)\,dx = \int_0^1 (\sqrt{x} - x^2)\,dx$$

Another way to answer this question is to construct a typical rectangular strip of width Δx within this region; its height is $\sqrt{x} - x^2$, so its area is $(\sqrt{x} - x^2)\Delta x$.

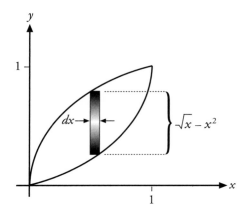

When we add the areas of all these strips (calling the sum S), and pass to the limit as the widths of the rectangles approach zero, we get

$$S = \Sigma(\sqrt{x} - x^2)\Delta x \rightarrow \int_0^1 (\sqrt{x} - x^2)\,dx$$

as before. Notice that the Riemann sum on the left becomes the definite integral on the right once we pass to the limit, where the widths of the rectangles approach zero. (In fact, the integral sign itself is simply an elongated S, which is meant to symbolize that the limit of a *sum* is being computed.) We can abbreviate this method even further, if we start by letting dx denote the width of the rectangle, and add up—that is, integrate—the areas of the rectangles. To illustrate this approach in a slightly different way, imagine constructing a horizontal rectangular strip of height dy and width $\sqrt{y} - y^2$—and thus, area of $(\sqrt{y} - y^2)dy$—within the region:

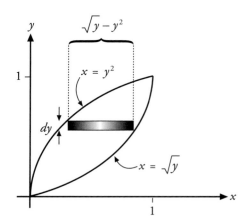

Allowing this strip to sweep through the region, by integrating from $y = 0$ up to $y = 1$, will give us the region's total area:

$$A = \int_0^1 (\sqrt{y} - y^2)\,dy$$

which is the same as the integral given earlier in the variable x (since x and y are just dummy variables). The value of A is shown below:

$$A = \int_0^1 (\sqrt{y} - y^2)\, dy = \frac{2}{3} y^{3/2} - \frac{1}{3} y^3 \Bigg]_0^1 = \frac{1}{3}$$

Volumes of Solids of Revolution

Imagine that we have a portion of a curve, $y = f(x)$ from $x = a$ to $x = b$, in the x-y plane, and we revolve it around a straight line—the x-axis, for example:

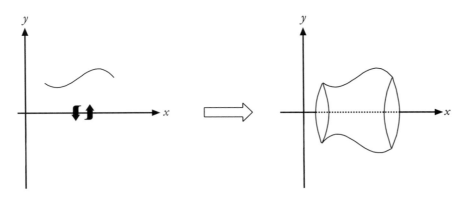

The result is called a **solid of revolution**. In this section, we'll develop techniques for finding the volumes of solids of revolution.

As we've done before, let's construct a narrow rectangle of base width dx and height $f(x)$, sitting under the curve. When this rectangle is revolved around the x-axis, we get a disk whose radius is $f(x)$ and whose height is dx. The volume of this disk is $dV = \pi \left[f(x) \right]^2 dx$, so the total volume of the solid is as follows:

$$V = \int_a^b dV = \int_a^b \pi [f(x)]^2\, dx$$

If the curve is revolved around a vertical line (such as the y-axis), then horizontal disks are used. If the curve can be solved for x in terms of y, $x = g(y)$, the formula above becomes as follows:

$$V = \int_c^d \pi [g(y)]^2\, dy$$

These equations illustrate the **disk method** for finding the volume of a solid of revolution.

Sometimes the region between two curves is revolved around an axis, and a gap is created between the solid and the axis. A rectangle within the rotated region will become a disk with a hole in it—also known as a washer. If the rectangle is vertical and extends from the curve $y = g(x)$ up to the curve $y = f(x)$, then when it's rotated around the x-axis, it will result in a washer with volume equal to

$$dV = \pi \left\{ \left[f(x) \right]^2 - \left[g(x) \right]^2 \right\} dx$$

which gives us

$$V = \int_a^b \pi \{[f(x)]^2 - [g(x)]^2\} dx$$

Similarly, if the region is revolved around a vertical axis, we'll get horizontal washers and the formula above will involve the variable y. This is the **washer method** for finding the volume of a solid of revolution.

The curve $x = y^2 + 3$ is the "inside" curve and the line $x = 4y$ is the "outside" curve (that is, for $1 \le y \le 3$, the curve $x = y^2 + 3$ is closer to the y-axis than is the line $x = 4y$), so the washer method gives us the following:

$$V = \int_c^d \pi \{[f(y)]^2 - [g(y)]^2\} dy$$
$$= \int_1^3 \pi[(4y)^2 - (y^2 + 3)^2] dy$$
$$= \pi \int_1^3 [10y^2 - y^4 - 9] dy$$
$$= \pi \left[\frac{10}{3} y^3 - \frac{1}{5} y^5 - 9y \right]_1^3$$
$$= \pi \left[\left(\frac{10}{3} \cdot 3^3 - \frac{1}{5} \cdot 3^5 - 9 \cdot 3 \right) - \left(\frac{10}{3} \cdot 1^3 - \frac{1}{5} \cdot 1^5 - 9 \cdot 1 \right) \right]$$
$$= \frac{304}{15} \pi$$

Arc Length

The length of a smooth curve (also called an arc) can also be found by integration. To establish the formula we need, let's consider the portion of the curve $y = f(x)$ from (a, c) to (b, d):

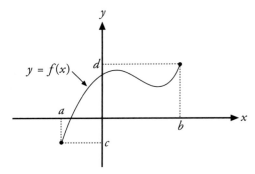

We can construct a differential right triangle with sides of lengths dx and dy, and hypotenuse ds along the curve:

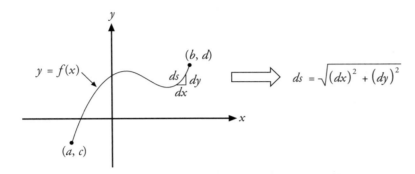

By adding up—that is, by integrating—the contributions ds, we get the following formula for s, the length of the curve:

$$s = \int ds = \int \sqrt{(dx)^2 + (dy)^2} = \int_a^b \sqrt{1 + \left(\frac{dy}{dx}\right)^2}\; dx \quad \text{or} \quad \int_c^d \sqrt{\left(\frac{dy}{dx}\right)^2 + 1}\; dy$$

The Natural Exponential and Logarithm Functions

Although we've already included the functions e^x and $\log x$ in the tables of differentials and integrals, we also want to include some other important information about these functions and the choice of the base, e.

The function e^x arises from the attempt to find a nonzero function that equals its own derivative. The derivative of every exponential function of the form $f(x) = a^x$ (with a positive) is equal to a multiple of itself, as the following calculation shows:

$$f'(x) = \lim_{h \to 0} \frac{f(x+h) - f(x)}{h} = \lim_{h \to 0} \frac{a^{x+h} - a^x}{h} = a^x \cdot \left(\lim_{h \to 0} \frac{a^h - 1}{h} \right)$$

If we can find the value of a that makes the expression in parentheses equal to 1, we will have satisfied the equation $f'(x) = f(x)$. This value of a is denoted by e. To obtain a numerical value for e, we notice that, by definition,

$$\lim_{h \to 0} \frac{e^h - 1}{h} = 1$$

so for small values of h, we can write

$$e^h - 1 \approx h \quad \Rightarrow \quad e^h \approx 1 + h \quad \Rightarrow \quad e \approx (1 + h)^{1/h}$$

If we replace h by $\frac{1}{n}$, then

$$e \approx \left(1 + \frac{1}{n}\right)^n$$

and the approximation gets better as *n* gets larger. In fact, the number *e* is often *defined* as

$$e = \lim_{n \to \infty} \left(1 + \frac{1}{n} \right)^n$$

We can now approximate *e* as closely as we wish; to 15 decimal places, the value of *e* is

$$e = 2.718281828459045 \ldots$$

This real number is not only irrational, but it's also transcendental, which means that no polynomial with integer coefficients has *e* as a zero. Although the number looks messy, it's specifically chosen to provide the equation $f'(x) = f(x)$ with the simplest possible solution. Also notice that, of all the exponential functions ($f(x) = a^x$), only when $a = e$ will the slope of this curve at $x = 0$ be equal to 1. For these reasons, the function $f(x) = e^x$ is called the **natural exponential** function.

The **natural logarithm** function, $f(x) = \log_e x = \log x$, is the inverse of the natural exponential function.

The most important property of the natural logarithm function is that it provides an antiderivative of the function $g(x) = \frac{1}{x}$. We can prove this easily. If $y = \log x$, then $x = e^y$; these two equations are equivalent. If we differentiate the equation $x = e^y$ implicitly with respect to *x*, we get

$$1 = e^y \frac{dy}{dx} \quad \Rightarrow \quad \frac{dy}{dx} = \frac{1}{e^y} = \frac{1}{x}$$

It's also useful to know that, because of the fundamental theorem of calculus and the fact that $\log 1 = 0$, the expression $\log x$ can be written as

$$\log x = \int_1^x \frac{1}{t}\, dt$$

In fact, $\log x$ can be defined by this equation from the start, and all the properties of the logarithm, and of its inverse function, $f(x) = e^x$, can then be derived.

L'Hôpital's Rule

You should know **L'Hôpital's rule.** L'Hôpital's rule provides us with one of the most useful techniques for evaluating limits.

Let's start by considering this example:

$$\lim_{x \to 1} \frac{x-1}{\sqrt{x}-1}$$

If we attempt to substitute $x = 1$ into this expression, we get the meaningless fraction $\frac{0}{0}$; this is called an **indeterminate form**, since it has no unique value. L'Hôpital's rule gives us an easy way to handle this situation; it says that if $f(x)$ and $g(x)$ are functions that are differentiable in an open interval, I, containing a (except possibly at a itself) such that $g'(x) \neq 0$ for all $x \neq a$ in I, and $f(a) = g(a) = 0$, then

$$\lim_{x \to a} \frac{f(x)}{g(x)} = \lim_{x \to a} \frac{f'(x)}{g'(x)} \quad (*)$$

provided that the limit on the right exists. Applying this rule to the limit problem above, we'd differentiate the numerator and denominator (separately!) and find

$$\lim_{x \to 1} \frac{x-1}{\sqrt{x}-1} = \lim_{x \to 1} \frac{1}{\frac{1}{2\sqrt{x}}} = \frac{1}{\frac{1}{2 \cdot 1}} = 2$$

The statement of L'Hôpital's rule remains valid if "$x \to a$" is replaced by either the left-hand limit "$x \to a-$" or the right-hand limit "$x \to a+$." It also applies when "$x \to a$" is replaced by "$x \to \infty$" or "$x \to -\infty$." Furthermore, the rule can take care of the indeterminate form $\frac{\infty}{\infty}$, which arises when both $f(x)$ and $g(x)$ become infinite, as $x \to a$. And finally, the statement of $(*)$ is still valid even when the right-hand side of $(*)$ is $+\infty$. L'Hôpital's rule is truly powerful!

Improper Integrals

Up to now, the only definite integrals we've looked at have been integrals over a bounded interval, $[a, b]$. But we will now begin to work with **improper integrals**, one type of which is integrals over unbounded intervals, of the form $[a, \infty)$, $(-\infty, b]$, or $(-\infty, \infty)$. The definition of such an integral is easy to give. For example,

$$\int_a^\infty f(x)\,dx = \lim_{b \to \infty} \int_a^b f(x)\,dx$$

provided that the limit on the right exists; if it does, then we say that the integral **converges**. Similarly, we define

$$\int_{-\infty}^b f(x)\,dx = \lim_{a \to -\infty} \int_a^b f(x)\,dx$$

For an improper integral over the entire real line, $(-\infty, \infty)$, we agree that, if both

$$\int_{-\infty}^{c} f(x)\,dx \qquad \text{and} \qquad \int_{c}^{\infty} f(x)\,dx$$

converge for some number c, then $\int_{-\infty}^{\infty} f(x)\,dx$ converges, and $\int_{-\infty}^{\infty} f(x)\,dx = \int_{-\infty}^{c} f(x)\,dx + \int_{c}^{\infty} f(x)\,dx$.

For example, let's determine the value of

$$\int_{0}^{\infty} \frac{2}{1+x^2}\,dx$$

By definition, we would write

$$\int_{0}^{\infty} \frac{2}{1+x^2}\,dx = \lim_{b\to\infty} \int_{0}^{b} \frac{2}{1+x^2}\,dx = \lim_{b\to\infty} \left[2\arctan x\right]_{0}^{b}$$
$$= 2\lim_{b\to\infty}[\arctan b]$$
$$= 2\left(\frac{\pi}{2}\right)$$
$$= \pi$$

As an example of a divergent improper integral, notice that

$$\int_{1}^{\infty} \frac{1}{x}\,dx = \lim_{b\to\infty} \int_{1}^{b} \frac{1}{x}\,dx = \lim_{b\to\infty}\left[\log x\right]_{1}^{b} = \lim_{b\to\infty}[\log b] = \infty$$

This type of integral is called *improper* because one or both of the limits of integration are infinite; these are sometimes referred to as *improper integrals of the first kind*. Another type of integral that's also called improper has finite limits of integration, but the integrand becomes infinite at one or both of the limits of integration or at a point between them. (These are *improper integrals of the second kind*.) For example,

$$\int_{0}^{1} \frac{1}{\sqrt{1-x^2}}\,dx$$

is an improper integral (of the second kind) because the integrand, $1/\sqrt{1-x^2}$, goes to infinity as $x \to 1$, the upper limit of integration. This kind of improper integral is also defined as a limit; in this case, we would write

$$\int_{0}^{1} \frac{1}{\sqrt{1-x^2}}\,dx = \lim_{b\to1} \int_{0}^{b} \frac{1}{\sqrt{1-x^2}}\,dx = \lim_{b\to1}\left[\arcsin x\right]_{0}^{b} = \lim_{b\to1}[\arcsin b] = \frac{\pi}{2}$$

CALCULUS DRILL

1. If $f'(x) = 2x + 1$ and the curve passes through the point (2, 5), what is the value of the integral constant C ?

   A. –5
   B. –1
   C. 0
   D. 11

2. The acceleration, in m/s² of a body is given by

   $\dfrac{dv}{dt} = \dfrac{2}{t+1}$, $t \geq 0$. The particle has an initial speed of

   6 m/s. What is the equation of velocity of the body?

   A. $v = \dfrac{-4}{(t+1)^2} + 10$

   B. $v = 2\ln(t + 1) + 6$

   C. $v = \dfrac{-4}{(t+1)^2} + 2$

   D. $v = 2\ln(t + 1) + 4$

3. To find the upper bound approximation for the area under the curve $y = 9x^2 + 2$ between $x = 0$ and $x = 1$, a student uses 10 rectangles. As shown in the diagram given below.

   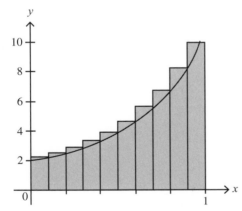

   Which expression should the student use to find the upper bound **approximation**?

   A. $0.9\sum\limits_{n=1}^{10}(0.1n)^2 + 20$

   B. $\sum\limits_{n=1}^{10}(0.9n)^2 + 20$

   C. $0.9\sum\limits_{n=1}^{10}(0.1n)^2 + 2n$

   D. $\sum\limits_{n=1}^{10}(0.9n)^2 + 2n$

4. What is the value of $\int_{0}^{2}(4-x)^3 dx$?

   A. 4
   B. 56
   C. 60
   D. 80

5. What is the value of the integral $\int_{0}^{\ln 3}e^{2u+1}du$?

   A. $3e$
   B. $4e$
   C. $8e$
   D. $16e$

6. What is the area of the region bounded by the curve $y = x^2 + 3$ and the line $y = 3x + 1$?

   A. $\dfrac{1}{6}$

   B. $\dfrac{2}{3}$

   C. $\dfrac{5}{6}$

   D. $\dfrac{3}{2}$

7. The graph of a function $f(x)$ is shown below.

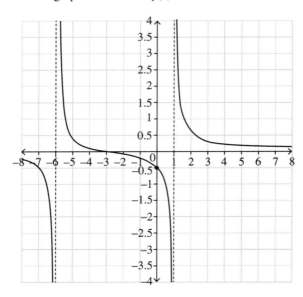

At what points of the graph does the function have infinite discontinuities?

A. $(1, -6)$
B. $(-1, 6)$
C. $(1, 6)$
D. $(-1, -6)$

8. At which point does the function $y = 54x - 9x^2$ have the **maximum** value?

A. $(-3, 81)$
B. $(3, 81)$
C. $(-9, 81)$
D. $(9, 81)$

9. The path traced by a ball is modeled by the equation $h(t) = 7.2t - 3.6t^2$, where t is the time in seconds and h is the height of the ball in meters. What is the **maximum** height the ball would reach?

A. 1.8 m
B. 2.0 m
C. 3.6 m
D. 14.4 m

10. What are the complex zeros of the function $f(x) = x^2 - 10x + 34$?

A. $x = -3 + 5i, -3 - 5i$
B. $x = -5 + 3i, -5 - 3i$
C. $x = 3 + 5i, 3 - 5i$
D. $x = 5 + 3i, 5 - 3i$

Want More Practice?
Register your book online for more drill questions!

CHAPTER 13 KEY TERMS

abscissa
absolute maximum
absolute minimum
Associative Law
asymptotes
average
average value
axis
bar graph
base
binomial
box-and-whisker plot
branches
center
Chain Rule
change-of-base formula
circle
common
commutative law for addition
complex conjugates
conic sections
definition of the derivative
denominator
dependent variable
difference quotient
directrix
discriminant
disk method
distributing
Distributive Law
dividend
divisors
domain
eccentricity
ellipse
essential discontinuity
even
exponent, or power
factorization
factors
five-number summary
focal axis
foci
focus
foiling or factoring

function
Fundamental Theorem of Calculus
graph
histogram
horizontal basis vector
horizontal scalar component
hyperbola
image
improper integrals
independent variable
indeterminate form
inequality
interquartile range
inverse function
inverse-function rule
jump discontinuity
left-hand limit
L'Hôpital's rule
linear equation
logarithm
major axis
maximum
mean
mean-value theorem for integrals
median
minimum
minor axis
mode
multiple
natural exponential
natural logarithm
natural logarithm function
numerator
odd
ordinate
outlier
parabola
percentage
percent change
point discontinuity
point-slope form
Power Rule
pre-image
prime factorization
probability

Product Rule
quadratic functions
quartiles
Quotient Rule
radius
range
ratio box
reflection
reflections
related rates
removable discontinuity
Riemann sum
right-hand limit
roots
scalar
scalar components
scale
scatterplot
secant line
slope
solid of revolution
standard deviation
statistics
symmetric with respect to the line

symmetric with respect to the origin
symmetric with respect to the x-axis
symmetric with respect to the y-axis
tangent line
tip-to-tail method
transformation
trend line
two-dimensional vectors
union symbol
unit vectors
vector
vector components
vertex
vertical and horizontal scaling
vertical and horizontal translations
vertical basis vector
vertical line test
vertical scalar component
vertices
washer method
whiskers
x-intercept
y-intercept
zero of a function

Answers and Explanations

1. **B** $\int f'(x) = \int (2x+1)dx + C$. $f(x) = 2\dfrac{x^2}{2} + x + C$. So, $f(x) = x^2 + x + C$. Substituting the

    point (2, 5), $5 = 4 + 2 + C$. Hence, $C = -1$. The answer is choice (B).

2. **B** On integrating, you get $\int \dfrac{dv}{dt} = \int \dfrac{2}{t+1} dt$; $v = 2\ln(t+1) + C$; when $t = 0$, $v = 6$m/s. This gives

    $6 = 2\ln(0+1) + C$, which gives $C = 6$. So, the velocity equation is $v = 2\ln(t+1) + 6$. The

    answer is choice (B).

3. **A** The width of each rectangle is $\dfrac{1-0}{10} = 0.1$. To find the height of each rectangle for the

    upper bound, find the values of y at $x = 0.1, 0.2, 0.3,$ and 1. Thus, the sum of the areas of the

    rectangles is as follows:

    $$0.1\begin{bmatrix} 9(0.1)^2 + 2 + 9(0.2)^2 + 2 + 9(0.3)^2 + 2 + 9(0.4)^2 + 2 + 9(0.5)^2 + 2 \\ +9(0.6)^2 + 2 + 9(0.7)^2 + 2 + 9(0.8)^2 + 2 + 9(0.9)^2 + 2 + 9(1)^2 + 2 \end{bmatrix}$$

    $$= (0.1)(9)\left\{ \left[\begin{array}{c} (0.1)^2 + 2 + (0.2)^2 + (0.3)^2 + (0.4)^2 + (0.5)^2 \\ +9(0.6)^2 + (0.7)^2 + (0.8)^2 + (0.9)^2 + (1)^2 \end{array} \right] + 10(2) \right\}$$

    $$= 0.9\sum_{n=1}^{10}(0.1n)^2 + 20]$$

    The answer is choice (A).

4. **C** Using the substitution method for integration, let $u = 4 - x$. Therefore, $du = -dx$. Evalu-

    ating u at the integration boundaries gives $u(0) = 4 - 0 = 4$ and $u(2) = 4 - 2 = 2$. Thus,

    $$\int_0^2 (4-x)^3 dx = -\int_4^2 u^3 du = \int_2^4 u^3 du = \left[\frac{1}{4}u^4\right]_2^4 = \left[\frac{(256-16)}{4}\right] = \frac{1}{4} \times 240 = 60.$$

    The answer is choice (C).

13.5

5. **B** $\int_0^{\ln 3} e^{2u+1} du = \int_0^{\ln 3} e^{2u} \times e^1 du = e^1 \int_0^{\ln 3} e^{2u} du$.

Integrating, $e^1 \int_0^{\ln 3} e^{2u} du = e\left[\dfrac{e^{2u}}{2}\right]_0^{\ln 3} = e\left[\dfrac{e^{2\ln 3} - e^0}{2}\right] = 4e$. The answer is choice (B).

6. **A** Solve the given equations as follows:

$3x + 1 = x^2 + 3$

$\Rightarrow x^2 - 3x + 2 = 0$

$\Rightarrow x^2 - 3x + 2 = 0$

$\Rightarrow x = 1, 2$

Calculate the area as follows

$\int_1^2 \left[(3x+1) - (x^2+3)\right] dx$

$= \int_1^2 \left[-x^2 + 3x - 2\right] dx$

$= \left[-\dfrac{x^3}{3} + \dfrac{3x^2}{2} - 2x\right]_1^2$

$= -\dfrac{4}{6} + \dfrac{5}{6} = \dfrac{1}{6}$. The answer is choice (A).

7. **A** Since the graph has the vertical asymptotes at $x = 1$, $y = -6$, the function has infinite discon-

tinuities at $(1, -6)$. The answer is choice (A).

8. **B** Simplify the equation as $y = -(9x^2 - 54x + 81) + 81 \Rightarrow y = -(3x - 9)^2 + 81$ and solve for x as $3x - 9 = 0 \Rightarrow x = 3$. Therefore, the function attains the maximum value at $(3, 81)$. The answer is choice (B).

9. **C** Solve the equation as $h(t) = -\dfrac{1}{10}(36t^2 - 72t) = -\dfrac{1}{10}(36t^2 - 72t + 36) + 3.6$. Therefore,

the ball reaches a maximum height of 3.6 meters. The answer is choice (C).

10. **D** Solve the equation as $x^2 - 10x + 34 = 0 \Rightarrow x^2 - 10x + 25 = -9 \Rightarrow (x - 5)^2 = -9 \Rightarrow x - 5 = \pm 3i \Rightarrow x = 5 \pm 3i$. The answer is choice (D).

Quick Review

- On the PCAT, square roots must be positive. However, exponents have both positive and negative roots.

- The eight main topics of arithmetic are

  - order of operations

  - fractions

  - decimals

  - percentages

  - ratios

  - averages

  - charts and graphs

  - combinations

- Arithmetic operations must be performed in a particular order. Here's an easy way to remember the order of operations: **P**lease **E**xcuse **M**y **D**ear **A**unt **S**ally. First, you do operations enclosed in **p**arentheses; then you take care of **e**xponents; then you **m**ultiply, **d**ivide, **a**dd, and **s**ubtract.

- Factors are numbers that divide into your original number. Multiples are numbers that your original number divides into.

  - Factors are smaller than or equal to your original number.

  - Multiples are larger than or equal to your original number.

- When you add or multiply a group of numbers, you can put them in any order that suits you. This is called the associative law.

- The distributive law states that $a(b + c) = ab + ac$ and that $a(b - c) = ab - ac$. On the PCAT, if you see a problem in one form, you will make the problem much easier by immediately putting it in the other form.

- A fraction can be thought of as a $\frac{\text{part}}{\text{whole}}$.

- You must know how to reduce, multiply, divide, compare, add, and subtract fractions. The Bowtie is a great method for doing the last three items mentioned, but your calculator is even better—if you know how to use it.

- Every fraction implies another fraction—what is left over. If a glass is $\frac{3}{5}$ empty, it is $\frac{2}{5}$ full.

- A decimal is just another way to express a fraction.

- You must know how to add, subtract, multiply, and divide decimals as well as be familiar with scientific notation.

- A percentage is just a fraction in which the denominator is equal to 100. Most percentage problems can be set up to look like this: $\frac{part}{whole} = \frac{x}{100}$.

- On word problems dealing with percentages, you can use the percent translation table to create a calculator-friendly equation.

- There are two formulas for percent change:

  - The basic formula for percent change is

$$\%\,Change = \frac{Amount\ Change}{Original} \times 100$$

  - The formula for repeated percent change is: Final = Original $\times$ [1 $\pm$ Rate]$^{\#\ of\ changes}$. If it's a repeated percent increase, you add Rate. If it's a decrease, you subtract Rate.

- In average questions, you should immediately think

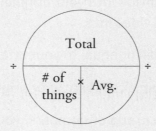

- The PCAT has a particular fondness for weighted averages. Be on the lookout for them.

- Raising a number greater than 1 to a power greater than 1 results in a bigger number. For example, $2^2 = 4$.

- Know the rules for multiplying and dividing exponents, raising a power to a power, and expressing fractional and negative exponents.

- Raising a fraction that's between 0 and 1 to a power greater than 1 results in a smaller number. For example, $\left(\dfrac{1}{2}\right)^2 = \dfrac{1}{4}$.

- A negative number raised to an even power becomes positive. For example, $(-2)^2 = 4$, because $(-2)(-2) = 4$.

- A negative number raised to an odd power remains negative. For example, $(-2)^3 = -8$, because $(-2)(-2)(-2) = -8$.

- A number raised to a negative power is equal to 1 over the number raised to the positive power. For example, $2^{-2} = \dfrac{1}{2^2} = \dfrac{1}{4}$.

- A number raised to the 0 power is 1, no matter what the number is. For example, $1,000^0 = 1$. Note, however, that 0 to the 0 power is undefined.

- A number raised to the first power is ALWAYS the number itself. For example, $1,000^1 = 1,000$.

- Inequalities get solved just like equations, but when you multiply or divide by a negative number, flip the sign.

- Absolute value questions often have two answers. Write out and solve both equations created by the absolute value.

- Simultaneous equation questions don't require solving one variable in terms of another. Just stack 'em and add or subtract to find what you need. Remember that you can multiply or divide before or after you add or subtract to get to what you want.

- The general form for a quadratic equation is $ax^2 + bx + c = 0$. To find the factors, just reverse FOIL the equation. There are three special quadratics that you should keep an eye out for to save time and brainpower. They are

  - $(x + y)^2 = x^2 + 2xy + y^2$
  - $(x - y)^2 = x^2 - 2xy + y^2$
  - $(x + y)(x - y) = x^2 - y^2$

- You can use Plugging In whenever

  - you see variables, percents, or fractions (without an original amount) in the answers
  - you're tempted to write and then solve an algebraic equation
  - you see the phrase "in terms of" in the question
  - there are unknown quantities or variables in the question

- Plug in the answer choices when you have numbers in the answers but don't know where to start or you are still tempted to write an algebraic equation. Don't forget to start with choice (C)!

- If you have a quadratic equation that you can't factor, try using the quadratic formula:

$$x = \frac{-b \pm \sqrt{b^2 - 4ac}}{2a}$$

- Probability is the number of ways to get what you want divided by the total number of possible outcomes.

- The probability of multiple events occurring can be calculated either by writing them all out or by multiplying the individual probabilities together.

- The number of possible combinations is the product of the number of things of each type from which you have to choose.

- Ratios are another way to show the relationship between two quantities.

- When using the Ratio Box, always add the ratio parts to find the ratio whole.

- All the ratio numbers are multiplied by the same factor to convert ratios to actual numbers; your job is to find the factor that connects a ratio number to the actual number.

- Statistics is about working with large groups of numbers and looking for patterns and trends in those numbers.

  ○ The mean is the average value of a set.

  ○ The median is the middle value of a set when the values of the set are in chronological order.

  ○ The mode is the value that occurs the most in a set.

  ○ The range of a set in statistics is the difference between the set's highest and lowest values.

  ○ The interquartile range is the range of the middle 50 percent of the data, the difference between the third quartile and the first quartile.

  ○ Standard deviation is a measure of a set's variation from its mean.

- Charts and graphs present data for you to analyze.

  - In a bar graph each value for the variable at the bottom of the graph is represented by a bar.

  - If the bars in a graph represent ranges of data, rather than distinct categories, the graph is a histogram.

  - In a scatterplot, each dot represents one data point. Sometimes, a trend line or curve "of best fit" will be drawn to represent the equation that most closely matches the data.

  - A box-and-whisker plot presents information from a five-number summary— [1] the minimum value, [2] the lower quartile, [3] the median value, [4] the upper quartile, and [5] the maximum value— of the data set.

  - Outliers are unusual observations that skew the data in a data set.

- To find the derivative of a function, use the following list of derivative rules!

- The definite integral gives the total algebraic area bounded by the curve $y = f(x)$. Memorize the following rules regarding integration for the PCAT!

- To find the derivative of a function, use the following list of derivative rules!

  - $\log_b(x_1 x_2) = \log_b x_1 + \log_b x_2$

  - $\log_b \dfrac{x_1}{x_2} = \log_b x_1 - \log_b x_2$

  - $\log_b(x^a) = a \log_b x$

  - $b^{\log_b x} = x$

  - $(\log_b a)(\log_a x) = \log_b x$ [this is the change-of-base formula, with $a \neq 1$]

- The definite integral gives the total algebraic area bounded by the curve $y = f(x)$. Memorize the following rules regarding integration for the PCAT!

1. $\int_b^a f(x)dx = -\int_a^b f(x)dx$

   This rule says that reversing the limits of integration changes the sign of the integral. Notice that if $a = b$, then this rule implies:

   $\int_a^a f(x)dx = 0$

2. $\int_a^c f(x)dx = \int_a^b f(x)dx + \int_b^c f(x)dx$

   This rule says that the integral from a to c is equal to the integral from a to b plus the integral from b to c.

3. $\int_a^b kf(x)dx = k\int_a^b f(x)dx$ (where k is a constant)

   This rule says that the integral of kf is equal to k times the integral of f, so a constant may be moved outside the integral sign.

4. $\int_a^b [f(x) \pm g(x)]dx = \int_a^b f(x)dx \pm \int_a^b g(x)dx$

   The integral of a sum (or difference) is equal to the sum (or difference) of the integrals.

5. If $f(x) \le g(x)$ for all $x \in [a, b]$, then $\int_a^b f(x)dx \le \int_a^b g(x)dx$

   This rule says that if one function is always greater than another function over a defined interval, then the integral is also greater.

Chapter 14

Writing

14.1   ABOUT CRITICAL THINKING ESSAYS

About the Writing Subtest

The first subsection of the PCAT test is Writing, which will present one writing topic. It is the last chapter of this book because it is generally the least of PCAT students' worries, however, it is still important for your overall score. In the Writing subtest, you will get 30 minutes to plan your response and write your solutions to the problem presented. The Writing will be scored on "conventions of language" and "problem solving." Even though the length of your essay will not necessarily be a factor in what score you get, you should make sure that your essay is of sufficient length to adequately explain your solutions to the problem.

Writing Topics

All of the PCAT writing prompts will state a problem that may involve either a health issue; a science issue; or a social, cultural, or political issue. You will be asked to present a solution (or more than one) to a problem presented. You will be scored on how well you write an essay that sufficiently explains and supports your solutions to the problem.

Here are some sample prompts.

Health Issues
- Discuss solutions to problems resulting from insufficient supplies of donated blood and plasma.
- Discuss solutions to the problem of providing adequate health care for undocumented persons.
- Discuss solutions to the problem of promoting healthy eating habits to children.

Science Issues
- Discuss solutions to the problem of dealing with sorting through garbage for recyclable materials.
- Discuss solutions to the problem of disappearing glaciers.
- Discuss solutions to the problem of protecting the diminishing amount of potable water.

Social, Cultural, and Political Issues
- Discuss solutions to the problems resulting from lack of funding for local government offices.
- Discuss solutions to the problem of protecting children from online predators.
- Discuss solutions to the problem of promoting face-to-face communication in a digital culture.

Expectations of Writing Scorers

For the problem presented in the prompt, you will be expected to:

- Provide a minimum of one solution to the problem presented.
- State a clear thesis.
- Present relevant support for your thesis from credible references that relate to academic or personal experience, reading, or studies.
- Discuss and evaluate possible alternative solutions to your primary solution.
- Use appropriate and conventional grammar, punctuation, word usage, and writing style.

How Does the Word-Processing Program Work?

Compared to any of the commercial word-processing programs, the one provided for the PCAT will seem extremely limited, but it does allow the basic functions: you can move the cursor with the arrow keys, and you can delete, copy, and paste. You won't have a dictionary, spell-check, or any reference materials handy, but for the most part, you will be able to use the computer like a regular word-processing program.

Scoring

The Writing section will be scored on a scale from 0 to 6.0, where 0 indicates a writing sample that is either left blank, not written in English, or that is off-topic. The scores concerning your conventions of language and problem solving will represent an average of scores assigned by two scorers, rounded to the nearest tenth, that will comprise your final earned Writing score.

Along with the earned Writing score, you will also receive a mean score. It represents the average of all Writing scores from the same testing window. It is for comparison purposes only so that you can compare your performance to the average score of other test-takers who took the same test that you did.

Explanations for Writing Scores

The descriptions below show the characteristics of each division of the Writing score. "Conventions of Language" is a measure of how well you wrote your essay, whereas "Problem Solving" measures whether or not you understood the problem, whether you presented clear and logical solutions, and whether you used appropriate examples to support your position. Keep these criteria in mind as you write practice essays.

Conventions of Language
- 6.0   (Superior)
  - Full command of the conventions of language
  - Few mistakes in grammar, sentence formation, word usage, and writing mechanics
  - Evidence of advanced or innovative writing techniques
- 5.0   (Proficient)
  - Proficient in applying the conventions of language
  - Some mistakes in grammar, sentence formation, word usage, and writing mechanics, but none serious enough to interfere with the meaning
  - Sophisticated structure
  - A clear beginning, middle, and end

4.0 (Effective)
- Mostly correct application of conventions of language
- Several mistakes in grammar, sentence formation, word usage, and writing mechanics
- Some disruption of overall flow but no interference with meaning
- Basic structure of multiple paragraphs (beginning, middle, and end)

3.0 (Satisfactory)
- Marginal success in applying conventions of language
- Patterns of mistakes in grammar, sentence formation, word usage, and writing mechanics that interfere with the understanding of the response
- Multiple paragraphs with a beginning, middle, and end

2.0 (Marginal)
- Little success in applying conventions of language
- Frequent and serious mistakes in grammar, sentence formation, word usage, and writing mechanics, making the response hard to understand

1.0 (Inadequate)
- Limited ability to apply the conventions of language
- Frequent mistakes in grammar, sentence formation, word usage, and writing mechanics make the content difficult to understand

0 (Invalid)
- Section left blank, written in a language other than English, or written unintelligibly
- Indicates an inability or refusal to attempt a response

Problem Solving

6.0 (Superior)
- Thoughtful care to avoid questionable reasoning
- Powerful and sophisticated argument
- Elegant composition style showing advanced rhetorical techniques
- Solution that shows direct correlation to the problem
- Solution fully detailed with relevant and convincing support, such as facts, examples, and anecdotes
- Main principles of the problem and solution described and defined
- Alternative or multiple solutions are proposed and analyzed
- Logical (or creative) organizational structure throughout

5.0 (Proficient)
- Reasoning that is slightly questionable
- Strongly persuasive argument
- Advanced composition techniques
- Solution that appears to be clearly connected to the problem
- Solution appropriately supported with some degree of depth
- Main principles of the problem and solution discussed and explained
- One or more alternative solutions are mentioned with some attempt at analysis or evaluation
- Logical organization with some minor flaws

4.0   (Effective)
- Effective composition techniques
- General presentation of solution with clear discussion of problem and solution
- Lacking in persuasiveness
- Solution clearly related to the problem with support that is appropriate and relevant
- Logical progression of writing, but loosely organized with digressions or unnecessary redundancies

3.0   (Satisfactory)
- Composition is fairly successful and effective
- Solution that is loosely related to problem with connections that are too general to be convincing
- Most support for solution is appropriate
- Flow is interrupted with redundancies, digressions, irrelevancies, and issues not clearly related to problem

2.0   (Marginal)
- Composition techniques are marginally effective
- Solution is not related to problem
- Support for solution is implicit and not clearly stated
- Arguments contain redundancies, digressions, and irrelevancies
- Chaotic organization

1.0   (Inadequate)
- Elements of effective composition are missing
- Discussion is not related to the problem stated
- Support contains contradictions, digressions, redundancies, and irrelevancies
- Chaotic organization
- No solution can be ascertained

0   (Invalid)
- Section left blank, written in a language other than English, or written unintelligibly
- Indicates an inability or refusal to attempt a response related to topic
- Problem solved addresses topic other than the one assigned

Stay Calm

The Writing section always seems daunting, especially since it will be the first task you'll be asked to do when you sit down. Though PCAT scores are important factors in the decision process of the admissions committees of pharmacy schools, remember that the Writing section will probably *not* be the most important aspect of your score that they'll be looking at. So take the first 30 minutes of the test that is assigned to writing and use that time to settle those nerves about the rest of the test. Think about the problem put forth in the prompt instead of the impending calculus questions. Take one section at a time and do your best. And now that you know the basics about the Writing section, we'll show you how to strengthen your writing skills and strategies so that you can make the most of the 30 minutes you have for each prompt.

For more information about the PCAT Writing section, refer to the current PCAT Candidate Information Booklet that is available to download as a PDF file from the PCAT website: www.PCATweb.info.

14.2 WRITING STRATEGY

Goals and Planning

The best essays will display the following hallmarks:

If you're still struggling with grammatical errors and sentence structures, check out our book *Writing Smart, 3rd Edition* for insightful exam writing tips to help you score well on the PCAT writing section!

Precision and Confidence

Don't use wishy-washy or vague wording in presenting your analysis. Project confidence in what you have to say.

Completeness

You must address all the tasks that accompany the prompt. No matter how brilliant your response, if it does not take great care to provide solutions and examples to the problem presented, your score will suffer. To cover the required aspects of the prompt in depth, you will need to take time and organize your thoughts. While it's quality—not quantity—that matters, an essay that is too brief gives the impression that you don't have much to say.

Clarity

Think before you write. Convoluted wording and pointless repetition will not score you points. Clear and concise analysis is much better than long and rambling paragraphs that continually repeat the same ideas or that are difficult for the reader to follow.

Consistency

Make sure all of your points and counter-points actually address the issue in the prompt.

Comprehensibility

Pay attention to spelling, grammar, and sentence construction. Don't use big words if you are not absolutely sure that they mean what you think they mean. Use simple, direct language.

Concrete and Fully Explained Examples

Realistic, specific, and concrete examples work better than vague hypothetical examples. If you must use a hypothetical example, make it as specific and detailed as possible. Don't make the reader guess at why you chose the examples you cite; explain the relevance of your examples to the themes of the prompt.

Originality

Catch the reader's attention. Your central mission is to give a complete and logically consistent response. If you can add to that unique examples, thoughtful and insightful analysis that gets below the surface of the question, and a direct and intriguing introduction to grab a reader's attention and to draw the grader into the essay, your score will be higher.

Three Basic Steps

Because you have only 30 minutes to write the essay, you'll need to have a pretty good idea of how you're going to attack it as soon as you sit down at the computer on test day. Our approach to the essay involves three steps. These are:

1. **Think**. Before you start writing, take a moment to brainstorm some thoughts about the topic.
2. **Organize**. Take the ideas you've come up with and fit them into the assignment for the prompt.
3. **Write**. Once you've completed the first two steps, the final step should be a snap.

You do not have a lot of time to write an essay, so you have to get it right the first time out. While you should leave enough time to proofread and edit your essay, it simply isn't feasible to expect to make any significant changes to it during the final minutes of the section. Furthermore, if you get halfway through your essay and realize you're stuck or you're not saying what you need to say, you'll be hard-pressed to fix it in the time you have left.

It is essential, therefore, to make sure you spend time planning your essay before you start writing. You have to figure out what it is you want to say before you begin; otherwise, you run the risk of writing an incoherent, rambling response. The first two steps are actually more important to a successful PCAT essay than the final step; by spending a little time planning your response, the actual writing part should be relatively painless.

> The keys to the essay: Think, Organize, Write.

Prewriting: A Four-Step Process

Effective prewriting consists of the following four-step process. You don't have to perform these steps in one particular order. In fact, you'll probably find that your prewriting process is recursive; that is, you cycle through the steps a few times, with ideas from one step giving you new ideas for another step.

Outlining

- ### Step 1: Brainstorm Examples and Ideas.
- ### Step 2: Identify and Define Key Topics.
- ### Step 3: Determine the Statement's Central Question.
- ### Step 4: Outline the Three Tasks.

Step 1:   **Brainstorm Examples and Ideas.**

After reading the entire prompt carefully, use your erasable noteboard to jot down relevant thoughts that come to mind. Write down possible examples and issues that appear to be important to the topic. Focus on the heart of the problem presented. Also brainstorm about alternative examples and solutions you could suggest that would not work as well as your primary solutions.

It's crucial not to censor yourself at this stage. Much of what you write down will not be usable, but by letting your mind work freely, you'll uncover those great examples and ideas now, instead of leaving them to work their way to the surface hours later.

Step 2:   **Identify and Define Key Terms.**

Identify the terms in the prompt that might be defined in several different ways. Abstract terms (e.g., "freedom," "duty," "justice") are some likely candidates. Think of all possible definitions and then narrow them down to the definition you want to use in your essay. For example, "the law" in a prompt could be all written laws, federal but not state or local laws, or unwritten laws and social norms that make up our "national culture." You might want to pick the most straightforward definition—all written laws.

Choose reasonable, common-sense definitions. Keep your definitions consistent throughout the essay; don't base your examples on defining key terms in two different ways.

Step 3:   **Determine the Statement's Central Question.**

Think about what important themes, debates, or political, social, or scientific controversies might have inspired the test-writers to come up with this particular prompt. The prompt might ask you to think about democratic principles (equality, freedom of speech and religion, representative government, etc.). Or, it may center on humanistic issues or social problems (How does technology affect people? How can our society improve? How do we address issues like crime, poverty, or illiteracy?). Finally, it may be generated by basic moral questions (When is it right or wrong to commit certain actions or hold particular beliefs?). Decide what core issues are involved in the prompt statement. Think about how these issues are embodied in the examples you choose and how they relate to the contrast between those examples.

Step 4:   Outline the Three Tasks.

Organize your thoughts so you can create a rough outline. Good organization is one of the most important aspects of a high-scoring essay. The essay graders read and evaluate each essay in only a few minutes. A poorly organized essay is difficult to follow, and the readers will not take extra time to piece together your ideas.

From your brainstorming session, select examples that are the best solutions to the problem presented in the prompt, then select another potential solution that you can suggest and evaluate. Have a third solution that is less-than-ideal to include if you have the time.

Next comes the outline, which is the most significant element in an essay's creation. If you spend the time to stitch all the elements into a viable structure, the essay will be much easier to compose. Graders love organization and have so little time to look for it, so make life easy for them. Once your reader sees that, he or she knows you took the time to organize your thoughts before you started writing your essay. This structure jumps out at the reader right away, and it makes a good impression.

Some people find it useful and time-effective to write quite detailed outlines, while others effectively use much briefer versions. Discover what works best for you.

What follows is a basic outline for you to use as a template, with a sample prompt to get you started. Use this basic outline while you research current education, scientific, social, cultural, and political issues when you are preparing for the test.

Sample Outline Template

Prompt: Discuss a solution to the problem of assuring national security while protecting the privacy of individual citizens.

1. **Brainstorm solutions.**
    Current examples of national security threats related to individual privacy:

    - _____

    - _____

    - _____

    Current examples of privacy issues:

    - _____

    - _____

    - _____

    - _____

    - _____

Potential solutions with reasoning behind why or why not each one would work:

- _____

- _____

- _____

- _____

Ways to implement solutions (Examples: education, intervention, legislation, or enforcement):

- _____

- _____

2. **Identify and define key terms.**
    "national security": _____

    _____

    "privacy": _____

    _____

    "individual rights": _____

    _____

3. **Determine the statement's central question.**
    Is there ever a time when it is OK to cross the line? Under what circumstances?

    _____

    _____

4. **Outline**
    Statement of Problem

    _____

    _____

    _____

Example: _____

_____

_____

Solution #1 and implementation

_____

_____

_____

Solution #2 and implementation

_____

_____

_____

Potential solution #3 with probable problems

_____

_____

_____

Conclusion

_____

_____

_____

Writing Clearly: Style

Simplifying—and thus clarifying—your writing will improve your Writing score. In order for your readers to understand exactly what you want to say, your argument must not be hidden in ponderous sentence construction. You don't want readers to have to do hard labor just to figure out what you are trying to communicate. You want to strip every sentence to its cleanest components. Here are some suggestions that will help clarify your writing.

Address One Idea at a Time

Don't try to put too much information into one sentence. If you're ever uncertain whether a sentence needs three commas and two semicolons or two colons and a dash, just make it into two separate sentences. Two simple sentences are better than one long, convoluted one.

Use Fewer Words to Express an Idea

In a 30-minute essay, you don't have time to experiment. In an attempt to sound important, many of us "pad" our writing. Always consider whether there's a shorter way to express your thoughts. We are all guilty of some of the following types of clutter:

Cluttered	Clear
due to the fact that	because
with the possible exception of	except
until such time as	until
for the purpose of	for
referred to as	called
at the present time	now
at all times	always

Table 1

Use Fewer Qualifiers

A qualifier is a little phrase we use to cover ourselves. Over-qualifying weakens your writing. Prune out these words and expressions wherever possible: kind of, a bit, sort of, pretty much, rather, basically, practically, essentially, in a way, quite.

Another type of qualifier is the *personal qualifier*, where instead of stating the truth, I state the truth "in my opinion." Face it: Everything you state (except perhaps for scientific or historical facts) is your opinion. Personal qualifiers like the following should be avoided: to me, in my opinion, in my experience, I think, it is my belief, it is my contention, the way I see it.

Avoid the over-used phrases "obviously" or "of course." If it's obvious, why do you need to say it? These phrases can be interpreted as condescending.

Use Fewer Adverbs

If you choose the right verb or adjective to begin with, an adverb is often unnecessary. Use an adverb only if it does useful work in the sentence. It's fine to say "the politician's campaign ran smoothly up to the primaries," because the adverb "smoothly" tells us something important about the running of the campaign. The adverb could be eliminated, however, if the verb were more specific: "the politician's campaign sailed up to the primaries." The combination of the strong verb *and* the adverb, as in "the politician's campaign sailed smoothly up to the primaries," is unnecessary because the adverb does no work.

Limit Your Use of Passive Voice

Consistently writing in the active voice and limiting your use of the passive voice will make your writing more forceful, authoritative, and interesting. Look at the sentences below. They convey essentially the same basic idea, but they have very different effects on the reader.

- The Tobacco Industry deliberately withheld data about the dangers of second-hand smoke.
- Data about the dangers of second-hand smoke was deliberately withheld by the Tobacco Industry.

The first sentence is in the active voice; the second, in the passive voice.

The active voice has a clear subject-verb relationship which illustrates that the subject is doing the action. A sentence is in the passive voice when the subject of the sentence, instead of acting, is acted upon. By distancing the subject from the verb, the passive voice makes it appear that the action is being done to the subject. Instead, own the action.

The passive voice uses a form of *be* (is, am, are, was, were, been) plus the main verb in past participle form. The "do-er" of a passive voice sentence is either absent or relegated to the end of the sentence in a "by" phrase.

Avoid Clichés Like the Plague

Clichés are comfortable. When we're stuck for the next word, a cliché will suddenly strike us, and we'll feel lucky. We write something like "this *tried and true* method" or "he was one of the *best and brightest.*" A cliché may let the writer off the hook, but the reader will be turned off. The reason a cliché is a cliché is because it is overused. Try something original instead.

Your Style of Writing

Now that we've covered the grammar and writing basics, let's talk a little about style. The term *style* is hard to define; it could involve all of the points we're about to discuss, or none of them. Style is the difference between "It was the best of times, it was the worst of times" and "Times were great, but they were bad too."

Your own style will evolve as you practice, but there are a few ways to add a little bit of style to your writing and increase an essay's value in the eyes of the reader.

Let Every Word Tell

No primer on the virtues of writing is complete without some pompous Shakespearean quote, so here's one that's especially relevant. As Polonius told Claudius in *Hamlet*, "brevity is the soul of wit."

Pointless repetition drags too many essays into the morass of mediocrity. If you've made your point, don't linger on it. You'll be tempted to make it again, and you'll weaken your message.

Word Variety

You don't have to have an encyclopedic vocabulary to vary your choice of words. No one's asking you to study a thesaurus, but adding a synonym now and then will help you avoid paragraphs like this:

> Communication is as important as creativity because no idea is worth anything unless it can be communicated to someone else. Communication starts at an early age, when we first learn to communicate with our parents. And let us not forget the quality of communication; an idea that is poorly communicated is not worth much more than one that is not communicated at all.

Without being too florid in your word choice, you can make a few strategic substitutions and turn that paragraph into this one:

> Communication is as important as creativity because no idea is worth anything unless **someone can convey it** to someone else. Communication starts at an early age, when we first learn to **talk** with our parents. And let us not forget the quality of communication; an idea that is poorly **expressed** is not worth much more than one that is not **expressed** at all.

It's okay to repeat a word once or twice within the same paragraph, especially a word like *communication* that has few appropriate synonyms. And it's also a good idea to use it twice in the same sentence (like *expressed* in the last sentence) for the sake of parallelism. But if you use the same word over and over and over and over and over (like now, for instance), your reader will likely be unimpressed.

Sentence Variety

As you write more, you'll also develop an appreciation for good rhythm. A paragraph that contains only identically constructed sentences sounds monotonous.

With some more descriptive words and a few connectors here and there, though, you can construct a paragraph with sentences that have different constructions and thus are more pleasant to read.

Just be careful, though, because no matter how sophisticated the sentence structure is, you can always overdo a good thing, so make sure you vary the length of your sentences instead of having them all sound the same with the same rhythm.

Distinguish Yourself

Remember the plight of the essay readers: hundreds of essays to read in a very short amount of time. If you can make your essays stand out (in a positive way, that is) from the others, you'll definitely benefit.

Feel the Burn!

Your writing ability is a lot like a muscle. If you use it often and keep in shape, your ability and endurance will improve, but in disuse it will atrophy and wither. While you're preparing for the PCAT on your own, make sure you write at least one essay each week. After a month or so, compare your most recent essays to the ones from the beginning. If you've kept up a brisk writing regimen, you should see improvements that you didn't even know were happening.

Writing

Now that we know how to prepare for the essays, we'll show you how you can pre-construct certain portions of your essay. Before we do that though, let's review what the readers are looking for from your writing.

What the Readers Want to See

The essay readers will be looking for four characteristics as they skim your essay. According to the PCAT, an outstanding essay:

- avoids faulty reasoning and contains a powerful and sophisticated solution to the problem
- describes and evaluates multiple solutions with convincing examples, facts, and anecdotes
- is clear and well organized
- demonstrates superior facility with the conventions of standard written English

To put it more simply, the readers are looking for good organization, good supporting examples for whatever solutions you've offered, and command of the English language. We've hopefully taken care of the first two parts, so now we'll deal with the next two.

Essay Essentials

As you learned in sixth-grade composition class, a basic essay has three parts: an introduction, some body paragraphs, and a conclusion. Each of these parts has a specific role to play.

1. The **Introduction** should introduce the topic of the essay, discuss the issues surrounding it, and present the essay's thesis.
2. The **Body Paragraphs,** each with a topic sentence, should use examples to support the thesis of the essay.
3. The **Conclusion** should summarize the major points of the issue, reiterate the thesis, and perhaps consider its implications.

Basically, if you try to think of each paragraph as having a specific job to do, you can pretty much preconstruct each type of paragraph and then fill in the specific details on test day.

Preconstruction: The Introduction

A good introduction accomplishes the following tasks:

1. clearly establishes the thesis statement and serves as a mini outline of the essay
2. previews both sides of the issue at hand
3. presents a transition to the next paragraph

We want the reader to know what issue the essay is going to talk about. Even though the grader will see the prompt you're writing about, he or she should be able to figure out the prompt just from reading the introduction of your essay. The introduction gives the reader a preview of how your essay will take shape.

Preconstruction: Body Paragraphs

A body paragraph should do the following:

1. use a good transition/topic sentence
2. present an example
3. explain how the example supports the thesis

Body paragraphs are a little harder to preconstruct because they are the most specific part of the essay. Still, there are some handy tips for creating body paragraphs that an essay grader will love.

Transition/Topic Sentence

Essay graders love organized essays that flow well. The best way to write an essay like this is to use strong topic sentences and good transitions for each of your body paragraphs. Your topic sentence should serve as a gentle reminder to the reader of what the thesis of the essay is. Avoid using simple transitions like "the first example," and "the second example." You can make your writing stronger by leading with the example and making the transition a little more subtle.

The important point is that each sentence introduces the example and reminds the reader of its purpose. It's important that you remember to link the example to your thesis.

Explain How Your Example Supports Your Thesis

Don't get so caught up in providing details for your example that you forget to explain to the reader how or why your example helps your thesis. The purpose of the essay is not to just list out some examples; the purpose is to develop and support solutions to a problem.

Just as a reader should be able to figure out what the topic of the paper is from the introduction, a reader should be able to figure out the thesis from each paragraph.

Don't forget to make sure you have a good topic/transition sentence, specific details for the example, and an explanation of how or why the example is relevant to the thesis.

Preconstruction: Conclusion Paragraphs

Your essay should always have a conclusion, for two reasons. First, a conclusion paragraph is evidence of good organization. It shows the reader that you knew exactly what points you wanted to make, you made them, and now you're ending the essay. And second, an essay that lacks a conclusion seems incomplete, almost as if your writing abruptly ends before it should. This can give the grader a negative impression of your essay. Fortunately, conclusion paragraphs are easy to write. A good conclusion basically:

1. alerts the reader that the essay is ending
2. summarizes the main points of the essay

Some test-takers even prefer to write their introduction and conclusion first and then fill in the body paragraphs. This strategy has the advantage of making your essay seem complete even if you happen to run out of time writing the body paragraphs.

Alert the Reader

Conclusion paragraphs have their own topic/transition sentences, which generally should contain a word or phrase that tells the reader he or she is reaching the end. Here are some examples of phrases that signify a conclusion:

In conclusion…
Ultimately…
As the bulk of the evidence shows…
Clearly…
The examples above all support the idea that…

Summarize Main Points

Your conclusion should also summarize the main points of the essay, meaning that it should mention the thesis and how the examples support it. Additionally, you can briefly consider the implications of the thesis.

Other Helpful Tips

1. Brush Up on Your Typing.

Writing under pressure is tense enough; you don't want to add to the headache by hunting and pecking around for the right letter.

If you can type the following in about 15 seconds without looking at your keyboard, you'll do just fine:

The quick brown fox jumps over the lazy dog.

This sentence contains all 26 letters in the alphabet, so use it to warm up when you practice writing essays. You'll be better prepared for the real thing.

2. Go for the Bookends First.

The paragraphs that will make the biggest impression on your essay grader are the first and last, otherwise known as the bookends. Because you have to use a word processor on the PCAT, why not use it to its greatest advantage? Most students start out okay on essays, but they tend to finish hurriedly when they see the time dwindling. Starting out with the bookends ensures that your essay will finish strong (especially if you take the time to read the whole thing at the end—see tip 10). If you can knock your reader's socks off with a strong introduction and conclusion, these paragraphs will stick in the reader's mind as he or she calculates your grade.

There is a saying that the easiest way to walk a straight line is to keep your eyes fixed on a faraway object on the horizon and walk toward it. That's the case with essays as well. If you know what you're going to conclude before you start writing, your essay will be much more cohesive. You would be surprised at the percentage of writers who just start typing and rambling when the timer starts, hoping that their theses will make more sense as time elapses.

3. Acknowledge Other Solutions.

Your ideas about a solution to the problem in the prompt become much more compelling if you show an understanding for other potential solutions that are less likely to be successful. This illustrates that you've considered more than one approach to an issue (whether or not you actually have) and can talk about the solutions and examples in an informed matter.

4. Refer to Books and/or Current Events.

Reading a lot is a great way to help you write better, but keeping up with your reading has a dual purpose. It also provides the foundation for using specific examples from current events in your essays.

5. Aim for Length.

Readers can't help themselves. If they look at an essay that's short, they will assume (subconsciously or otherwise) that the thesis is inadequately developed. Right away, your score will probably be slightly lower. On the other hand, if you go on and on with no concern for brevity or conciseness, your essay will appear verbose and rambling. Neither too short nor too long is what will get you a high score. Your goal should be to write at least four or five good-sized paragraphs.

6. Cater to a Short Attention Span.

If you've had any experience writing essays in high school and college, you know that one of the best ways to make an essay look longer is to break the information into paragraphs instead of simply rambling in one long paragraph. Don't forget to use a short sentence every once in a while to give your paragraph some variation and your reader a break. Alternating your essay's structure has a dual effect, though—it also makes the essay easier to read. Think of critical reading passages; each new paragraph offers you a chance to rest before you begin reading again.

Indentations in the passage make the text look less immense and ponderous. They also make the very important impression that you're not likely to repeat yourself as you make your points.

7. Say It Once and Move On.

The most common trap you will likely encounter is the feeling that you need to keep repeating your points. It may be because you could think of only one pertinent thought and figured you'd do your best to string it out until it looked long enough. This is akin to adding water to soup so that it will feed more people. All you have is a big vat of watery soup.

More often, repetition comes from the stress of the time limit. Once you decide that you have a good point to make, you want to emphasize it by saying it again, only in different words. (Some writers don't even bother to change the words, and that's an even worse transgression. Don't do this.)

8. Be Resolute.

Your job as a writer is to compel your reader to share your beliefs. Therefore, it's very important not to use weak persuasive words. If you don't seem convinced of your viewpoint, how can you persuade others?

Your writing should be sure of itself. Therefore, minimize the use of words such as *would*, *might*, and *possibly*, and replace them with stronger words such as *is* and *will*. Don't worry; you won't lose points for sounding too liberal or too conservative.

9. Write in the Present Tense.

One of the most common grammatical errors that students make on essays is using improper verb-tense shifts. You should be writing in the present tense throughout the essay—and you should shift to the past tense only if you are relating historical facts.

10. Save Time for a Final Read.

Even though the computer gives you 30 minutes to create literary magic, you really should use only 28 or so. As you practice these essays, you may notice that you lose flow if you work on different parts of your essay at different times. Ideally, you should save a couple of minutes to give your essay a final read-through, looking for typos, grammatical glitches, and any other issue that doesn't make any sense.

If All Else Fails

Take a deep breath. It is an important test, but the Writing portion is probably not going to make or break your chances of getting into a Pharmacy program, so it is not worth fretting over. Just take your time, do the best you can, and don't let the first Writing section (and the first 30 minutes) put you in a defeated mindset before you even get to the rest of the exam (which is much more important).

Your Examples

In many ways, the examples will be the most important part of your essay. Without strong, relevant examples you cannot expect to achieve a high score on the Writing section. In general, the more specific your examples are, the better your essay score. And examples from history or current events are better than personal observations or experiences. Are they specific? Are they relevant to the topic? Do they support your solutions to the problem in the prompt? The strength of your examples will determine the strength of your solutions and your argument for those solutions. It's hard to write a convincing paper with weak examples. Avoid hypothetical examples—the more specific your example is, the better.

> Good examples are relevant to the topic and contain specific details.

Revising

How to Critique Your Essay

Now it's time to put on your essay-scoring hat and prepare to critique your own essay. After you write the essay on the real exam, you'll have only a few precious minutes to review what you have written, so while you are actually writing, take a few seconds to make sure you are following your outline.

When you are studying for the exam, and you're practicing your essay writing, take the time to evaluate each of your practice essays. Check for smooth transitions and the strength of your examples. If you're lucky enough to have a friend who is also preparing for the PCAT, you could switch essays and grade each other's. You'll need to be objective during this process. Remember, the only way to improve is to honestly assess your weaknesses and systematically eliminate them.

Set a timer for two minutes. Read the essay carefully but quickly, so that you do not exceed the two minutes on the timer.

Now ask yourself the following questions about the essay you wrote and measure your success:

1. Overall, did it make sense?
2. Did you address the topic directly?
3. Did you address the topic thoroughly?
4. Did your introduction paragraph repeat the issue to establish the topic of the essay?
5. Did you consider alternate solutions to the problem?
6. Did your examples make sense?
7. Did you flesh out your examples with details?
8. Did you explain how your examples supported your thesis?
9. Did your essay have a strong concluding paragraph?
10. Was your essay well organized, using transitions and topic sentences?
11. Did you use language that made the organization of the essay obvious?
12. Did you use correct grammar, spelling, and language?

If you could answer "yes" to all or almost all of these questions, congratulations! Your essay would probably receive a strong score. If you continue to practice, and write an essay of similar quality on the real Writing section of the real test, you should score very well.

If you answered "yes" to fewer than 12 of the questions, you have room for improvement. Fortunately, you also know which areas you need to strengthen as you continue to practice.

If you answered "yes" to fewer than 6 of the questions, your essay would probably not score very well on the real PCAT. You need to continue to practice, focusing on the areas of weakness that you discovered during this scoring process.

Final Thought: Read More!

Writing better comes from a better appreciation of the process and from better acquaintance with the best writing you can find. If you're a native English speaker, you learned to speak English not by reading a textbook, but by mimicking whoever raised you. Mimicry is still the best way to learn any new language (to which anyone who has spent any time as an exchange student will attest) as well as to improve your grasp on the language you currently speak.

So spend as much extra time as you can reading the work of professional writers. Sources of the best reading material include:

- **News Outlets:** You'll want what you write on your essay to have the same formal tone that most daily newspapers and credible news websites project. Granted, you'll want your writing style to have a bit more flair than the choppy, no-nonsense style of basic print journalism, but it's still an excellent example of writing that states its case once and moves on.
- **Magazines:** You probably have a few favorite weeklies and monthlies, so be sure to read them before you bundle them all up to recycle, or peruse their websites for content.
- **Books:** You'll want to go for the nonfiction titles, not the best "beach reads."

Quick Review

- The best essays avoid vague wording, provide solutions and examples, show clear and concise analysis, address the issues, use simple and direct language, use concrete examples, and show originality.

- Follow these three simple steps: Think, Organize, Write.

- Begin your writing by brainstorming—write down possible examples and issues that are important to the topic. Make sure your examples are relevant solutions to the problem and are as specific as possible.

- Identify key terms in the writing prompt and write down reasonable, common-sense definitions you want to use in your essay.

- Decide which core issues are involved in the prompt statement, how they are embodied in the examples you choose, and how they relate to each other.

- Organize your thoughts by creating a rough outline. Don't wait until after you've begun to write the essay itself.

- Clarity is a primary goal in your writing. Address one idea at a time without putting too much information into one sentence.

- Use fewer, more concise words to express a thought, and avoid using qualifiers, such as *in my opinion*, and over-used phrases, such as *obviously*.

- Limit the use of adverbs by making the verb more specific.

- Consistently write in the active voice, avoid using the passive voice, and use an original phrase rather than a cliché.

- Avoid lingering on a point you've already made. Make sure you stick to the issue of the prompt without going off on a tangent.

- Substitute word choices to add variety to your writing style. Write paragraphs with sentences that have different constructions to add interest.

- Readers are looking for good organization, good supporting examples for the solutions offered, and command of the English language. Make it easy for the grader to follow your logic and your ideas.

- An essay has three parts: an introduction, body paragraphs, and a conclusion.

- An introduction establishes the thesis statement and provides a general outline of the essay, it previews the different perspectives presented, and it provides a transition to the body paragraphs.

- Body paragraphs have transition and topic sentences, present an example, and explain the example's significance by linking it to your thesis.

- Conclusion paragraphs provides an ending and summarize the main points of the essay and any implications of the thesis.

- First write the essay's introduction and conclusion to ensure that you stay within the allotted time.

- Acknowledge other solutions and refer to specific examples from current events, personal observations, or relevant experiences.

- Vary your sentence structure and write four or five good-sized paragraphs. Avoid redundancies, use persuasive words, and write in the present tense.

- Allow time to proofread, correcting grammar, spelling, and language.

- You can enhance your writing score by adhering to these rules:

  - Learn the rules for comma usage and practice them until you gain proficiency. Skillful placement of commas will help to make your meaning clear.

  - Avoid fragmented and run-on sentences. They make it difficult for the reader to follow your line of thought.

  - Use nonsexist language.

  - Spell out words in full. Avoid abbreviations, shortcut words, symbols, and "cute" spellings—they give the impression that you don't care about your writing.

Index of Key Terms

Index of Key Terms

Symbols

A

E

M

N

NOTES

NOTES

NOTES

NOTES

NOTES